Manual of I.V. Therapeutics

Manual of I.V. Therapeutics

third edition

Lynn Dianne Phillips
RN, MSN, CRNI
Director, Nursing Department
Butte Community College
Oroville, California

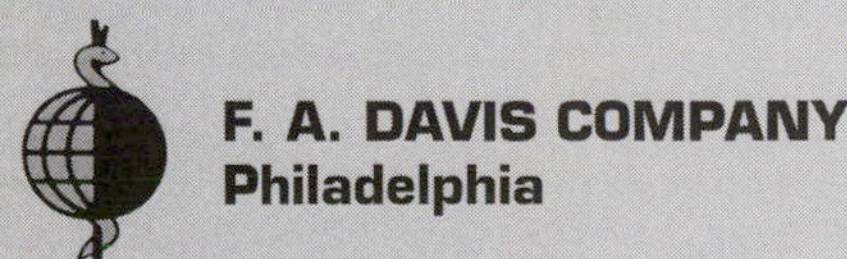

F. A. Davis Company
1915 Arch Street
Philadelphia, PA 19103
www.fadavis.com

Printed in the United States of America

Last digit indicates print number: 10 9 8 7 6 5

Acquisition Editor: Joanne P. DaCunha, RN, MSN
Developmental Editor: Diane Schweisguth
Production Editor: Jessica Howie Martin
Cover Designer: Louis J. Forgione

As new scientific information becomes available through basic and clinical research, recommended treatments and drug therapies undergo changes. The author and publisher have done everything possible to make this book accurate, up to date, and in accord with accepted standards at the time of publication. The author, editors, and publisher are not responsible for errors or omissions or for consequences from application of the book, and make no warranty, expressed or implied, in regard to the contents of the book. Any practice described in this book should be applied by the reader in accordance with the professional standards of care used in regard to the unique circumstances that may apply in each situation. The reader is advised always to check product information (package inserts) for changes and new information regarding dose and contraindications before administering any drug. Caution is especially urged when using new or infrequently ordered drugs.

Library of Congress Cataloging-in-Publication Data

Phillips, Lynn Dianne, 1947-
Manual of I.V. Therapeutics / Lynn Dianne Phillips.—3rd ed.
p. ; cm.
Includes bibliographical references and index.
ISBN 0-8036-0808-X (pbk.)
1. Intravenous therapy—Handbooks, manuals, etc. I. Title: Manual of IV therapeutics. II. Title.
[DNLM: 1. Infusions, Intravenous—methods—Examination Questions. 2. Infusions, Intravenous—methods—Handbooks. 3. Infusions, Intravenous—nursing—Examination Questions. 4. Infusions, Intravenous—nursing—Handbooks. WB 39 P561m 2001]
RM170 .P48 2001
615'.6—dc21 00-065837

This book is dedicated to the memory of
Leslie Jean Baranowski
1958-1998

Thank you for your dedication to the nursing
specialty of infusion therapy,
for your talent to mentor,
and for your dear friendship.
You are missed.

Preface

Infusion-related skills are performed by nurses in many settings, including acute, home care, clinic, and extended-care units. During many years of educating nurses about techniques in infusion therapy, I have heard this question asked over and over again: "Why don't we have more of this information about I.V.s in nursing school?" Another common question is, "Why doesn't our staff development department have more classes so that we can keep up our competency skills in infusion-related therapies?" Lack of time is the answer. With time as a valued resource, this manual can be used by the student, novice, or advanced practitioner in any setting where infusion-related skills are necessary.

This self-paced, comprehensive text is presented in a modular-experiential format. *Manual of I.V. Therapeutics,* 3rd edition, provides a text from which instruction builds from simple to complex, incorporating theory into clinical application. The skills of recall, nursing process, critical thinking, and patient education, along with detailed summaries, provide the foundation to produce a knowledgeable practitioner. The psychomotor skills associated with infusion therapy are presented in step-by-step recurring displays based on standards of practice. Competency criteria at the end of each chapter detail performance-based criteria with critical action statements. The cognitive knowledge necessary to perform the task is identified in each performance-based model, and the links to other competencies are identified. Suggestions for evaluation criteria are also presented in each model.

This book uniquely combines a workbook, text, and pocket guide. Each chapter has accompanying objectives, defined glossary terms, a pre-test and a post-test, key points summary, and critical thinking activities. Icons are used throughout the text to identify key points. Included in this new edition are focus spots on key nursing implications, web sites, patient education, home care issues, and cultural considerations using recurring icons. The icons used in this third edition are as follows:

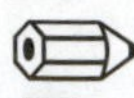 **NOTE:** Identifies key points and nursing implications

 Identifies web sites

 Identifies key patient education

 Identifies home care issues

Standards of practice are emphasized using the guidelines of the Occupational Safety and Health Administration (OSHA), Intravenous Nursing Standards of Practice (INS), and Centers for Disease Control and Prevention (CDC). Intravenous Nursing Standards are identified throughout the text with the following icon:

This manual is divided into three units. Unit One lays the foundation for practice; Unit Two provides basics of infusion therapy; and Unit Three covers advanced practice. Unit One provides four chapters designed to give in-depth information to the reader on risk management, legal responsibilities, steps of continuous quality assessment and competency criteria, infection control practices related to infusion therapy, and fundamentals of fluid and electrolyte balance.

Unit Two provides the essential five chapters for a solid foundation in infusion therapy practice. This third edition has incorporated recurring displays for procedures, cultural issues, and web sites, plus increased photos and other illustrations. Unit Two provides the reader with comprehensive information on parenteral solutions, infusion equipment, techniques for peripheral infusion therapy, complications, and the special needs of the geriatric and pediatric populations.

Unit Three includes five chapters encompassing the advanced topics of infusion medication delivery, management of central lines, transfusion therapy, antineoplastic therapy, and nutritional support.

The appendixes include CDC Standard Precautions; OSHA Guidelines for Controlling Occupational Exposure to Hazardous Drugs; a resource list of national organizations; and a summary of recommended procedures for maintenance of intravenous catheters, administration sets, and parenteral fluids by the CDC.

The CD-ROM accompanying this textbook contains 300 questions based on INS Standards of Practice and follows the guidelines of the INS Core Curriculum for certification.

I hope this new edition provides you, whether you are a practicing health care professional or student, with valuable insight into the safe practice of infusion therapy and a reference for this rapidly advancing field.

Lynn D. Phillips

Acknowledgments

The author would like to acknowledge the following:

The nurses in the specialty practice of infusion therapy

The nursing department at Butte Community College for their support and encouragement during this revision.

At F. A. Davis:

Joanne P. Da Cunha, Nursing Acquisitions Editor, who assisted in the final development of this manual.

Diane Schweisguth, Developmental Editor, who helped bring this vision to reality.

Robert Butler, Director of Production, for guiding this manuscript through the production process.

Robert G. Martone, Publisher, Nursing, whose foresight brought the project to F. A. Davis.

Jessica Howie Martin, Production Editor, who assisted in the final editing and production of this manuscript.

Consultants

JEANNIE CAPEL, RN, OCN, CRNI, CNSN, CCM
Director, Clinical Management
Gentiva Health Services
Tampa, Florida

LYNDA S. COOK, BSN, CRNI
Infusion Therapy Nurse Consultant
PharmMerica
Greensboro, North Carolina

JULIE EDDINS, MSN, CRNI
Clinical Nurse Educator, Johnson & Johnson
Medical Vascular Access
Johnson & Johnson Medical
A Division of Ethicon, Inc.
Arlington, Texas

BETH FABIAN, RN, BA, CRNI
Vice President, Clinical Operations
Ivonyx, Inc.
Livonia, Michigan

MARTHA HANN, RN, CRNI
Clinical Nurse Consultant
B. Braun Medical, Inc.
Columbus, Ohio

PAMELA HOCKETT, RN, BSN, OCN, CRNI
Cancer Center Coordinator
Enloe Medical Center
Chico, California

BRENDA BRADLEY JOHANSSON, RN,C, MSN, CCRN
Faculty
Nurse Educator
Butte Community College
Oroville, California

ROXANNE R. PERUCCA, MSN, CRNI
I.V. Therapy Nurse Manager
University of Kansas Hospital
Kansas City, Kansas

CHRISTINE PIERCE-BROCKETTI, RNCS, MSN, CHCE
Administrative Director, Cleveland Clinic Home Care
Cleveland Clinic Health System
Cleveland, Ohio

OFELIA SANTIGO, BSN, CRNI
Director of Clinical Services and Case Management Care IV, Inc.
Home Infusion and Disease Management Services
Wichita, Kansas

ALIVIA STRAWN, RN, BS, CIC
Manager, Epidemiology and Safety
Enloe Medical Center
Chico, California

MELISSA WARTHEN, RN, MSN, CCRN
Consultant, Clinical Support
Electronic Drug Delivery Systems
Abbott Laboratories
Hospital Products Division
North Chicago, Illinois

Contents

UNIT TWO
Basic Infusion Practice 177

Tables

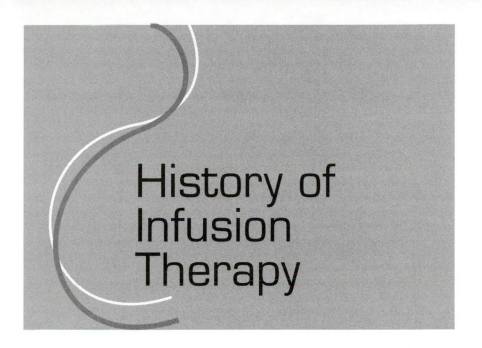

History of Infusion Therapy

The foundation for intravenous (I.V.) therapy began slowly with contributions from chemists, physicians, and architects. The specialty practice of I.V. therapy as we know it today has many heroes and heroines who have made an imprint on this area of medicine. The history of I.V. therapy is woven with individuals aided by advances in technical development. Five hundred years have elapsed since the discovery of the circulation of blood to today's state-of-the-art tunneled catheters, implanted ports, and blood component therapy. A review of the roots of I.V. therapy helps nurses understand how far we have come.

The history of I.V. therapy began with the discovery of the circulation of blood by Sir William Harvey in 1616. Until the late Renaissance period, it was known that the arteries and veins both contained blood, but it was believed that blood ebbed and flowed "like the human breath."

In 1660, Sir Christopher Wren, the famous architect of St. Paul's Cathedral in London, worked with a chemist to produce the first hypodermic needle. Wren inserted a hollow pipe in the blood vessel of a dog and injected wine, ale, opium, scammony, liver of antimony, and other substances directly into the bloodstream and studied their effects. He was thus credited for using a quill and bladder to inject the first I.V. substance.

A German physician, Johann Majors, was the first to use Wren's discovery of the hypodermic needle. He injected unpurified compounds into humans in 1662. The disastrous consequences of this early experimental work were compounded by the fact that infections occurred at the site of injection, resulting in death.

In 1667, the first well-documented transfusion from an animal to a human was performed. The Parisian physician Jean Baptiste Denis infused lamb's blood directly into the circulation of a 15-year-old boy. The boy quickly died. Of course, this early experiment was not well received, and in 1687, animal-to-human transfusions were prohibited in Europe by edict of the Church and Parliament. Because of this edict, 150 years passed before injecting substances into the circulation again became of interest.

ASEPTIC TECHNIQUE ADVANCE

During the latter part of the 19th century, accelerated knowledge regarding bacteriology, pathology, and pharmacology revealed new approaches to problems of medicine.

One new approach was the use of nitrous oxide and ether as a form of anesthesia by Horace Wells. A chemist, Charles Jackson, assisted W.T.G. Morton in his first surgical operations with ether at Massachusetts General Hospital in Boston on October 16, 1846. This method of anesthesia quickly spread throughout America and Europe, but chloroform soon came to be preferred to ether.

In 1847, a Viennese obstetrician, Ignaz Semmelweis, noted that physicians moving from autopsies to the obstetrical unit were communicating highly pathogenic substances between the two departments. He was the first to require physicians to wash their hands in a solution of chlorine before obstetrical examinations. Semmelweis reduced the death rate in maternity wards by more than 90 percent between 1846 and 1848 through this simple procedure of cleanliness.

Louis Pasteur, a chemist, later demonstrated the scientific basis for Semmelweis' theory, proving that bacteria were living microorganisms. However, Pasteur's ideas were challenged, and it was not until Lister's work in 1867 that the germ theory was accepted and the war won. Lister's work focused on sterility in the operating room and led to the practice of asepsis. His aseptic technique came to replace older antiseptic methods and was universally accepted.

In 1889, William Halsted of Johns Hopkins Hospital, in cooperation with the Goodyear Rubber Company, introduced the use of gloves for surgical procedures. By 1899, the use of rubber gloves became popular, not only to protect patients but to also protect practitioners from corrosive hand rinses.

The primitive state of medical knowledge and practice in the 1880s had an influence on the morbidity or mortality of infants and young children of the time. The infant mortality rate during this time varied from 250 to 500 of 1000 live births. The worldwide high morbidity and mortality rates of the late 19th century accounted for the average life span's remaining at 35 to 38 years. Enteric disorders, malnutrition, and common respiratory and contagious diseases were the major causes of death during the 19th century.

INFUSION ADVANCES

In 1831, the Anatomy Act was designed to regulate human dissection. An outbreak of cholera, the second pandemic, was spreading across Asia and Europe from India. In that same year, Brooke O'Shaughnessy, a 22-year-old recent Edinburgh graduate, wrote his first paper on cholera. He became engrossed in the cause and cure of cholera. O'Shaughnessy described cholera and studied the blood drawn from patients with the disease. He wrote to *The Lancet* on February 4, 1832: "The blood drawn in the worst cases . . . is unchanged in its anatomical or globular structure. . . . It has lost a large proportion of its water. . . . It has lost also a great proportion of its neutral saline ingredients. . . . Of the free alkali contained in healthy serum, not a particle is present."

The first practical application of O'Shaughnessy's observations was Dr. Thomas Latta, who used infusions of saline to treat the intractable diarrhea of cholera. He published his results in *The Lancet* on June 2, 1832. However, there were no previous records of water and salts being given deliberately to restore constituents of the blood. Of the first 25 reported cases treated by saline, eight patients survived. There was severe criticism of this method of treatment, and when the pandemic spread to America in 1852 to 1863, the use of intravenous saline was not accepted.

Until Florence Seibert discovered pyrogen substances (proteins foreign to the blood) in distilled water, there were many problems related to pyrogens within solutions. Researchers worked to eliminate those pyrogens, and the administration of parenteral solutions became safer. Until 1925, the most frequently used parenteral solution was 0.9 percent sodium chloride solution because of its isotonic relationship to blood. After 1925, dextrose was used extensively to provide a source of calories. I.V. solutions, however, were used only for critically ill patients.

Great strides were made at Massachusetts General Hospital, the first place where certain nurses were designated as I.V. nurses . The services of I.V. nurses consisted of administering I.V. solutions and transfusions, cleaning infusion sets, and cleaning and sharpening needles.

In the mid-1950s, I.V. therapy was used for two main purposes: major surgery and dehydration. Solutions of 5 percent dextrose and water or 0.9 percent sodium chloride for surgical patients were infused over 3 to 4 hours and discontinued at night.

Fewer than 20 percent of hospital patients received I.V. therapy in the mid-1950s. The site most frequently used by nurses during this period was the antecubital vein. A 16- to 18-gauge steel reusable needle was used and stabilized with leather restraints. Disposable plastic sets became available and replaced reusable rubber tubing. Frequent infiltrations that occurred with the use of metal needles led to the development of the flexible plastic catheter for insertion using the cut-down method.

In 1950, the Rochester needle was introduced. This device consisted of a resinous catheter on the outside of a steel needle; the catheter was slipped off the needle into the vein and the needle removed. In 1958, the Intracath (Deseret Pharmaceutical Co.), a plastic catheter lying within the lumen of the needle, was introduced in individual sterile packaging. This type of catheter reduced the need for surgical cut-down for placement of the 1940s-type catheter. The first change in the steel needle appeared in 1957, when McGaw Laboratories introduced small vein sets with foldable wings as grips.

The momentum for change in the I.V. therapy field occurred during the 1960s. A variety of solutions were marketed, expanding the choice to approximately 200. Piggyback medications were used, and filters and electronic infusion devices flooded the market.

Since the 1980s, tunneled catheters, such as Hickman-Broviac and Groshong, have provided a means of central venous access for delivery of total parenteral nutrition (TPN) and cytoxic therapy.

In the 1990s, totally implanted access devices, consisting of a subcutaneous reservoir connected to a catheter positioned in the central circulation, provided alternatives for patients requiring long-term access. The changes in management of patients needing long-term I.V. therapy with permanent central venous lines have expanded the field of I.V. therapy.

TRANSFUSION ADVANCES

During the 19th century, there were many advances in medicine. One of the first was human-to-human transfusion, first performed by James Blundell in London in 1834. Blundell is credited with the correlation between blood loss and hypoxemia during hemorrhage.

In 1900, Karl Landsteiner proved that all human blood was not alike with the discovery of three of the four main blood groups. This led the way to compatible blood transfusions and the development of blood banks. In 1911, Dr. Reuben Ottenberg of New York demonstrated that it was safe to use a donor whose serum agglutinated the recipient's red blood cells but unsafe to use a donor whose red blood cells were acted on by the recipient's serum. This work originated the idea of the universal donor. Until 1914, there was no way to prevent the coagulation of blood, and every transfusion was performed with the direct method, donor to recipient. However, with the discovery of sodium citrate, blood could be stored and blood banking began.

Many advances in transfusion practices occurred during wartime. Between 1936 and 1939 during the Spanish Civil War, the practicality of supplying stored blood from the civilian population to wounded men on the front was proved. During World War I, criteria for transfusion were established. During World War II, the donor criteria were established and the closed collection system used.

Additional advances include the use of packed red blood cells in the United States during the 1940s, the discovery of the Rh factor on red blood cells in 1940, and the establishment of the American Association of Blood Banking (AABB) in 1947 to meet civilian needs.

Component therapy began when Stanley Cohen designed the first cell separator in 1951.

In 1968, RhoGAM was manufactured and made available to physicians for Rh-negative mothers to prevent hemolytic disease of newborns. In 1970, blood components and the prescribing of selected components for individual situations, such as packed cells for the anemic patient, were instituted.

NUTRITIONAL SUPPORT ADVANCES

Claude Bernard, a French physiologist, experimented with injecting sugar solution into dogs in 1834. He continued his work for the next two decades, injecting egg whites and milk into animals with some success. Bernard also discovered that cane sugar injected intravenously soon appeared in the urine, whereas ingested sugar did not because of breakdown by the digestion process.

Further advances in nutritional support came in 1869 when Menzel and Perco of Vienna wrote a paper on the use of fat, milk, and camphor injected subcutaneously. By 1878, the use of oil and protein extract to treat patients suffering from anorexia nervosa was reported, and cow's milk was injected for nutritional support. In Canada, Hodder experimented with the use of cow's milk to correct fluid and nutritional losses caused by cholera. The results were considered good. His colleagues, however, barred Hodder from the practice of medicine, and further work in nutritional support was abandoned.

The first I.V. hydrolyzed protein and fat infusion was administered to animals during the early 20th century, leading the way to today's nutritional support solutions. In 1937, W.C. Rose identified amino acids and led to the development of protein hydrolysates for infusion into humans.

In 1963, at the Harrison Department of Surgical Research at the University of Pennsylvania, a young surgical resident, Stanley Dudrick, conducted the first experiment to determine definitely whether or not long-term total I.V. nutrition was feasible. Dudrick's experiments were quickly applied to starving adult patients, who would probably not have survived without TPN. Stanley Dudrick's name is now synonymous with parenteral nutrition. Because of Dudrick's work, patients receive total nutrition and survive diseases and conditions that had formerly resulted in death.

During the 1970s, fat emulsion (Intralipid, Abbott Pharmaceuticals) was instituted as an adjunct to nutritional support. In 1977, the formation of nutritional support teams began. The American Society for Parenteral and Enteral Nutrition (ASPEN) was formed and held its first clinical congress in Chicago.

In the 1980s, TPN evolved into a science, providing nutrients by vein in sufficient amounts to achieve anabolism. Disease-specific formulas were developed to address the particular needs of patients with renal, cardiac, or hepatic disease. In 1983, TPN moved to the home (home parenteral nutrition [HPN]).

Research continues in this sophisticated field, with further work on the role of amino acids; indications for medium-, short-, and long-chain triglycerides; and the use of antioxidants, or "free radical scavengers."

MEDICATION ADMINISTRATION ADVANCES

Medications during the transition from the 19th to the 20th century were limited primarily to coal tar products, which were used to treat febrile illnesses and influenza. The 10 most commonly administered compounds during the 19th century were ether, morphine, digitalis, diphtheria antitoxin, smallpox vaccine, iron, quinine, iodine, alcohol, and mercury.

As the 20th century progressed, medications were not routinely administered by the I.V. route; sometimes they were given intramuscularly. For seriously ill patients with diseases such as meningitis, penicillin or chloraphenicol was given by continuous I.V. drip. When patients required medication added to their infusions, an intern carried out this procedure, often using medication that had not been refrigerated for long periods of time. When blood was needed, the patient received whole blood that was contained in a glass bottle, and the intern administered the blood with assistance from the nursing staff.

The cut-down procedure continued to be used until the mid-1970s for severely ill patients to prevent the complication of infiltration. Catheter sites were changed only when they were not functioning. It was not until the early 1970s that the Centers for Disease Control and Prevention (CDC) developed recommendations for infection control related to I.V. therapy.

During the 1970s, alternative routes expanded the administration of pain medication. In 1976, Yaks and Rudy demonstrated successful administration of morphine directly into the subarachnoid space of animals. In 1977, Wang proved that an intrathecal injection of morphine provided profound relief of pain in humans. Today the intrathecal and epidural routes have proved effective for administering specific medication therapies.

EDUCATIONAL ADVANCES

In the 1970s, there was a scarcity of information about I.V. therapy in nursing journals, and I.V. therapy journals were nonexistent until the late 1970s. Nursing schools presented I.V. therapy in a limited manner, with more theory than practical management.

The past 10 years have been the fastest ever in growth for the I.V. therapy field. The National Intravenous Therapy Association (NITA) published recommendations for practices in the early 1980s. On October 1, 1980, the U.S. House of Representatives recognized and nationalized I.V. Nurse Day throughout the country. It was "resolved, that I.V. Nurse Day be nationally celebrated in honor of the National Intravenous Therapy Association Inc. on January 25 of each year . . ." according to a portion of the proclamation as presented by the Honorable Edward J. Mackey from the Fifth Congressional District of Massachusetts.

NITA's first national Certification Examination for Intravenous Nurses was offered in March 1985. In 1987, NITA changed its name to the Intravenous Nursing Society (INS).

TRENDS FOR THE 21ST CENTURY

In the 21st century, it is inconceivable that nurses will be limited to the responsibilities they hold today. Nurses are assuming more healthcare responsibilities. Changes in expenditures for healthcare, hospital costs, and seriously ill patients have made and continue to make a serious impact on the nursing profession.

Nurses now play a major role in healthcare reform because they can provide 60 to 80 percent of primary healthcare traditionally provided by physicians.

A shift in focus from high-tech, hospital-based care to primary healthcare has already begun. This trend has accelerated with nurses in the present decade cognizant of terms such as "global budgeting," "managed care," and "total quality management."

Occupational exposure to bloodborne pathogens is a risk to nurses, especially those working in I.V. therapy. Safety will continue to be an issue, with focus on product features. Legislation on product design for practitioner protection has affected clinical standards of practice.

Technology continues to evolve in healthcare. Patients are finding treatment, and nurses today routinely provide services in noninstitutional settings such as outpatient centers, diagnostic centers, self-care centers, and health-related shopping centers. It is projected that patients will become more capable of matching their diseases or illnesses with the appropriate care settings and will have more autonomy in preventing and treating illnesses. The Internet has connected consumers to the "information superhighway" in disease treatment options.

New roles are emerging, with nurses developing interdependent, collaborative, and peer relationships with physicians. I.V. therapy is just one of the interdependent roles that needs a sound foundation in basic as well as advanced theory.

The roles of licensed nurses are well defined in the initiation, maintenance, and therapeutic modalities identified in each state's nursing practice act. Standards of practice established by the INS and the CDC have set guidelines for the role of registered nurses (RNs) and licensed vocational/practical nurses (LVNs/LPNs) in all aspects of I.V. therapy and nutritional support.

UNIT ONE

Fundamental Foundations of Practice

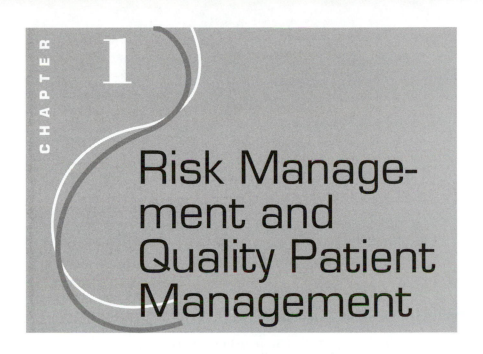

Risk Management and Quality Patient Management

The world, more especially the Hospital world, is in such a hurry, is moving so fast, that it is too easy to slide into bad habits before we are aware.

Florence Nightingale, 1873

CHAPTER CONTENTS

LEARNING OBJECTIVES

Upon completion of this chapter, the reader will be able to:

1 Define the terminology related to risk management and quality patient management.

2 Identify the sources of laws.

3 Differentiate between standards of care and standards of practice.

4 Identify the areas of breach of duty in I.V. nursing.

5 State the key points in an unusual occurrence report.

6 Identify three occupational risks for the I.V. nurse.

7 State the definition of quality management.

8 State the three parts of a competency-based program.

9 Differentiate between performance improvement and total quality management.

10 Identify the role of the nurse as an expert witnesss.

GLOSSARY

Audit A review of care using defined criteria

Civil law Laws that affect the legal rights of private persons or corporations

Competent Being capable or able; knowing how to function

Competency Integrated behaviors derived from an explicit set of desired outcomes

Competency validation program (CVP) System developed by Clinical Center Nursing Department at the National Institutes of Health to identify, describe, validate, and document the nursing competencies required for safe and effective nursing practice

(CQI) Continuous quality improvement

Criminal law Offense against the general public; effects on welfare of society as a whole

Criteria Elements necessary to define and measure quality
Data collection Gathering information through interviewing, observing, and inspecting
Dimensions of performance Characteristics of what is done and how well it is done
Documentation A recording, in written or printed form, containing original, official, or legal information
Evaluation Inspection, examination, and quality judgment
Expert testimony Witness from the same professional specialty explaining to the court what the standard of care should be in the situation at hand
Goal Broad statement of a desired outcome
Implementation Carrying out a plan
Intervention Interference that may affect outcome
Liable Legally responsible for damages, answerable
Malpractice Negligent conduct of a professional person
Negligence Not acting in a reasonable or prudent manner
Nursing standard Specific statement about the quality of some facet of nursing care
Outcome The result of the performance (or nonperformance) of a function or process(es)
Performance improvement (PI) The continuous study and adaptation of functions and processes of a healthcare organization to increase the probability of achieving desired outcomes and to better meet the needs of patients and other users of services; the third segment of the performance measurement, assessment, and improvement system
Process A goal-directed, interrelated series of actions, events, mechanisms, or steps
(QA) Quality assessment
Quality assurance (QA) The determination of the degree of excellence through monitoring and evaluating to detect and resolve problems
Quality management An ongoing, systematic process for monitoring, evaluating, and problem solving
Risk management Process that centers on identification analysis, treatment, and evaluation of real and potential hazards
Standards of care Focuses on the recipient of care and describes outcomes of care that patients can expect to receive
Standards of practice Focuses on the provider and defines the activities and behavior needed to achieve patient outcomes
Statutes Written laws enacted by the legislature
Structure Standard that refers to conditions and mechanisms that provide support for the delivery of care (e.g., policy and resources)
Tort Private wrong, by act or omission, that can result in a civil action by the harmed person
(TQM) Total quality management

PRE-TEST

1. Which of the following is an example of malpractice in I.V. therapy?
   - **a.** Failure to document
   - **b.** Starting an I.V. on a coherent patient against the patient's wishes
   - **c.** Refusing to wear gloves for a venipuncture
   - **d.** Failure to report product defect
2. Sources of law include all of the following **EXCEPT**:
   - **a.** Constitution
   - **b.** Statutes
   - **c.** Common law
   - **d.** Joint commission standards
3. Performance improvement is:
   - **a.** The adaptation of functions and processes to increase the probability of achieving desired outcomes
   - **b.** The determination of the degree of excellence through monitoring
   - **c.** The carrying out of a plan
   - **d.** A goal-directed, interrelated series of actions, events, mechanisms, or steps
4. The definition of standards of care is:
   - **a.** Focus on the provider and defines the activities and behaviors needed
   - **b.** Focus on the recipient of care and describes outcomes of care
   - **c.** Written laws enacted by the legislature
   - **d.** Result of the performance of a function or process
5. The following are all occupational risks associated with I.V. therapy **EXCEPT:**
   - **a.** Latex allergy
   - **b.** Needlestick injuries
   - **c.** Chemical exposure
   - **d.** Falls
6. According to the Intravenous Nursing Revised Standards of Practice, expert I.V. therapy nurses should possess which of the following credentials?
   - **a.** Masters in Science in Nursing
   - **b.** Certification in Critical Care
   - **c.** Certification in Intravenous Nursing
   - **d.** Licensed Vocational or Practical Nurse
7. A risk management tool that is a proactive strategy is:
   - **a.** Unusual occurrence reports
   - **b.** Informed consents
   - **c.** Documentation records
   - **d.** Professional liability insurance
8. All of the following should be reported to the Food and Drug Administration (FDA) under the Medical Device Act **EXCEPT**:
   - **a.** Outdated medication
   - **b.** Misleading packaging

c. Cracked or leaking I.V. solution bag
d. Defective infusion pump tubing

9. The elements of I.V. nursing competency include all of the following **EXCEPT**:
   a. Accountability
   b. Communication
   c. Autonomy
   d. Risk assessment
10. The three parts to a competency-based program include:
   a. Competency statement, goal, and return demonstration
   b. Competency statement, criteria for learning, and evaluation
   c. Goal, evaluation, and feedback
   d. Assessment, problem statement, and case-based review

SOURCES OF LAW

In the United States, there are four primary sources of law: (1) constitutional law, (2) statutory law, (3) administrative law, and (4) common law. The Constitution is the basic framework on which our government is built. The Constitution, however, has little direct involvement in the area of **malpractice**.

Statutes are laws enacted by the legislature and passed by the House of Representatives and the Senate as basic rules for society. There were a minimal number of statutes dealing with malpractice before the malpractice crisis of the mid-1970s. Today only a few federal statutes deal with malpractice; however, there are many state laws that deal with it.

Administrative law is a form of law made by administrative agencies, such as the National Labor Relations Board and the Interstate Commerce Commission. These agencies have limited effect on malpractice.

The final source of law is common law. This is court-made law. Most law in the area of malpractice is court-made law. The courts are responsible for interpreting the statutes. Most malpractice law is not addressed by statute but is established by the courts (Sharpe, 1999).

Legal Terms

Legal terms that nurses should become familiar with are criminal law, civil law, tort, malpractice, and the rule of personal liability. **Criminal law** relates to an offense against the general public caused by the potential harmful effect to society as a whole. A government authority prosecutes criminal actions, and punishment includes imprisonment, fine, or both. The administration of I.V. therapy, if performed in an unlawful manner, can involve a nurse in a criminal offense. Violation of the Nurse Practice Act or the Medical Practice Act by an unlicensed person is considered a criminal offense.

Civil law affects the legal right of private persons and corporations. When harm occurs, the guilty party may be required to pay damages to the injured person.

A private wrong, by act or omission, is referred to as a **tort**. Most tort law is found in common law. There are two types of tort, intentional and unintentional. Intentional torts include assault, battery, false imprisonment, restraints as a form of false imprisonment, defamation, and breach of confidentiality (Sharpe, 1999). When dealing with a rational patient who refuses treatment, it is best to explain the treatment, verbally reassure the patient, and then notify the physician of refusal.

NOTE: Coercion of a rational adult patient to place an I.V. cannula device constitutes assault and battery.

Negligence occurs when a nurse does not act in a reasonable and prudent manner, with resultant damage to a person or a person's property.

Malpractice is the negligent conduct of a professional person. However, carelessness is not synonymous with negligence. Medical malpractice is generally defined as "a departure from the accepted standards of practice which the average qualified healthcare provider of the same or similar specialty as the defendant would deliver at the time and under the circumstances with consideration for the resources available and advances in medical science" (Sharpe, 1999).

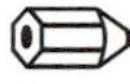

NOTE: If an act of malpractice does not create harm, legal action cannot be initiated.

The rule of personal liability is "every person is **liable** for his own tortuous conduct" (his own wrongdoing). A physician cannot protect a nurse from an act of negligence by bypassing this rule with verbal assurance. Nurses are liable for their own wrongdoings in carrying out physicians' orders. This rule is relevant to nurses in the areas of medication errors (the most common cause of malpractice claims) and administration of I.V. fluids. Nurses have a legal and professional responsibility to be knowledgeable regarding the I.V. fluids and medication that are administered (Weinstein, 1997).

WEB SITES:

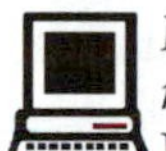

Medical Malpractice Resource Page: *www.helpquick.com/medmal.htm*

Internet Legal Resource Guide: *www.ilrg.com*

Others: ______________________________

STANDARDS OF PRACTICE AND STANDARDS OF CARE

EVOLUTION OF STANDARDS

In 1912, the Third Clinical Congress of Surgeons of North America resolved that "some system of standardization of hospital equipment and hospital work should be developed. Institutions having the highest ideals may have proper recognition before the profession, and those of inferior standards should be stimulated to raise the quality of their work. In this way patients will receive the best type of treatment, and the public will have some means of recognizing those institutions devoted to the highest ideals of medicine." From 1919 to 1970, the adopted standards referred to the minimum level "considered essential to proper care and treatment of patients in the hospital."

At the national level, the American Nurses Association (ANA) and The Joint Commission on Accreditation of Healthcare Organizations (JCAHO), along with various specialty organizations, establish the standards of nursing practice. At the state level, the various Nurse Practice Acts are the authority by which nurses can practice. At the local level, specific standards are set forth in hospital and agency procedure manuals (Sharpe, 1999).

STANDARDS OF PRACTICE

Nursing standards of practice are specific statements about the quality of some facet of nursing care. The focus is on the provider of care. Standards are the criteria for measuring performance against the optimal achievable degree of clinical excellence and are formulated to communicate expectations of nursing practice. Several agencies are influential in developing standards of practice.

WEB SITES:
JCAHO: *www.jcaho.org*
Intravenous Nurses Society: *www.ins1.org*
Others: ____________________________________

STANDARDS OF CARE

Standards of nursing care reflect the missions, values, and philosophy of the agency. Nursing **processes**, professional accountability, fiscal responsibility, and other areas of care are included within these standards. **Standards of care** describe the results or outcomes of care and focus on the patient. These are called **performance standards** and should (1) include the minimum acceptable behavior for the nurse congruent with department standards and standards of practice; (2) define performance in observable, measurable behaviors; (3) be specific to the staff nurse role and job description; (4) include all aspects of nurses' roles, including leadership and organizational expectations; and (5) serve as the basis for employee selection decisions and performance appraisal system.

There are three types of standards in nursing:

1. Standards of structure, which consider the organizational framework
2. Standards of process, which encompass patient procedures in healthcare settings
3. Standards of outcome, which consider the objectives or goals of patient care

The National Institutes of Health (NIH) Clinical Center Nursing Department has developed structure standards that define the physical and organizational characteristics needed to operate, direct, and control the nursing delivery system. Standards of care include:

1. Standard of Care I: Protection from Harm
2. Standard of Care II: Provision of Comfort
3. Standard of Care III: Promotion and Maintenance of Equilibrium
4. Standard of Care IV: Foster Autonomy and Dignity
5. Standard of Care V: Maximizing Knowledge and Understanding (National Institutes of Health, 1995).

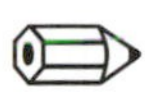

NOTE: For nurses who practice predominantly in the area of infusion therapy, certification is advisable. Certification is the granting of special recognition to nurses who have practiced and pursued an advanced role in a particular area of nursing. A nongovernment agency or private organization confers certification on nurses who have a higher level of competency than that mandated by state licensure. Membership in the Intravenous Nurses Society (INS) and certification (CRNI) by the Intravenous Nurses Certification Corporation (INCC) are options to be considered (Josephson, 1999).

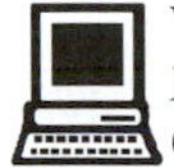

WEB SITES:
National Institutes of Health: *www.cc.nih.gov/nursing/nsgstand.html*
Others: ______________________________

BREACH OF DUTY

After the standard of care has been established and legal duty shown in negligence cases, the injured party must prove that breach of duty has occurred. In negligence cases, breach of duty often involves the matter of foreseeability. Forseeability is the legal requirement that the case must be judged on the unique facts as they were at the time of the occurrence because it is always easier to state what should have been done in retrospect. Certain events may foreseeably cause a specific result. The following is a list of breach of duties related to I.V. therapy nursing:

1. Delay in the administration of medication
2. Unfamiliarity with the drug
3. Route of administration not clarified
4. Failure to qualify orders
5. Negligence in patient teaching

Nurses must be aware at all times that failure to observe, failure to intervene, and verbal rather than written orders are potential risks for all nursing areas. Nurses must assess each patient and formulate a nursing diagnosis to meet the specific patient's needs. At this time, the courts have not extended the concept of nursing diagnosis to the liability of a nurse's practice.

Malpractice cases are most frequently based on negligence in physical care. There are many documented cases of malpractice related to all procedures performed on patients. Sometimes the breach of duty occurs because a nurse fails to perform a procedure according to proper standards of care.

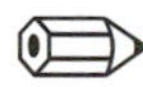

NOTE: Because of the risk of malpractice, policy and procedure manuals are vitally important in all aspects of physical nursing care. Practicing and performing specific physical care based on the policies and procedures ensure quality care.

The practice of using verbal orders rather than written orders potentially places nurses at higher liability risks.

INS STANDARDS Infusion therapy is initiated with a physician's order or on the order of a prescriber authorized by state Nurse Practice Acts using the nursing process. An order shall be complete and written in the patient's medical record. (INS 2000, 10)

THE I.V. NURSE'S ROLE AS EXPERT WITNESS

Studies indicate that 70 to 80 percent of all civil litigation involves medical and scientific evidence and the testimony of experts. In the profession of nursing, especially the specialty of I.V. therapy, the likelihood of being involved in some legal matter, directly or indirectly, is great (Masoorli, 1995).

In every negligence or malpractice proceeding, the injured party or plaintiff must prove that the defendant did not act in the way that a reasonably prudent professional would have acted in the same or similar circumstance.

Historically, care rendered by a malpractice defendant was measured legally against the professional standards of the locality where the defendant practiced. Holding a practitioner to local standards was meant to protect rural general practitioners who otherwise might be held to the same standards of practice as urban clinicians who had substantially greater access to technology, research, and consultative opinions (Dowd, 1999). The "locality rule" is the foundations for an expert witness familiar with standards of practice in specialty clinical practice. An expert is required to explain the appropriate standard of care and to indicate the deviation from standard care. An expert called to testify against a defendant clinician is required to be from the same locality and, therefore, familiar with the existing standards in the region.

The role of the expert is *NOT* to establish standards of care. Rather, the expert's role is to educate the judge and jury regarding the standards already established by the profession. **Expert testimony** increases with the technical complexity of a case. An expert witness is usually selected from the same area of experience as the defendant nurse. Additional expertise, such as national I.V. certification or research experience, is also important (Fiesta, 1994).

INS STANDARDS 2000 Revised Intravenous Nursing Standards of Practice state that an expert nurse is certified in I.V. therapy: Certified Registered Nurse Intravenous (CRNI). An expert nurse gives advice and consultation throughout the litigation process.

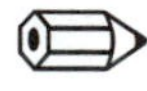

NOTE: The specialty area of I.V. therapy is a high-risk technical area.

RISK MANAGEMENT AND RISK ASSESSMENT

The Revised Intravenous Standards of Practice (1998) define **risk management** as "a process that centers on identification, analysis, treatment and evaluation of real and potential hazards." Risk assessment is the scientific process of asking how risky something is. It is a process of collecting and analyzing scientific data "to describe the form, dimension, and characteristics of risk." Risk assessment and risk management are equally important but different processes, with different objectives, information content, and results (Patton, 1993).

Risk management concepts include the concerns that organizations face with exposure to losses. Organizations handle the chances of losses or risks by financing, purchasing insurance, or practicing loss control. Loss control is preventive and protective activities that are performed before, during, and after losses are incurred. Risk management involves all medical and facility staff. It provides for the review and analysis of risk and liability sources involving patients, visitors, staff, and facility property. Risk management consists of the following components:

- Identification and management of clinical areas of actual and high risk
- Identification and management of nonclinical (i.e., visitor, staff) areas of actual and high risk
- Identification and management of probable claims events
- Management of property loss occurrences
- Review and analysis of customer surveys and patient complaints
- Review and analysis of risk assessment surveys
- Operational linkages with hospital **quality management**, safety, and **performance improvement** programs
- Provision of risk management education
- Compliance with state risk management and applicable federal statutes, including the Safe Medical Devices Act (Clinical Orientation Manual, 1998)

Risk assessment is performed by government agencies such as the Environmental Protection Agency (EPA). Risk assessment takes different approaches depending on available information. Some assessments look back to try to assess effects after an event. They may also look ahead before a new product is approved for use.

The Joint Commission on Accreditation of Health Care Organizations (JCAHO) advocates establishing an integrated risk management and quality assurance program.

Risk management strategies combine the elements of both loss reduction and loss prevention. Risk management strategies that may decrease the risk of potential liability are as follows:

- Informed consent
- Unusual occurrence reports
- Documentation

- Professional liability insurance
- Patient relations
- Quality management (Baldwin & Mantel, 1995).

INFORMED CONSENT

One of the most effective proactive strategies taken in risk management is informed consent. The purpose of informed consent is to provide patients with enough information to enable them to make a rational decision regarding whether to undergo treatment. The focus is on a patient's understanding the procedure, not just signing a consent to perform a procedure (Goldman, 1991).

According to Hogue (1986), three conditions must be met for consent to be valid: (1) the patient must be capable of giving consent; (2) the patient must receive the necessary information to make an informed decision; and (3) the consent must not be coerced. Getting the consent form signed may be a nurse's responsibility and is defined by policy. If the patient does not give informed consent, there may be grounds for liability. The consent form is actually a **risk management** tool designed to avoid charges of malpractice, along with protecting the consumer. Table 1–1 identifies the necessary component parts to informed consent.

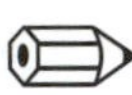

NOTE: The consent form helps to establish a good relationship with a patient and to protect everyone, including the nurse, doctor, hospital, and patient. Informed consent forms are used when inserting peripheral central lines and placing implanted ports or tunneled catheters.

TABLE 1–1

KEY COMPONENTS OF INFORMED CONSENT

Process	1. Accurate and complete information 2. An understanding of: ● Risks ● Benefits ● Alternatives 3. An understanding of: ● Language idioms ● Intelligence ● Hearing loss 4. Opportunity for dialogue
Consent	1. After consideration of all options 2. Agreed to in verbal and written word 3. Documentation of consent obtained

Source: Kathleen Sazama, M.D., J.D. Associate Medical Director, Center for Blood Research, Sacramento, CA; with permission.

UNUSUAL OCCURRENCE REPORTS

Unusual occurrence reports should be filed every time there is a deviation from the standard. These reports are simple records of an event and are considered an internal reporting mechanism for quality assurance. They should be reported to the superior staff member and the episode must be objectively charted, but reference to the report should not appear in the legal patient record.

The occurrence report should contain the following 10 key points:

1. Patient's admitting diagnosis
2. Date when the incident occurred
3. Patient's room number
4. Age of the patient
5. Location of the incident
6. Type of incident
7. Nature of incident (e.g., medication error, mislabeling, misreading, policy and procedure not followed, overlooked order on chart, patient identification not checked). It should be noted (on the unusual occurrence report) if a physician's order was needed after the occurrence.
8. Factual description of the incident
9. Patient's condition before the incident
10. Results of the incident or injury

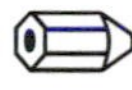

NOTE: Unusual occurrence reports are meant to be nonjudgmental, factual reports of the problem and its consequences.

Unusual occurrence reports are useful for identification of patterns of I.V. medication errors or potentially dangerous situations. Trend analysis monitors patterns of their occurrences. Nursing staff members must feel free to file reports; a report is not an admission of negligence. These reports have the potential for saving lives by identifying unsafe practices. More than ever before, risk may be managed by prevention. In 1996, the JCAHO implemented five indicators on medication use for its Indicator Measurement System, a performance measurement system intended to help to evaluate the performance of healthcare organizations as part of its survey and accreditation process. Table 1–2 presents risk-management screens for I.V. therapy.

DOCUMENTATION

Another strategy for risk management is **documentation**, which should be an accurate, timely, complete written account of the care rendered to the patient. The healthcare record charts the patient's history, health status, and **goal** achievement (Baker, 1990). It should be objective and completed promptly. Documentation should be legible and include only standard abbreviations. Nurses and other healthcare providers

TABLE 1–2

I.V. THERAPY RISK-MANAGEMENT SCREENS

The unusual occurrence report should be given to the supervisor or quality assurance director or risk manager.

1. Medication error
2. Intravenous fluid error
3. Anaphylaxis or severe allergic reaction
4. Severe irritation or breakdown at site
5. Site infection
6. Phlebitis stage +2 or +3 (INS Standards)
7. Needlestick to patient, family member, or healthcare personnel
8. Neurologic deficit, sign, or symptom not present before I.V. therapy
9. Patient withdraws consent for treatment or refuses treatment
10. Equipment failure or malfunction with potential impact on patient care
11. Patient complaint related to I.V. therapy
12. Other adverse or unexpected event (specify)
13. Break in policy or procedure (specify)
14. Particulate or other observable contaminant of I.V. fluid or medication
15. Severe infiltration or extravasation of vesicant agent

For home infusion services add these additional screens:

1. Diarrhea, fever, dysrhythmia, sudden weight loss or gain, and infections other than site infections
2. Questioned safety of home environment for continued home I.V. therapy
3. Rehospitalization for I.V. therapy

Source: Adapted from Tan (1990). Occurrence screens: A risk and quality control tool for intravenous nurses. *Journal of Intravenous Therapy*, 13(5), 308–311; with permission.

should keep charts free of criticism or complaints. There should be no vacant lines in charts, and every entry should be signed. In an office or home care environment, chart dates of return visit, canceled or failed appointments, all telephone conversations, and all follow-up instructions.

Since the 1990s, the emphasis has been on quality improvement, with a focus on evaluating organizational and clinical performance outcomes. Documentation is one way of evaluating **outcomes**. The many formats for charting include problem-oriented medical record, pie charting, focus charting, narrative charting, and charting by exception. Regardless of the format developed for documenting I.V. therapy, basic requirements of the plan of care exist, including goals, actual and potential problems, and nursing interventions and outcomes.

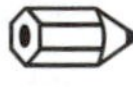

NOTE: Patient complaints of vascular access device discomfort should include the date and time, name of vein-specific insertion location, gauge and length of the device, brand and style of the device, the I.V. solution or intermittent injection device infused by gravity or pump, the rate of flow, and patient comments (Masoorli, 1995).

DEVELOPING AND PARTICIPATING IN PRODUCT EVALUATION

PRODUCT PROBLEM REPORTING

The FDA regulates products in the United States, including over-the-counter and prescription drugs and pharmaceuticals, food, cosmetics, veterinary products, biologic devices, and medical devices. Nurses use many medical devices and are usually the primary reporters of device problems.

In 1990, the Medical Device Act was amended to clearly place responsibility for ensuring that medical devices in domestic commercial distribution are safe and effective for their intended purposes.

Nurses are the best judges of product integrity by inspecting equipment before use. Examples of medical device problems related to I.V. therapy practice are:

- Loose or leaking catheter hubs
- Occluded cannulae
- Defective infusion pump tubing
- Contaminated infusates
- Misleading labeling
- Inadequate packaging
- Cracked or leaking I.V. solution bag

When to Report

Participation in product evaluation is an ongoing responsibility of professional practitioners. Inappropriate use of medical devices may contribute to pain and suffering. The FDA evaluates approximately 2000 medical devices a month. Devices are inspected on three levels:

1. Good manufacturing controls
2. Application for a device existing before 1976 and in common use
3. Implantable or hazardous devices

The simple act of "gerryrigging" or otherwise manipulating a device to overcome a small problem results in the liability for that piece of equipment residing with the institution (Weinstein, 1996). The law states that the responsibility shifts to the institution when a practitioner interferes with the design of a piece of equipment (Abbey, 1993).

What to Report

Report any problems with medical devices if the event observed involves, or has the potential to cause, a death, serious injury, or life-threatening malfunction. In 1992, a congressional hearing focused on needle safety, a needleless system, and safe medical devices. Since this hearing, Occupational Safety and Health Administration (OSHA) and the Centers for Disease Control and Prevention (CDC), along with the FDA, have been collaboratively reviewing the issue of safe medical devices. OSHA expects hospitals to have an ongoing system in place to evaluate safer medical devices (Williams, 1995).

Report a complete description of the problem and information regarding the device needs to be submitted, including:

- Product name
- Manufacturer's name and address
- Identification numbers of the device (lot number, model number, serial number, expiration date)
- Problem noted
- Name, title, and practice specialty of the device's user

How to Report

Report serious adverse events and product problems with all medical products to MedWatch using their postage-paid form or contacting them by telephone (800-FDA-1088), fax (800-FDA-1088), or via their Web site (*www.fda.gov/medwatch/report/hcp.htm*).

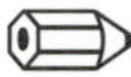

NOTE: Use facilities under the Safe Medical Device Act (SMDA) of 1990 are legally required to report suspected medical device related deaths to both the FDA and manufacturer, if known, and serious injuries to the manufacturer or the FDA if the manufacturer is unknown. Health professionals within a user facility should familiarize themselves with their institution's procedures for SMDA reporting. The MedWatch form can be downloaded from the FDA's Web site.

DEVELOPING NURSING COMPETENCY STANDARDS

COMPETENCY STANDARDS

Competency is the demonstration of knowledge and skills in meeting professional role expectations (ANA, 1994). A **competent** nurse in I.V. therapy is well qualified by education and capable of performing I.V. therapy in an exact and effective manner using the appropriate knowledge of nursing, technical expertise, and specialized skills (Dugger, 1997). Within the educational context, competency may be defined as a simultaneous integration of the knowledge, skills, and attitudes required for performance in a designated role and setting. In developing standards, it is important to have a clear understanding of terms such as *competent* and *competency*.

The practice setting for I.V. therapy delivery is as varied as the patient populations served by this specialty practice. From hospitalized neonates to elderly persons in extended care facilities or private homes, the competencies of nurses and the combination of knowledge, skills, and abilities necessary to fulfill the role of a nurse administering I.V. therapy, spans all ages and disease processes. Basic competencies are intended to serve as guidelines for practicing nurses and to assist in designing orientation and continuing education programs (Pierce, 1995).

I.V. nursing is defined as using the nursing process relating to fluids, electrolytes, infection control, oncology, pediatrics, pharmacology, quality assurance, technology and clinical applications, parenteral nutrition, and transfusion therapy. The practice of I.V. nursing encompasses the nursing management and coordination of care to the patient in accordance with:

1. State statutes
2. INS standards of practice
3. Established institutional policy
4. JCAHO requirements

Elements

Elements of I.V. nursing competency include:

- Accountability: The role of I.V. nurses implies that nurses are astute and knowledgeable enough to adjust their **interventions** (i.e., interferences that may affect outcome) to accomplish short- and long-term care goals.
- Communication: Exchange of information allows everyone involved in the patient's care to make intelligent decisions based on complete data and professional collaboration.
- Collaboration: JCAHO demands multidisciplinary involvement at all levels of patient care. I.V. leaders must develop the skills of collaboration, consultation, and negotiation to achieve positive patient outcomes.
- Autonomy: Nurses can have increased autonomy by being allowed to make certain decisions independently (Dugger, 1997).

COMPETENCY-BASED EDUCATIONAL PROGRAMS

Competency-based educational programs establish specific goals, accountability, individualization, and behaviors for practitioners by defining clear expectations for levels of performance. According to Scrima (1987), the licensing examination required for all nurses cannot be expected to accurately reflect knowledge in a profession in which the knowledge base exhibits a half-life of 5 years. Therefore, the responsibility of ensuring a competent staff often falls to the institution in which a nurse is practicing. A framework for developing staff competencies and ensuring that the institution is delivering safe care includes:

- Development of standards
- Development of skills test
- Assessment of learning needs
- Establishment of a plan of educational programs

- Presentation of educational programs
- Evaluation of learning outcomes

Competencies should be directed toward essential mandatory aspects of performance, have measurable clinical behaviors, include **evaluation** mechanisms, and test cognitive performance **criteria**. A competency program can consist of self-assessment, skill checklist, self-study modules, written examinations, and program evaluation. (Rudzik, 1999).

Three-Part Competency Model

A three-part competency model includes:

1. Competency statement: Statement that reflects a measurable goal
2. Domains of learning criteria: Cognitive criteria (knowledge base) and performance criteria (psychomotor skills: observed behaviors)
3. Evaluation and learning outcomes: Written tests, return demonstrations, and precepted clinical experience

Table 1–3 presents an example of a three-part competency model with example. This model will be used in each chapter of this book as a framework for assessing competency of I.V. practitioners.

All professional nurses are accountable and responsible for all parts of the tasks associated with I.V. therapy and for tasks that are delegated to the licensed practical nurse or technician for care rendered to the patient while under care (Dugger, 1997). The three-part competency model is an effective tool for ensuring competent practice. A competency-based educational model requires developing the three major parts of the model: the competency statement, the performance criteria, and the evaluation and learning options.

COMPETENCY VALIDATION PROGRAM

The **competency validation program** (CVP) is based on current literature related to competency programs and reflects the work of Nursing Department Shared Governance Committees, the Nursing Department Education Center, and other Nursing Department staff. The CVP presumes that both professional and nonprofessional direct care providers are responsible and accountable for their practices and the outcomes of their patient care and other work (NIH, 1995). The CVP is available on the NIH's Web site.

OCCUPATIONAL RISKS

Two types of occupational hazards are associated with I.V. therapy: physical hazards and biological hazards. In the past, healthcare workers were not mandated to report work-related injuries to a risk manager.

TABLE 1–3

JCAHO'S COMPETENCY REQUIREMENTS

1. The organization's leaders define the qualifications and performance expectations for all staff positions.
   A. Leaders have a published mission statement that is communicated to staff members
   B. Job descriptions that include the required qualifications and competencies are developed and used in the competence assessment process.
   C. The hospital's departments study the job that needs to be done and define the qualifications competencies and number of staff members needed to fulfill its mission.
2. Departments provide an adequate number of staff members with the experience and training needed to serve and fulfill the department's part of the hospital's mission.
   A. Education and training are consistent with applicable legal and regulatory requirements.
   B. The individual is licensed, certified, or registered.
   C. The individual's knowledge and experience are appropriate for the assigned responsibilities.
3. The leaders ensure that the competence of all staff members is assessed, maintained, demonstrated, and improved continually.
   3.1 The hospital encourages and supports self-development and learning for all staff.
      A. Personnel receive feedback on performance.
      B. Improvement opportunities related to processes rather than individual issues are reflected in the "Improving Organization Performance" chapter of the manual.
4. The orientation process provides initial job training and information and assesses the staff's ability to fulfill specific responsibilities.
   3.1 The hospital orients and educates staff about their responsibilities related to patient care.
   3.2 The hospital provides ongoing in-service and other education and training to maintain and improve staff competence.
   3.3 The hospital regularly collects aggregate data on competence patterns and trends to identify and respond to the staff's learning needs.

Source: Joint Commission on Accreditation of Health Care Organizations. (1998). *Accreditation Manual for Hospitals,* Section 2, Human Resources, pp 355–371.

Reporting of exposure to blood or body fluid or other occupational risks was voluntary, and only 50 percent were reported.

PHYSICAL HAZARDS

Physical hazards associated with I.V. therapy include (but are not limited to) needlestick injuries, abrasions, contusions, chemical exposure, and latex allergy.

Needlestick Injuries

An important risk to all healthcare workers is exposure to bloodborne pathogens. Needlestick injuries are associated with recapping the needle, improperly discarding the needle, carelessness, and accidents while performing tasks. Needlestick injuries can lead to exposure to human immunodeficiency virus (HIV), hepatitis B virus (HBV), hepatitis C virus (HCV), and cytomegalovirus (CMV).

According to OSHA (1999), needlestick injuries account for approximately 80 percent of all accidental exposures to blood, with 20 percent occurring before or during the use of needles and up to 70 percent after use and before disposal. Most needlestick injuries result from using unsafe needle devices rather than carelessness by healthcare workers. Safer needle devices have been shown to significantly reduce needlestick injuries and exposures to potentially fatal bloodborne illnesses (CDC, 1997; Jagger & Perry, 1999).

During the past decade, many have worked to put safer needles in the hands of healthcare workers. A safer needle device has built-in safety controls to reduce needlestick injuries before, during, or after use and to make needlestick injuries less likely.

Properly designed safer needle devices provide:

- A barrier between the hands and the needle after use
- A means to allow or require the worker's hands to remain behind the needle at all times
- Safety features integral to the device itself rather than as accessories
- A feature that is in effect before disassembly
- Simple and easy operation with little or no training
- Minimum interference with the delivery of patient care

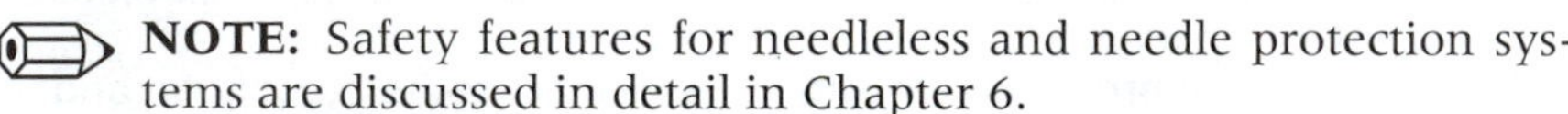

NOTE: Safety features for needleless and needle protection systems are discussed in detail in Chapter 6.

At this time, the OSHA Bloodborne Pathogens Standard does not require employers to institute the use of specific devices, but it does require that employers evaluate the effectiveness of existing controls and review the feasibility of instituting more advanced engineering controls.

California legislated regulations in January of 1999 to substantially revise the state's bloodborne pathogens standard. The Safer Needle Bill AB 1208 required the California Occupational Safety and Health Administration (CAL-OSHA) to amend the state's bloodborne pathogens standard. The Migden bill (named after the legislator who introduced the bill) requires the following:

1. Revise the definition of "engineering controls" to include needleless systems and needles with engineered sharps injury protection.
2. Require that sharps prevention technology be included as engineering or work practice controls.

3. Require that written exposure control plans include an effective procedure for identifying and selecting existing sharps prevention technology.
4. Require that information concerning exposure incidents be recorded in a sharps injury log. (Fig. 1–1 provides an example of a sharps injury log.)
5. Make available a list of needleless systems and needles with engineered needlestick protection (CAL-OSHA Resource Package, 1998).

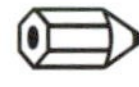

NOTE: Exposure Prevention Information Network (EPINet) is a program that includes manuals and software, data collection tools, and tracking and reporting systems for surveillance of bloodborne exposures tracking device injuries, and evaluating the efficacy of safer needle devices. EPINet can be reached at 800-528-9803.

WEB SITES:

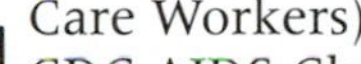

OSHA: *www.osha.gov* (See Safer Needle Devices, Protecting Health Care Workers)
CDC AIDS Clearinghouse: *www.cdcac.org*
CDC Hepatitis Branch: *www.cdc.gov/ncidod/disease/hepatitis/hepatitis.htm*
Epinet: *www.med.virginia.edu*
Others: ____________________________________

Abrasions and Contusions

Abrasions and contusions can be caused by needlesticks and contact with broken glass, sharp edges of containers, or any jagged-edge item. Small or undetected skin abrasions can be potential portals for microorganisms or viruses such as *Staphylococcus aureus*, herpes simplex, and HIV. Use caution when assembling and manipulating I.V. equipment. Excellent handwashing practices and use of barrier precaution prevent the invasion of microorganisms.

Chemical Exposure

The Occupational Safety and Health Administration published guidelines for the management of cytotoxic (antineoplastic) drugs in the workplace in 1986. Since that time, surveys indicated further clarification was needed in management of exposure to chemicals. OSHA revised its recommendations for hazardous drug handling in 1995. To provide recommendations consistent with current scientific knowledge, the information was expanded to cover hazardous drugs, in addition to the cytotoxic (see Appendix D for list). The recommendations apply to all settings where employees are occupationally exposed to hazardous drugs (OSHA, 1995).

Hazardous drugs (HDs) have demonstrated the ability to cause chromosome breakage in circulating lymphocytes and mutagenic activity

SAMPLE SHARPS INJURY LOG

Injury ID (please leave blank) | Facility ID (please leave blank)

Please complete a Log for each employee exposure incident involving a sharp.

Fill in the one circle corresponding to the most appropriate answer. Use block print and avoid touching lines.

Institution:	Department:
Address:	Page # of
City:	State: Zip code:
Date filled out: by:	Phone number: ( )

Facility injury ID#

Date of injury: month / day / year

Time of injury: : ○ am ○ pm

optional
Sex: ○ Male ○ Female
Age

Description of the exposure incident:

Job classification:
○ MD ○ Nurse
○ Medical assistant
○ Phlebotomist/Lab tech
○ Housekeeper/Laundry
○ CNA/HHA
○ Student, type ________
○ Other ________

Department/Location:
○ Patient room ○ Emergency dept.
○ Operating room ○ Procedure room
○ CCU/ICU ○ Home
○ Clinical laboratory
○ Medical/outpatient clinic
○ Service/utility area (disp. rm./laundry)
○ Other ________

Procedure:
○ Draw venous blood ○ Heparin / saline flush
○ Draw arterial blood ○ Cutting
○ Injection, though skin ○ Suturing
○ Start IV / set up heparin lock
○ Unknown / not applicable
○ Other ________

Did the exposure incident occur:
○ During use of sharp ○ Disassembling
○ Between steps of a multistep procedure
○ After use and before disposal of sharp
○ While putting sharp into disposal container
○ Sharp left, inappropriate place (table, bed, etc)
○ Other ________

Body part: check all that apply
○ Finger ○ Face / head
○ Hand ○ Torso
○ Arm ○ Leg
○ Other ________

Identify sharp involved: (if known)
Type: ________
Brand: ________
Model: ________
e.g. 18g needle / ABC Medical / "no stick" syringe

Did the device being used have engineered sharps injury protection?
○ yes ○ no ○ don't know
Was the protective mechanism activated?
○ yes-fully ○ yes-partially ○ no
Did the exposure incident occur:
○ Before ○ During ○ After activation

Exposed employee: If sharp had no engineered sharps injury protection, do you have an opinion that such a mechanism could have prevented the injury? ○ yes ○ no
Explain: ________

Exposed employee: Do you have an opinion that any other engineering, administrative or work practice control could have prevented injury? ○ yes ○ no
Explain: ________

Based on propos revisions to 8CC 5193 effective 1/15/99 & 8/1/99

Sharps Injury Control Program (Sharps), Department of Health Services, Occupational Health Branch / University of Calif.

FIG. 1–1. Sample sharps injury log. (From Sharps Injury Control Program (Sharps), Department of Health Services, Occupational Health Branch, University of California. Reprinted with permission.)

in urine, along with causing skin necrosis after surface contacts with abraded skin or damage to normal skin. It is recommended that nurses preparing HDs wear surgical latex gloves (double gloves if they do not interfere with techniques) and wear a protective disposable gown made of lint-free, low-permeability fabrics with closed front, long sleeves, and elastic or knit-closed cuffs when indicated. Because surgical masks do not protect against the breathing of aerosols, a biologic safety cabinet or an air-purifying respirator should be used when preparing HDs. A plastic face shield or splash goggles should be worn if a biologic safety cabinet is not used.

See Chapter 13, Antineoplastic Agents, and Appendix C for further information on OSHA Guidelines Controlling Occupational Exposure to Hazardous Drugs.

Latex Allergy

Natural rubber latex allergy is a serious medical issue for healthcare workers. Latex allergy develops with exposure to natural rubber latex, a plant cytosol that is used extensively to manufacture medical gloves and other medical devices. Allergic reactions to latex range from asthma to anaphylaxis that can result in chronic illness, disability, career loss, and death. There is no treatment for latex allergy except complete avoidance of latex. Patients and healthcare providers must be assured safety from sensitization and allergic reaction to latex (ANA, 1997).

Researchers have hypothesized that allergy outbreak is the result of multiple factors, including deficiencies in manufacturing processes, increased latex exposure, hand care practices, immunologic cross reactivity, and changes in agricultural practices (Truscott, 1995; Charous, 1994; Slater, 1992). Many persons who have experienced a latex allergy have a history of atopy, a genetic predisposition for allergic conditions such as asthma, eczema, or hay fever (Brown, 1998).

Latex allergy affects between 8 and 12 percent of workers in all health disciplines regularly exposed to latex. In the healthcare industry, workers at risk of latex allergy from ongoing latex exposure include physicians, nurses, aides, dentists, dental hygienists, operating room employees, laboratory technicians, and housekeeping personnel (NIOSH, 1997).

Two types of allergies are associated with rubber: chemical contact dermatitis and latex immediate hypersensitivity, which is termed latex allergy.

Chemical contact dermatitis is a delayed cell-mediated type IV localized allergy that is caused by chemicals used to manufacture rubber products. The most common contact sensitizers are the accelerators: thiurams, mercapobenzothiazols (MBTs), and carbamates (Truscott, 1995).

Latex allergy is a type I IgE-mediated hypersensitivity reaction that involves systemic antibody formation to proteins in products made of natural rubber latex. Natural rubber latex is harvested commercially from the rubber tree, *Hevea brasiliensis,* and used to manufacture rubber products. Natural rubber latex contains up to 240 potentially allergenic protein fragments (Alenius, Kurup, & Kelly, 1994).

Those sensitive to latex should take the following precautions:

- Avoid all contact with latex.
- Carry auto-injectable epinephrine.
- Wear a medical identification bracelet.
- Negotiate with hospitals and providers in advance for latex-safe healthcare delivery.

Providers must be prepared to identify sensitized patients, provide emergency treatment, and use nonlatex medical devices in an environment that is free of contamination (Kelly, 1996).

To reduce the risk of an allergic response, avoid using hand lotions or lubricants that contain mineral oil, petroleum salves, and other hydrocarbon-based gels or lotions to prevent the breakdown of the glove material and maintain barrier protection. Do not reuse disposable examination gloves because disinfecting agents can damage the barrier properties of gloves. Handwashing is recommended after gloves are removed and before a new pair is applied. Gloves should not be stored where they will be subjected to excessive heat, direct ultraviolet or fluorescent light, or ozone.

On July 30, 1999, the FDA issued a proposed rule announcing significant changes in the requirement for all medical gloves. Highlights of the proposed rule are:

- All medical gloves will be classified as class II medical devices subject to special controls. Medical gloves will also now be classified into four different categories: powdered surgeon's, powder-free surgeon's, powdered patient examination, and powder-free patient examination.
- Special controls applicable to all medical gloves include expiration dating and labeling requirements. (All gloves containing natural rubber latex or powder will be required to bear new caution statements depending on the actual protein and powder content of the gloves.)

More information about requirements for medical gloves can be found in the Medical Glove Guidance Manual (publication FDA 99-4257) formerly known as Guidance for Medical Gloves: A Workshop Manual (Center for Devices and Radiological Health, 1999). The manual is available in the July 30, 1999, Federal Register, or you can obtain the rules from the Center for Devices and Radiological Health's Fact on Demand system (800-899-0381).

WEB SITES:

Medical Glove Guidance Manual: *www.fda.gov/cdrh/manual/glovmanl.pdf*

Latex Allergy: *www.latexallergyrn.com*

Others: ________________________________

Nurses working in I.V. therapy are at risk because of the common routes of exposure. The routes of exposure for latex reaction for I.V. nurses include aerosol and glove contact. Aerosolized latex exposure may be the greatest danger for those with type I latex allergy caused by respiratory distress (Gritter, 1999). For healthcare workers, the exposure can be to powder released in the air during the removal of powdered latex gloves. Latex proteins are carried on the powder from gloves and latex balloons and can remain airborne for as long as 5 to 12 hours (Beezhold et al., 1996). Frequent use of gloves during the insertion and maintenance of I.V. therapy increases the risk of sensitization.

INS STANDARDS Latex exposure should be minimized. Healthcare workers and patients are provided education regarding latex allergy or sensitivity and methods to minimize risk of exposure. Nonlatex personal protective equipment is provided to latex-sensitive individuals. Nonlatex supplies and equipment shall be used on patients who have or may have latex allergy or sensitivity. (INS, 2000, 34)

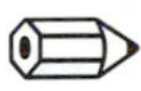

NOTE: Radioallergosorbent testing (RAST) immunoassay is a blood test that measures the serum level of latex-specific IgE (Burt, 1998).

BIOLOGIC HAZARDS

Hazards of bloodborne pathogens must be communicated to I.V. nurses during training. Training should occur during information on bloodborne pathogens, as well as OSHA regulations and employers' exposure control plan (Brooke, 1997). Healthcare employees face a significant risk as the result of occupational exposure to materials that may contain bloodborne pathogens, including HBV, which causes hepatitis B (a serious liver disease) and HIV, which causes AIDS. I.V. therapy nurses potentially incur the highest risk of blood and hollow-bore needlestick injury caused by repeated procedures to access patients' vascular systems.

Factors that significantly increase I.V. therapy nurses' potential for exposure to HIV, HBV, and hepatitis C virus (HCV) include:

- The increasing use of central line catheters in the hospital and home environment
- The increasing number of nurses placing peripherally inserted central catheters (PICC) in various settings
- The expanding application of implantable vascular access catheters with manipulation of needles to access and de-access these devices (Brooke, 1996).

Exposure can be minimized or eliminated using a combination of engineering and work practice controls, personal protective clothing and equipment, training, medical surveillance, hepatitis B vaccination, signs and labels, and other provisions (OSHA, 1991). Percutaneous injury with exposure to HIV-infected blood in healthcare workers has accounted for 80 percent of occupational exposures (CDC, 1995).

The following are cases reported to CDC from 1985 to 1996 of bloodborne pathogen transmission to healthcare workers:

- HIV: 54 documented transmissions; 132 possible transmissions
- HBV: estimate of annual incidence of transmissions was 17,000 in 1983 and 400 in 1995
- HCV: estimate of less than 4 percent of all acute HCV infections occupationally related

Nurses should follow standards established by OSHA regarding glove wearing and handwashing practices. All bodily secretions, and therefore fluids from patients, can be potentially infectious. All personnel who have contact with patients must adhere to strict guidelines.

The Occupational Safety and Health Administration's Rules for Occupational Exposure to Bloodborne Pathogens enforces new regulations regarding standard precautions. OSHA's new standard makes universal (standard) precautions fully enforceable for the first time and spells out what inspectors will look for. Healthcare workers should be aware of how the rules are observed in each agency. The CDC established an additional system of isolation precautions. This new concept was adopted in 1996. Unlike universal precautions, which list "certain" body fluids as posing possible risks for transmission of bloodborne pathogens, standard precautions take a broader approach to the protection of medical staffs and patients. These standards set infection control precautions that will be standard for all patients (West & Cohen, 1997). These new guidelines contain two tiers of precautions: standard and transmission based. Standard precautions combine the major features of universal precautions and body substance isolation (CDC, 1995).

For further information on infection control practices, see Chapter 2. Appendix A lists OSHA's rules for Occupational Exposure to Bloodborne Pathogens, and Appendix B lists in detail Applications of Standard Precautions.

PERFORMANCE IMPROVEMENT AND QUALITY PATIENT MANAGEMENT

Whereas risk management handles "errors," **quality assurance (QA)** seeks "perfection." Both are mutually compatible and interdependent. QA works at preventing malpractice claims and promoting better patient outcomes. All hospital departments are involved in both QA and risk management activities (Fiesta, 1994).

Risk Management + Quality Assurance = Quality Management

Quality management is a systematic process to ensure desired patient outcomes. A quality management program includes both risk management and quality assurance and is established to objectively identify, evaluate, and solve problems associated with I.V. patient treatment modalities.

Quality assurance requirements have always been a part of the JCAHO's accreditation process, but introduction of the Agenda for Change in 1986 shifted the emphasis from problem-solving endeavors to continuous improvement of quality. With this shift, JCAHO initiated the transition from QA to **continuous quality improvement (CQI)**. The goal was to create **outcome** monitoring and evaluation processes to assist organizations in improving the quality of care. QA frequently focuses solely on the clinical aspects of care rather than the interrelated managerial, governance, support, and clinical processes that affect patient care outcomes. Quality cannot be assured; it can only be assessed, managed, or improved. Dennis O'Leary, JCAHO president, has admitted that, in retrospect, quality assurance was an "unfortunate semantic selection because it does not accurately reflect JCAHO's vision of quality."

Beginning in the 1980s, healthcare consumers, third-party payers, and healthcare providers began looking at positive patient outcomes as a measure of quality. JCAHO was the driving force in this movement, along with peer review organizations (PROs), Medicare and Medicaid reimbursement regulations, federal and state laws, and court interpretations of liability and private health insurers' standards (Cassidy & Friesen, 1990). In the early 1980s, guidelines initiated by JCAHO were formed to provide a nursing quality assurance (NQA) committee. This committee recognized that QA had to be ongoing to ensure high-quality patient care. The committee in each facility should include management, chief nursing officers, and staff members (O'Brien, 1988). NQA focuses on two endeavors: checking achievement of standards and solving patient care problems.

JCAHO (1995) has changed the wording of continuous quality improvement to **performance improvement (PI).** The goal of improving organization performance is to continuously improve patient health outcomes.

APPROACHES TO QUALITY MANAGEMENT

Assessing the achievement of nursing care standards involves measuring the quality of care provided. This is part of the nursing process: observing care delivered, assessing patient satisfaction, documenting care received, and evaluating outcomes based on short- and long-term goals. Involving staff in quality assessments can increase their awareness of standards, as well as enhance their assessment skills. Three approaches to outcome are CQI, total quality management (TQM), and the newest approach, PI.

PERFORMANCE IMPROVEMENT

The use of outcomes and other performance measures complements the application of standards and completes the quality equation. Performance results usually validate the fact that an organization did the right things and provide the baseline stimulus for future quality improvement activities (JCAHO, 1998).

Performance is what is done and how well it is done to provide healthcare. Characteristics of what is done and how well it is done are called **dimensions of performance**.

Doing the right thing includes:

- The *efficacy* of the procedure or treatment in relation to the client's condition
- The a*ppropriateness* of a specific test, procedure, or service to meet the client's need

Doing the right thing well includes:

- The *availability* of a needed test, procedure, treatment, or service to the client who needs it
- The *timeliness* with which a needed test, procedure, treatment, or service is provided to the client
- The *effectiveness* with which tests, procedures, treatments, and services are provided.
- The *continuity* of the services provided to the client with respect to other services, practitioners, and providers and overtime
- The *safety* of the client and others to whom the care and services are provided
- The *efficiency* with which care and services are provided (JCAHO, 1998)
- The *respect and caring* with which care and services are provided.

In 1998, JCAHO established standards, scoring, and aggregation rules for improving organization performance. The standards can be downloaded off their Web site.

WEB SITES:
JCAHO: *www.jcaho.org/standard/Itc-pi.html*
Others: ______________________________

CONTINUOUS QUALITY IMPROVEMENT

I.V. therapy CQI includes compliance with policy and procedure manuals, documentation of I.V. therapy-related complications, equipment evaluation, and chart documentation.

Continuous quality improvement is an approach to quality management that builds on the traditional QA models. This approach was first introduced in 1992 as an effective way to improve the quality of healthcare. In 1992, JCAHO first introduced standards that mandated CQI methodology from hospitals receiving accreditation surveys (LaRochelle & Shahinpour, 1995). CQI broadens the focus to all facets of an organization that affect patient outcomes, not just to those that affect the clinical aspects of care. An essential characteristic of CQI is that it is continuous; outcomes are never optimized but may be constantly improved. A distinctive feature of CQI is that it emphasizes improvement in the interdisciplinary processes involved in patient care delivery. CQI incorporates leadership principles from total quality management and has become the central theme or standard in healthcare.

TOTAL QUALITY MANAGEMENT

Total quality management (TQM) is an outgrowth of several healthcare organizations that have adopted a management system fostering continuous improvement at all levels and for all functions by focusing on maximizing customer satisfaction. TQM and CQI share many characteristics; however, unlike CQI, TQM is not unique to healthcare. It requires that those in top management be committed to the program and provide clear vision for the organization; employees must participate actively in the quality improvement process. TQM contributes to a positive work environment, fosters collaboration, and promotes teamwork to enhance interdepartmental communication (Milakovich, 1991).

In healthcare, the most widely used and accepted format for assessing quality is the 10-step monitoring and evaluation process outline by JCAHO (JCAHO, 1998). These standards emphasize the importance of planned, systematic, and ongoing monitoring and evaluation activities. Table 1–4 presents this 10-step process.

The quality improvement process may be performed by lengthy studies, short-term sampling, or problem solving with documentation and reporting (Weinstein, 1997). Three categories are used to create a model for quality management, and each is linked as a measurement of quality patient care. The three categories are structure, process, and outcome.

TABLE 1–4

JCAHO 10-STEP MONITORING AND EVALUATION PROCESS

1. Assign responsibility
2. Delineate the scope of care and service
3. Identify important aspects of care and service
4. Identify indicators
5. Establish thresholds for evaluation
6. Perform data collection
7. Evaluate
8. Take action
9. Assess actions and document improvement
10. Communicate relevant information

Source: Joint Commission on the Accreditation of Healthcare Organizations (1992). *Accreditation Manual for Hospitals.*

Structure

Structure is the conditions and mechanisms that provide support for the actual provision of care. This is defined as evaluation of resources, both material and human. Material resources are classified as facilities, equipment, mission, philosophy, goals of organization, and financial resources. Human resources include the number and qualifications of nurses performing I.V.-related procedures.

Process

Process denotes what is actually done in giving and receiving care. Process is a goal-directed, interrelated series of actions, events, mechanisms, or steps. It includes a patient's activities in seeking care, **data collection,** and a practitioner's activities in making a nursing diagnosis, along with evaluation of actual performance of procedures. This link sets the standards by which evaluation can take place. Process standards focus on job descriptions, performance standards, procedures, and protocols.

Outcome

Outcome denotes the effect of care on the health status of patients. The result of the performance (or nonperformance) of a function or process is the outcome. Improvements in a patient's knowledge and changes in his or her health status are components of outcome criteria. The assessment of outcomes is a method by which quality of care is established. Outcome in the practice of I.V. therapy should reflect final results of the therapy, including patient recovery and rates of complications. Table 1–5 presents an example of a quality management model for catheter-related sepsis.

In summary, the goals of continuous quality improvement are to (1)

TABLE 1–5

EXAMPLE OF QUALITY MANAGEMENT MODEL: CATHETER-RELATED SEPSIS

Structure (equipment)

- Aseptic equipment available for insertion of I.V. therapy
- Experience of clinician inserting line

Process

- Before line insertion, the site is prepared per policy and procedure by nurse
- I.V. lines are assessed for continued need after 72 hours

Outcome

- The rate of catheter-related sepsis will be less than X%
  (Percentage determined by hospital, patient population, and experience of clinician inserting lines.)

prevent complications, (2) decrease morbidity and mortality, (3) decrease cost, (4) shorten hospital stays, (5) increase patient comfort, and (6) increase patient knowledge.

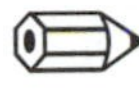

NOTE: Helpful guidelines for evaluation of CQI include the following:

Centers for Disease Control (CDC), Guidelines for Prevention of Intravascular Infections

Intravenous Nurses Society (INS), Revised Standards of Practice, 1998

Joint Commission on Accreditation of Healthcare Organizations (JCAHO) Performance Standards for I.V. Therapy

American Association of Blood Banking (AABB)

PATIENT EDUCATION

State nursing boards mandate patient education by including it in their rules and regulations. Failure to adhere to these stipulations constitutes a violation of state law. JCAHO also has measurement criteria for evaluation of hospitals and home care agencies on patient education practices. (Josephson, 1999)

Although detailed instructions and explanations are presented to a patient, the patient may refuse treatment.

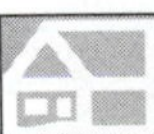

HOME CARE ISSUES

Creating a safe home care environment for a nurse visiting a patient is part of the risk management for home care. Nurses in alternative settings must be aware that they have the same occupational risks as hospital-based nurses: biologic hazards, latex allergy, needlestick injury, and chemical exposure, as well as the increased risks of physical hazards. The home care setting places nurses at risk of exposure to a variety of external hazards.

KEY POINTS

Primary sources of law include constitutional statues, administrative law, and common law (civil and criminal law are the two main classifications directly related to nursing practice)

Common torts in the nursing practice of I.V. therapy: Coercion of a rational adult patient to place an I.V. cannula device constitutes assault and battery

Nurses must understand the elements of malpractice (including duty, breach of duty, causation, and harm) to recognize situations of liability and litigation

EVOLUTION OF STANDARDS:

- National level: Standards of nursing practice established by the ANA and JCAHO
- State level: Nurse Practice Act
- Local level: Hospital and agency policy and procedure manuals

BREACHES OF DUTY RELATED TO INFUSION THERAPY INCLUDE:

- Delay in administration of medication
- Unfamiliarity with the drug
- Inappropriate route of administration
- Failure to qualify orders
- Negligence in patient teaching

I.V. NURSES TESTIFYING AS EXPERT WITNESSES SHOULD BE CERTIFIED IN INFUSION THERAPY (i.e., HAVE THEIR CRNI) CATEGORIES OF RISK MANAGEMENT INCLUDE:

- Using patterns of risk through internal audits and tracking
- Reporting individual risk-related incidents
- Developing and participating in product evaluation systems
- Monitoring patient care
- Preventing events most likely to lead to liability

STRATEGIES FOR RISK MANAGEMENT INCLUDE:

- Understanding laws that govern practice
- Establishing nursing standards of practice
- Informed consent
- Developing and participating in product evaluation
- Developing nursing competency standards
- Documentation

COMPETENCY STANDARDS

Competency-based educational programs establish goals, accountability, and behaviors for practitioners. The framework for developing staff competencies includes:

- Developing standards
- Developing skill lists
- Assessing learning needs
- Planning educational programs
- Presenting educational programs
- Evaluating learning outcomes

THREE-PART MODEL

- Step 1: Critical behaviors are identified and competency standards written
- Step 2: Steps of performance criteria are made
- Step 3: Evaluation and remediation

OCCUPATIONAL RISKS ASSOCIATED WITH INFUSION THERAPY INCLUDE:

- Needlestick injuries
- Abrasions and contusions
- Chemical exposure
- Latex allergy
- Biologic hazards of bloodborne pathogens

APPROACHES TO QUALITY MANAGEMENT INCLUDE:

- Performance improvement (PI)
- Continuous quality improvement (CQI)
- Total quality management (TQM)

CHAPTER ACTIVITIES

COMPETENCY CRITERIA: Application of Principles of Occupational Safety
COMPETENCY STATEMENT: The competent I.V. therapy nurse will be able to identify occupational risks associated with I.V. therapy and demonstrate risk management techniques.
Note: The cognitive (knowledge) information that is embedded within this performance-based competency includes aseptic technique.
This competency *links* to the competency of infection control.

Performance	Skilled	Needs Education
Critical Action Statements		
1. Uses needleless system in management of I.V. apparatus.		
2. Completes latex allergy screen for identification of risks to the healthcare professional.		
3. Uses OSHA guidelines for delivery of hazardous drugs (HD) A. Is aware of need for environmental protection B. Uses personal protective equipment C. Disposes of waste appropriately D. Cleans up spills using guidelines E. Transports and stores HD appropriately F. Implements and maintains written hazardous communication program		
4. Uses CDC guidelines for protection against bloodborne pathogens A. Gloves B. Handwashing C. Protective goggles, gown, and mask where appropriate		

(continued)

(continued)

Performance	Skilled	Needs Education
Critical Action Statements		
5. Demonstrates use of appropriate safety equipment when performing I.V. procedures A. Washes hands after removing latex gloves		
6. Incorporates Standard Precautions into daily delivery of patient care		

EVALUATION CRITERIA

1. Validation of handwashing and gloving by preceptor.
2. Validation of use of Standard Precautions in clinical setting.
3. Validation of use of OSHA standards for handling Hazardous Drugs in the clinical setting.

CRITICAL THINKING ACTIVITY

1. In your current work environment, what are some occupational risks that you encounter in performance of your job?

2. What is your best legal strategy to avoid litigation when practicing nursing?

3. Look up the competency criteria for I.V. therapy at your facility. What are the cognitive criteria and psychomotor criteria that are measured?

4. A registered nurse (RN) team leader is very busy and needs to administer a unit of blood to a patient and start several I.V.s on newly admitted patients, one of whom the RN anticipates will need a blood transfusion. A newly hired licensed vocational nurse (LVN) offers to start some of the I.V.s, saying, "I did it all the time where I worked before. I even started blood when the RNs were too busy." The RN decides to delegate the administration of a unit of blood. The LVN does not stay with the patient after starting the blood, and the patient has a severe blood reaction. What issues and legalities surround this case?

POST-TEST

1. The three parts of a competency-based program include:
   a. Competency statement, goal, and return demonstration
   b. Competency statement, criteria for learning, and evaluation
   c. Goal, evaluation, and feedback
   d. Assessment, problem statement, implementation
2. Occupational risks associated with I.V therapy include:
   a. Malpractice, documentation errors, negligence
   b. Latex allergy, exposure to bloodborne pathogens, burns
   c. Exposure to bloodborne pathogens, latex allergy, exposure to hazardous drugs
   d. Ingestion of chemicals, needlestick injuries, malpractice
3. The tool used to report critical incidents is:
   a. Performance improvement sheet
   b. Unusual occurrence report
   c. Competency validation tool
   d. Quality assurance report
4. The definition of standard of practice states that it:
   a. Defines activities and behaviors of the practitioner needed to achieve patient outcomes
   b. Focuses on the recipient of care and describes outcomes that the patient can expect to receive
   c. Is an ongoing systematic process for monitoring and problem solving
   d. Refers to conditions and mechanisms that provide support for the delivery of care
5. A nurse walks into a patient's room and finds the I.V. solution container dry. The bag had been hung 1 hour earlier. The nurse informs the charge nurse and the physician that this has occurred. The nurse is instructed to complete an unusual occurrence report. The report allows the analysis of adverse patient events by:
   a. Evaluating quality care and the potential risks for injury to the patient
   b. Determining the effectiveness of nursing interventions
   c. Providing a method of reporting injuries to local, state, and federal agencies
   d. Providing clients with necessary stabilizing treatments
6. A product evaluation is part of a nurse's responsibility to ensure product integrity. Examples of medical device problems related to I.V. therapy practice include all of the following **EXCEPT:**
   a. Defective infusion pump tubing
   b. Misleading labeling
   c. Cracked or leaking I.V. solution bag
   d. Outdated medication
7. The Safe Medical Device Act requires that medical device related deaths be reported to the:
   a. FDA
   b. OSHA

c. JCAHO
d. CDC

8. A program that tracks and provides an avenue for reporting bloodborne exposures is:
   a. OSHA
   b. CDC
   c. EPINET
   d. NIOSH
9. Characteristics of performance improvement (doing the right thing well) include all of the following **EXCEPT**:
   a. Availability of a needed test
   b. Documenting the quality of care received
   c. Timeliness with which test, procedure, and treatment are provided
   d. Continuity of the services provided
10. The definition of a tort is:
    a. A written law enacted by the legislature
    b. A private wrong, by act or omission, that can result in a civil action by the harmed person
    c. An offense against the general public
    d. Being capable or able; knowing how to function

REFERENCES

American Nurses Association (1997). Position statement: latex allergy (Internet). Available: *www.nursingworld.org* (1997, Sept 15).

Center for Devices and Radiological Health (1999). Letter to the medical glove industry (Internet). Available: *www.fda.gov/cdrh/dsma/glovelet.html* (1999, July 30).

Beezhold, D.H., Sussman, G.L., Liss, G.M., et al. (1996). Latex allergy can induce clinical reactions to specific foods. *Clinical Exp Allergy, 26*, 416–422.

Brooke, P.S. (1997). What is OSHA and how does it impact IV nurses? *Journal of Intravenous Nursing Supplement, 20*(6S), 45–53.

Brown, R.H., Schauble, J.F., & Hamilton, R.G. (1998). Prevalence of latex allergy among anesthesiologists. *Anesthesiology, 89*, 292–299.

Burt, S. (1998). What you need to know about latex allergy, *Nursing, 98*(10), 33–39.

California OSHA. (1999). California OSHA safety needle law: compliance & implementation guide (Internet). Available: *www.vanishpoint.com* (1999, May 15).

Centers for Disease Control and Prevention, Division of HIV/AIDS Prevention, National Center for HIV, STD and TB Prevention. (1997). *Surveillance Report*, 9(1): Atlanta, GA.

Clinical orientation manual. (1998). *Risk management* (Internet). Available: *www3.kumc.edu/comanual/risk.htm* (1998, April), 1–3.

Dowd, J.A. (1999). Expert testimony in malpractice litigation. (Internet). Available: *www.afip.org/legalmed/expert.html* (1999, Oct 10).

Dugger, B. (1997). Intravenous nursing competency: Why is it important? *Journal of Intravenous Nursing, 6* (20), 287–299.

Fiesta, J. (1994). 20 Legal Pitfalls for Nurses to Avoid. Albany: Delmar Publishers; 10–25.

Food and Drug Administration. (1996). Latex-containing devices; user labeling; proposed rules, Federal Register 1996, *61*, 32618–36121.

Gritter, M. (1998). The latex threat. *American Journal of Nursing, 98*, 23–26.

Gritter, M. (1999). Latex allergy: Prevention is the key. *Journal of Intravenous Nursing, 22*(5), 281–285.

Hibberd, P.L. (1995). Patients, needles and health care workers. *Journal of Intravenous Nursing, 18*(2), 65–76.

Jagger, J., & Perry, J. (1999). Power in numbers: Reducing your risk of bloodborne exposures. *Nursing, 99*(1), 51–52.

Joint Commission of the Accreditation of Healthcare Organizations. (1998). *Comprehensive Accreditation Manual for Hospital.* Chicago, JCAHO, 239–273, 397–404.

Intravenous nursing (2000). *Revised standards of practice, 21*(1S):7–19.

Josephson, D.L. (1999). Intravenous infusion therapy for nurses: Principles and practice. Albany: Delmar Publishers; 46–57.

Kelly, K.J., Sussman, G.I., & Fink, JN. (1996). Stop the sensitization. *Journal of Allergy Clinical Immunology, 98,* 857–858.

LaRochelle, D.R., & Shahinpour, N. (1995). Total quality management guest editorial. *Nursing Clinics of North America, 30*(1).

Masoorli, S. (1995). Infusion therapy lawsuits. *Journal of Intravenous Nursing, 18*(2), 88–91.

National Institute of Health (1995). Clinical center nursing department nursing standards (Internet). Available: www.cc.nih.gov/nursing/nsgstand.html (1998, May 19).

National Institute for Occcupational Safety and Health. NIOSH (1997). *Alert: Preventing allergic reactions to natural rubber latex in the workplace.* Washington, DC: National Institute for Occupational Safety and Health. Publication 97–135.

OSHA National News Release (1995). OSHA lists 18 priority safety and health hazards as result of priority planning process (Internet). Available: *www.osha.gov/media/oshnews/dec95/osha95517.html* (1995, December 13).

Occupational Safety and Health Administration. (1999). How to prevent needlestick injuries: Answers to some important questions. (Internet) Available: www.osha.gov (no date).

OSHA (1991). OSHA work-practice for personnel dealing with hazardous drugs. *American Journal of Hospital Pharmacy, 43,* 1193.

Pierce, C. (1995). Intravenous nursing as a specialty. *In Intravenous Therapy Clinical Principles and Practices.* Philadelphia: W.B. Saunders; 6–14.

Rudzik, J. (1999). Establishing and maintaining competency. *Journal of Intravenous Nursing, 22*(2), 69–73.

Sharpe, C. (1999). *Nursing malpractice: Liability and risk management.* Connecticut: Auburn House; 1–16, 160.

Truscott, W. (1995). The industry perspective on latex. *Immunology and Allergy Clinics of North America, 15*(1):89–121.

Weinstein, S. (1997). *Plumer's Principles and Practices of Intravenous Therapy.* (6th ed). Philadelphia: J.B. Lippincott.

Weinstein, S. (1996). Legal implications/risk management. *Journal of Intravenous Nursing Supplement, 19*(3S):16–18.

West, K., & Cohen, M.L. (1997). Standard precautions: A new approach to reducing infection transmission in the hospital setting. *Journal of Intravenous Nursing, 20*(6S):7–10.

Williams, H.F. (1995). Integrating the occupational safety and health administration mandates on bloodborne pathogens in the practice setting. *Journal of Intravenous Nursing, 18*(6S):9–16.

ANSWERS TO CHAPTER 1

Pre-Test

1. b, **2.** d, **3.** a, **4.** b, **5.** d, **6.** c, **7.** b, **8.** a, **9.** d, **10.** b

Post-Test

1. b, **2.** c, **3.** b, **4.** a, **5.** a, **6.** d, **7.** a, **8.** c, **9.** b, **10.** b

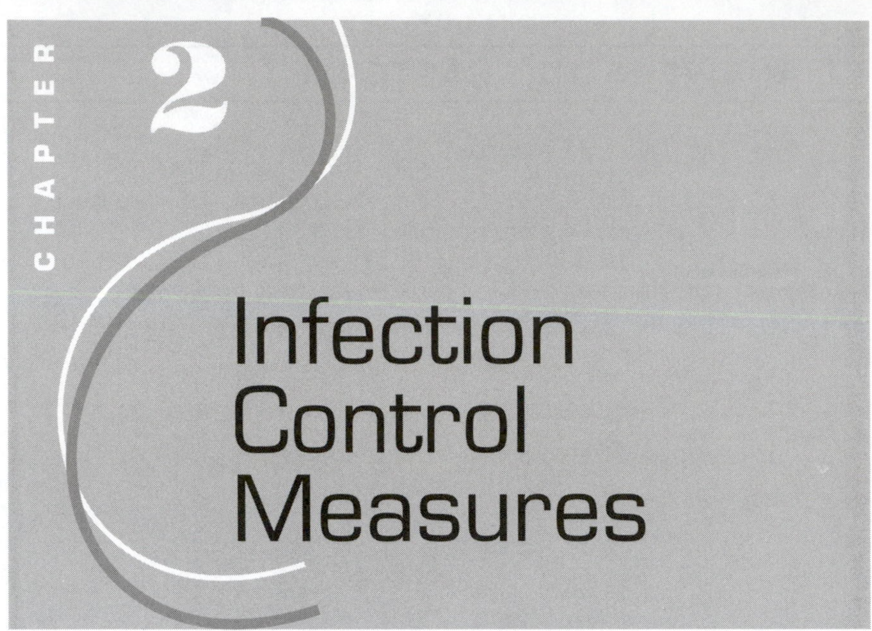

Infection Control Measures

It may seem a strange principle to enunciate as the very first requirement in a Hospital that it should do the sick no harm. It is quite necessary to lay down such a principle.

Florence Nightingale, 1859

CHAPTER CONTENTS

LEARNING OBJECTIVES

Upon completion of this chapter, the reader will be able to:

1. State the definitions of the glossary terms.
2. Discuss the function of the immune system.
3. Identify the organs involved in the immune system.
4. Identify the factors important for maintaining the well-being of the host.
5. State the four clinical symptoms of an impaired host.
6. State the causes of secondary immune deficiencies.
7. Identify the three carrier states.
8. Discuss the links in the chain of infection.
9. Identify strategies to prevent infection.
10. State the factors that influence formation of infusion phlebitis.
11. State the Intravenous Nurses Standards of Practice for preventing infection.
12. Discuss sources of intravenous (I.V.) cannula-related infections.
13. State the most prevalent microorganisms found in I.V.-related infections.
14. Relate the critical nursing interventions for infection control.

GLOSSARY

Antigens Microbic invaders that bombard the body and trigger immune response

Asepsis Freedom from infection or infectious material, absence of viable pathogenic organisms

Bloodborne pathogen Pathogenic microorganisms that are present in human blood and can cause disease in humans.

Colonization Growth of microorganisms in a host without overt clinical symptoms or detected immune reaction

Contamination Microorganisms present on a body surface without tissue invasion or physiologic reaction

Dissemination Movement of microorganisms from an individual into the immediate environment or movement of microorganisms from a confined site (e.g., skin, kidney) to the bloodstream to other parts of the body

Endogenous Produced within or caused by factors within the organism

Epidemiology Branch of science concerned with the study of the factors determining and influencing the frequency and distribution of disease, injury, and other health-related events and their causes in a defined human population for the purpose of establishing programs to prevent and control their development and spread

Exogenous Developed or originating outside the organism

Extrinsic contamination Of external origin

Hematogenous Produced by or derived from the blood; disseminated through the bloodstream or by the circulation

Host The organism from which a microorganism obtains its nourishment

Immunosuppression Inhibition of the formation of antibodies to antigens that may be present

Intrinsic contamination Contamination during manufacture

Leukopenia Reduction of the number of leukocytes in the blood to a count of 5000 or less

Nosocomial infection Hospital-acquired infection, which was not present or incubating at the time of admission

Passive acquired immunity Transient immunity that develops from a person-to-person passage of immune cells or from gamma-globulin infusion

Pathogens Any disease-producing agent or microorganism

Phlebitis Inflammation of a vein

Resident flora Microorganisms that are indigenous to each individual and are present mainly on the skin and in the respiratory, gastrointestinal, and reproductive systems

Reservoir The place where the organism maintains its presence, metabolizes, and replicates

Septicemia The presence of pathogenic microorganisms or their toxins in the blood or other tissues; the condition associated with such presence

Transient flora Microorganisms that are picked up, usually on the skin, that can be removed fairly easily with handwashing

Transmission The movement of an organism from the source to the host

Virulence Relative power and degree of pathogenicity possessed by organisms to produce disease

PRE-TEST

1. The purpose of the immune system is to provide:
   - **a.** The body with a way to recognize and destroy invading antigens
   - **b.** The body with antigens
   - **c.** A way to inhibit the formation of antibodies to antigens
   - **d.** A way for the movement of an organism from the source to the host
2. All of the following are organs of the immune system **EXCEPT:**
   - **a.** Thymus
   - **b.** Bone marrow
   - **c.** Heart
   - **d.** Lungs
3. An immunosuppressed host has all of the following characteristics **EXCEPT:**
   - **a.** Frequent infections
   - **b.** Infections that are more severe than usual
   - **c.** Incomplete response to treatment
   - **d.** Leukocyte count of 5000 to 10,000
4. Which of the following cutaneous antiseptics is used for preventing I.V. device-related septicemias?
   - **a.** Alcohol
   - **b.** Povidone-iodine
   - **c.** Acetone
   - **d.** Polyantibiotic ointment
5. Which of the following is the **MOST** prevalent microorganism found in I.V.-related infections?
   - **a.** *Staphylococcus* spp.
   - **b.** *Klebsielleae* spp.
   - **c.** *Pseudomonas* spp.
   - **d.** *Yersinia* spp.
6. All of the following are factors that can contribute to the contamination of infusion equipment **EXCEPT:**
   - **a.** Faulty handling of equipment
   - **b.** Injection ports
   - **c.** Antibiotics
   - **d.** Three-way stopcocks
7. Which of the following is a nursing intervention when caring for a patient with an infusion-related infection?
   - **a.** Monitoring for signs and symptoms of sepsis
   - **b.** Monitoring for dysrhythmias
   - **c.** Use of full barrier protection
   - **d.** Educating the patient on good handwashing techniques
8. The definition of colonization is:
   - **a.** Any disease-producing agent
   - **b.** Originating outside the organism

c. Growth of microorganisms in a host without overt clinical symptoms
d. Place where the organism maintains its presence

9. Examples of bloodborne organisms include all of the following **EXCEPT:**
   a. Hepatitis B
   b. Human immunodeficiency virus
   c. Hepatitis A
   d. Hepatitis C

10. Dissemination is:
    a. The movement of microorganisms from an individual into the immediate environment
    b. The movement of an organism from source to the host
    c. Produced within or caused by factors within the organism
    d. Developed outside the organism

"Because the intravenous system provides a direct access into the vascular system, an understanding of basic epidemiology principles and common causative organisms due to infusion therapy is imperative" (INS, 1998, S15). In the United States, the following organizations set standards and guidelines for infection control related to infusion therapy:

- Centers for Disease Control and Prevention (CDC), which is a division of the Department of Health and Human Services and sets standards for infection control practices.
- Occupational Safety and Health Administration (OSHA), which is the enforcing agency that provides the mandates to protect employees of all fields.
- Intravenous Nurses Society (INS), which sets standards for practice and provides a framework for the development of infusion policies and procedures in all practice settings along with the Association of Vascular Access Network (NAVAN) and the Association of Practitioners in Infection Control and Epidemiology, Inc. (APIC).

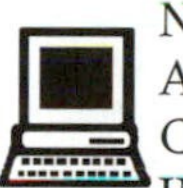

WEB SITES:
NAVAN: *www.navan.org*
APIC: *www.apic.org*
CDC: *www.cdc.org*
INS: *www.ins1.org*
Others: ____________________

To be a competent practitioner, it is important to have an understanding of the functioning of the immune system, the principles of epidemiology, infectious disease processes, and infections caused by infusion therapy.

IMMUNE SYSTEM FUNCTION

The immune system provides the body with a way of distinguishing itself from foreign invaders. These invaders constantly bombard the body and trigger immune responses. They are termed **antigens** and can include microbes such as viruses, bacteria, and parasites (Gurka, 1989). Appropriate immune response occurs when the immune system recognizes and destroys invading antigens.

The immune system also acts as a "clean-up crew" that disposes of used, mutant, or damaged cells that result from catabolism, growth, and injury (Grady, 1988).

ORGANS

The organs and cells involved in the immune system form a complex when antigens and immune system cells are constantly moving through the lymph system, blood circulation, and lymphatic organs. The primary organs of the immune system are the thymus and bone marrow. Secondary organs include lymph nodes, spleen, liver, Peyer's patches, appendix, tonsils and adenoids, and lungs. Table 2–1 shows the locations and functions of these organs.

TABLE 2–1

ORGANS OF THE IMMUNE SYSTEM

Organs	Location	Function
	Primary	
Thymus	Mediastinal cavity	Provides immune function in early years: T-cell development
Bone marrow	Ribs, sternum, long bones	Produces stem cells, which are precursors to leukocytes and lymphocytes
	Secondary	
Lymph nodes	Interconnected system of vessels and modes; chains of pathway of lymph drainage	Stores T cells. B cells, macrophages; circulates leukocytes; drains and filters waste products (celluar debris)
Spleen	Left upper abdominal quadrant beneath diaphragm	Stores red cells, leukocytes, platelets, lymphocytes; serves as hematopoietic organ; filters out antigens
		Kupffer's cells filter out antigens
Liver	Right upper abdominal quadrant	Areas of lymphoid tissue that contain B cells and T cells
	Small intestine	
Peyer's patches, appendix	Right lower abdominal quadrant	Unknown
	Pharynx	Filter antigenic material and cellular debris
Tonsils and adenoids	Thoracic cavity	
Lungs		

Source: Frey, A.M. (1991). The immune system and intravenous administration of immune globulin. Part I. *Journal of Intravenous Nursing,* 14(5), 316.

MECHANISMS OF DEFENSE

A mutual compatibility exists between a healthy host (human) and environmental microbes. The factors most important in maintaining the well being of the host are nonspecific responses and specific immune response. The natural immune response consists of nonspecific defenses present at birth. These mechanisms function without prior exposure to an antigen. Nonspecific mechanisms include:

First-line mechanisms:

- Physical: Skin, mucous membranes, epiglottis, respiratory tract cilia, sphincters
- Chemical: Tears, gastric acidity, vaginal secretions
- Mechanical: Lacrimation, intestinal peristalsis, urinary flow

Second-line mechanisms

- Phagocytosis, complement cascade

Nonspecific Immune Response

Physical nonspecific mechanisms of defense against infections include intact skin and mucosal barriers. The skin forms the first barrier against infection; it is a physical barrier that contains secretions with antibacterial actions. This tight network of cells provides an impenetrable physical barrier against invasion by microbes that reside on the external or internal environment (Brachman, 1998).

Chemical barriers inhibit growth and invasion by environmental microbes. Chemical barriers include acid secretion by mucus, urine acidity, and variety of lipids secreted in the skin. There are also physiologic mechanisms. The large airway of the lungs secretes mucus that traps inspired particles; the inspired debris is removed by epithelium and expectorated.

Through mechanical action, peristalsis in the gastrointestinal (GI) tract and urinary tract expel organisms from the internal environment of the host (Hudak & Gallo, 1994).

Age influences nonspecific factors and is associated with decreased resistance at either end of the age spectrum—the very young and the very old. Factors such as surgery and the presence of chronic disease (e.g., diabetes, blood disorders, certain lymphomas and collagen diseases) alter host resistance, which influences nonspecific factors (Massanari, 1989).

Specific Immune Response

Acquired or specific host defense mechanisms function most efficiently when there has been prior exposure to invading antigens. Passive acquired immunity is transient and develops by passage of immune cells from one person to another or by gamma-globulin infusion. Active acquired immunity develops from direct contact with antigens by disease. The key players in specific immune response are leukocytes, T-cell lymphocytes, B lymphocytes, immunoglobulin, and the complement cascade.

Leukocytes make up one of the most important components of the immune system. A differential white blood cell (WBC) count provides specific information related to infections and disease. **Leukopenia** is defined as a reduction of the number of leukocytes in the blood to a count less than $5000/mm^3$. Normal WBC count ranges from 5000 to 10,000/mL. Other components of the immune system are the B and T lymphocytes, which form the specific immune response system. Lymphocytes have specific antigen recognition and can neutralize toxin and phagocytize invading bacteria and viruses (DiJulio, 1991). Lymphocytes recognize an antigen because of genes known as human leukocyte antigen (HLA) genes.

Immunoglobulin circulates through the body, aiding in the destruction of microorganisms and neutralizing toxin. Immunoglobulins are divided into five major classes: IgA, IgD, IgE, IgG, and IgM. The absence of one or more of these substances has been linked to infection or disease processes.

The phagocytic cells provide a first line of defense against invasion by bacteria and selected fungi. These cells circulate in the bloodstream until summoned by chemical mediators to sites of infections. The immune system provides a surveillance network that enables the host to monitor and identify foreign material and generate specific protection against invading pathogens. Immunologic responses are mediated through the production of antibodies that circulate in the plasma.

The complement system consists of a complex of about 17 different proteins that are responsible for several steps in the inflammatory process, including summoning phagocytic cells to the site of infection. Complement also attaches to the infectious agent and promotes ingestion by the phagocyte. The complement proteins are numbered C1 through C9 and act in a cascade fashion to initiate action of the next protein. These proteins are part of the nonspecific and specific response system. As a nonspecific immune response, C3 and C5 increase vascular permeability and chemically attract granulocytes (Grady, 1988). As part of the specific response, the normally inactive proteins are activated by specific antibodies in two pathways: the classic pathway requires interaction of C1 with the antigen–antibody complex, or the alternative pathway occurs with the absence of a specific antibody (Frey, 1991).

IMPAIRED HOST RESISTANCE

Many factors can result in impaired host defense. Persons who acquire an infection because of a deficiency in any of their multifaceted host defenses are referred to as compromised hosts. Persons with major defects related to specific immune responses are referred to as **immunosuppressed** hosts. These two terms often are used interchangeably.

The following is a general clinical picture of immune dysfunction:

- Infections occur frequently.
- Infections are more severe than usual.
- Unusual infecting agents or infections with opportunistic organisms occur.
- There is an incomplete response to treatment without complete elimination of the infecting agent.

Primary immunodeficiency disorders are congenital or inherited. B-cell immunodeficiencies account for about 50 percent of primary immunodeficiencies, and T-cell immunodeficiencies account for about 40 percent (Frey, 1991).

Secondary immunodeficiencies arise from disease processes or therapies that decrease immune system organ or cell function. These deficiencies are acquired. Causes of secondary immune deficiency are age, stress, trauma, poor nutritional status, and drug therapy. Often these types of immunodeficiencies are transient and respond well to antibody therapy with IgG or a removal of the cause (Gurka, 1989).

BASIC PRINCIPLES OF EPIDEMIOLOGY

Epidemiology is the "study of things that happen to people." Historically, it involves the study of epidemics. Epidemiology is the study of determinants, occurrence, and distribution of health and disease in a population (Patterson & Hierholzer, 1992).

COLONIZATION

Infection is the replication of organisms in the tissue of a host and development of clinical signs and symptoms. **Colonization** is the presence of a microorganism in or on a host, with growth and multiplication of the microorganisms with no clinical symptoms or detected immune reaction at the time of isolation.

A carrier (or colonized person) is an individual colonized with a specific microorganism and from whom the organism can be recovered but who shows no signs and symptoms of presence of the microorganism. A carrier may have a history of previous disease. The carrier state may be transient (short term), intermediate (on occasion), or chronic (long term, permanent, or persistent).

DISSEMINATION

Dissemination is the shedding of microorganisms from a person carrying them into the immediate environment. Cultures of air samples, surfaces, and objects reveal dissemination or shedding of microorganisms.

Some facilities routinely culture all or selected asymptomatic staff in an attempt to identify carriers of certain organisms; however, such surveys lack practical relevance unless related to a specific outbreak of disease. Usually only a fraction of colonized persons are disseminating; therefore, nondisseminators are not associated with the actual spread of infection.

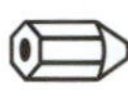

NOTE: The risk of dissemination is generally greater from individuals with disease caused by that organism than from individuals with subclinical infection or who are colonized with the organism.

NOSOCOMIAL INFECTIONS

Nosocomial infections develop within a hospital or are produced by organisms acquired during hospitalization. Infections incubating at the time of a patient's admission to the hospital are not nosocomial; rather, they are community acquired unless they are from a previous hospitalization. Community-acquired infections, however, can be a source of infection for other patients or personnel and must be considered in the total scope of hospital-related infections (Brachman, 1998). These infections may involve anyone in contact with the hospital environment, including staff, volunteers, visitors, and workers. Nosocomial infections are preventable, and their sources can be endogenous or exogenous.

Endogenous infections are caused by a person's own flora. **Exogenous infections** are from sources outside a person's body.

CHAIN OF INFECTION

Infections result from interaction between infectious agents and susceptible hosts. This interaction is called **transmission.** The chain of infection refers to agent, transmission, and host; the links interrelate (Fig. 2–1.)

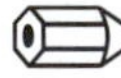

NOTE: To control a nosocomial infection, the chain of infection must be attacked at its weakest link.

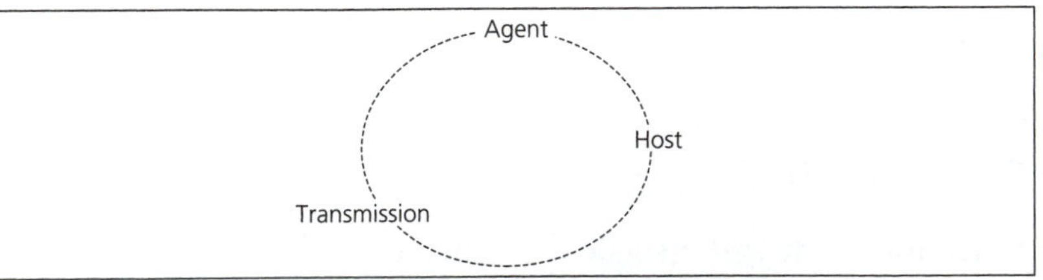

FIG. 2–1. Chain of infection.

INFECTION CONTROL

FIRST LINK: AGENT

The first link in the chain of infection is the microbial agent or source, which may be a bacterium, fungus, virus, or parasite. Most nosocomial infections are caused by bacteria and viruses (Brachman, 1998). The ability of the organisms to induce disease is called its **virulence** or invasiveness.

All organisms have a reservoir and a source; these may be the same or different. It is important to distinguish between the reservoir and the source. The **reservoir** is the place where the organism maintains its presence, metabolizes, and replicates. Viruses survive better in human reservoirs; whereas the reservoir of gram-positive bacteria is usually a human, gram-negative bacteria may have either a human or animal reservoir or an inanimate reservoir. The source is the place from which the infectious agent passes to the host. This may occur either by direct contact or indirect contact through a vehicle as the means of **transmission.** Sources can be animate or inanimate (Brachman, 1998).

The exit site is important in transmission of infection. Organisms from humans usually have a single portal of exit. The major portals of exit are the respiratory tract, GI tract, and skin (e.g., in wounds). In addition, blood may be a portal of exit and is a concern for I.V. nurses.

SECOND LINK: TRANSMISSION

The second link in the chain of infection involves the movement of organisms from source to host (i.e., the mechanisms of transmission). There are four different routes of transmission: contact, common vehicle, airborne, and vector borne. An organism may have a single route of transmission or two or more routes.

Contact

In contact transmission, the host has contact with the source, which occurs directly, indirectly, or by droplets. Direct contact transmission is spread by physical person-to-person contact between source and host. Indirect contact transmission involves participation of an intermediate object (usually inanimate) that is passively involved in transmission of the infectious agent from source to host. The intermediate object may become contaminated from an animate or inanimate source. An example of an indirectly transmitted infection is one that is caused by the use of a tourniquet on an infected person that is reused on another person.

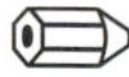

NOTE: Intact skin is the best defense against infection; for transmission spread in this manner, you must have a portal of exit and reentry with nonintact skin.

Droplet transmission refers to the brief passage of the infectious agent through the air when the source and host are relatively near each other (usually within several feet). The transmission generally occurs by coughing or sneezing. Examples of droplet-spread infections are influenza and streptococcal pharyngitis.

Common Vehicle

In common vehicle transmission of infection, a contaminated inanimate vehicle serves as the vector for transmission to many people. The hosts become infected after contact with the common vehicle. The organisms replicate while in the vehicle; an example is when *Salmonella* spp. is replicated in food or is passively carried by a vehicle such as hepatitis A in food.

Arborne

Airborne transmission involves organisms that have an airborne phase in their route of dissemination. Airborne precautions (or the equivalent) should be used for patients known or suspected to be infected with microorganisms transmitted by airborne droplet nuclei of evaporated droplets containing microorganisms that remain suspended in the air and that can be dispersed by air currents. The primary diseases in this category include tuberculosis, varicella, and measles.

Vector Borne

Vector-borne transmission of infection includes external and internal vector transmission. External vector-borne transmission is the mechanical transfer of microorganisms on the body or appendages of the vector (e.g., *Shigella* and *Salmonella* spp. are transferred by flies). Internal vector-borne transmission includes harborage and biologic transmission. In transmission by harborage, there is no biologic action between vector and agent. In biologic transmission, the agent goes through biologic changes within the vector, as when malarial parasites change within a mosquito.

THIRD LINK: HOST

The third link in the chain of infection is the host. Note that disease does not always follow the transmission of infectious agents to a host. This may be caused by certain host factors that influence the development of infections. Such factors include the site of deposition of the agent and the host's defense mechanisms.

BREAKING THE CHAIN OF INFECTION

New Microbiologic Methods

New laboratory methods can determine strains of bacterial organisms at the molecular level. Current standard nosocomial outbreak investigations often involve some type of molecular analysis.

Advancement of Epidemiologic Methods

At one time, epidemiologic methodology was descriptive and analytical; now sophisticated methods include relative risk, risk ratios, regression analysis, and correlation coefficients to study nosocomial infections. Computerization of infection control surveillance has expanded epidemiology databases.

Continuous Quality Improvement Programs

The linking of hospital reimbursement to quality of care and assessment has been a strong incentive to expand the model and methods of hospital epidemiology to continuous quality improvement surveillance. Quality assessment of noninfectious risks requires risk and outcome definitions.

Risk Management

Formal programs have been established to deal with poor outcome evaluation and control in patients with liability-centered and malpractice-related risk management programs.

Antibiotic Use

The Joint Commission on Accreditation of Healthcare Organizations (JCAHO) requires medical staffs to develop a systematic process for evaluating empiric, therapeutic, and prophylactic use of drugs; this process includes programs for review of antibiotic use. Each hospital should provide support for a group concerned with the appropriate use of antibiotics. This team should be headed by an infectious disease physician. Strategies to improve antibiotics use include education, ordering policies, drug utilization review, restriction policies, control of laboratory susceptibility testing, and limitation of contact time between physician and pharmaceutical representatives (Patterson & Hierholzer, 1992). Table 2–2 presents strategies to improve the use of antibiotics.

To break the chain of infection, antimicrobial therapy is used in three stages. Stage 1 therapy is used when an infection is diagnosed or suspected and broad-spectrum therapy by I.V. route is initiated. Stage 1 is guided by a report of sample microscopy (e.g., morphology or Gram stain). Stage 1 patients are usually unstable from the standpoint of the infection process. The causative organisms should be cultured before the patient is treated with antibiotics. Table 2–3 presents a list of antibiotics and their effectiveness against certain pathogens at this stage.

Stage 2 therapy is adjusted to antimicrobial agents active against the isolated organism. Results of antibiotic sensitivity testing are used to guide therapy. Antimicrobial agents with a narrower spectrum of activity are often used. A third and final stage is reached when the patient shows signs of successful treatment and is converted to oral therapy before the patient is discharged.

TABLE 2–2

STRATEGIES TO IMPROVE ANTIBIOTIC USE

Strategy	Advantages	Disadvantages
Education	Palatable; does not encroach the practice of medicine	Requires reinforcement; effectiveness difficult to document
Hospital formulary	Immediate impact; enables generic and therapeutic equivalency substitutions	Requires strong Pharmacy and Therapeutics Committee; perception that patient care is being compromised
Ordering practices	Special order sheets shown to be effective; automatic stop orders also useful	Extra paperwork; physicians may be resentful; automatic stop orders may, at times, compromise patient care
Drug utilization review	Provides feedback to physicians; ongoing, comprehensive review enables intervention	Labor intensive; requires contact time between reviewers and physician
Restriction policies	Enables tight control, especially of the newer, more expensive agents	Limits freedom of physicians; may arouse resentment against the "antibiotic police"
Control of laboratory susceptibility testing	Easily accomplished; can influence prescribing habits	May hinder appropriate use, especially of the newer agents
Limitation of contact time between physician and pharmaceutical representatives	Probably effective in the teaching setting; minimizes confusion among residents	Probably ineffective in the private practice setting

Source: Bryan, C.S. (1989). Strategies to improve antibiotic use. *Infectious Disease Clinics of North America,* 1, 723.

TABLE 2–3

ANTIMICROBIAL AGENTS EFFECTIVE AGAINST CERTAIN NOSOCOMIAL PATHOGENS

Organism	Antimicrobial Agents
Gram Positive	
Staphylococci (methicillin sensitive)	First-generation cephalosporin, nafcillin
Staphylococci (methicillin resistant)	Vancomycin
Enterococci	Ampicillin or vancomycin with or without aminoglycoside
Clostridium difficile (diarrhea, colitis)	Oral vancomycin, oral metronidazole
Gram Negative	
Klebsiella spp.	Cephalosporin, quinolone
Escherichia coli	Imipenem or third-generation cephalosporin with or without aminoglycoside
Enteric bacilli (*Enterobacter, Citrobacter, Serratia* spp.)	Ceftazidime, aztreonam, or extended-spectrum penicillin with or without aminoglycoside, ciprofloxacin
Pseudomonas aeruginosa	Imipenem, ciprofloxacin
Acinebacter spp.	Erythromycin with or without imipenem
Legionella spp.	
Other	
Candida spp.	Amphotericin B, fluconazole, ketoconazole
Aspergillus spp.	Amphotericin B, itraconazole
Anaerobes	Clindamycin, metronidazole, ticarcillin/clavulanate, ampicillin/sulbactam

Source: Perruca, R., Hedrick, C., Terry, J., & Johnson, J. (1995). Infection control. In Terry, J., Baranowski, L., Lonsway, R., & Hedrick, C. (eds.): *Intravenous Therapy: Clinical Principles* and *Practice.* Philadelphia: W.B. Saunders, p. 145.

Pharmacoepidemiology

The JCAHO requires that hospitals have the capacity to document and evaluate adverse drug reactions in their patients. The link between antibiotic use issues and adverse drug reactions has involved epidemiologists in pharmacoepidemiology (i.e, study of both the beneficial and adverse effects of drugs).

Emporiatics

Physicians involved in infection control are often asked for travel advice. It is relevant for hospital epidemiologists to stay apprised of current infectious disease events worldwide. This study of disease in travelers is called emporiatics.

STRATEGIES FOR PREVENTING INFECTION

Nurses involved in maintaining vascular access devices must have the knowledge base and competency to initiate infusion-related protocols to prevent infection. The principles of infection control provide the foundation for the delivery of I.V. therapy. Prevention begins with knowledge regarding the techniques used to prevent infection. These techniques include (1) using the correct handwashing procedure; (2) knowing what is clean, disinfected, and sterile; (3) knowing what is dirty (contaminated); (4) correcting contamination immediately; and (5) following CDC Standard Precautions guidelines.

FOLLOW HANDWASHING PROCEDURE

Handwashing reduces nurses' and patients' risks of infection. Good handwashing with ordinary soap removes dirt, organic material, and **transient flora.** A vigorous 10- to 15-second scrub with antiseptic soap using friction removes most microbes and should be used when placing invasive devices, when persistent antimicrobial activity is desired, and when it is important to reduce the numbers of **resident skin flora** in addition to transient microorganisms. Using gloves should not replace handwashing and does not provide complete protection (Crow, 1996).

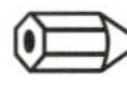

NOTE: The combination of wearing gloves and washing hands after their removal markedly reduces the risk of contamination. Handwashing is the single most important means of preventing the spread of infection. Sterile gloves are recommended when inserting peripheral I.V. cannulae in high-risk patients, such as those with leukemia (Maki, 1989).

KEY POINTS OF STRATEGIES FOR PREVENTING INFECTION

1. Wash hands before and after touching patients or patient care items, especially before and after handling patients' body fluids.
   - Wash hands after touching any area of a patient's body.
2. Wash all areas of hands, including wrists, for at least 10 seconds between the care of different patients.

There is some degree of noncompliance among nursing staff regarding this simple and inexpensive technique to prevent infections. The following reasons have been suggested to account for this low level of compliance:

1. Lack of priority over other required procedures
2. Insufficient time to accomplish handwashing
3. Inconvenient placement of sinks or other handwashing tools
4. Allergy or intolerance to the handwashing solutions

5. Lack of leadership
6. Lack of personnel commitment to the routine of handwashing

KNOW WHAT IS CLEAN, DISINFECTED, AND STERILE

Items are considered clean when they have been thoroughly washed and dried. Appropriately attired personnel should clean items in a controlled area. The use of an instrument cleaner is recommended. Items that are cleaned, dried, and soaked in disinfectant solution such as glutaraldehyde are considered disinfected. An item is sterile when it has been cleaned, dried, packaged, and processed in steam or gas sterilizers. The process of disinfection is not sufficient to kill spores. Steam or gas sterilization kills all microbes, including resistant bacterial spores (Crow, 1996).

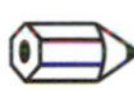

NOTE: Disinfectants used for cleaning equipment can be toxic to personnel.

KNOW WHAT IS DIRTY

The words "dirty" and "contaminated" tend to be synonymous in relation to infection control. Any instrument used to enter a patient's body is considered contaminated. It is important to clean and process items contaminated from patient's excreta immediately after use. Items that do not enter the body, such as sphygmomanometers, may be used from patient to patient unless contaminated. (Disposable sphygmomanometers are now used more frequently.)

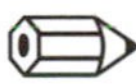

NOTE: Contaminated items should be stored separately from clean equipment.

CORRECT CONTAMINATION IMMEDIATELY

If contamination has occurred, immediate action must be taken. Nurses are patient advocates and must speak up the moment they notice a break in technique. Too often the incident is reported to the infection control department or reported by means of an unusual occurrence report, which simply delay corrective action and possibly jeopardize a positive patient outcome.

FOLLOW CENTERS FOR DISEASE CONTROL AND PREVENTION STANDARD PRECAUTIONS GUIDELINES

In 1996, the Hospital Infection Control Practice Advisory Committee (HICPAC) of the CDC developed new isolation guidelines that better addressed the growing concerns of the transmission of resistant organisms. The new system for isolation blends body substance isolation, category isolation, and disease-specific isolation into a two-tiered approach.

Tier One: Standard Precautions

Standard precautions incorporate the fundamentals of universal precautions (designed to reduce exposure risks to bloodborne pathogens) and body substance isolation (designed to reduce risk of exposures to pathogens residing in moist body fluids) and requires consistent use of these precautions on all patients regardless of their infection status.

Standard precautions are imposed when (1) there is risk of exposure to blood; (2) there is risk of exposure to all other body fluids, including secretions and excretions (not including sweat), whether or not there is evidence of blood present; (3) nonintact skin is present; (4) there will be contact with any mucous membranes.

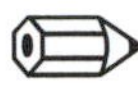 **NOTE:** The primary barrier to protect healthcare workers from blood and or body fluid exposures are gloves in conjunction with appropriate handwashing practices, eye protection, and mucous membrane protection (i.e., face shield or goggles and mask) (Garner, 1996).

Tier Two: Transmission-Based Precautions

Transmission-based precautions are the second tier of the isolation precautions. These additional precautions are based on the known or suspected infectious state of the patient and the possible routes of transmission. There are three categories of transmission-based precautions:

1. Airborne precautions, which require special air handling and ventilation to prevent the spread of these organisms. They also require additional respiratory protection (HEPA or N95 respirators for patients with tuberculosis). Examples are tuberculosis, varicella, and measles
2. Droplet precautions, which require the use of mucous membrane protection (eye protection and masks) to prevent transmission of infectious organism from contacting the conjunctivae or mucous membranes of the nose or mouth. Examples are mumps, rubella, influenza, and pertussis.
3. Contact precautions, which require the use of gloves and gowns when direct skin-to-skin contact or with contaminated environment is anticipated. Examples are *Clostridium difficile* enteritis, methicillin-resistant *Staphylococcus aureus,* and vancomycin-resistant *Enterococcus* spp. (Garner, 1996).

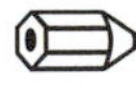 **NOTE:** Implementation of standard precautions has implications for I.V. therapy nurses: (1) Use of I.V. therapy carts and trays may be limited for patients who are on contact transmission precautions

(especially for methicillin-resistant *S. aureus* and vancomycin-resistant *Enterococcus* spp.); and (2) glove usage will increase; and (3) there is a need to develop compliance-monitoring tools for members of the I.V. team to ensure compliance with new procedures (West, 1997).

I.V.-RELATED INFECTIONS

Death rates from infections are the third leading cause of death in the United States (after cardiovascular disease and cancer) and the number one cause of deaths worldwide (Kidder-Ridder News Service, 1998). Each year in the United States, hospitals and clinics purchase approximately 150 million intravascular devices. Most are peripheral venous catheters; however, 5 million central venous devices of various types are sold in the United States annually (Maki, 1998). More than 50 percent of all epidemics of nosocomial bacteremia or candidemia reported in the world literature between 1965 and 1991 were derived from vascular access in some form (Maki, 1990).

INFUSION PHLEBITIS

Infusion **phlebitis** is a common cause of pain and discomfort for the millions of patients who receive I.V. therapy through peripheral cannulae. Infusion phlebitis is primarily a physiochemical phenomenon, and studies have shown that the following influence phlebitis formation:

- Cannula material
- Length of cannula and bore size
- Operator skill on insertion
- Anatomic site of cannulation
- Duration of cannulation
- Frequency of dressing changes
- Character of the infusate
- Host factors such as patient age, ethnic background, gender, and the presence of underlying disease (these factors significantly influence the risk of infusion phlebitis)

In a study by Maki and associates (1991), the risk for phlebitis exceeded 50 percent by the fourth day after cannula placement. Also according to Maki and associates (1991), the factors influencing the development of infusion phlebitis include I.V. antibiotics, female gender, catheterization for longer than 48 hours, and catheter material. Table 2–4 gives a complete list of risk factors for infusion phlebitis.

The three major types of phlebitis are mechanical, chemical, and bacterial, all of which are described in Chapter 8. Bacterial phlebitis (or septic phlebitis) occurs when an I.V. infusate becomes contaminated, allowing bacteria to enter and proliferate; this, in turn, leads to septicemia.

TABLE 2–4

RISK FACTORS FOR INFUSION PHLEBITIS

- Catheter material
  - Polypropylene > Teflon
  - Silicone elastomer > polyurethane
  - Teflon > polyetherurethane
  - Teflon > steel needle
- Catheter size
  - Large bore > smaller bore
  - 8-inch Teflon > 2-inch Teflon
- Insertion in emergency room > inpatient units
- Disinfection of skin with antiseptic before catheter insertion
  - None > chlorhexidine-alcohol
- Experience, skill of person inserting catheter
  - House offices, nurses > hospital I.V. team
  - House officers, nurses > decentralized unit I.V. nurse educator
- Increasing duration of catheter placement in site
- Subsequent catheters beyond the first infusate
  - Low pH solutions (e.g., dextrose-containing solutions)
  - Potassium chloride
  - Hypertonic glucose, amino acids, lipid for parenteral nutrition
  - Antibiotics (especially β-lactams, vancomycin, metronidazole)
  - High rate of flow of I.V. fluid (>90 mL/h)
- Frequent I.V. dressing changes
  - Daily >every 48 hours
- Catheter-related infection
- Host factors
  - "Poor quality" peripheral veins
  - Insertion site
  - Upper arm, wrist > hand
- Age
  - Children: older > younger
  - Adults: younger > older
- Gender
  - Female > male
- Ethnicity
  - European American > African American
- Underlying medical disease
- Individual biologic vulnerability

NOTE: The > symbol denotes a significantly greater risk of phlebitis.

Source: Maki, D.G. & Mermel, L.A. (1998). Infections due to infusion therapy. In Bennett, J., & Brachman, P. (eds.). *Hospital Infections* (4th ed.). Philadelphia: Lippincott, p. 690, with permission.

Bacterial phlebitis can occur because of compromised aseptic technique during admixture of fluids, inadequate skin preparation, failure to inspect containers for cracks or leaks, and improper cleansing of injection sites before administration of medications.

SEPTICEMIA AND FUNGEMIA

Infusates are parenteral fluids, blood products, or I.V. medications administered through an intravascular device. Infusion-related **septicemia** and fungemia are more likely than cannula-related infections to culminate in frank shock and are often unrecognized. Fortunately, there is a low incidence of bloodstream infection (<1%) (Maki, 1998). Of 30 million patients in the United States receiving infusions each year, this translates to 50,000 to 100,000 cases of septicemia (Maki, 1990).

Most infusion-related septicemia is caused by gram-negative bacilli introduced by intrinsic contamination (i.e., by manufacturer) or by extrinsic contamination (i.e., during its preparation and administration). Table 2–5 lists the microorganisms most frequently encountered in various forms of intravascular-related infections. Intravascular device–related sepsis is preventable. To prevent this type of sepsis, nurses must be aware of the reservoirs of nosocomial pathogens, modes of transmission to patients' infusion, and the rationale and effect guidelines for prevention.

The two major sources of bloodstream infections associated with any intravascular device are infection of cannulae and contamination of infusate.

In one study (Beck-Sague, Jarvis, & National Nosocomial Infections Surveillance System, 1993), nosocomial fungemia were more than three times as likely to appear in patients with central intravascular catheters compared with those who did not have a central intravascular catheter. Patients with bloodstream infections receiving total parenteral nutrition or in intensive care units were more likely to have fungemia compared with those not receiving total parenteral nutrition and not in intensive care units.

Factors that contribute to contamination and infection include:

1. *Faulty handling.* Glass containers can become cracked or damaged and plastic bags punctured; bacteria and fungi may invade a hairline crack in an I.V. container.

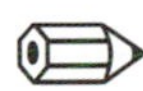

NOTE: Before use, containers of fluid should be examined against light and dark backgrounds for cracks, defects, turbidity, and particulate matter. Any glass container lacking a vacuum when opened should be considered contaminated.

2. *Admixtures.* The risk of contamination when admixtures are prepared is decreased when trained personnel prepare mixtures under laminar flow hoods. The use of a strict aseptic technique is vital.
3. *Manipulation of in-use I.V. equipment.* Faulty technique in handling equipment can lead to contamination. When an administration set is inserted into the container and the container is inverted, the fluid tends to leak from the vent onto the nonsterile surface of the container. Regurgitation of the contaminated fluid can occur.

TABLE 2–5

MICROORGANISMS MOST FREQUENTLY ENCOUNTERED

Source	Pathogens
Catheter related Peripheral I.V. catheter	Coagulase-negative staphylococci* *Staphylococcus aureus* *Candida* spp.*
Central venous catheters	Coagulase-negative staphylococci *Staphylococcus aureus* *Candida* spp. *Corynebacterium* spp. (especially JK-1) *Klebsiella* and *Enterobacter* spp. *Mycobacterium* spp. *Trichophyton beigelii* *Fusarium* spp. *Malassezia furfur**
Contaminated I.V. infusate	Tribe *Klebsiella* *Enterobacter cloacae* *Enterobacter agglomerans* *Serratia marcescens* *Klebsiella* spp. *Burkholderia cepacia* *Bukrholderia acidovorans, Burkholderia picketti* *Stenotrophomonas maltophilia* *Citrobacter freundii* *Flavobacterium* spp. *Candida tropicalis*
Contaminated blood products	*E. cloacae* *S. marcescens* *Ochrobactrum anthropi* *Flavobacterium* spp. *Burkholderia* spp. *Yersinia* spp. *Salmonella* spp.

*Also seen with peripheral I.V. catheters in association with the administration of lipid emulsion for parenteral nutritional support.

Source: Maki, D.G. & Mermel, L.A. (1998). Infections due to infusion therapy. In Bennett, J., & Brachman, P. (eds.): *Hospital Infections* (4th ed.). Philadelphia: Lippincott, p. 690. with permission.

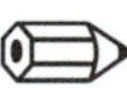

NOTE: To prevent regurgitation of fluid and minimize the risk of contamination, squeeze the drip chamber of the administration set before inserting it into the container and release it when the container is inverted.

4. *Injection ports.* Aseptic technique must be maintained when injection ports are used for "piggyback," or secondary infusions. The injection port located at the distal end of the tubing can expose the patient to excreta and drainage.

INS STANDARDS Latex injection and access ports should be aseptically cleansed before access. (INS, 2000, 41)

5. *Three-way stopcocks.* These adjunct devices are potential sources of transmission of bacteria because their ports, unprotected by sterile covering, are open to moisture and contaminants. These devices are usually connected to central venous catheters (CVCs) and arterial lines and are frequently used for drawing blood. Using an aseptic technique is vital.

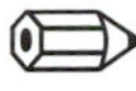

NOTE: Whenever fluid is seen leaking at injection sites, connections, or vents, the I.V. set should be replaced.

CANNULA-RELATED INFECTIONS

Approximately 200,000 nosocomial bloodstream infections occur yearly in the United States, and 90 percent of them can be attributed to central lines (Maki, Stolz & Wheeler, 1997). Over the past two decades, there has been a change in the number of gram-positive, rather than gram-negative, species reported as the cause of bloodstream infections. The majority of intravascular catheter-related bloodstream infections are caused by microorganisms that colonize the skin of hospitalized patients: staphylococci (both coagulase-negative and coagulase-positive *S. aureus*), *Candida* spp., *Corynebacterium* spp., and *Bacillus* spp. (Maki & Mermel, 1998).

Staphylococcus epidermidis (coagulase-negative staphylococci) has become the most frequently isolated pathogen, accounting for 28 percent of all nosocomial bloodstream infections reported from 1986 to 1989 (Schaberg, Culver, & Gaynes, 1991). *S. aureus* now accounts for 16 percent of reported nosocomial bloodstream infections; before 1986, it was the leading cause. Approximately 8 percent of infections are caused by enterococci. However, the emergence of the vancomycin-resistant enterococci (VRE) is more alarming. From 1989 to 1993, 3.8 percent of the blood isolates from bloodstream infections reported to CDC were vancomycin resistant (CDC, 1993). Fungal pathogens represented an increasing proportion of nosocomial infections during 1980 to 1990. *Candida albicans* accounted for more than 75 percent of all nosocomial fungal infections reported (Voss, et al, 1994).

Sources of Cannula-Related Infections

The major sources of cannula-related infections are the skin flora, contamination of the catheter hub, contamination of infusate, and hematogenous colonization of the device (Fig. 2–2).

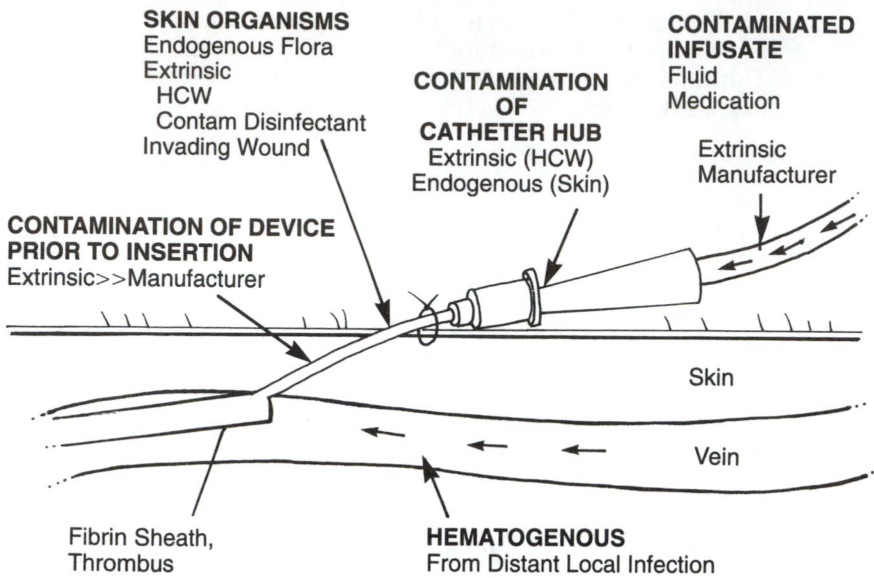

FIG. 2-2. Sources of I.V. cannula-related infections.

Use of short-term devices such as the steel needle or Teflon or polyurethane catheters indicate the lowest rate of infection. Conversely, the polyvinyl chloride or polyethylene catheter has been associated with bloodstream infections (Maki & Ringer, 1991).

Primary risk factors associated with central I.V. line infections include duration of catheterization (number of catheter days), multiple lines, colonization of catheter insertion site by skin organisms, location of catheter subclavian placement, aseptic dressing changes, and aseptic insertion technique. Factors contributing to a lesser degree to central line infections include secondary bacteremia, host defense status, contaminated infusate, and number of catheter lumina (single versus triple lumen) (Cunha, 1998). The CDC and INS guidelines for changing catheters, administration sets, and catheter site care is presented in Appendix E.

Recent studies note that peripherally inserted central catheters (PICC) pose a lower risk of causing catheter-related bloodstream infections (Dietrich, & Lobos 1988; Graham, et al., 1991). However, further studies are needed to adequately determine how long PICCs can be safely left in place. The CDC (1995) recommends change at least every 6 weeks with no recommendation for frequency of change when the duration of therapy is expected to exceed 6 weeks.

Central venous catheters in all their forms pose the greatest risk of causing septicemia today (Wey et al., 1989; Trilla et al., 1991). The lowest rate of infection with CVCs has been with surgically implanted Hickman or Broviac catheters that incorporate a Dacron cuff. The totally implantable intravascular devices have the lowest reported rates of catheter-related blood septicemias, possibly because they are located beneath the skin with no orifice for ingress of microorganisms (Groeger, Lucas, & Thaler et al., 1993). In their current recommendations, the CDC states: "Because insertion and maintenance of intravascular catheters by inexperienced staff may increase the risk of catheter colonization and catheter related bloodstream infections, many institutions have established infusion therapy teams. Available data suggest that trained personnel designated with the responsibility for insertion and maintenance of intravascular devices provide a service that effectively reduced catheter related infections and overall costs" (CDC, 1995).

Culturing Techniques

If the I.V. catheter is in any way compromised, it should be cultured. The recommended method for culturing a catheter, is the semiquantitative culture technique (Procedures Display 2–1). Semiquantitative culture technique involves thoroughly cleaning the area around the insertion site with 70 percent alcohol and permitting the area to air dry. Alcohol is recommended because the residual antimicrobial activity of iodine-containing solutions may kill organisms on the catheter when it is removed. After the catheter is withdrawn, at least 5 cm of the tip and the catheter segment, beginning 1 to 2 mm inside the skin–catheter junction point, is clipped off with sterile scissors and dropped into a sterile specimen tube or cup. Purulent drainage at the site should be cultured before the site is cleaned.

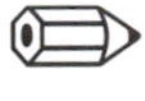

NOTE: A positive, semiquantitative culture of 15 or more colony-forming units (CFUs) confirms a local cannula infection (Maki & Mermel, 1998).

Disadvantages of this semiquantitative method are (1) this method may fail to detect bacteremia of the internal lumens of the catheter tip and (2) the catheter must be removed for culturing and may not be actually be the source of infection.

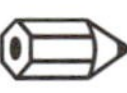

NOTE: Culture any purulent drainage from the site. If the I.V. solution is the suspected source of infection, send the fluid container and tubing to a laboratory for analysis (Castle, 1983).

Blood cultures drawn through a peripheral vein and through the I.V. cannula can be a helpful alternative to culturing the cannula. If the results of the catheter blood sample are five times the peripheral blood sample, a catheter-related infection is suspected and the catheter should be removed.

INFUSATE-RELATED INFECTIONS

The occurrence of epidemic gram-negative bacteremia in the United States in 1970 and 1971 brought awareness that fluids given in I.V. infu-

PROCEDURE 2–1. STEPS IN CATHETER CULTURING

When an I.V.-related infection is suspected, obtain culture from suspected source.

Procedure: Catheter Culturing

Patient Assessment:

- Verify patient identity.
- Obtain physician's order.
- Place patient in a comfortable position.
- Assess I.V. site.

Equipment needed:

- Sterile scissors
- Sterile gloves
- 70% alcohol swab
- Sterile specimen container
- Label

Instructions to Patients:

- Inform patient of purpose of culture.
- Inform patient that there is no discomfort or pain associated with this procedure.

Procedure

1. Explain procedure to patient.
2. Remove dressing over I.V. site.
3. Wash hands and put on sterile gloves.
4. Wipe skin around puncture site with 70% alcohol to cleanse area of any blood or antimicrobial ointment.
5. Withdraw catheter carefully. Be sure to direct the removed portion of the catheter upward to keep it away from the patient's skin.
6. Hold catheter over specimen container; with sterile scissors, cut half the length of the catheter and drop it into the container.
7. Close container and label.

Documentation:

Document all relevant information:

- Record on the patient's chart the taking of the specimen and source.
- Include the date and time; the appearance of the exudate; the color, consistency, amount, and odor of any drainage; and any discomfort experienced by the patient.

sions also are vulnerable to contamination (Maki, 1976). From 1965 to 1978, 28 of the 30 epidemics of infusion-related bacteremia were traced to containers of infusates contaminated during manufacturing. Most epidemics of infusion-related septicemia have been traced to contamination of infusate by gram-negative bacilli that was introduced during manufacture (i.e., intrinsic contamination) or during its preparation and administration in the hospital (i.e., extrinsic contamination) (Maki, 1990).

The proliferation of microbes in 5 percent dextrose in water is most commonly related to tribe *Klebsiella* spp.: *Pseudomonas cepacia, Acinetobacter* spp., and *Serratia* spp. Most bacteria grow in 0.9 percent sodium chloride fluids, but *Candida. Candida* species flourish in synthetic amino acids and 25 percent dextrose solutions (Maki & Mermel, 1998).

Mechanisms of Fluid Contamination

Parenteral fluids can become contaminated during administration owing to the duration of uninterrupted infusion through the same administration set and to the frequency with which the set is manipulated. Microorganisms gain access from air entering bottles, from entry points into administration set, from the I.V. device through the line, or at the junction between the administration set and the catheter hub.

Molds gain access into glass I.V. bottles through microscopic cracks long before the bottle is hung for use; visible cloudiness or filmy precipitates and "fungus balls" in an I.V. bottle are visible to nurses.

Total parenteral nutrition fluids should be used as soon as possible after preparation and stored at 4°C for growth of *C. albicans* to be suppressed.

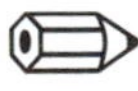

NOTE: Manipulations of the delivery system, especially the administration set, provide means for access of microorganisms to in-use infusate (Maki & Mermel, 1998).

Key points to remember include:

- Inspect all infusates before administering.
- Observe stringent asepsis during preparing and compounding admixtures in the central pharmacy or on individual patient care units.
- Follow good aseptic techniques when handling infusions, such as when injecting medications or changing bags or bottles of fluids.
- Replace the administration set at periodic intervals to prevent the buildup of dangerous introduced contaminants and to further reduce the risk of related septicemia (Maki, 1993).

REPORTING

If intrinsic contamination of a commercially distributed product is identified or even strongly suspected, especially if clinical infections have occurred as a consequence, the local, state, and federal (e.g., CDC and

FDA) public health authorities must be contacted immediately. The unopened lot or lots should be quarantined and saved for analysis (Maki & Mermel, 1998).

Aseptic Technique

Vigorous handwashing along with antiseptic-containing preparation and the use of gloves must always precede the insertion of a peripheral I.V. cannula. The use of sterile gloves is recommended during routine placement of peripheral I.V. cannulae in high-risk patients, such as those with severe burns (Pearson, 1996).

Inappropriate catheter care is an independent risk factor for catheter-related infections. The use of special I.V. therapy teams (consisting of trained nurses to ensure a high level of aseptic technique during catheter insertion and in follow-up care of patients with catheters) has been associated with substantially lower rates of catheter-related infections (Goetz, Miller, & Squier, 1993; Tomford & Hershey, 1985).

Cutaneous Antiseptic Agents

It is important to use cutaneous antiseptic agents because many I.V. device–related infections result from cutaneous colonization at the insertion site. A study by Maki and associates (1991) used povidone–iodine, 70 percent alcohol, or 2 percent aqueous chlorhexidine for disinfecting the site before insertion and for site care every other day. Chlorhexidine was associated with the lowest incidence of catheter-related infection and catheter-related bacteremia.

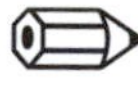

NOTE: The use of acetone to defat the skin was found to be of no benefit (although it is still practiced) and actually added to the inflammation and discomfort of patients (Maki & McCormick, 1987).

Topical Antimicrobial Ointments

The use of topical polyantibiotic ointments on peripheral venous catheters has shown only moderate or no benefit (Maki, 1981), and the use of polyantibiotic ointments has been associated with an increased incidence of *Candida* infection (Maki & Band, 1981; Flowers et al., 1989). Use of topical povidone–iodine ointment applied to CVC sites has shown no benefit.

Dressings

The purpose of an I.V. site dressing is prevention of trauma to catheter wounds and cannulated vessel and prevention of extrinsic contamination of wounds. Transparent dressings permit continuous inspection of the site, secure the device reliably, and generally are more comfortable than gauze and tape. Transparent dressings permit patients to bathe and shower without saturating the dressing. Factors that affect cutaneous floral growth beneath the dressings include differences in physical properties such as moisture, vapor transmission rate, oxygen transmission, and cutaneous adherence. Transparent polyurethane dressings are more expensive than gauze and tape.

Innovative Technologies

Innovations in the design and construction of the infusion apparatus are being developed. These innovations attempt to deny access of microorganisms into the system or prevent organisms that might gain access from proliferating to high concentrations. Some technologic advances under development are:

- The incorporation of an antiseptic (povidone–iodine) into a transparent catheter dressing to suppress subcutaneous colonization under the dressing (at this time not effective).
- Chlorhexidine over povidone–iodine for cutaneous disinfection of vascular catheter sites (incorporating chlorhexidine into dressing's adhesive, which is possibly more effective than povidone–iodine alone).
- A chlorhexidine-impregnated urethane sponge composite (Biopatch; Johnson & Johnson, Arlington, Texas) has been shown to significantly reduce catheter colonization.
- A tissue-interface barrier (VitaCuff; Vitafore Corporation, San Carols, California) has been developed that consists of a detachable cuff made of biodegradable collagen to which silver ion is chelated.
- A catheter material resistant to colonization, which binds a nontoxic antiseptic or antimicrobial to the catheter surface, is being developed by Kamal and associates (1991).
- Catheters coated with minocycline and rifampin have been shown to significantly reduce the incidence of catheter colonization and bloodstream infection (Raad & Darouiche, 1995).

NOTE: Widespread use of these devices is of concern because of the risk of developing resistance to these valuable antibiotics.

- A new test CVC in which the catheter material, polyurethane, is impregnated with minute quantities of silver sulfadiazine and chlorhexidine (Arrowgard; Arrow International, Reading, PA) and reduced the incidence of catheter-related infection.
- Strategies related to reducing hub-related bloodstream infection have been devised (Segura, Alvarez-Lerma & Tellado, 1996).
- Addition of nontoxic, biodegradable antiseptic to I.V. fluid or I.V. admixtures may eliminate the hazard of fluid contamination and reduce the risk of hub contamination.

NURSING PLAN OF CARE

INFECTION CONTROL

Focus Assessment

Subjective

- History of risk factors: fever, diarrhea

Objective

- Baseline immunologic studies: T-cell count, WBC count, differential
- Vital signs, especially temperature
- Redness, inflammation, purulent drainage, tenderness, and warmth of insertion site

Patient Outcome Criteria

Patient will:

- Be free from nosocomial infection.
- Maintain adequate oxygenation.
- Verbalize understanding of precautions for catheter care.
- Report any need for additional dressing changes.
- Not contaminate healthcare team, other patients, or family.

Nursing Diagnoses

- Risk for infection related to immunodeficiency and malnutrition
- Risk for impaired gas exchange related to alveolar capillary membrane changes with infection
- Risk for altered thought processes related to HIV or opportunistic infection of central nervous system
- Risk for knowledge deficit related to illness and impact on patient's future
- Risk for infection transmission

Nursing Management

1. Use standard precautions.
2. Use aseptic technique and follow appropriate protocols when changing catheter dressing, I.V. tubing, and solutions.
3. Use sterile technique when inserting and removing catheter and when maintaining system.
4. Ensure complete skin preparation before insertion.
5. Ensure peripheral catheter removal within 72 and 96 hours.
6. Change insertion site dressing when wet, soiled, or nonocclusive.
7. Secure proximal I.V. connections with a Luer locking set, if possible.
8. Monitor for signs and symptoms of sepsis (fever, hypotension, positive blood cultures).
9. Monitor oxygen saturation with oximetry.
10. Observe handwashing techniques between patients.
11. Use proper insertion and maintenance of invasive devices.
12. Use sterile equipment and aseptic technique appropriately.
13. Give attention to proper skin care.
14. Use needleless I.V. systems.

Pediatric infection control practices are covered in Chapter 9; infection control issues related to blood products are covered in Chapter 12; CVC infections are discussed further in Chapter 11; and issues of infection control related to parenteral nutrition are covered in Chapter 14.

PATIENT EDUCATION

In all healthcare environments, patient education is an important component for preventing catheter-related complications. Education regarding vascular access management is crucial. Information regarding catheter management should be individualized to meet the patient's needs but remain consistent with established polices and procedures for infection control (Perucca et al., 1995).

Education should include:

- Instructions on handwashing; aseptic technique; and concept of dirty, clean, and sterile
- Proper methods for handling equipment
- The judicious use of antibiotics is a major role of the nurse in order to slow the epidemic of drug-resistant infections
- Importance of complying with directions for prescribed antibiotics
- Written information on steps for dressing changes
- Assessment of the site and the key signs and symptoms to report to the home care agency, hospital healthcare worker, or physician

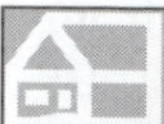

HOME CARE ISSUES

It is generally believed that at-home risk factors for developing a catheter-related infection should be somewhat reduced from risk factors in a hospital setting. Research and study are needed to describe infection risks in the home setting.

The Environmental Protection Agency (EPA) has developed many advisory committees regarding infectious waste disposal in the home care setting. The Medical Waste Tracking Act of 1988 mandated to the EPA the investigation and development of guidelines for handling home-generated medical waste. The home care provider should establish policies and procedures for handling waste (Weinstein, 1997). Prepackaged kits are available from a number of manufacturers and include sharps disposal systems and the CHemBLOC spill kit.

Each home healthcare nurse or aide needs appropriate equipment and supplies related to infection control. OSHA requires that handwashing and eyewash stations are available to employees who are exposed to blood and body fluids. The stations may not be available in the home setting; it is important to provide an alternative until the employee has access to them. It is important to have antiseptic wipes to clean hands, a spill kit in event of a large amount of blood or body fluid is spilled on the floor or a surface, and appropriate containers for disposal and transport of medical waste and contaminated sharps.

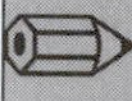

NOTE: Rubbermaid tubs with a sealing lid work well for transporting medical waste from homes to home healthcare agency. Sharps containers must be used for all contaminated sharps (Thomas, 1997).

When in an alternative site where running water is not accessible, healthcare workers should use an alcohol-based hand rinse or foam, rubbing vigorously to cover all parts of the hands until dry. If hands are visibly soiled, the nurse may have to go out of the way to find a source of running water because alcohol does not remove soil or organic matter (APIC, 1996).

KEY POINTS

In the United States, the CDC, a division of the Department of Health and Human Services, is the agency that investigates, develops, recommends, and sets standards for infection control practices.

The purpose of the immune system is to recognize and destroy invading antigens. Organs include primary (thymus and bone marrow) and secondary (lymph nodes, spleen, liver, Peyer's patches, appendix, tonsils and adenoids, and lungs).

Impaired host resistance includes:

- B-cell immunodeficiencies (50% of primary immunodeficiencies)
- T-cell immunodeficiencies (40% of primary immunodeficiencies)

The epidemiologic triangle consists of:

- The host: The living person or animal that provides the atmosphere in which organisms are able to live
- The agent: The organism that is capable of eliciting a disease process
- The environment: The interacting group of conditions, surroundings, and influences in which the host and agent coexist

Strategies for preventing infection include:

- Follow handwashing procedure
- Know what is dirty
- Correct contamination immediately
- Follow isolation guidelines
- Use culturing techniques

A nosocomial infection is one that develops in a patient during or after, but as a result of, his or her stay in a healthcare setting.

One of the main complications of infusion therapy is sepsis (septicemia), a pathologic state, usually accompanied by fever, that is the result of microorganisms in the bloodstream. The staphylococci organisms are responsible for the majority of nosocomial I.V.-related infections.

Risk factors for infection include:

- Percutaneously inserted, noncuffed CVCs used for hemodialysis (highest risk)
- Peripherally inserted CVCs (lower risk)
- Surgically implanted CVCs (lowest risk)
- CVCs in all forms pose greatest risk of septicemia; skin site is the most common source of organism colonization

CHAPTER ACTIVITIES

COMPETENCY CRITERIA: INFECTION CONTROL
COMPETENCY STATEMENT: Competent I.V. therapy nurses will be able to use CDC guidelines for infection control practices in the management of peripheral and central intravenous catheters.
Note: The cognitive (knowledge) information that is embedded within this performance-based competency includes principles of aseptic technique and understanding of the chain of infection.
This competency *links* to management of dressing, administration set changes, initiation of peripheral I.V. therapy.

Performance	**Skilled**	**Needs Education**
Critical Action Statements		
1. Demonstrates handwashing technique before handling I.V. equipment A. Uses antimicrobial soap B. Demonstrates thorough handwashing 15 to 20 seconds		
2. Demonstrates standard precautions A. Tier one: Standard precaution Universal precautions B. Tier two: Airborne precautions Droplet precautions Contact precautions		
3. Demonstrates sterile technique when changing dressing on central line A. Dons sterile gloves B. Uses mask C. Opens dressing tray in correct manner		
4. Uses biohazard waste bags		

EVALUATION CRITERIA

A. Observation of application of standard precautions in caring for individual patients.
B. Demonstration of sterile technique with dressing change.
C. Observation of handwashing procedure before I.V. procedures.

CRITICAL THINKING ACTIVITY 2-1

1. Do you know where to locate the infection control policies and procedures for your agency? List the location.

2. Does your agency have a policy regarding reporting of contaminated infusates or I.V. equipment? Is that information accessible to you?

3. Describe a situation in which you cared for a patient with a suspected nosocomial infection.

4. You observe a healthcare worker enter a private room of a patient with a known diagnosis of tuberculosis who is not using appropriate personal protective equipment (PPE). What do you do?

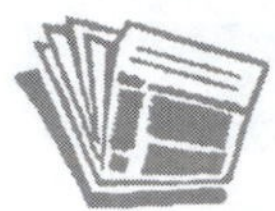

POST-TEST

1. Which of the following constitute the first line of nonspecific defense mechanisms?
   - **a.** Phagocytosis, complement cascade
   - **b.** Leukocytes, proteins
   - **c.** Physical and chemical barriers
   - **d.** Immune system and phagocytes
2. The complement system consists of 17 different:
   - **a.** Glucose molecules
   - **b.** Proteins
   - **c.** Fatty acids
   - **d.** Immune responses
3. The most common immunodeficiency disorders are:
   - **a.** B-cell immunodeficiencies
   - **b.** T-cell immunodeficiencies
   - **c.** Induced by drug therapy
   - **d.** Caused by poor nutritional status
4. All of the following are carrier states **EXCEPT:**
   - **a.** Transient
   - **b.** Intermediate
   - **c.** Chronic
   - **d.** Acute
5. Which of the following describes dissemination?
   - **a.** Shedding of microorganisms from a person carrying them into the environment
   - **b.** Infections that develop within a hospital or are produced by organisms during hospitalization
   - **c.** Infections caused by a patient's own flora
   - **d.** The first link in the chain of infections
6. All of the following describe the movement of organisms from source to host **EXCEPT:**
   - **a.** Contact spread
   - **b.** Airborne
   - **c.** Dissemination
   - **d.** Vector borne
7. Factors that influence formation of phlebitis include all of the following **EXCEPT:**
   - **a.** Cannula material
   - **b.** Frequency of dressing changes
   - **c.** Character of the infusate
   - **d.** Low flow rates of I.V. solutions
8. Microorganisms frequently found in contaminated blood products include all of the following **EXCEPT:**
   - **a.** *Pseudomonas* spp.
   - **b.** *Salmonella* spp.

c. *Enterobacter cloacae*
d. *Staphylococcus aureus*

9. All of the following can contribute to the contamination of I.V. equipment and lead to sepsis EXCEPT:
   a. Electronic infusion devices
   b. Faulty handling of equipment
   c. Injection ports
   d. Three-way stopcocks
10. Standard Precautions is the CDC guideline that says the blood and body fluids that are to be considered potentially harmful come from:
   a. Persons known to have HIV
   b. Persons known to have HBV
   c. Persons with suspected HIV or AIDS
   d. All persons

REFERENCES

Association for Professionals in Infection Control and Epidemiology (APIC). (1996). *APIC Infection Control and Applied Epidemiology: Principals and Practices*. St Louis, MO: Mosby.: 68.

Beck-Sague, Jarvis, & National Nosocomial Infections Surveillance System, 1993.

Brachman, P.S. (1998). Epidemiology of nosocomial infections. In Bennett, J.V., & Brachman, P.S. (eds.): *Hospital Infections* (4th ed.). Philadelphia: Lippincott-Raven.

Centers of Disease Control and Prevention (1995). *Intravascular Device-Related Infections Prevention Guideline Availability;* Notice. Federal Register. Centers for Disease Control. Atlanta, GA, 49993–49996.

Crow, S. (1996). Prevention of intravascular infections ways and means. *Journal of Intravenous Nursing,* 19(4), 175–179.

Cunha, B.A. (1998). Intravenous line infections. *Critical Care Clinics,* 4(2), 239–345.

Garner, J.S. (1996). Hospital infection control practices advisory committee: Guideline for isolation precautions in hospitals. *Infection Control Hospital Epidemiology,* 17, 53–80.

Joint Commission on the Accreditation of Healthcare Organization's (1999). *1999 Comprehensive Accreditation Manual for Hospitals.* Chicago: JCAHO.

Maki, D.G., & Mermel, L.A. (1998). Infection due to infusion therapy. In Bennett, J.V., & Brachman, P.S. (eds.): *Hospital Infections* (4th ed.). Philadelphia: Lippincott-Raven.

Maki, D.G., Stolz, S.M., & Wheeler, S. (1997). Prevention of central venous catheter-related bloodstream infection by use of an antiseptic-impregnated catheter: a randomized, controlled trial. *Annals of Internal Medicine,* 127, 257–266.

Pearson, M.L. (1996). The hospital infection control advisory committee. Guideline for prevention of intravascular-device-related infections. *Infection Control Hospital Epidemiology,* 17, 438–473.

Perruca, R., Hedrick, C., Terry, J., & Johnson, J. (1995). Infection control. In Terry, J., Baranowski, L., Lonsway, R., & Hedrick, C. (eds.): *Intravenous Therapy: Clinical Principles and Practice.* Philadelphia: W.B. Saunders.

Raad, I., & Darouiche, R. (1995). Central venous catheters (CVC) coated with minocycline and rifampin for the prevention of catheter-related bacteremia (abstract). In Programs and abstracts of the thirty-fifth interscience conference on antimicrobial agents and chemotherapy. September, San Francisco: California American Society for Microbiology: 258.

Segura, M., Alvarez-Lerma, F., Ma Tellado, J., et al. (1996). A clinical trial on the prevention of catheter-related sepsis using a new hub model. *Ann Surgery,* 223, 363–369.

Thomas, C.S. (1997). Management of infectious waste in the homecare setting. *Journal of Intravenous Nursing,* 20(4), 188–192.

Weinstein, S.W. (1997). *Plumer's Principles & Practices of Intravenous Therapy* (6th eds). Philadelphia: J.B. Lippincott.

West, K.H., & Cohen, M.L. (1997). Standard Precautions: A new approach to reducing infection transmission in the hospital setting. *Journal of Intravenous Nursing,* 20 (6S), 7–10.

ANSWERS TO CHAPTER 2

Pre-Test

1. a, **2.** c, **3.** d, **4.** b, **5.** a, **6.** c, **7.** a, **8.** c, **9.** c, **10.** a

Post-Test

1. c, **2.** b, **3.** a, **4.** d, **5.** a, **6.** c, **7.** d, **8.** d, **9.** a, **10.** d

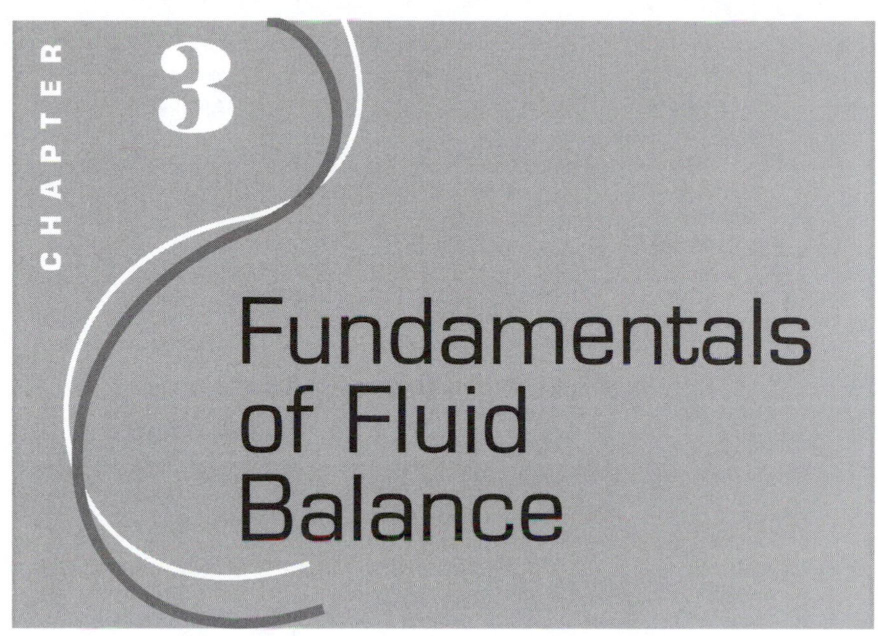

Fundamentals of Fluid Balance

"Chinese say that water is the most powerful element, because it is perfectly nonresistant. It can wear away rock and sweep all before it."

Florence Scovel Shinn

CHAPTER CONTENTS

LEARNING OBJECTIVES

Upon completion of this chapter, the reader will be able to:

1 Define terminology related to fluids and electrolytes.

2 Identify the three fluid compartments within the body.

3 Identify the mechanisms of daily intake and daily output.

4 State the functions of body fluids.

5 Differentiate between active and passive transport.

6 Define the concept of osmosis and delineate examples of this concept.

7 State the average insensible loss for 24 hours.

8 Recall the homeostatic organs.

9 Compare and contrast the movement of water in hypotonic, hypertonic, and isotonic solutions.

10 Summarize the major fluid balance disorders.

11 List the six major body systems assessed for fluid balance disturbances.

12 Identify patients with fluid volume deficit and fluid volume excess using the nurses' quick assessment guide.

13 Determine the nursing diagnosis appropriate for care of patients experiencing fluid balance disturbances.

GLOSSARY

Active transport The passage of a substance across a cell membrane by an energy-consuming process that permits diffusion to take place

Antidiuretic hormone (ADH) A hormone secreted from the pituitary mechanism that causes the kidney to conserve water; sometimes referred to as the "water-conserving hormone"

Body fluid Body water in which electrolytes are dissolved

Diffusion The passage of molecules of one substance between the molecules of another to form a mixture of the two substances

Extracellular fluid (ECF) Body fluid located outside the cells

Filtration The process of passing of fluid through a filter using pressure

Fingerprinting A condition in which imprints are made on the hands, sternum, or forehead when pressed firmly by the fingers

Homeostasis The ability to restore equilibrium under stress

Hypertonic Having an osmotic pressure greater than that of the solution with which it is compared

Hypotonic Having an osmotic pressure less than that of the solution with which it is compared

Insensible loss Output that is difficult to measure, such as perspiration

Isotonic Having an osmotic pressure equal to that of blood; equivalent osmotic pressure

Interstitial fluid Body fluid between the cells

Intracellular fluid (ICF) Body fluid inside the cells

Intravascular fluid The fluid portion of blood plasma

Oncotic pressure The osmotic pressure exerted by colloids (proteins), as when albumin exerts oncotic pressure within the blood vessels and helps to hold the water content of the blood in the intravascular compartment

Osmolarity A measure of solute concentration; the concentration of a solution in terms of osmoles of solutes per liter of solution

Osmosis The movement of water from a lower concentration to a higher concentration across a semipermeable membrane

Syndrome of inappropriate antidiuretic hormone (SIADH) secretion A condition in which excessive ADH is secreted, resulting in hyponatremia

Sensible loss Output that is measurable

Solute The substance that is dissolved in a liquid to form a solution

PRE-TEST

1. What are the three fluid compartments related to body fluid?
   a. Intracellular, interstitial, intravascular
   b. Interstitial, extravascular, intravascular
   c. Extracellular, extravascular, interstitial
2. What is (are) the function(s) of body fluid?
   a. Maintain blood volume
   b. Transport material to and from cells
   c. Assist digestion of food through hydrolysis
   d. Regulate body temperature
   e. All of the above
3. Water is passively transported within the body by:
   a. Osmosis
   b. Adenosine triphosphate (ATP) in cell membrane
   c. Diffusion
   d. The sodium-potassium pump
4. Which of the following is the range of milliosmoles (mOsm/liter) for an isotonic solution?
   a. 150 to 250
   b. 250 to 375
   c. 320 to 460
   d. 350 to 500
5. Which of the following may be signs and symptoms of fluid volume deficit?
   a. Bounding pulse, decreased blood pressure, and moist crackles
   b. Increased respiratory rate; warm, moist skin; and decreased body temperature
   c. Increased pulse rate, decreased blood pressure, and poor skin turgor
   d. Dyspnea, jugular vein distention, and sternum fingerprinting
6. A patient has the following signs and symptoms: moist crackles (rales), increased respiratory rate, dyspnea, and 3 plus edema of the ankles. What is the appropriate nursing diagnosis?
   a. Fluid volume deficit
   b. Fluid volume excess
   c. Tissue integrity impaired
   d. Tissue perfusion altered, renal
7. What is the range of the average insensible loss in an adult?
   a. 200 to 400 mL/d
   b. 400 to 600 mL/d
   c. 500 to 1000 mL/d
   d. 800 to 1200 mL/d
8. Diffusion is a passive process in which molecules move from:
   a. An area of low concentration to one of high concentration
   b. An area of high concentration to one of low concentration
   c. A region of low pressure to one of high pressure, using hydrostatic pressure

FLUID FUNCTION

Fluids within the body have several important functions. The ECF transports nutrients to the cells and carries waste products away from the cells by means of the capillary bed. Body fluids are in constant motion, maintaining living conditions for body cells (Metheny, 2000). The fluid within the body also has the following functions:

1. Maintains blood volume
2. Regulates body temperature
3. Transports material to and from cells
4. Serves as aqueous medium for cellular metabolism
5. Assists digestion of food through hydrolysis
6. Acts as solvent in which solutes are available for cell function
7. Serves as medium for the excretion of waste

FLUID TRANSPORT

Movement of particles through the cell membrane occurs through four transport mechanisms: passive transport consisting of diffusion, osmosis, and filtration; and active transport. Materials are transported between the ICF and the extracellular compartment by these four mechanisms.

PASSIVE TRANSPORT

Passive transport is also referred to as non–carrier-mediated transport. It is the movement of solutes through membranes without the expenditure of energy. It includes passive diffusion, osmosis, and filtration (Josephson, 1999).

Passive Diffusion

Passive diffusion is the passive movement of water, ions, and lipid-soluble molecules randomly in all directions from a region of high concentration to an area of low concentration (Josephson, 1999). Diffusion occurs through semipermeable membranes by either passing through pores, if small enough, or dissolving in the lipid matrix of the membrane wall. If there is no force opposing diffusion, particles distribute themselves evenly. Many substances can diffuse through the cell membrane, and these substances diffuse in both directions. Influencing factors in the diffusion process are concentration differences, electrical potential, and pressure differences across the pores. The greater the concentration, the greater the rate of diffusion. An increase in the pressure on one side of the membrane increases the molecular forces striking the pores, thus creating a pressure gradient. Other factors that increase diffusion include:

- Increased temperature
- Increased concentration of particles
- Decreased size or molecular weight of particles
- Increased surface area available for diffusion
- Decreased distance across which the particle mass must diffuse

Osmosis

Osmosis is the passage of water from an area of lower particle concentration toward a higher particle concentration across a semipermeable membrane. For a membrane to be semipermeable, it has to be more permeable to water than to solutes. This process tends to equalize the concentration of two solutions.

Osmosis governs the movement of body fluids between the intracellular and ECF compartments, therefore influencing the volumes of fluid within each. Through the process of osmosis, water flows through semipermeable membranes toward the side with higher concentration of particles (thus from lower to higher).

Pressure Gradients

Osmotic pressure develops as **solute** particles collide against each other. Osmotic pressure is the amount of hydrostatic pressure needed to draw a solvent (water) across a membrane and develops as a result a high concentration of particles colliding with one another. As the number of solutes increases, there is less space for them to move; therefore, they come in contact with one another more frequently. This results in increased osmotic pressure, which causes the movement of fluid. The concentration of a solution containing more solute particles increases the collisions creating a greater osmotic pressure (Josephson, 1999). Osmotic pressure is measured in milliosmoles (mOsm). Whereas **osmolality** is the total number of osmotically active particles per liter of solution, osmolarity refers to the concentration of a solute in a volume of solution. The two terms are very similar and are often used interchangeably. The term osmolarity will be used within this text. The normal osmolarity of body fluids is between 280 and 295 mOsm/L, and the osmolarity of ICF and ECF is always equal.

Tonicity

Tonicity reflects the concept and effects of hypotonic, hypertonic, and isotonic solutions on body cells. Figure 3–3 shows the movement of water by osmosis in hypotonic, isotonic, and hypertonic solutions.

Isotonic solutions, such as 0.9 percent sodium chloride (NaCl) and 5 percent dextrose in water, have the same osmolarity as that of normal body fluids. Solutions that have an osmolarity of 250 to 375 mOsm/L are

HYPOTONIC
Less than body less 250 mEq/kg

A
Na⁺
H_2O
H_2O
H_2O
H_2O
Na⁺
Dehydrated Cell
H_2O

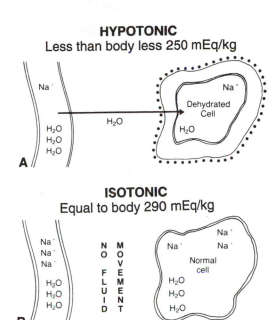

ISOTONIC
Equal to body 290 mEq/kg

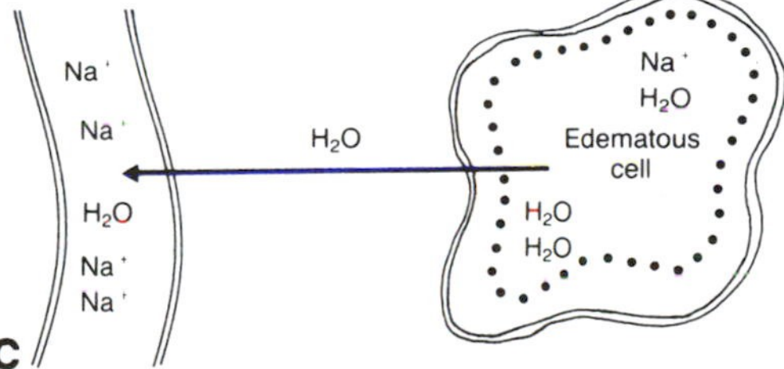

HYPERTONIC
More than body greater 375 mEq/kg

C
Na⁺
Na⁺
H_2O
Na⁺
Na⁺
H_2O
Na⁺
H_2O
Edematous cell
H_2O
H_2O

FIG. 3–3. Effects of fluid shifts in isontonic, hypertonic, and hypotonic states. From Kuhn, M. Pharmacotherapeutics: A Nursing Process Approach, 4th ed. F.A. Davis, Philadelphia, 1998, p. 128, with permission.

considered isotonic solutions and have no effect on the volume of fluid within the cell; the solution remains within the ECF space. Isotonic solutions are used to expand the ECF compartment.

Hypotonic solutions contain less salt than the intracellular space, and when infused, have an osmolarity below 250 mOsm/L, and move water into the cell, causing the cell to swell and possibly burst. By lowering the serum osmolarity, the body fluids shift out of the blood vessels into the interstitial tissue and cells. Hypotonic solutions hydrate cells and can deplete the circulatory system. An example of a hypotonic solution is 2.5 percent dextrose in water.

Hypertonic solutions, conversely, cause the water from within a cell to move to the ECF compartment, where the concentration of salt is greater, causing the cell to shrink. Hypertonic solutions have an osmolarity of 375 mOsm/L and above. These solutions are used to replace electrolytes.

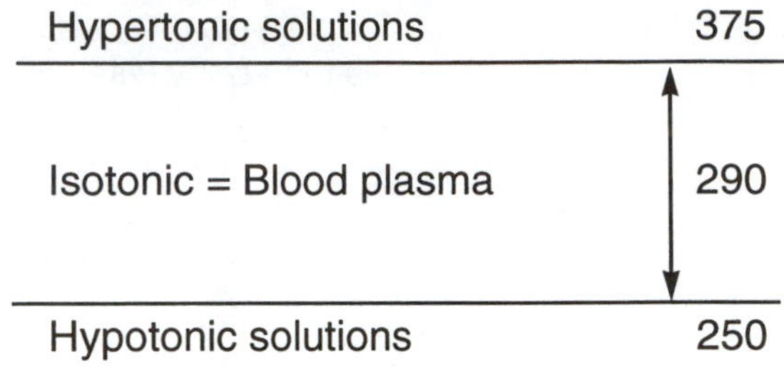

FIG. 3–4. Tonicity/osmolarity ranges of solutions.

When hypertonic dextrose solutions are used alone, they also are used to shift ECF from interstitial tissue to plasma. Examples of hypertonic solutions are 5 percent dextrose and 0.9 percent NaCl, or 5 percent dextrose and Normosol M. Figure 3–4 illustrates tonicity (osmolarity) ranges.

The osmotic pressure exerted by plasma colloids (or solutes) is called the colloid osmotic pressure, or oncotic pressure. For example, albumin, a plasma protein, exerts oncotic pressure within the blood vessels and helps to hold the water content of the blood in the intravascular space. Proteinates are concentrated in the intracellular (55 mEq/L) and intravascular (16 mEq/L) spaces.

Filtration

Filtration is the transfer of water and a dissolved substance from a region of high pressure to a region of low pressure; the force behind it is hydrostatic pressure (i.e., the pressure of water at rest). The pumping heart provides hydrostatic pressure in the movement of water and electrolytes from the arterial capillary bed to the interstitial fluid. Diffusion moves in either direction across a membrane; filtration moves in one direction only because of the hydrostatic, osmotic, and interstitial fluid pressure. Filtration is likened to pouring a solution through a sieve: the size of the opening in the sieve determines the size of the particle to be filtered (Josephson, 1999).

The plasma compartment contains more protein than the other compartments. Plasma protein, composed of albumin, globulin, and fibrinogen, creates an osmotic pressure at the capillary membrane, preventing fluid from the plasma from leaking into the interstitial spaces. Osmotic pressure created within the plasma by the presence of protein (mainly albumin) keeps the water in the vascular system.

Starling's Law of the Capillaries maintains that under normal circumstances, fluid filtered out of the arterial end of a capillary bed and reabsorbed at the venous end is exactly the same, creating a state of near equilibrium. However, it is not exactly the same because of the difference in hydrostatic pressure between the arterial and venous capillary beds. The pressure that moves fluid out of the arterial end of the network amounts to a total of 28.3 mm Hg. The pressure that moves fluid back into circulation at the venous capillary bed is 28 mm Hg. The small amount of excess remaining in the interstitial compartment is returned to the circulation by way of the lymphatic system (Josephson, 1999).

ACTIVE TRANSPORT

Active transport is similar to diffusion except that it acts against a concentration gradient. Active transport occurs when it is necessary for ions (electrolytes) to move from an area of low concentration to an area of high concentration. By definition, active transport implies that energy expenditure must take place for the movement to occur against a concentration gradient. Adenosine triphosphate (ATP) is released from the cell to enable certain substances to acquire the energy needed to pass through the cell membrane. For example, sodium concentration is greater in ECF; therefore, sodium tends to enter by diffusion into the intracellular compartment. This tendency is offset by the sodium-potassium pump, which is located on the cell membrane. In the presence of ATP, the sodium-potassium pump actively moves sodium from the cell into the ECF. Active transport is vital for maintaining the unique composition of both the extracellular and intracellular compartments (Lee, 1996).

HOMEOSTATIC MECHANISMS

Regulation of body water is maintained through exogenous sources, such as the intake of food and fluids and endogenous sources, that are produced within the body through chemical oxidation process. Several homeostatic mechanisms are responsible for the balance of fluid and electrolytes within the body. When homeostasis is compromised and imbalance occurs, the nurse is responsible for managing the exogenous source of fluid replacement via the intravenous route. The endogenous sources of balancing fluid and electrolytes is through various body systems such as the renal, cardiovascular, lymphatic, respiratory, nervous, and endocrine systems.

RENAL SYSTEM

The kidneys are vital to control fluid and electrolyte balance. They normally filter 170 L of plasma per day in the adult, and excrete only 1.5 L of urine. They act in response to bloodborne messengers such as aldosterone and antidiuretic hormone (ADH). Functions of the kidneys in fluid balance are:

- Regulation of fluid volume and osmolarity by selective retention and excretion of body fluids

- Regulation of electrolyte levels by selective retention of needed substances and excretion of unneeded substances
- Regulation of pH of ECF by excretion or retention of hydrogen (H^+) ions
- Excretion of metabolic wastes (primarily acids) and toxic substances (Metheny, 2000).

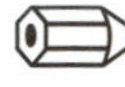

NOTE: Renal failure can result in multiple fluid and electrolyte imbalances.

CARDIOVASCULAR SYSTEM

The pumping action of the heart provides circulation of blood through the kidneys under pressure, which allows urine to form. Renal perfusion makes renal function possible. Blood vessels provide plasma to reach the kidneys in sufficient volume (20% of circulating blood volume) to permit regulation of water and electrolytes. Baroreceptors located in the carotid sinus and aortic arch respond to the degree of stretch of the vessel wall, which has been generated by the body's reaction to hypovolemia. The response is to stimulate fluid retention.

LYMPHATIC SYSTEM

The lymphatic system serves as an adjunct to the cardiovascular system by removing excess interstitial fluid (in the form of lymph) and returning it to the circulatory system. Fluid overload in the interstitial compartment would result if it were not for the lymphatic system. The lymphatic system carries the excess fluid, proteins, and large particulate matter that cannot be reabsorbed by the venous capillary bed out of interstitial compartment. This minute excess (0.3 mm Hg) accounts for 1.7 mm/min of fluid. If the lymphatic system were not continually removing this small amount of fluid, there would be a buildup of 2448 m in the interstitial compartment over a 24-hour period of time (Josephson, 1999).

RESPIRATORY SYSTEM

The lungs are vital for maintaining homeostasis and constitute one of the main regulatory organs of fluid and acid–base balance. The lungs regulate acid–base balance by regulation of the hydrogen (H^+) ion concentration. Alveolar ventilation is responsible for the daily elimination of approximately 13,000 mEq of H^+ ions. The kidneys excrete only 40 to 80 mEq of hydrogen daily. Under influence from the medulla, the lungs act promptly to correct metabolic acid–base disturbances by regulating the level of carbon dioxide (a potential acid) in the ECF. Functions of the lungs in body fluid balance are:

- Regulation of metabolic alkalosis by compensatory hypoventilation, resulting in carbon dioxide (CO_2) retention and increased acidity of the ECF
- Regulation of metabolic acidosis by causing compensatory hyperventilation, resulting in CO_2 excretion and thus decreased acidity of the ECF
- Removal of 300 to 500 mL of water daily through exhalation (i.e., insensible water loss)

NERVOUS SYSTEM

The nervous system is the master controller in fluid and electrolyte balance through the regulation of sodium and water. It does this by stimulating various endocrine glands.

ENDOCRINE SYSTEM

The glands responsible for aiding in homeostasis are the adrenal, pituitary, and parathyroid glands. The endocrine system responds selectively to the regulation and maintenance of fluid and electrolyte balance through hormonal production.

Antidiuretic Hormone

The pituitary hormone influencing water balance is ADH. This hormone, which affects renal reabsorption of water, is also referred to as the "water-conserving" hormone. Functions of ADH are to maintain osmotic pressure of the cells by controlling renal water retention or excretion and control of blood volume. Excessive secretion of ADH results in syndrome of inappropriate antidiuretic hormone secretion (SIADH).

Numerous drugs (e.g., alcohol, narcotic antagonists) can block ADH activity or reduce tubular responsiveness to ADH (e.g., lithium, demeclocycline), which results in increased water loss, causing dehydration and hypernatremia. Increased ADH secretion may be the result of disease (hormone-secreting tumor, head injury) or may be related to administration of drugs such as chlorpropamide, Vinca alkaloids, carbamazepine, cyclophosphamide, tricyclic antidepressants, and narcotics (Klotz, 1998).

Pathologic changes that affect ADH productions include head trauma, anesthesia and surgery in general, tumors of the brain or lung, and certain drugs (e.g., barbiturates, antineoplastics, and nonsteroidal anti-inflammatory agents [NSNA, 1997]).

Parathyroid Hormone

The parathyroid gland is embedded in the corners of the thyroid gland and regulates calcium and phosphate balance. The parathyroid gland influences fluid and electrolytes, increases serum calcium levels, and lowers serum phosphate levels. A reciprocal relationship exists between extracellular calcium and phosphate levels. A decrease in parathyroid hormone (PTH) lowers serum calcium levels and increases serum phosphate levels. Another hormone that regulates calcium is calcitonin, a substance secreted by the thyroid gland. Calcitonin's action on calcium is opposite to that of PTH: calcitonin reduces plasma calcium concentrations.

Aldosterone

The adrenal cortex is important in fluid and electrolyte homeostasis. The primary adrenocortical hormone influencing the balance of fluid is aldosterone. Aldosterone is responsible for the renal reabsorption of sodium, which results in the retention of chloride and water and the excretion of potassium. Aldosterone also regulates blood volume by regulating sodium retention.

Epinehrine

Epinephrine, another adrenal hormone, increases blood pressure, enhances pulmonary ventilation, dilates blood vessels needed for emergencies, and constricts unnecessary vessels.

Cortisol

When produced in large quantities, the adrenocortical hormone cortisol can produce sodium and fluid retention and potassium deficit.

PHYSICAL ASSESSMENT

A body systems approach is the best method for assessing fluid and electrolyte imbalances related to I.V. therapy. The I.V. nurse should begin by assessing vital signs, infusion rate of any I.V. infusions, and intake and output. Nurses should follow this with assessing body systems at the beginning of each shift and as needed to monitor the patient's reactions to infusions.

NEUROLOGIC

There is a progressive loss of central nervous system (CNS) cells with advancing age, along with decreases in the sense of smell and tactile sense. The thirst mechanism in elderly people may be diminished and is a poor guide for fluid needs in older patients. An ill patient may not be able to verbalize thirst or to reach for a glass of water. Sensation of thirst depends on excitation of the cortical centers of consciousness. The use of antianxiety agents, sedatives, or hypnotic agents can lead to confusion and disorientation, causing the patient to forget to drink fluid. Changes in orientation can also be an indicator of fluid volume deficit.

Fluid volume changes, along with serum sodium levels, affect the CNS cells, resulting in confusion, stupor, seizures, or coma. CNS cells shrink in sodium excess and expand when serum sodium levels decrease. Assessment of neuromuscular irritability is particularly important when imbalances in calcium, magnesium, and sodium are suspected.

CARDIOVASCULAR

The quality and rate of the pulse are indicators of how the patient is tolerating the ECF volume. The peripheral veins in the extremities provide a way of evaluating plasma volume. Examination of hand veins can evaluate the plasma volume. Peripheral veins empty in 3 to 5 seconds when the hand is elevated and fill in the same amount of time when the hand is lowered to a dependent position. Peripheral vein filling takes longer than 3 to 5 seconds in patients with sodium depletion and extracellular dehydration (Metheny, 2000). Slow emptying of the peripheral veins indicates overhydration and excessive blood volume (Fig. 3–5).

A 20-mm Hg fall in systolic blood pressure when shifting from the lying to the standing position (postural hypotension) usually indicates fluid volume deficit. The jugular vein provides a built-in manometer for evaluation of central venous pressure (CVP). Changes in fluid volume are reflected by changes in neck vein filling.

The external jugular veins, with the patient supine, fill to the anterior border of the sternocleidomastoid muscle. Flat neck veins in the supine position indicate a decreased plasma volume. When the patient is in a 45-degree position, the external jugular distends no higher than 2 cm above the sternal angle. Neck veins distending from the top portion of the sternum to the angle of the jaw indicate elevated venous pressure (Fig. 3–6).

Edema indicates expansion of interstitial volume. Edema can be localized (usually caused by inflammation) or generalized (usually related to capillary hemodynamics). Edema should be assessed over bony surfaces of the tibia or sacrum and rated according to severity 1+ to 4+ (Fig 3–7; Horne & Swearingen, 1993). The presence of periorbital edema suggests significant fluid retention.

RESPIRATORY

A key to the assessment of circulatory overload is an assessment of the lung fields. Changes in respiratory rate and depth may be a

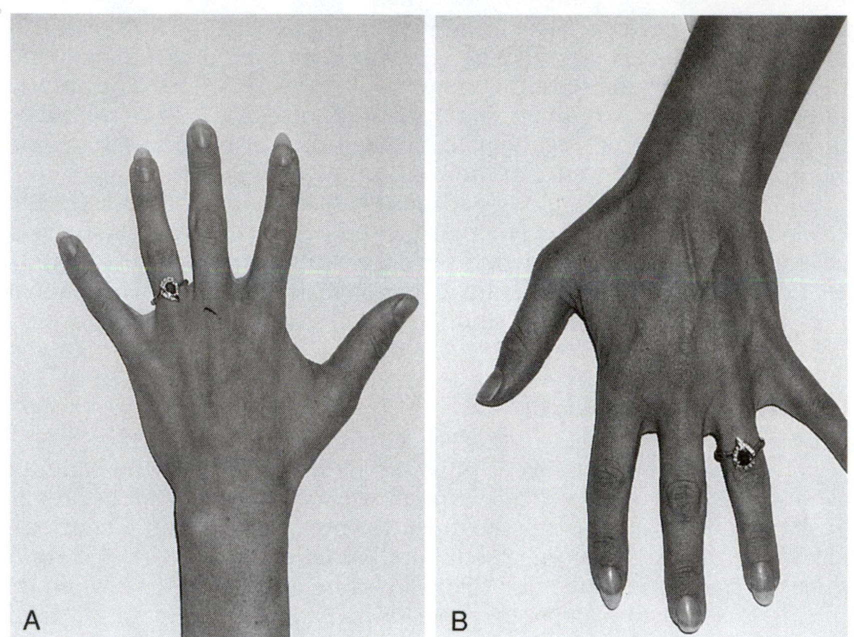

FIG. 3–5. Hand vein assessment. Peripheral vein filling takes longer than 3 to 5 seconds in patients with sodium depletion and dehydration. Slow emptying of hand veins indicates overhydration and excessive blood volume.

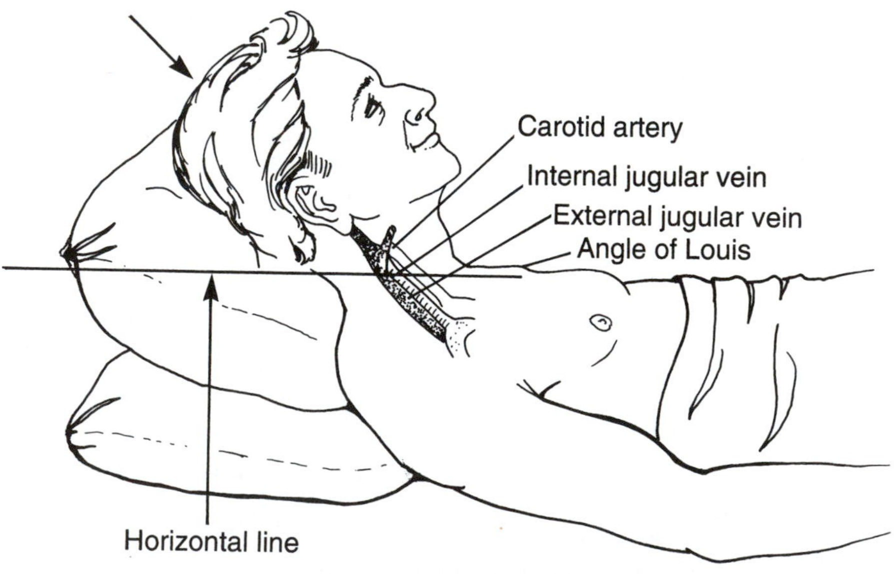

FIG. 3–6. Jugular venous distention.

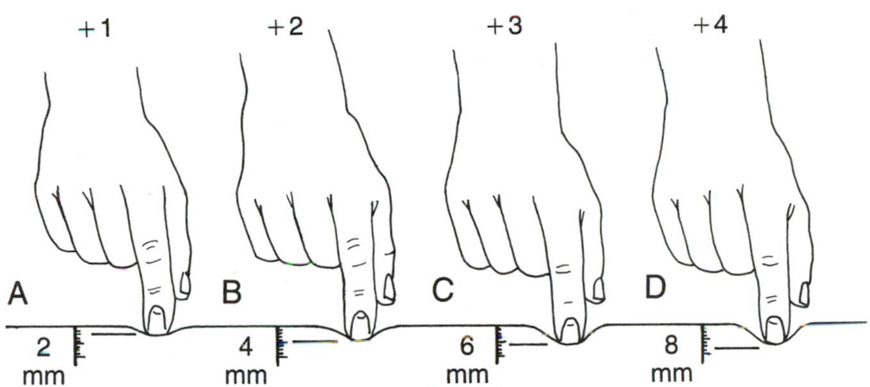

FIG. 3–7. Edema scale.

compensatory mechanism for acid–base imbalance. Moist crackles in the absence of cardiopulmonary disease indicate fluid volume excess. Shallow, slow breathing may indicate metabolic alkalosis or respiratory acidosis. Deep, rapid breathing may indicate respiratory alkalosis or metabolic acidosis. See Chapter 4 for further information on acid–base imbalances.

INTEGUMENTARY

Assessments of temperature and skin surface are key in determining fluid volume changes. Skin turgor can be assessed by pinching the area over the hand, sternum, or forehead. In a normal person, the pinched skin immediately falls back to its normal position when released. This elastic property, referred to as turgor, is partially dependent on interstitial fluid volume. In a person with a fluid volume deficit, the skin may remain slightly elevated for many seconds. In persons older than age 55 years, skin turgor is generally reduced because of loss of elasticity, particularly in areas that have been exposed to the sun. A more accurate assessment can be made on the skin over the sternum. A condition in which placement of fingers firmly on the patient's skin leaves finger imprints is called fingerprinting and is associated with fluid volume excess. Fingerprint edema is demonstrated by pressing a finger firmly over the sternum or other body surface for a period of 15 to 30 seconds. Upon removal of the finger, a positive sign is a visible fingerprint similar to that seen when a fingerprint is made on paper with ink.

SPECIAL SENSES

The eyes, mouth, lips, and tongue are also key indicators of fluid volume imbalances. The absence of tearing and salivation in a child is a sign of fluid volume deficit. In a healthy person, the tongue has one

TABLE 3–2

QUICK ASSESSMENT GUIDE FOR FLUID IMBALANCE

Body System Assessed	Fluid Volume	
	Excess	**Deficit**
Neurologic		Changes in orientation Confusion
Cardiovascular	Bounding pulse Increased pulse rate Jugular vein distention Overdistended hand veins that are slow to empty (> 3 s)	Increased pulse rate Decreased blood pressure Narrow pulse pressure Slow hand filling (> 3 s) Decreased pulse volume
Respiratory	Moist crackles Respiratory rate >20 bpm Dyspnea Pulmonary edema	Lungs clear
Integument	Warm, moist skin Fingerprinting over sternum	Decreased turgor over sternum and forehead Decreased skin temperature
Eyes	Periorbital edema (suggests significant fluid retention)	Dry conjunctiva Sunken eyes Decreasing tearing
Mouth		Sticky, dry mucous membranes
Lips		Dry, cracked
Tongue		Extralongitudinal furrows
Body weight	Mild: <5% over normal Moderate: 5% to 10% over normal Severe: >15% over normal	Mild: <5% less than normal Moderate: 5% to 10% less than normal Severe: >15% less than normal

longitudinal furrow. In the person with fluid volume deficit, the tongue has additional longitudinal furrows and is smaller because of fluid loss (Metheny, 2000).

Mucous membranes often show the first sign of dehydration; as fluid volume decreases, the mouth becomes dry and sticky and the lips dry and cracked. In fluid volume deficit, the patient's eyes tend to appear sunken; in significant fluid volume excess, periorbital edema is present.

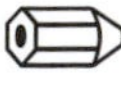

NOTE: Good oral hygiene is imperative with mouth-breathing patients. If the patient is receiving good oral care and the crusted, dry, furrowed tongue is not improving, fluid volume deficit must be restored to aid in solving this problem.

BODY WEIGHT

Taking daily weights of patients with potential fluid imbalances is an important clinical tool. Accurate body weight measurement is a better indicator of gains or losses than intake and output records. A loss or gain of 1 kg (2.2 lb) reflects a loss or gain of 1 L of body fluid. Generally, fluid volume excess is considered severe when body weight is more than 15 percent higher than the person's normal body weight. Severe fluid volume deficit occurs when body weight is more than 15 percent less than the person's normal body weight. Table 3–2 provides a summary of assessment findings that indicate altered fluid status.

FLUID VOLUME IMBALANCES

Fluid volume imbalances may reflect an increase or a decrease in total body fluid or an altered distribution of body fluids. There are two major alterations in ECF balance: fluid volume deficit and fluid volume excess (Table 3–3).

FLUID VOLUME DEFICIT

Extracellular fluid volume deficit reflects a contracted vascular compartment caused by either a significant ECF loss or by an accumulation of fluid in the interstitial space. ECF deficit is also referred to as dehydration. It may be caused by an actual decrease in body water; excessive fluid loss or inadequate fluid intake; or a relative decrease in which fluid (plasma) shifts from the intravascular compartment to the interstitial space, a process called "third spacing" (Lee, 1996).

Etiology

Gastrointestinal dysfunction is the most common cause of ECF deficit. Other common causes include overzealous use of diuretics and diaphoresis. Third spacing is caused by peritonitis, intestinal obstruction, postoperative conditions, thrombophlebitis, acute pancreatitis, ascites, fistulous drainage, and burns.

Fluid volume deficit occurs when there is either an excessive loss of body water or an inadequate compensatory intake. The ECF consists predominantly of the electrolytes, sodium and chloride, both of which tend to attract water; loss of these electrolytes also leads to loss of water. Table 3–3 lists common causes of dehydration.

AGE-RELATED CONSIDERATIONS 3–1

Infants and small children are prone to dehydration.

TABLE 3–3

EXTRACELLULAR FLUID DISORDERS: DEFICIT AND EXCESS

	Fluid Volume Deficit	Fluid Volume Excess
Definition (causes)	Hypovolemia Fever with diaphoresis GI dysfunction (most common) Fluid and electrolyte loss Diarrhea Overdose of cathartics Renal dysfunction Neurologic dysfunction Lethargy and coma Endocrine dysfunction Diabetes insipidus	Hypervolemia Too-rapid administration of I.V. fluids Cardiovascular dysfunction Congestive heart failure Pulmonary edema Renal dysfunction Serum protein depletion and hyponatremia Cirrhosis with ascites and portal hypertension Endocrine dysfunction Hyperaldosteronism
Clinical picture	Acute weight loss Neurologic Changes in mental status, disorientation, lethargy, seizures Cardiovascular Postural hypertension, dizziness, syncope, vertigo, weak pulse, absence of neck vein distention, decreased central venous pressure, decreased cardiac output GI Nausea, vomiting, anorexia Fluid intake versus output Increased thirst, decreased urine output, poor skin turgor over sternum and forehead, dry skin and mucous membranes, sunken eyeballs, hyperthermia	Acute weight gain Neurologic Changes in mental status and level of consciousness, seizures Cardiovascular Hypertension, tachycardia, bounding pulse, increased central venous pressure, neck vein distention Fluid intake versus output True pitting edema, taut and shiny skin Respiratory Shortness of breath, tachypnea, dyspnea, cough, crackles, pulmonary edema Renal Urine output disproportionately less than fluid intake

(Continued)

Clinically, ECF deficit is characterized by acute weight loss, altered cardiovascular function that reflects the underlying ECF volume deficit, and complaints of nausea and vomiting. The cardiovascular assessment is the most important part of the process to determine plasma volume changes. In a patient who is hypovolemic, the heart rate increases, the blood pressure decreases, and the peripheral pulses are weak. Symptoms

TABLE 3–3

EXTRACELLULAR FLUID DISORDERS: DEFICIT AND EXCESS *(Continued)*

	Fluid Volume Deficit	Fluid Volume Excess
Laboratory data	Electrolyte parameter (by itself) indicative of fluid deficit Serum Hematocrit: Increased Hemoglobin: Increased Proteins: Increased Osmolarity: Normal BUN: >20 mg/100 mL Urine Sodium: <50 mEq/L Osmolarity: >500 mOsm/L Specific gravity: 1:030	Electrolyte parameter (by itself) indicative of fluid excess Serum Hematocrit: Normal to low Hemoglobin: Normal to low Proteins: Normal to low Osmolarity: Normal BUN: Normal to low Urine Sodium: Reduced Osmolarity: <500 mOsm/L Specific gravity: 1:010
Treatment	Restore fluid and electrolyte balance using I.V. isotonic saline Treat underlying cause	Reduce fluid retention by salt and fluid restriction Diuretics to increase fluid excretion Treat underlying cause

Source: Adapted from Ruppert, S.D., et al. (1996). *Dolan's Critical Care Nursing: Management through the Nursing Process* (2nd ed.). Philadelphia: F.A. Davis.

reflect a dehydrated state with sunken eyeballs, poor skin turgor, and oliguria commonly seen.

Laboratory findings in fluid volume deficit reflect hemoconcentration with the serum hemoglobin, hematocrit, and proteins increased. Blood urea nitrogen is elevated above 20 mg/100 mL. The urine specific gravity reflects high solute concentration of more than 1.030.

Treatment

Treatment for patients with an ECF volume deficit entails fluid replacement (orally or intravenously) until the oliguria is relieved and the cardiovascular and neurologic systems stabilize. Isotonic electrolyte solutions such as 0.9 percent NaCl or lactated Ringer's solution are used to treat hypotensive patients with a fluid volume deficit. A hypotonic electrolyte solution (0.45% NaCl) is often used to provide electrolyte and free water for renal excretion of metabolic wastes (Metheny, 2000).

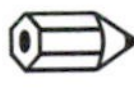

NOTE: Extreme caution must be exercised in fluid replacement therapy to avoid fluid overload.

NURSING PLAN OF CARE

FLUID VOLUME DEFICIT

Focus Assessment

Subjective

- History of contributing factors and cause, such as diabetes mellitus, cardiac disease, or GI disorder
- Recent weight loss
- History of laxative, enema, or diuretic overuse
- Fluid intake (amount and type)

Objective

- Present weight
- Changes in mentation
- Dry skin and mucous membranes
- Poor skin turgor
- Decreased pulse rate
- Decreased blood pressure
- Slow vein filling
- Decreased urine output
- Increased urine specific gravity

Patient Outcome Criteria

The Patient Will:

- Increase fluid intake to a minimum of 2000 mL/d unless contraindicated.
- Relate the need for increased fluid intake during stress or heat.
- Maintain a urine specific gravity within normal range.
- Demonstrate no signs and symptoms of dehydration.

Nursing Diagnoses

- Fluid volume deficit related to failure or regulatory mechanisms
- Fluid volume deficit related to loss of body fluid and inadequate fluid intake
- Fluid volume deficit related to high-solute tube feedings
- Altered oral mucous membrane related to dehydration
- Altered tissue perfusion: cardiopulmonary, renal, and peripheral related to hypovolemia
- Risk of injury related to confusion

(continued)

(continued)

Nursing Management

1. Monitor fluid status, including intake and output.
2. Monitor specific gravity.
3. Monitor trends of daily weights.
4. Monitor hemodynamic status (central venous pressure when appropriate).
5. Observe for indicators of dehydration (e.g., poor skin turgor, delayed capillary refill, weak or thready pulse, severe thirst, dry mucous membranes, decreased urine output, and hypotension).
6. Monitor fluid loss (e.g., bleeding, vomiting, diarrhea, and perspiration tachypnea).
7. Administer isotonic solutions for extracellular rehydration, if appropriate.
8. Administer hypotonic solutions for intracellular rehydration, if appropriate.
9. Monitor hemoglobin and hematocrit.
10. Monitor serum sodium levels.
11. Encourage oral fluid intake.
12. Promote skin integrity (monitor areas at risk for breakdown).
13. Provide frequent oral hygiene.

Source: Sparks & Taylor, 1998.

FLUID VOLUME EXCESS

Extracellular fluid volume excess causes an expansion of the ECF compartment. The primary cause of ECF excess is cardiovascular dysfunction. Fluid volume excess is always secondary to an increase in total body sodium content, which causes total body water increase. Normally, the posterior pituitary decreases secretion of the ADH when excess water moves into the cells. This causes the kidney to eliminate excess fluid. However, if a patient has an excessive secretion of ADH, the water will be retained, placing the patient at risk for fluid volume excess. Excessive secretion of ADH can be caused by fear, pain, postoperative reaction 12 to 24 hours after surgery, and acute infections. Table 3–3 provides additional causes of ECF volume excess.

Etiology

Conditions that cause isotonic overhydration include excessive administration of oral or I.V. fluids, excessive irrigation of body cavities or organs and use of hypotonic fluids to replace isotonic fluid losses (Lee, 1996). Hypotonic fluid overload is also called water intoxication.

Conditions that cause hypotonic overload are SIADH, excessive water intake, and congestive heart failure.

AGE-RELATED CONSIDERATIONS 3–2

If a person has poor cardiac function, fluid overload can occur rapidly and lead to congestive heart failure. This is a common issue for older persons, who often have poor cardiac reserve and a history of cardiovascular disease.

Clinically, ECF volume excess has distinct signs and symptoms, the most prominent being weight gain. Edema is usually not apparent until 2 to 4 kg of fluid have been retained. Alterations in respiratory and cardiovascular function are present and include hypertension and tachycardia. In addition to common assessment finding, some patients also experience confusion, altered levels of consciousness, skeletal muscle weakness, and increased bowel sounds.

In fluid volume excess, the hematocrit may be decreased because of hemodilution. The serum sodium and serum osmolarity will be decreased if hypervolemia occurs as a result of excessive retention of water.

Treatment

Treatment of ECF volume excess is directed toward sodium and fluid restriction, administration of diuretics, and the treatment of the underlying cause (Dolan, 1995).

NURSING PLAN OF CARE

FLUID VOLUME EXCESS

Focus Assessment

Subjective

- History of symptoms, shortness of breath, or signs of fluid overload
- Recent weight gain
- History of contributing factors and causes, such as family or personal history of diabetes mellitus or cardiac or renal diseases
- Alcoholism
- Steroid therapy
- Excessive salt intake

(continued)

(continued)

Objective

- Excessive parenteral fluid replacement
- Weight gain
- Bounding pulse
- Increased respiratory rate
- Moist crackles in lungs
- Increased blood pressure
- Slow vein emptying
- Peripheral edema
- Neck vein distention

Patient Outcome Criteria

The Patient Will:

- Relate causative factors and methods of preventing edema
- Exhibit decreased peripheral and sacral edema.

Nursing Diagnoses

- Fluid volume excess related to infusion of sodium chloride solution
- Fluid volume excess related to compromised regulatory function secondary to renal failure, acute or chronic
- Fluid volume excess related to dependent venous pooling or venostasis
- Impaired skin integrity related to altered circulation, edema

Nursing Management

1. Monitor fluid status, including intake and output.
2. Monitor trends of daily weights.
3. Monitor specific gravity.
4. Monitor serum sodium levels.
5. Monitor hemodynamic status (central venous pressure when appropriate).
6. Monitor vital signs.
7. Maintain patent I.V. access.
8. Identify ways to decrease dependent edema, such as frequent position changes, avoiding constrictive clothing, elevating legs, wearing elastic support stocking.
9. Encourage decrease in salt intake.
10. Avoid infusion of I.V. fluid in limb with poor lymphatic drainage.
11. Provide passive range of motion of all extremities every 4 hours.
12. Monitor for edema in sacral area every 2 hours if patient is in high Fowler's position.
13. Inspect skin for redness and blanching.
14. Reduce pressure on skin areas by padding chairs and footstools.

Source: Sparks & Taylor, 1998.

PATIENT EDUCATION

- Explain to client and family the reasons for intake and output records.
- Teach the client to keep track of oral liquids consumed.
- Assess patient's understanding of the type of fluid loss being experienced.
- Give verbal and written instructions for fluid replacement (drink at least 3 quarts of liquid).
- Teach to increase the fluid intake during hot days, in the presence of fever or infection and to decrease activity during extreme weather.
- Teach how to observe for dehydration (especially in infants).
- Instruct to seek medical consultation for continued dehydration.
- Teach appropriate use of laxatives, enemas, and diuretics.
- Inform patient to notify physician if they have excessive edema or weight gain (more than 2 lbs/d) or increased shortness of breath.
- Provide literature concerning low-salt diets; consult with dietitian if necessary.
- Write instructions for diet.

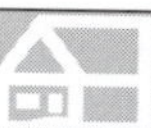

HOME CARE ISSUES

- Consider home care visit to follow up with patients with diabetes mellitus, cardiovascular disorders, and severe GI disorders.
- Follow up with home care for patients taking drug therapy (diuretics) for edema.
- Consider home care visit to follow up on diet and instructions on use of pressure stockings.

KEY POINTS

Fluid is distributed in three compartments: intracellular (40%), intravascular (5%), and interstitial (15%); total body weight in water is 60 percent for an average adult

Fluid is transported passively by filtration, diffusion, and osmosis

Electrolytes are actively transported by ATP on cell membranes and the sodium-potassium pump

Osmosis is the movement of water from a lower concentration to a higher concentration across a semipermeable membrane

The osmolarity of I.V. solutions has the following ranges:

- Isotonic solutions: 250 to 375 mOsm/L
- Hypotonic solutions: <250 mOsm/L
- Hypertonic solutions: >375 mOsm/L

The homeostatic organs that regulate fluid and electrolyte balance include the kidneys; heart and blood vessels; lungs; and adrenal, parathyroid, and pituitary glands

Nurses must remember that there are six areas to assess for fluid balance: neurologic status, cardiovascular, respiratory, integumentary, special senses, and body weight

Fluid imbalances fall into two categories:

1. Fluid volume deficit caused primarily by disorders of the GI system; signs and symptoms reflect a dehydrated individual; treatment is aimed at rehydration with isotonic sodium chloride
2. Fluid volume excess caused primarily by cardiovascular dysfunction, renal or endocrine dysfunction, and too-rapid administration of I.V. fluids; signs and symptoms reflect fluid overload; treatment is aimed at decreasing the sodium level, using diuretics to increase the excretion of fluids, and treating the underlying cause

CHAPTER ACTIVITIES

COMPETENCY CRITERIA: Patient Assessment of Fluid Balance
COMPETENCY STATEMENT: Competent intravenous therapy nurses will be able to monitor patients for signs and symptoms of fluid volume disturbances.
Note: The cognitive (knowledge) information that is embedded within this performance-based competency includes osmolarity, physiology of fluid balance within the body, movement of water from extracellular to intracellular compartments, homeostatic mechanisms, and interpretation of laboratory data related to electrolyte balance.This competency *links* to the competency of delivery of parenteral fluids and assessment of electrolyte balance.

Performance	Skilled	Needs Education
Critical Action Statements		
1. Performs physical assessment directed at identifying fluid volume abnormalities A. Cardiovascular system Pulse Edema scale Blood pressure Jugular vein distention Hand vein filling B. Pulmonary Lung sounds Rate C. Integumentary Skin turgor Skin surfaces Fontanelles sign (pediatric) D. Special senses Condition of conjunctiva Condition and characteristics of mucous membranes E. General data collection Accurate BP, pulse, and respirations Weight I & O Specific gravity		

(continued)

(continued)

Performance	Skilled	Needs Education
Critical Action Statements		
2. Demonstrates recording of data on appropriate documentation form A. Physical assessment B. Graphics C. Intake and output record		

EVALUATION CRITERIA

1. Validation of assessment skills performed at bedside with preceptor or in simulation laboratory on skills manikin.
2. Observation and review of documentation.
3. Implementation of nursing interventions (i.e., notification of physician) when appropriate.

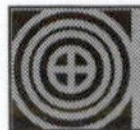

CRITICAL THINKING ACTIVITY

1. Within your work environment, identify the patients at risk for fluid volume deficit or excess. Remember that even outpatient units see patients at risk.

2. Using the six body systems to assess for fluid volume excess or deficit, choose four patients on your unit to assess and check for fluid volume changes.

3. Check I.V. solutions infusing on your patients and identify whether the solutions are isotonic, hypotonic, or hypertonic.

POST-TEST

1. A solution of 5 percent dextrose and 0.9 percent NaCl has an osmolarity of 559. By administering this, you know that fluid will move from the ____ space to the ___ space.
   a. Intracellular, vascular
   b. Vascular, interstitial
   c. Interstitial, cellular
2. A solution of 0.45 percent NaCl has an osmolarity of 154. By administering this, you know that fluid will move from the ___ space to the ___ space.
   a. Intracellular, vascular
   b. Vascular, intracellular
   c. Interstitial, cellular
3. Lactated Ringer's solution has an osmolarity of 273. By administering this, you know that fluid will:
   a. Move from the intracellular space to the vascular space
   b. Move from the vascular space to the cellular space
   c. Stay in the vascular space
4. Water is transported passively by:
   a. Diffusion
   b. Osmosis
   c. Filtration
   d. All of the above
5. You have just completed a physical assessment of a 68-year-old man. He knows who he is but is unsure of where he is (previous orientation normal). His eyes are sunken, his mouth is coated with an extra longitudinal furrow, and his lips are cracked. Hand vein filling takes more than 5 seconds, and tenting of the skin appears over the sternum. His vital signs are blood pressure of 128/60 mm Hg, pulse of 78, and respiratory rate of 16 (previously 150/78, 76, 16, respectively). Your assessment would lead you to suspect:
   a. Fluid volume deficit
   b. Fluid volume excess
6. If the external temperature is 101°F, which of the following age groups is at highest risk for fluid volume deficit?
   a. Infants
   b. School-age children
   c. Adolescents
   d. Middle-aged adults
7. All of the following could be the etiology for a nursing diagnosis of fluid volume excess **EXCEPT:**
   a. Excessive infusion of 0.9 percent sodium chloride solution
   b. Suppression of the parathyroid function
   c. SIADH
   d. Congestive heart failure
8. Which of the following lab values are consistent with fluid volume deficit?
   a. Urine specific gravity 1.10

b. Blood urea nitrogen 6
c. Hemoglobin 13
d. Serum osmolarity 305 mOsm/kg

9. All of the following conditions produce excess antidiuretic hormone **EXCEPT:**
   a. Head trauma
   b. Anesthesia
   c. Ovarian cancer
   d. Brain tumor
10. If a patient presents with peripheral edema, which of the following does he probably have?
    a. Fluid accumulation in the interstitial space
    b. Fluid accumulation in the vascular space
    c. Aldosterone insufficiency
    d. Pituitary insufficiency

REFERENCES

Adelman, R.D., & Solhung, M.J. (1996). Pathophysiology of body fluids and fluid therapy. In Behrman, R.E., Kliegman, R.M., & Arvin, A.M. (eds): *Nelson Textbook of Pediatrics* (15th ed.). Philadelphia: W.B. Saunders, 185–222.

Dolan, J.T. (1995). *Critical Care Nursing: Clinical Management Through the Nursing Process.* Philadelphia: F.A. Davis.

Kuhn, M. (1998). *Pharmacotherapeutics: A Nursing Process Approach* (4th ed.). Philadelphia: F.A. Davis.

Josephson, D.L. (1999). *Intravenous Infusion Therapy for Nurses Principles and Practice.* Albany, NY: Delmar Publishers.

Lee, C.A., Barrett, C., & Ignatavicius, D.D. (1996). *Fluid and Electrolytes: A Practical Approach* (4th ed.). Philadelphia: F.A. Davis.

Metheny, N.M. (2000). Fluid and Electrolyte Balance. In *Nursing Considerations* (4th ed.). Philadelphia: Lippincott-Williams & Wilkins.

National Student Nurses Association, Inc. (1997). *Fluids and Electrolytes.* Albany, NY: Delmar Publishers.

Sparks, S.M., & Taylor, C.M. (1998). *Nursing Diagnosis Reference Manual* (4th ed.). Springhouse, PA: Springhouse Corporation.

ANSWERS TO CHAPTER 3

Pre-Test

1. a, **2.** e, **3.** a, **4.** b, **5.** c, **6.** b, **7.** c, **8.** b, **9.** c, **10.** a

Post-Test

1. a, **2.** b, **3.** c, **4.** b, **5.** a, **6.** a, **7.** b, **8.** d, **9.** c, **10.** a

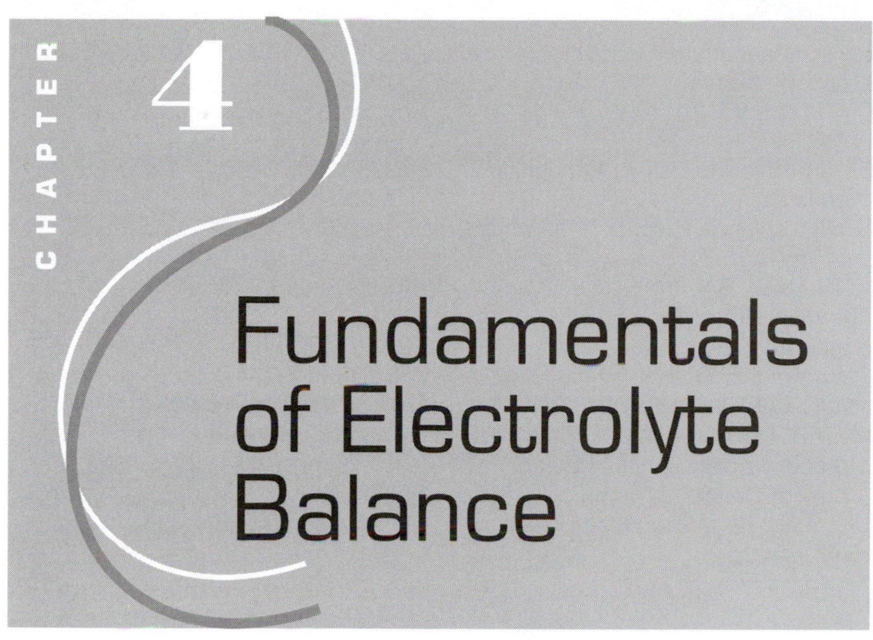

CHAPTER 4

Fundamentals of Electrolyte Balance

When they went ashore the animals that took up a land life carried with them a part of the sea in their bodies, a heritage which they passed on to their children and which even today links each land animal with its origin in the ancient sea.

Rachel Carson, 1961

CHAPTER CONTENTS

LEARNING OBJECTIVES

Upon completion of this chapter, the reader will be able to:

1. Define terminology related to electrolytes.
2. State the seven major electrolytes within the body fluids.
3. Differentiate between cations and anions.
4. Contrast each of the seven electrolytes and their major roles in body fluids.
5. Identify signs and symptoms of deficits of sodium, potassium, calcium, magnesium, chloride, and phosphate.
6. Identify signs and symptoms of excesses of sodium, potassium, calcium, magnesium, chloride, and phosphate.
7. Recognize patients at risk for electrolyte imbalances.
8. State the normal pH range of body fluids.
9. Compare clinical manifestations of metabolic acidosis and alkalosis.
10. Identify regulatory organs of acid–base balance.
11. Identify nursing diagnoses and interventions related to electrolyte balance.

GLOSSARY

Acidosis Blood pH below normal (<7.35)
Alkalosis Blood pH above normal (>7.45)
Anion Negatively charged electrolyte
Antidiuretic hormone (ADH) A hormone secreted from the pituitary mechanism that causes the kidney to conserve water; sometimes referred to as the "water-conserving hormone"
Cation Positively charged electrolyte
Chvostek's sign A sign elicited by tapping the facial nerve about 2 cm anterior to the earlobe, just below the zygomatic process; the response is a spasm of the muscles supplied by the facial nerve
pH Hydrogen ion (H^+) concentration
Syndrome of inappropriate antidiuretic hormone (SIADH) secretion A condition in which excessive ADH is secreted, resulting in hyponatremia
Tetany Continuous tonic spasm of a muscle
Trousseau's sign A spasm of the hand elicited when the blood supply to the hand is decreased or the nerves of the hand are stimulated by pressure; elicited within several minutes by applying a blood pressure cuff inflated above systolic pressure

PRE-TEST

1. Which of the following groups of electrolytes are all positively charged?
   a. Potassium, sodium, bicarbonate
   b. Potassium, sodium, calcium
   c. Bicarbonate, phosphate, chloride
   d. Chloride, magnesium, bicarbonate
2. Which of the following signs and symptoms indicate alkalosis (bicarbonate excess)?
   a. Kussmaul respirations, confusion, increased respiratory rate
   b. Tetany, soft tissue calcification
   c. Dizziness, tingling of fingers and toes, carpopedal spasm
3. You assess your patient and find the following signs and symptoms: fatigued muscles, complaints of nausea and anorexia, irritability and diminished deep tendon reflexes. You check serum electrolytes and find: chloride 92 mEq/L, potassium 3.1 mEq/L, and sodium 135 mEq/L. What would you suspect?
   a. Hyponatremia
   b. Hyperchloremia
   c. Hypokalemia
   d. Hypernatremia
4. Your patient has a nasogastric tube to continuous suction. What electrolyte deficit(s) is(are) the patient at risk for?
   a. Sodium
   b. Potassium
   c. Chloride
   d. All of the above
5. Which are the regulatory organs in acid–base balance?
   a. Lungs and liver
   b. Lungs and kidneys
   c. Pituitary glands and adrenal glands
6. A patient presents with the following: confusion, respiratory rate 30, blood pressure 100/70 mm Hg, previous admission for renal failure. ABG values are pH 7.32, HCO_3 20 mEq/L, $Paco_2$ 34 mm Hg. What would you suspect?
   a. Metabolic acidosis
   b. Metabolic alkalosis
   c. Respiratory acidosis
7. The most common cause of hypermagnesemia is:
   a. Nasogastric tubes to suction
   b. Renal failure
   c. Overzealous administration of I.V. potassium chloride
   d. Use of respirators
8. Patients in an oncology unit are at risk for which of the following electrolyte imbalances?
   a. Hypercalcemia, hyponatremia, hyperkalemia
   b. Hyperkalemia, hypernatremia, hyperchloremia
   c. Hyponatremia, hypocalcemia, hypophosphatemia

9. Cardiac arrest may occur if the serum potassium level is:
   a. 2.5 mEq/L
   b. 3.5 mEq/L
   c. 4.0 mEq/L
   d. 5.0 mEg/L
10. Metabolic acidosis may be manifested by:
   a. CNS stimulation, hyperactive reflexes, shallow breathing
   b. CNS depression, confusion, stupor, pH <7.35
   c. Irritability, seizures and pH >7.45

BASIC PRINCIPLES OF ELECTROLYTE BALANCE

Chemical compounds in solution behave in one of two ways: they separate and combine with other compounds, or they remain intact. One group of compounds remains intact; these are called nonelectrolytes (e.g., urea, dextrose, and creatinine). These compounds do not separate from their complex form when added to a solution. The second group of compounds, electrolytes, dissociates or separates in solution. These compounds break up into separate particles known as ions in a process called ionization. The major electrolytes in body fluid include sodium, potassium, calcium, magnesium, chloride, phosphorous, and bicarbonate.

Ions, which are the dissociated particles of an electrolyte, each carry an electrical charge, either positive or negative. Negative ions are called **anions** and positive ions are called **cations.**

TABLE 4–1

COMPARISON OF ELECTROLYTE COMPOSITION IN FLUID COMPARTMENTS

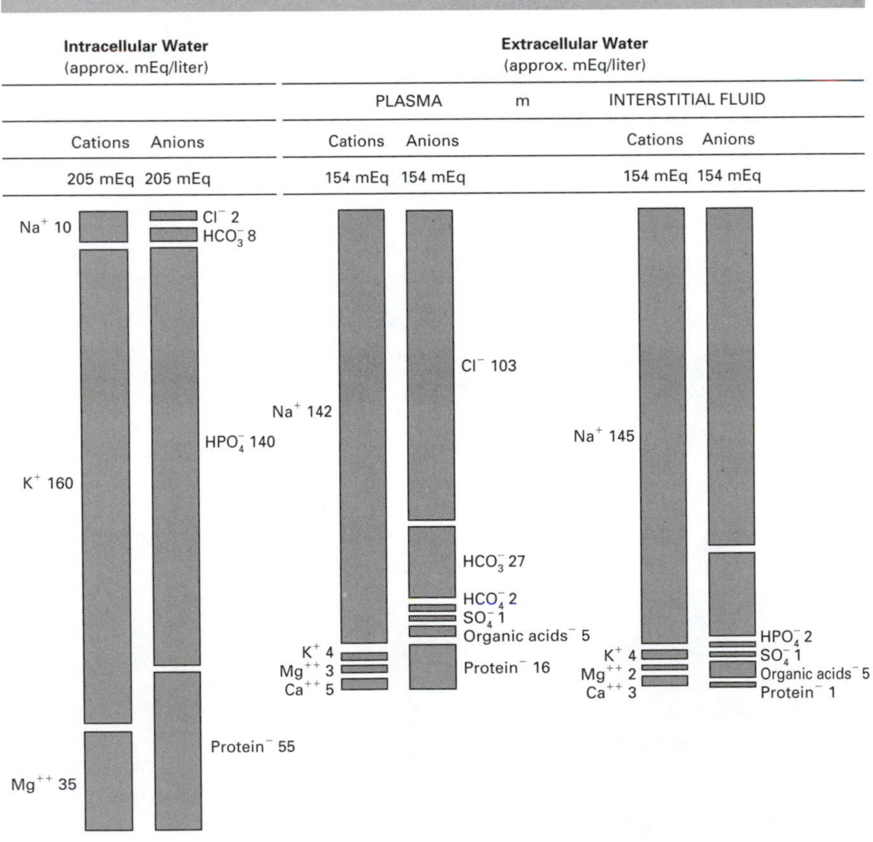

Electrolytes are active chemicals that unite. The ions are expressed in terms of milliequivalents (mEq) per liter rather than milligrams. A milliequivalent measures chemical activity or combining power rather than weight. For example, when a hostess creates a guest list for a party, she does not invite 1000 pounds of boys per 1000 pounds of girls; rather, she invites the same number of boys and girls. The total milliequivalents of cations and anions in a given compartment is equal. There are 154 mEq of anions and 154 mEq of cations in the plasma. Each water compartment of the body contains electrolytes. The concentration and composition of electrolytes vary from compartment to compartment. See Table 4–1 for a diagrammatic comparison of electrolyte composition in the fluid compartments.

Most of the electrolytes have more than one physiologic role; often several electrolytes work together to mediate chemical events. The physiologic role of electrolytes include:

- Maintaining electroneutrality in fluid compartments
- Mediating enzyme reactions
- Altering cell membrane permeability
- Regulating muscle contraction and relaxation
- Regulating nerve impulse transmission
- Influencing blood clotting time

The electrolyte content of intracellular fluid (ICF) differs from that of extracellular fluid (ECF). Usually only ECF plasma electrolytes are measured because of the special techniques required to measure the concentration of electrolytes in ICF. The serum plasma levels of electrolytes are important in the assessment and management of patients with electrolyte imbalances.

SODIUM (NA^+)

NORMAL REFERENCE VALUE: 135 TO 145 mEq/L

PHYSIOLOGIC ROLE

The physiologic role of sodium includes:

- Regulation of fluid distribution in the body: Water follows sodium
- Maintenance of body fluid osmolarity
- Promotion of neuromuscular response: Transmission of nerve and muscle impulses depends on sodium, gradient between ECF and ICF
- Regulation of acid–base balance: Sodium combines with chloride and bicarbonate to alter pH (NSNA, 1997)

The major function of sodium is to maintain ECF volume. Extracellular sodium level has an effect on the cellular fluid volume based on the principle of osmosis. Sodium represents about 90 percent of all the

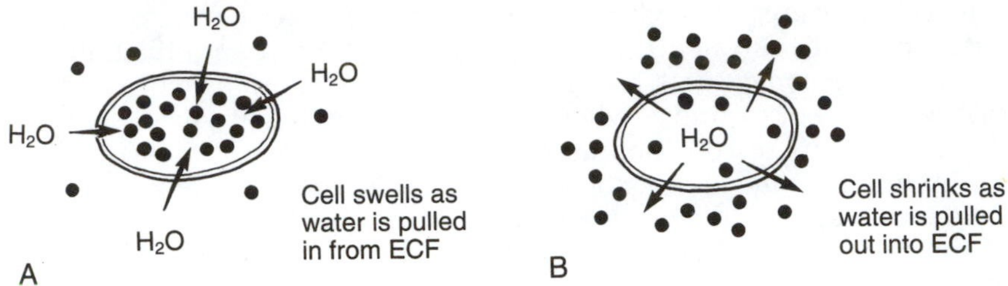

FIG. 4–1. Sodium and cellular fluid relationship. *(A)* Hyponatremia. The cell swells as water is pulled in from the extracellular fluid. *(B)* Hypernatremia. The cell shrinks as water is pulled out into the extracellular fluid.

extracellular cations. Sodium does not easily cross the cell wall membrane and is therefore the most abundant cation of ECF.

A low serum sodium level results in dilute ECF, therefore allowing water to be drawn into the cells (lower to higher concentration). Conversely if the serum sodium is high, water is drawn out of the cells, leading to cellular dehydration. Figure 4–1 shows the relationship between sodium and cellular fluid. The normal daily requirement for sodium in adults is approximately 100 mEq.

The kidneys are extremely important in the regulation of sodium. This regulation is primarily accomplished through the action of the hormone aldosterone. Hyponatremia is a common complication of adrenal insufficiency because of aldosterone and cortisol deficiencies. Elderly persons have a slower rate of aldosterone secretion, which places them at risk for sodium imbalances.

Three factors can create a sodium imbalance:

1. Change in the sodium content of the ECF such as a deficit caused by excessive vomiting
2. Change in the chloride content, which can affect both the sodium concentration and the amount of water in the ECF; when the ratio of chloride to sodium deviates from normal, it is reflected as an acid–base imbalance (Lee, 1996)
3. Change in the quantity of water in the ECF

SERUM SODIUM DEFICIT: HYPONATREMIA

Hyponatremia is a condition in which the sodium level is below normal (i.e., <135 mEq/L). A low sodium level can be the result of an excessive loss of sodium or an excessive gain of water; in either event, hyponatremia is caused by a relatively greater concentration of water than of sodium.

Pathophysiology and Etiology

The pathophysiology that contributes to sodium deficit (hyponatremia) is often a sign of a serious underlying disease; there are also many causes of hyponatremia.

All gastrointestinal (GI) secretions contain sodium; therefore, any abnormal loss of GI secretions can cause a sodium deficit. GI disorders such as vomiting, diarrhea, drainage from suction or fistulas, and excessive tap water enemas may also cause hyponatremia.

Other causes of hyponatremia are losses from skin in excessive sweating, combined with excessive water consumption and the use of thiazide diuretics (especially dangerous with low-salt diets).

Hormonal factors such as labor induction with oxytocin and the syndrome of inappropriate antidiuretic syndrome (SIADH) cause the amount of sodium per volume to be reduced, in turn causing a dilutional hyponatremia. Oxytocin has been shown to have an intrinsic antidiuretic hormone effect, acting to increase water reabsorption from the glomerular filtrate. Adrenal insufficiency (aldosterone deficiency) also can cause sodium loss (Metheny, 2000). Other factors include excessive parenteral hypo-osmolar fluids such as dextrose in water solutions.

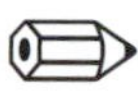

NOTE: SIADH has progressed from a rare occurrence to the most common cause of hyponatremia seen in general hospitals. It occurs in patients with inflammatory disorders such as pneumonia; tuberculosis; abscess; oat cell cancer of the lung; and central nervous system (CNS) disorders such as meningitis, trauma, stroke, and degenerative diseases (Metheny, 2000).

Chemical agents may also impair renal water excretion, leading to sodium deficit. Pharmacologic agents that contribute to sodium deficit include nicotine, chlorpropamide (Diabinese), cyclophosphamide (cytoxan), morphine, barbiturates, and acetaminophen.

Signs and Symptoms

Hyponatremia affects cells of the CNS. Patients with chronic hyponatremia may experience impaired sensation of taste, anorexia, muscle cramps, feeling of exhaustion, apprehension, feeling of impending doom (Na^+ <115), and focal weaknesses (e.g., hemiparesis, ataxia). Patients with acute hyponatremia caused by water overload experience the same symptoms as well as fingerprint edema (sign of intracellular water excess).

AGE-RELATED CONSIDERATIONS 4–1

Dehydration and chronic hyponatremia can lead to confusional states that interfere with fluid intake in elderly people, who are very susceptible to dehydration (Rolls & Phillips, 1990).

Because of the differences in cerebral metabolism, women (especially premenopausal women) seem to be at substantially greater risk than men for developing severe neurologic symptoms and irreversible brain damage related to hyponatremia. Young women account for most of the reported cases of fatalities secondary to hyponatremia.

Diagnostic Tests

- Serum sodium: <135 mEq/L
- Serum osmolarity: <280 mOsm/L
- Urine specific gravity: <1
- Urine sodium: Decreased (usually <20 mEq/L)
- Hematocrit: Above normal when fluid volume deficit (FVD) exists

Treatment and Management

Treatment of patients with hyponatremia aims to provide sodium by the dietary, enteral, or parenteral route. Patients able to eat and drink can easily replace sodium by ingesting a normal diet. Those unable to take sodium orally must take the electrolyte by the parenteral route. An isotonic saline or Ringer's solution may be ordered, such as 0.9 percent sodium chloride (NaCl), or lactated Ringer's solution.

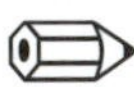

NOTE: When the primary problem is water retention, it is safer to restrict water than to administer sodium. An I.V. solution that can contribute to hyponatremia is excessive administration of 5 percent dextrose in water.

General treatment guidelines for patients with hyponatremia are:

1. Replace sodium and fluid losses through diet or parenteral fluids. (If serum sodium level is lower than 125 mEq/L, it is important to quickly bring the level up to more than 125 mEq/L, then to gradually continue to return the sodium to a normal level.)
2. Restore normal ECF volume.
3. Correct any other electrolyte losses such as potassium or bicarbonate.

Nursing Management

Nursing assessments include:

1. Obtaining a patient history of high-risk factors for hyponatremia (vomiting, diarrhea, eating disorders, low sodium diet).
2. Obtaining a history of medications with emphasis on those predisposing patients to hyponatremia (i.e., diuretics).
3. Assess for signs of hyponatremia.
4. Obtain baseline laboratory tests (e.g., serum sodium, serum osmolarity, serum potassium, serum chloride, and urinary specific gravity).

Key nursing interventions include:

1. Monitoring laboratory tests with emphasis on serum sodium.
2. Monitoring GI losses.
3. Keeping accurate records of fluid intake and output.
4. Monitoring for changes in central venous system symptoms.
5. Weighing the patient daily.

SERUM SODIUM EXCESS: HYPERNATREMIA

The physiologic role of potassium includes:

- Regulation of fluid volume within the cell
- Promotion of nerve impulse transmission
- Contraction of skeletal, smooth, and cardiac muscle
- Control of hydrogen ion (H^+) concentration, acid–base balance; when potassium moves out of the cell, hydrogen ions move in, and vice versa
- Role in enzyme action for cellular energy production

The serum level of sodium is elevated to above 145 mEq/L in patients with hypernatremia. This elevation can be caused by a gain of sodium without water or a loss of water without loss of sodium.

Pathophysiology and Etiology

Increased levels of serum sodium can occur with deprivation of water, occurring when a person cannot respond to thirst; during hypertonic tube feeding with inadequate water supplements; with excessive parenteral administration of sodium-containing solutions; and when a person is drowning in sea water. Sodium is lost with watery diarrhea (a particular problem in infants), increased insensible loss, ingestion of sodium in unusual amounts, profuse sweating, heat stroke, and diabetes insipidus when water intake is inadequate.

AGE-RELATED CONSIDERATIONS 4–2

In aging adults, there is a diminished thirst response that may lead to inadequate fluid intake. Infants are unable to obtain fluid independently and may be at risk of inadequate fluid intake, especially in warmer weather.

Signs and Symptoms

Patients with hypernatremia may experience marked thirst; elevated body temperature; swollen tongue; red, dry, sticky mucous membranes;

severe hypernatremia; disorientation; and irritability or hyperactivity when stimulated.

Diagnostic Tests

- Serum sodium: >145 mEq/L
- Serum osmolarity: >295 mOsm/kg
- Urine specific gravity: >1.015 (except for those with diabetes insipidus)
- Dehydration test: Water is withheld for 16 to 18 hours; serum and urine osmolarity are checked 1 hour after administration of antidiuretic hormone (ADH); this test is used to identify the cause of polyuric syndromes (central versus nephrogenic diabetes insipidus)

Treatment and Management

The goal of treatment of patients with hypernatremia is to gradually lower the serum sodium level, infusing a hypotonic electrolyte solution such as 0.45 percent normal saline or 5 percent dextrose in water. Gradual reduction is necessary to decrease the risk of cerebral edema. The sodium level should not be lowered more than 15 mEq/L in an 8-hour period of time for adults (Weldy, 1996).

Generally, treatment guidelines for hypernatremia are:

1. Infusion of an isotonic solution (0.9% NaCl) or hypotonic electrolyte solution (0.45% NaCl or 5% dextrose in water).
2. Sodium levels can also be decreased by use of diuretics, which induce excretion of water and sodium.

Nursing Management

Nursing assessment includes:

1. Obtaining a patient history of high-risk factors for hypernatremia (e.g., increased sodium intake, water deprivation, increased adrenocortical hormone production, use of sodium-retaining drugs).
2. Assessing for signs of hypernatremia.
3. Obtaining baseline values of laboratory tests, especially serum sodium.

Key nursing interventions include:

1. Monitoring laboratory test results with emphasis on serum sodium and serum osmolarity.
2. Keeping accurate fluid intake and output records.
3. Monitoring for signs of pulmonary edema when the patient is receiving large amounts of parenteral sodium chloride.

POTASSIUM (K^+)

NORMAL REFERENCE VALUE: 3.5 TO 5.5 mEq/L

PHYSIOLOGIC ROLE

The physiologic role of potassium includes:

- Regulation of fluid volume within the cell
- Promotion of nerve impulse transmission
- Contraction of skeletal, smooth, and cardiac muscle
- Control of hydrogen ion (H^+) concentration, acid–base balance; when potassium moves out of the cell, hydrogen ions move in, and vice versa
- Role of enzyme action for cellular energy production.

Potassium is an intracellular electrolyte with 98 percent in the ICF and 2 percent in the ECF. Potassium is a dynamic electrolyte. Cellular potassium replaces ECF potassium if it becomes depleted. Potassium is acquired through diet and must be ingested daily because the body has no effective method of storage. The daily requirement is 40 mEq. Potassium influences both skeletal and cardiac muscle activity. Alterations in the concentration of plasma potassium changes myocardial irritability and rhythm. Potassium moves easily into the intracellular space when the body is metabolizing glucose. It moves out of the cells during strenuous exercise, when cellular metabolism is impaired, or when the cell dies. Potassium, along with sodium, is responsible for transmission of nerve impulses. During nerve cell innervation, these ions exchange places, creating an electrical current (Metheny, 2000).

There is a relationship between acid–base imbalances and potassium balance. Hypokalemia can cause alkalosis, which in turn can further decrease serum potassium. Hyperkalemia can cause acidosis, which in turn can further increase serum potassium.

The regulation of potassium is related to several other processes, including:

- Sodium level: Enough sodium must be available for exchange with potassium.
- Hydrogen ion excretion: When there is an increase in hydrogen ion excretion, there is a decrease in potassium excretion.
- Aldosterone level: An increased level of aldosterone stimulates and increases excretion of potassium.

Potassium imbalances are common in clinical practice because of their association with underlying disease, injury, or ingestion of certain medications.

SERUM POTASSIUM DEFICIT: HYPOKALEMIA

Hypokalemia is a serum potassium level below 3.5 mEq/L. It usually reflects a real deficit in total potassium stores; however, it may occur in patients with normal potassium stores when alkalosis is present. Hypokalemia is a common disturbance; many factors are associated with this deficit, and many clinical conditions contribute to it.

Pathophysiology and Etiology

Many conditions can lead to potassium deficit, including GI and renal loss, increased use of increased perspiration, shifting of extracellular potassium into the cells, and poor dietary intake.

Gastrointestinal loss includes diarrhea or laxative overuse, prolonged gastric suction, and protracted vomiting.

Renal loss includes potassium-wasting diuretic therapy; excessive use of glucocorticoids; ingestion of drugs such as sodium penicillin, carbenicillin, or amphotericin B; excessive ingestion of European licorice (which mimics the action of aldosterone); and excessive steroid administration.

Sweat loss includes heavy perspiration in persons acclimated to the heat.

Shifting into the cells can occur with total parenteral nutrition therapy without adequate potassium supplementation, alkalosis, and excessive administration of insulin.

Poor dietary intake can occur with anorexia nervosa, bulimia, and alcoholism.

Signs and Symptoms

Patients with hypokalemia may experience neuromuscular changes such as fatigue, muscle weakness, diminished deep tendon reflexes, and flaccid paralysis (late). Other symptoms include anorexia, nausea, vomiting, irritability (early), increased sensitivity to digitalis, electrocardiographic (ECG) changes, and death (in those with severe hypokalemia) caused by cardiac arrest.

Diagnostic Tests

- Serum potassium: <3.5 mEq/L
- Arterial blood gas (ABG): May show metabolic alkalosis (increased pH and bicarbonate ion)
- ECG: ST segment depression, flattened T wave, presence of U wave, and ventricular dysrhythmias (Fig. 4–2)

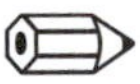 **NOTE:** Clinical signs and symptoms rarely occur before the serum potassium level has fallen below 3 mEq/L.

Treatment and Management

Replacement of potassium is the key concept in treating patients with potassium deficit. General treatment guidelines include:

1. Mild hypokalemia is usually treated with dietary increases of potassium or oral supplements.

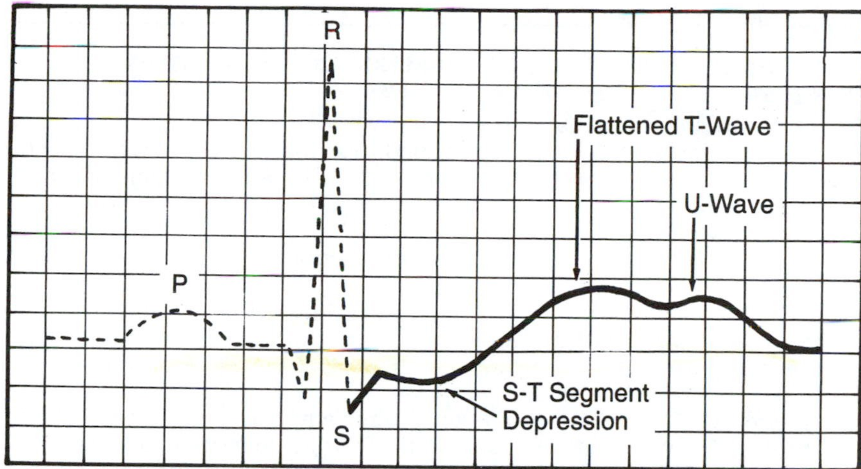

FIG. 4–2. Sample ECG tracing: hypokalemia. The ECG tracing for hypokalemia has ST-segment depression, flattened T wave, and the presence of a U wave.

2. Salt substitutes (e.g., Morton Salt Substitute, Co-Salt, Adolph's Salt Substitute) contain potassium and can be used to supplement potassium intake.
3. If the serum potassium is below 2 mEq/L, monitor the patient's ECG and administer potassium by means of a secondary piggyback set in a volume of 100 mL (Metheny, 2000).

Table 4–2 gives critical guidelines for nursing in I.V. administration of potassium.

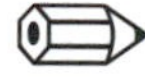 **NOTE:** Potassium replacement must take place slowly to prevent hyperkalemia. Extreme caution should be used when potassium chloride replacement exceeds 120 mEq in 24 hours. The patient must be monitored for dysrhythmias.

Nursing Management

Nursing assessment includes:

1. Obtain history of high-risk factors for hypokalemia such as vomiting, renal disease, and diuretic use.
2. Assess for signs of hypokalemia.
3. Obtain baseline laboratory test values such as ECG reading, serum potassium, and serum osmolarity.

Key nursing interventions include:

1. Monitoring the laboratory test results, especially serum potassium

TABLE 4–2

CRITICAL GUIDELINES FOR ADMINISTRATION OF POTASSIUM

Never give a potassium I.V. push.

Potassium chloride (KCl) should be added to a nondextrose solution such as isotonic saline to treat severe hypokalemia because administration of KCl in a dextrose solution may cause a small reduction in the serum potassium level.

Never administer concentrated potassium solutions without first diluting them as directed.

KCl preparations greater than 60 mEq/L **should not** be given in a peripheral vein. Concentrations greater than 8 mEq/100 mL can cause pain and irritation of peripheral veins and lead to postinfusion phlebitis (Rapp, 1987).

When adding KCl to infusion solutions, especially plastic systems, make sure the KCl mixes with the solution thoroughly. Invert and agitate the container to ensure mixing. ***Do not add KCl to a hanging container!***

For patients with any degree of renal insufficiency or heart block, Zull (1989) recommends reducing the infusion by 50 percent. For example, 5 to 10 mEq/h rather than 10 to 20 mEq/h.

Administer potassium at a rate not to exceed 10 mEq/h through peripheral veins (Kokko & Tannen, 1990; Gahart, 1994).

For patients with extreme hypokalemia, rates should be no more than 40 mEq/h while ECG is constantly monitored (Kokko & Tannen, 1990).

If KCl is administered into the subcutaneous tissue (infiltration), it is extremely irritating and can cause serious tissue loss. Use extravasation protocol in this situation.

2. Keeping accurate intake and output records
3. Monitoring for changes in cardiac response
4. Monitoring for signs of phlebitis (potassium irritates veins) when given by I.V. route

SERUM POTASSIUM EXCESS: HYPERKALEMIA

Hyperkalemia occurs less frequently than hypokalemia, but it can be more dangerous. It seldom occurs in patients who have normal renal function. Hyperkalemia is defined as a serum plasma level of potassium above 5.5 mEq/L. The main causes of hyperkalemia are (1) increased intake of potassium (oral or parenteral), (2) decreased urinary excretion of potassium, and (3) movement of potassium out of the cells and into the extracellular space.

Pathophysiology and Etiology

High levels of serum potassium can be caused by either a gain of potassium body or shift of potassium from the ICF to the ECF (NSNA, 1997). Hyperkalemia can be caused by excessive administration of

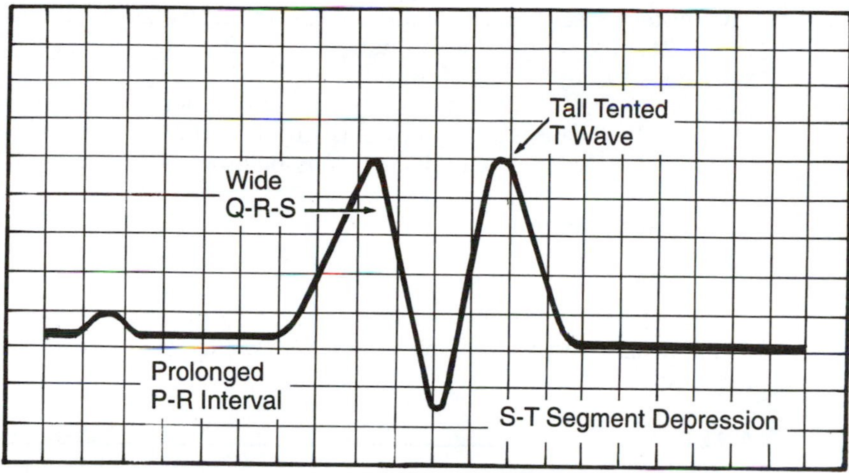

FIG. 4–3. Sample ECG tracing: Hyperkalemia. The ECG tracing for hyperkalemia shows progressive changes; tall, thin T waves; prolonged PR intervals; ST-segment depression; widened QRS; and loss of P wave.

potassium parentally or orally; severe renal failure resulting in reduced potassium excretion; release of potassium from altered cellular function, such as with burns or crush injuries; and acidosis.

Drugs that can cause a predisposition to hyperkalemias include potassium penicillin, indomethacin, amphetamines, nonsteroidal anti-inflammatory drugs, alpha agonists, beta-blockers, succinylcholine, cyclophosphamide, and potassium-sparing diuretics. Pseudohyperkalemia can occur with prolonged tourniquet application during blood withdrawal.

Signs and Symptoms

Patients with hyperkalemia may experience changes shown on ECGs, vague muscle weakness, flaccid paralysis, anxiety, nausea, cramping, and diarrhea.

Diagnostic Tests

- Serum potassium: >5.5 mEq/L
- ABG values: Metabolic acidosis (decreased pH and bicarbonate ion)
- ECG: Widened QRS, prolonged PR, and ventricular dysrhythmias (Fig. 4–3)

Treatment and Management

The following are guidelines for the treatment of patients with hyperkalemia:

1. Restrict dietary potassium in mild cases.
2. Discontinue supplements of potassium.

3. Administer I.V. calcium gluconate if necessary for cardiac symptoms.
4. Administer I.V. sodium bicarbonate, which alkalinizes the plasma and cause a temporary shift of potassium into the cells.
5. Administer regular insulin (10 to 25 U) and hypertonic dextrose (10%), which causes a shift of potassium into the cells.
6. Peritoneal dialysis or hemodialysis may be ordered.

Nursing Management

Nursing assessment includes:

1. Obtain client history relative to high-risk factors for hyperkalemia (renal disease, potassium-sparing diuretics, excessive salt substitute use)

TABLE 4–3

CRITICAL GUIDELINES FOR REMOVAL OF POTASSIUM

Treatment Guidelines
● **Sodium polystyrene sulfonate** is a cation exchange resin that removes potassium from the body by exchanging sodium for potassium in the intestinal tract. This method should not be the sole treatment for severe hyperkalemia because of its slow onset.
Oral sodium polystyrene sulfonate (15 to 30 g); may repeat every 4 to 6 hours as needed; it removes potassium 1 to 2 hours.
Rectal sodium polystyrene sulfonate (50 g) as retention enema; when administered, use an inflated rectal catheter to ensure retention of the dissolved resin for 30 to 60 minutes; it removes potassium in 30 to 60 minutes; each enema can lower the plasma potassium concentration by 0.5 to 1.0 mEq/L (Rose, 1989)
● **Dialysis** is used when more aggressive methods are needed. Peritoneal dialysis is not as effective as hemodialysis. Whereas peritoneal dialysis can remove approximately 10 to 15 mEq/h, hemodialysis can remove 25 to 35 mEq/h (Kokko & Tannen, 1990).
● **Glucose and insulin**
Insulin facilitates potassium movement into the cells, reducing the plasma potassium level. Glucose administration in nondiabetic patients may cause a marked increase in insulin release from the pancreas, producing desired plasma potassium-lowering effects (Rose, 1989).
500 mL of 10 percent dextrose with 15 to 10 U of regular insulin over 1 hour: The potassium-lowering effects are delayed about 30 minutes but are effective for 4 to 6 hours (Zull, 1989).
● **Emergency measures**
Calcium gluconate: 10 mL of 10 percent calcium gluconate administered slowly over 2 to 3 minutes. Administer only to patients who need immediate myocardial protection against toxic effects of severe hyperkalemia. Protective effect begins within 1 to 2 minutes and lasts only 30 to 60 minutes (Spital, 1989).
Sodium bicarbonate: 45 mEq (1 ampule of 7.5% sodium bicarbonate) infused slowly over 5 minutes. This temporarily shifts potassium into the cells and is helpful in patients with metabolic acidosis.

2. Assess for signs of hyperkalemia
3. Obtain baseline ECG; assess for altered T waves
4. Obtain baseline serum potassium

Key nursing interventions include:

1. Monitoring the laboratory test results especially serum potassium
2. Keeping accurate intake and output records
3. Monitoring for changes in cardiac response
4. Monitoring vital signs, with special attention to tachycardia and bradycardia

Table 4–3 provides critical guidelines for nursing in treatment of patients with potassium excess.

CALCIUM (CA^{++})

NORMAL REFERENCE VALUE: 8.5 TO 10.5 mg/dL

PHYSIOLOGIC ROLE

The physiologic role of calcium includes:

- Maintaining skeletal elements; calcium is needed for strong, durable bones and teeth
- Regulating neuromuscular activity
- Influencing enzyme activity
- Converting prothrombin to thrombin, a necessary part of the material that holds cells together

The calcium ion is most abundant in the skeletal system, with 99 percent residing in the bones and teeth. Only 1 percent is available for rapid exchange in the circulating blood bound to protein. The parathyroid hormone (PTH) is responsible for transfer of calcium from the bone to plasma. PTH also augments the intestinal absorption of calcium and enhances net renal calcium reabsorption. Calcium is acquired through dietary intake. Adults require approximately 1 g of calcium daily, along with vitamin D and protein, which are required for absorption and utilization of this electrolyte.

Calcium is instrumental in activating enzymes and stimulating essential chemical reactions. It plays an important role in maintaining the normal transmission of nerve impulses and has a sedative effect on nerve cells. Calcium plays its most important role in the conversion of prothrombin to thrombin, a necessary sequence in the formation of a clot.

Calcium and phosphate have a reciprocal relationship; that is, an increase in calcium level causes a drop in the serum phosphorus concentration, and a drop in calcium causes an increase in phosphorus level.

Calcium is present in three different forms in the plasma: (1) ionized (50% of total calcium); (2) bound (<50% of total calcium); and (3) complexed (small percentage that combines with phosphate). Only ionized calcium (i.e., calcium affected by plasma pH, phosphorus, and albumin levels) is physiologically important. A relationship between ionized calcium and plasma pH is reciprocal; an increase in pH decreases the percentage of calcium that is ionized. The relationship between plasma phosphorus and ionized calcium is also reciprocal. Albumin does not affect ionized calcium, but it does affect the amount of calcium bound to proteins.

SERUM CALCIUM DEFICIT: HYPOCALCEMIA

A reduction of total body calcium levels or a reduction of the percentage of ionized calcium causes hypocalcemia.

Pathophysiology and Etiology

Total calcium levels may be decreased because of increased calcium loss, reduced intake secondary to altered intestinal absorption, and altered regulation, as in those with hypoparathyroidism.

The most common cause of hypocalcemia is inadequate secretion of PTH caused by primary hypoparathyroidism or surgically induced hypoparathyroidism. It can also result from calcium loss through diarrhea and wound exudate, acute pancreatitis, hyperphosphatemia usually associated with renal failure, inadequate intake of vitamin D or minimal sun exposure, prolonged nasogastric tube suctioning resulting in metabolic alkalosis, and infusion of citrated blood (citrate-phosphate-dextrose).

Drugs that predispose an individual to hypocalcemia include potent loop diuretics and dioxin.

Signs and Symptoms

Patients with hypocalcemia may experience neuromuscular symptoms such as numbness of the fingers, cramps in the muscles (especially the extremities), hyperactive deep tendon reflexes, and a positive **Trousseau's sign** (Fig. 4–4) and **Chvostek's sign** (Fig. 4–5).

Other symptoms include irritability, memory impairment, delusions, seizures (late), prolonged QT interval, and altered cardiovascular hemodynamics that may precipitate congestive heart failure. In patients with hypocalcemia caused by citrated blood transfusion, the cardiac index, stroke volume, and left ventricular stroke work values have been found to be lower.

The most dangerous symptom associated with hypocalcemia is the development of laryngospasm and tetany-like contractions. A low mag-

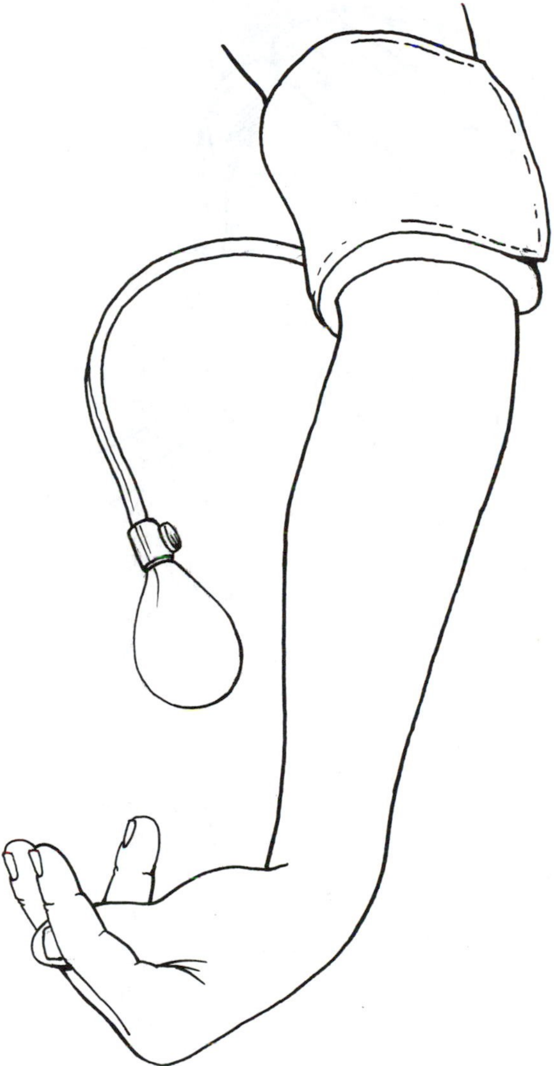

FIG. 4–4. Positive Trousseau's sign. Carpopedal attitude of the hand when blood pressure cuff is place on the arm and inflated above systolic pressure for 3 minutes. A positive reaction is the development of carpal spasm.

nesium level and a high potassium level potentiate the cardiac and neuromuscular irritability produced by a low calcium level. However, a low potassium level can protect patients from hypocalcemic tetany (Lee, 1996).

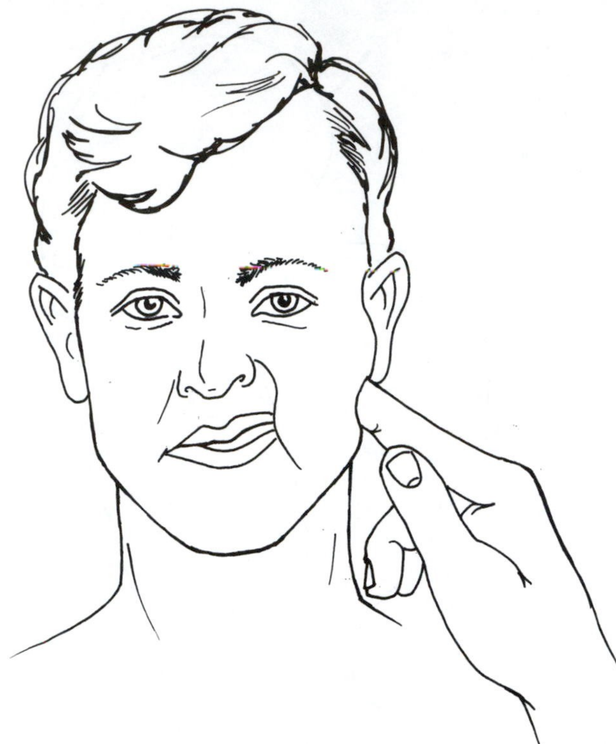

FIG. 4–5. Positive Chvostek's sign, which occurs after tapping the facial nerve approximately 2 cm anterior to the earlobe. Unilateral twitching of the facial muscle occurs in some patients with hypocalcemia or hypomagnesemia.

Treatment and Management

The goal of treatment is to alleviate the underlying cause.

Treatment of patients with hypocalcemia consists of administration of calcium gluconate, either orally (preferred) with calcium supplements, 1000 mg/d, to raise the total serum calcium level by 1 mg/dL, or intravenously, 10 to 20 mL of a 10 percent solution in 5 percent dextrose in water for 20 minutes.

Nursing Management

Nursing assessments include:

1. Obtain history relative to potential causes of hypocalcemia, such as low-calcium diet, lack of vitamin D, low protein diet, chronic diarrhea, or hormonal disorders.
2. Obtain history of drugs that could predispose the patient to hypocalcemia, such as furosemide (Lasix) or cortisone.

AGE-RELATED CONSIDERATIONS 4–3

There are two types of hypocalcemia in newborn infants. The first occurs early after birth during the first 3 days of life; this is attributed to parathyroid immaturity or maternal hyperparathyroidism. This resolves within the first week of life (Metheny, 2000). The second type of neonatal hypocalcemia occurs about 1 week after birth and is associated with hyperphosphatemia and hypomagnesemia. Providing milk with a high phosphorus level can lead to hyperphosphatemia and then hypocalcemia (Narins, 1994).

3. Assess for signs of hypocalcemia.
4. Obtain baseline values for serum calcium, ionized calcium serum albumin, and acid–base status.

Key nursing interventions include:

1. Taking safety precautions and preparing to adopt seizure precautions if hypocalcemia is severe.
2. Monitoring laboratory test results with emphasis on serum and ionized calcium.
3. Monitoring ECGs for changes in pattern.
4. Monitoring for irritation of subcutaneous tissue and tissue sloughing when calcium is given parenterally.
5. Monitoring for signs of cardiac arrhythmias in patients receiving digitalis and calcium supplements.
6. Monitoring for hypocalcemia in patients receiving massive transfusion of citrated blood.

SERUM CALCIUM EXCESS: HYPERCALCEMIA

Hypercalcemia is caused by excessive release of calcium from the bone, almost always from malignancy, hyperparathyroidism, thiazide-diuretic use, or excessive calcium intake.

Pathophysiology and Etiology

Most symptoms of hypercalcemia are present only when serum calcium is greater than 12 mg/dL and tend to be more severe if hypercalcemia develops quickly. Causes of hypercalcemia include hyperparathyroidism, Paget's disease, multiple fractures, and overuse of calcium-containing antacids. Patients with solid tumors that have metastasized, such as breast, prostate, and malignant melanomas, and hematologic tumors, such as lymphomas, acute leukemia, and myelomas, are also at risk for developing hypercalcemia.

Drugs that predispose an individual to hypercalcemia include calcium salts, megadoses of vitamin A or D, thiazide diuretics (potentiate action of PTH), androgens or estrogen for breast cancer therapy, I.V. lipids, lithium, and tamoxifen.

Signs and Symptoms

Patients with hypercalcemia may experience neuromuscular symptoms such as muscle weakness, incoordination, lethargy, deep bone pain, flank pain, pathologic fractures (caused by bone weakening). Other symptoms include constipation, anorexia, nausea, vomiting, polyuria or polydipsia leading to uremia if not treated, and renal colic caused by stone formation. Patients taking digitalis must take calcium with extreme care because it can precipitate severe dysrhythmias.

Diagnostic Tests

- Total serum calcium: May be more than 10.5 mg/dL
- Serum ionized calcium: 5.5 mg/dL
- Serum parathyroid hormone: Increased levels in primary or secondary hyperparathryoidism
- Radiography: May reveal osteoporosis, bone cavitation, or urinary calculi

Treatment and Management

Hypercalcemia should be treated according to the following guidelines:

1. Treat the patient's underlying disease.
2. Administer saline diuresis. Fluids should be forced to help eliminate the source of the hypercalcemia. A solution of 0.45 percent NaCl or 0.9 percent NaCl I.V. dilutes the serum calcium level. Rehydration is important to dilute the Ca^+ ion and promote renal excretion.
3. Give inorganic phosphate salts orally (Neutra-Phos) or rectally (Fleet Enema).
4. Provide hemodialysis or peritoneal dialysis to reduce serum calcium levels in life-threatening situations.
5. Use furosemide, 20 to 40 mg every 2 hours, to prevent volume overloading during saline administration.
6. Administer calcitonin, 4 to 8 U/kg intramuscularly or subcutaneously every 6 to 12 hours. This will temporarily lower the serum calcium level by 1 to 3 mg/100 mL.
7. Give biphosphonates to inhibit bone reabsorption. Pamidronate is effective, 60 to 90 mg in 1 L of 0.9 percent NaCl or 5 percent dextrose in water is infused over 24 hours.
8. Administer plicamycin (Mithramycin), which inhibits bone reabsorption and reliably lowers serum calcium. It is used only in those with malignant hypercalcemia because of its toxicity. A

single dose of 25 μg/kg in 500 mL of 5 percent dextrose in water is infused intravenously over 4 to 6 hours (Phillips & Kuhn, 1999).

Nursing Management

Nursing assessment includes:

1. Obtain a patient history of probable cause of hypercalcemia, such as cancer; excessive use of calcium supplements, antacids, or thiazide diuretics; or steroid therapy.
2. Assess for signs of hypercalcemia.
3. Obtain baseline values for serum calcium and serum phosphate.
4. Obtain baseline ECG.
5. Assess client's fluid volume status and mental alertness.

Key nursing interventions include:

1. Monitoring changes in vital signs and laboratory tests.
2. Encouraging the patient to drink 3 to 4 L of fluid per day.
3. Encouraging the patient to consume fluids (e.g., cranberry or prune juice) that promote urine acidity to help prevent formation of renal calculi.
4. Keeping accurate fluid intake and output records.
5. Monitoring for digitalis toxicity.
6. Handling the patient gently to prevent fractures.
7. Encouraging the patient to avoid high calcium foods.

MAGNESIUM

NORMAL REFERENCE VALUE: 1.5 TO 2.5 mEq/L

PHYSIOLOGIC ROLE

The physiologic role of magnesium includes:

- Enzyme action
- Regulation of neuromuscular activity (similar to calcium)
- Regulation of electrolyte balance, including facilitating transport of sodium and potassium across cell membranes, influencing the utilization of calcium, potassium, and protein.

Magnesium is a major intracellular electrolyte. The normal diet supplies approximately 25 mEq of magnesium. Approximately one third of serum magnesium is bound to protein; the remaining two thirds exists as free cations. The same factors that regulate calcium balance have an influence on magnesium balance. Magnesium balance is also affected by many of the same agents that decrease or influence potassium balance.

Magnesium acts directly on the myoneural junction and affects neuromuscular irritability and contractility, possibly exerting a sedative effect. Magnesium acts as an activator for many enzymes and plays a role in both carbohydrate and protein metabolism. Magnesium affects the cardiovascular system, acting peripherally to produce vasodilation. Imbalances in magnesium predispose the heart to ventricular dysrhythmias (Metheny, 2000).

SERUM MAGNESIUM (MG^{++}) DEFICIT: HYPOMAGNESEMIA

Hypomagnesemia is often overlooked in critically ill patients. This imbalance is considered to be one of the most underdiagnosed electrolyte deficiencies (Metheny, 2000). Symptoms of hypomagnesemia tend to occur when the serum level drops below 1.0 mEq/L.

Pathophysiology and Etiology

Hypomagnesemia can result from chronic alcoholism; malabsorption syndrome, especially if the small bowel is affected; prolonged malnutrition or starvation; prolonged diarrhea; acute pancreatitis; administration of magnesium-free solutions for more than one week; and prolonged nasogastric tube suctioning.

Drugs that predispose an individual to hypomagnesemia include aminoglycosides, diuretics, cortisone, amphotericin, digitalis, cisplatin, and cyclosporine. Infusion of collected blood preserved with citrate can also cause hypomagnesemia (Lee, 1996).

Signs and Symptoms

Patients with hypomagnesemia often experience neuromuscular symptoms, such as hyperactive reflexes, coarse tremors, muscle cramps, positive Chvostek's and Trousseau's signs (see Figs. 4–4 and 4–5), seizures, paresthesia of the feet and legs, and painfully cold hands and feet. Other symptoms include disorientation, dysrhythmias, tachycardia, and increased potential for digitalis toxicity.

Diagnostic Tests

- Serum magnesium: <1.5 mEq/L
- Urine magnesium: Helps to identify renal causes of magnesium depletion.
- Serum albumin: A decrease may cause a decreased magnesium level resulting from the reduction in protein-bound magnesium.
- Serum potassium: Decreased because of failure of the cellular sodium-potassium pump to move potassium into the cell and because of the accompanying loss of potassium in the urine.
- Serum calcium: May be reduced because of a reduction in the release and action of PTH.
- ECG: Findings of tachydysrhythmias, prolonged PR and QT intervals, widening of the QRS, ST segment depression, and

flattened T waves. A form of ventricular tachycardia (i.e., torsades de pointes) associated with all three electrolyte imbalances (i.e., magnesium, calcium, and potassium) may develop.

Treatment and Management

Treatment of patients with hypomagnesemia includes:

1. Administering oral magnesium salts.
2. Administering 40 mEq (5 g) magnesium sulfate added intravenously to 1 L of 5 percent dextrose in water or 5 percent dextrose/NaCl.
3. Administering 1 to 2 g of 10 percent solution of magnesium sulfate by direct I.V. push at a rate of 1.5 mL/min (Phillips & Kuhn, 1996).

Table 4–4 provides critical guidelines for nurses who are administering magnesium.

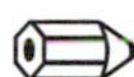

NOTE: Be aware that other CNS depressants could cause further depressed sensorium when magnesium sulfate is being administered. Therefore, be prepared to deal with respiratory arrest if hypermagnesemia inadvertently occurs during administration of magnesium sulfate.

Nursing Management

Nursing assessment includes:

1. Obtain a patient history, being alert to factors that predispose to hypomagnesemia such as alcoholism, laxative abuse, total parenteral nutrition (TPN), potassium-wasting diuretic use.
2. Assess for signs and symptoms of hypomagnesemia.
3. Obtain baseline values for laboratory tests, serum magnesium, serum calcium, and serum potassium.
4. Obtain baseline ECG.

TABLE 4–4

CRITICAL GUIDELINES FOR ADMINISTRATION OF MAGNESIUM

- Double check the order for magnesium administration to ensure that it stipulates the concentration of the solution to be used. Do not accept orders for "amps" or "vials" without further clarification.
- Use caution in patients with impaired renal function; watch urine output.
- Reduce other CNS depressants when five are given concurrently with magnesium preparations.
- Therapeutic doses of magnesium can produce flushing and sweating and occur most often if the administration rate is too fast.
- Closely assess patients receiving magnesium.

Key nursing interventions include:

1. Monitoring vital signs.
2. Monitoring closely for digitalis toxicity.
3. Keeping accurate intake and output records.
4. Taking safety precautions if a patient is mentally confused.

SERUM MAGNESIUM (MG^{++}) EXCESS: HYPERMAGNESEMIA

Hypermagnesemia occurs when a person's serum level is greater than 2.5 mEq/L. The most common cause of hypermagnesemia is renal failure in patients who have an increased intake of magnesium.

Pathophysiology and Etiology

Renal factors that lead to hypermagnesemia include renal failure, Addison's disease, and inadequate excretion of magnesium by kidneys.

Other causes include hyperparathyroidism; hyperthyroidism; excessive magnesium administration during treatment of patients with eclampsia; hemodialysis with excessively hard water with a dialysate inadvertently high in magnesium; or ingestion of medications high in magnesium, such as antacids and laxatives are iatrogenic causes of hypermagnesemia.

Signs and Symptoms

Patients with hypermagnesemia may experience neuromuscular symptoms such as flushing and sense of skin warmth, lethargy, sedation, hypoactive deep tendon reflexes, depressed respirations, and weak or absent cry in newborn. Other symptoms include hypotension, sinus bradycardia, heart block, and cardiac arrest (serum level >15 mEq/L) and increased susceptibility to digitalis toxicity, nausea, vomiting, and seizures.

Diagnostic Tests

- Serum magnesium: >2.5 mEq/L
- ECG: Findings of QT interval and atrioventricular block may occur (at levels >2.5 mEq/L)

Treatment and Management

Guidelines for treatment of patients with hypermagnesemia are:

1. Decrease oral magnesium intake.
2. Administer calcium gluconate to antagonize the action of magnesium.

3. Support respiratory function.
4. Order peritoneal or hemodialysis in severe cases of hypermagnesemia.

Nursing Management

Nursing assessment includes:

1. Evaluate possible causes of hypermagnesemia, including renal insufficiency and chronic laxative use.
2. Assess for signs of hypermagnesemia.
3. Obtain baseline values for serum magnesium and serum calcium.
4. Obtain baseline ECG.

Key nursing interventions include:

1. Monitoring vital signs.
2. Monitoring laboratory test values.
3. Monitoring for ECG changes.
4. Encouraging fluid intake if not contraindicated.
5. Being prepared to provide ventilatory assistance or resuscitation.

PHOSPHORUS (HPO_4^-)

NORMAL REFERENCE VALUE: 3.0 TO 4.5 mg/dL

PHYSIOLOGIC ROLE

The physiologic role of phosphorus is:

- Phosphorus is essential to all cells
- Role in metabolism of proteins, carbohydrates, and fats
- Essential to energy, necessary in formation of high-energy compounds adenosine triphosphate (ATP), and adenosine diphosphate (ADP)
- As a cellular building block, it is the backbone of nucleic acids and is essential to cell membrane formation
- Delivery of oxygen; functions in formation of red blood cell enzyme

Approximately 80 percent of phosphorus in the body is contained in the bones and teeth, and 20 percent is abundant in the ICF. PTH plays a major role in homeostasis of phosphate because of its ability to vary phosphate reabsorption in the proximal tubule of the kidney. PTH also allows for the shift of phosphate from bone to plasma.

Phosphorus plays an important role in delivery of oxygen to tissues by regulating the level of 2,3-diphosphoglycerate (2,3-DPG), a substance in red blood cells that decreases the affinity of hemoglobin for oxygen.

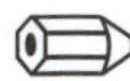

NOTE: Phosphorus and calcium have a reciprocal relationship: an increase in the phosphorus level frequently causes hypocalcemia.

SERUM PHOSPHATE DEFICIT: HYPOPHOSPHATEMIA

Phosphorus is a critical constituent of all the body's tissues. Hypophosphatemia occurs when the serum level is below the lower limit of normal (<2.5 mg/dL). This imbalance may occur in the presence of total body phosphate deficit or may merely reflect a temporary shift of phosphorus into the cells.

Pathophysiology and Etiology

Hypophosphatemia can result from overzealous refeeding, total parenteral nutrition administered without adequate phosphorus, malabsorption syndromes, or alcohol withdrawal. GI losses include vomiting, chronic diarrhea, and malabsorption syndromes.

Hormonal influences such as hyperparathyroidism enhance renal phosphate excretion. Drugs that predispose an individual to hypophosphatemia include aluminum-containing antacids (which bind phosphorus, thereby lowering serum levels), diuretics, androgens, corticosteroids, glucagon, epinephrine, gastrin, and mannitol. Other causes include treatment of patients with diabetic ketoacidosis (dextrose with insulin causes shift of phosphorus into cells).

Signs and Symptoms

Hypophosphatemia can affect the CNS, neuromuscular and cardiac status, and the blood. An affected patient may experience disorientation, confusion, seizures, paresthesia (early), profound muscle weakness, tremor, ataxia, incoordination, dysarthria, dysphagia, and congestive cardiomyopathy. Hypophosphatemia affects all blood cells, especially red cells. It causes a decline in 2,3-DPG levels in erythrocytes. 2,3-DPG in red cells normally interacts with hemoglobin to promote the release of oxygen. With reduced 2,3-DPG, oxygen delivery to peripheral tissues is impaired.

Diagnostic Tests

- Serum phosphorus: <2.5 mg/dL (1.7 mEq/L)
- Serum PTH: Elevated
- Serum magnesium: Decreased because of increased urinary excretion of magnesium

- Serum alkaline phosphate: Increased with increased osteoblastic activity
- Radiography: Skeletal changes of osteomalacia or rickets

Treatment and Management

Treatment should include the following regimen:

1. For mild to moderate deficiency, oral phosphate supplements, such as Neutra-Phos or Phospho-Soda, can be administered.
2. For severe hypophosphatemia, administer I.V. phosphorus solutions in severe deficiency.

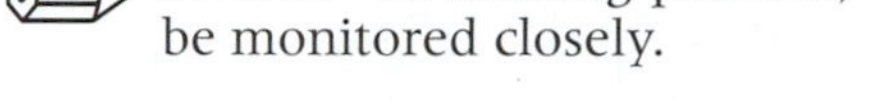

NOTE: In treating patients, be aware that calcium levels should be monitored closely.

Nursing Management

Nursing assessment includes:

1. Obtain a patient history with focus on factors that put patients at high risk for hypophosphatemia, such as alcoholism, use of TPN, and diabetic ketoacidosis.
2. Assess for signs of hypophosphatemia.
3. Obtain baseline laboratory values of serum phosphate, and serum calcium.

Key nursing interventions include:

1. Monitoring for cardiac, GI, and neurologic abnormalities.
2. Monitoring for changes in laboratory test values.
3. Keeping accurate intake and output records.
4. Taking safety precautions when a patient is confused.
5. Being alert to signs when feeding is restarted after prolonged starvation (refeeding syndrome).
6. Being alert to complications of I.V. administration of phosphorus (hypocalcemia, hyperphosphatemia).

SERUM PHOSPHATE EXCESS: HYPERPHOSPHATEMIA

A variety of conditions can lead to hyperphosphatemia, but the major disorder is renal disease.

Pathophysiology and Etiology

Hyperphosphatemia can result from renal insufficiency, hypoparathyroidism, or increased **catabolism.** It is also seen in patients with cancer states such as myelogenous leukemia and lymphoma.

Drugs that can predispose an individual to hyperphosphatemia include oral phosphates, I.V. phosphates, phosphate laxatives, and excessive vitamin D, tetracyclines, and methicillin. Other causes include massive blood transfusions caused by phosphate leaking from the blood cells.

Signs and Symptoms

Patients with hyperphosphatemia may experience many symptoms, including hypocalcemia; tetany (short-term); soft tissue calcification (long-term); mental changes, such as apprehension, confusion, and coma; and increased 2,3-DPG levels in red blood cells.

Diagnostic Tests

- Serum phosphorus: >4.5 mg/dL (2.6 mEq/L)
- Serum calcium: Useful in assessing potential consequences of treatment
- Serum PTH: Decreased in those with hypoparathyroidism
- Blood urea nitrogen: Assess renal function
- Radiography: Skeletal changes of osteodystrophy

Treatment and Management

Treatment should include the following regimen:

1. Identify the underlying cause of hyperphosphatemia.
2. Restrict dietary intake.
3. Administer the intake of phosphate-binding gels (e.g., Amphojel, Basaljel, and Dialume).

Nursing Management

Nursing assessment includes:

1. Obtain a patient history for factors that place patients at high risk for hyperphosphatemia, including renal insufficiency and laxative use.
2. Assess for signs and symptoms of hyperphosphatemia.
3. Obtain baseline laboratory values for serum phosphate.
4. Check urinary output; less than 600 mL/d increases serum phosphate levels.

Key nursing interventions include:

1. Monitoring for cardiac, GI, and neuromuscular abnormalities
2. Monitoring changes in laboratory test values
3. Keeping accurate intake and output records
4. Observing the patient for signs and symptoms of hypocalcemia; when phosphate levels increase, calcium levels decrease

CHLORIDE (CL^-)

NORMAL REFERENCE VALUE: 95 TO 108 mEq/L

PHYSIOLOGIC ROLE

The physiologic role of chloride is:

- Regulation of serum osmolarity
- Regulation of fluid balance when sodium is retained chloride is also retained, causing water retention and increase fluid volume
- Control of acidity of gastric juice
- Regulation of acid–base balance
- Role in oxygen–carbon dioxide exchange (chloride shift)

Chloride is the major anion in the ECF. Changes in serum chloride concentration are usually secondary to changes in one or more of the other electrolytes. Chloride has a reciprocal relationship with bicarbonate (HCO_3). For example, a decrease in HCO_3 concentrations results in a reciprocal rise in chloride level; when chloride decreases, HCO_3 level increases in compensation. Chloride exists primarily combined as sodium chloride or hydrochloric acid. Measurement of serum chloride is most frequently done for its inferential value.

Reabsorption of chloride by the renal tubules is one of the major regulatory functions of the kidneys. As sodium chloride is reabsorbed, water follows through osmosis. It is through this function that vascular blood volume is maintained.

Chloride plays its most important role in acid–base balance. Its role in the pH balance of the ECF is referred to as the "chloride shift." The chloride shift is an ionic exchange that occurs within red blood cells. This shift preserves the electrical neutrality of the red blood cells and maintains a 1:20 ratio of carbonic acid and HCO_3 that is essential for pH balance of the plasma.

SERUM CHLORIDE DEFICIT: HYPOCHLOREMIA

Loss of chloride ions occurs mainly through GI losses and significantly alters acid–base balance because of the reciprocal relationship with HCO_3.

Pathophysiology and Etiology

Hypochloremia results primarily from severe vomiting and diarrhea, pyloric obstruction, acute infection, and use of chlorothiazide diuretics. Other causes of hypochloremia include the prolonged use of I.V. 5 percent dextrose in water, which dilutes serum electrolytes.

Signs and Symptoms

Patients with hypochloremia may experience neuromuscular symptoms such as tetany and hypertonic reflexes. Other symptoms include depressed respiration and excessive loss of chloride, resulting in alkalosis because of an increase in HCO_3 level.

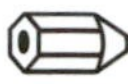 **NOTE:** A deficiency in chloride reflects a deficiency in potassium. When replacing potassium, use potassium chloride solution.

Diagnostic Tests

- Serum chloride: <96 mEq/L
- ABG values: Consistent with alkalosis
- ECG: May show dysrhythmias related to associated hyperkalemia

Treatment and Management

The principles of treating patients with hypochloremia are twofold: (1) treat the underlying cause (alkalosis) and (2) administer NaCl solutions.

Nursing Management

Nursing assessment includes:

1. Obtain a patient history of conditions that predispose an individual to hypochloremia, such as continuous vomiting.
2. Assess for signs and symptoms of hypochloremia.
3. Assess for signs of metabolic alkalosis.
4. Obtain baseline laboratory test values for serum chloride.

Key nursing interventions include:

1. Monitoring changes in laboratory test values for serum chloride and potassium
2. Monitoring for increased signs of hypochloremia
3. Monitoring serum carbon dioxide or arterial bicarbonate for metabolic alkalosis
4. Keeping accurate records of gastric secretions

SERUM CHLORIDE EXCESS: HYPERCHLOREMIA

Excessive Cl^- ions result from any condition that causes a decrease in HCO_3 and can also influence the acid–base balance.

Pathophysiology and Etiology

Trauma such as head injury causes retention of sodium and chloride ions. Hormonal factors affecting retention of chloride include excessive secretion of adrenal cortical hormone. Severe dehydration elevates serum

TABLE 4–5

PATIENTS AT RISK FOR ELECTROLYTE IMBALANCE

Patient Care Unit	Conditions That Can Lead to Imbalance	Potential Electrolyte Imbalances
Geriatric	Prolonged diarrhea Prolonged malnutrition Diuretic therapy	Fluid volume deficit Hypernatremia Hypokalemia
Medical	Anorexia nervosa Profuse sweating Overuse of antacids Gastroenteritis Hyperparathyroidism Diabetic ketoacidosis Alcoholism Renal failure SIADH	Fluid volume deficit Hyponatremia Hypomagnesemia Hypocalcemia Hypokalemia Hyperkalemia Hypermagnesemia
Surgical	Infections Surgical hypoparathyroidism Nasogastric suction Postoperative complications Use of pharmacologic agents: morphine, penicillin, and carbenicillin Ileus	Fluid volume deficit Fluid volume excess Hypokalemia Hypomagnesemia Hypocalcemia Hypochloremia Hyponatremia
Oncologic	Myelogenous leukemia Lymphoma Cytoxan Hypertonic tube feeding Neoplastic disease Solid tumors: Breast and prostate Malignant melanoma	Hypomagnesemia Hyponatremia Hypercalcemia Hypernatremia Hypermagnesemia Hypocalcemia* Hyperkalemia* Hyperphosphatemia*
Critical care	Crushing injuries Total parenteral nutrition administration Hypertonic tube feedings Burns Drowning in sea water Head injuries	Hypomagnesemia Hypophosphatemia Hyponatremia Hypercalcemia Hypernatremia Hyperkalemia

*Components of tumor lysis syndrome.

electrolytes, including chloride. As bicarbonate ions decrease, chloride ions increase in metabolic acidosis.

Signs and Symptoms

Patients with hyperchloremia may experience symptoms related to acidosis, such as drowsiness, lethargy, headache, weakness, tremors, dyspnea, tachypnea, Kussmaul respirations (with pH <7.20), hyperventilation, and dysrhythmias.

Diagnostic Tests

- Serum chloride: >106 mEq/L
- Serum carbon dioxide: <22 mEq/L when associated with acidosis
- Serum pH: <7.35 when associated with metabolic acidosis
- ECG: Presence of dysrhythmias

Treatment and Management

Nursing assessment includes:

1. Obtain history of predisposing conditions such as head injury or cortisone use.
2. Assess for signs and symptoms of hyperchloremia.
3. Obtain baseline laboratory test values for serum chloride and potassium.

Key nursing interventions include:

1. Monitoring changes in laboratory test values, especially serum chloride and serum potassium
2. Monitoring for increased signs of hyperchloremia
3. Monitoring serum carbon dioxide or arterial bicarbonate levels for metabolic acidosis
4. Keeping an accurate record of 24-hour urinary output

Table 4–5 summarizes common electrolyte imbalances that can occur in a variety of clinical settings.

ACID–BASE BALANCE

The regulation of the hydrogen ion concentration of body fluids is actually the key component of acid–base balance. The pH of a fluid reflects the hydrogen ion concentration of that fluid. The normal pH of arterial blood ranges from 7.35 to 7.45. A solution is either basic or acidic on the basis of the concentration of hydrogen ions in the solution, and the pH scale is used to describe the hydrogen ion concentration. The pH scale is a

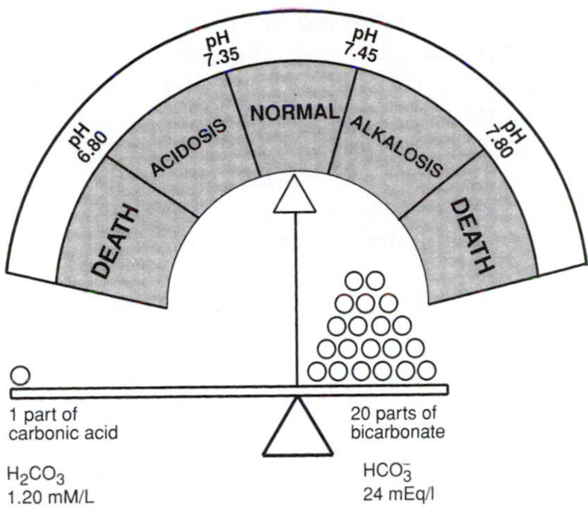

FIG. 4–6. Acid–base scale.

logarithmic scale with values from 0.00 to 14.00. A neutral solution (i.e., neither acidic or basic) has a pH of 7.00 (Lee, 1996).

The inverse proportion of the pH to the concentration of hydrogen ions is reflected in the concept that the higher the pH value, the lower the hydrogen ion concentration. Conversely, the lower the pH value, the higher the hydrogen ion concentration. Therefore, a pH below 7.35 reflects an acidic state, but a pH greater than 7.45 indicates alkalosis and a lower hydrogen ion concentration. A variation from 7.35 to 7.45 of 0.4 in either direction can be fatal. Figure 4–6 shows the pH scale.

Three mechanisms operate to maintain the appropriate pH of the blood:

1. Chemical buffer systems in the ECF and within the cells
2. Removal of carbon dioxide by the lungs
3. Renal regulation of the hydrogen ion concentration

CHEMICAL BUFFER SYSTEMS

The buffer systems are fast-acting defenses that provide immediate protection against changes in the hydrogen ion concentration of the ECF. The buffers also serve as transport mechanisms that carry excess hydrogen ions to the lungs.

A buffer is a substance that reacts to minimize **pH** changes when either acid or base is released into the system. There are three primary buffer systems in the ECF: the hemoglobin system, the plasma protein system, and the bicarbonate system. The capacity of a buffer is limited; therefore, after the components of a buffer system have reacted, they must be replenished before the body can respond to further stress.

The hemoglobin and deoxyhemoglobin found in red blood cells, together with their potassium salts, act as buffer pairs. The electrolyte chloride shifts in and out of the red blood cells according to the level of oxygen in the blood plasma. For each chloride ion that leaves a red blood cell, a bicarbonate ion enters the cell; for each chloride ion that enters a red blood cell, a bicarbonate ion is released.

Plasma proteins are large molecules that contain the acid (or base) and salt form of a buffer. Proteins then have the ability to bind or release hydrogen ions.

The bicarbonate buffer system maintains the blood's pH in the range of 7.35 to 7.45 with a ratio of 20 parts bicarbonate to 1 part carbonic acid by a process that is called hydration of carbon dioxide and is a means of buffering the excess acid in the blood. If a strong acid is added to the body, the ratio is upset. In this acid imbalance, the largest amount of carbon dioxide diffuses in the plasma to the red blood cells; carbon dioxide then combines with plasma protein. Carbon dioxide that is dissolved in the blood combines with water to form carbonic acid (Lee, 1996).

RESPIRATORY REGULATION

In healthy individuals, the lungs form a second line of defense in maintaining the acid–base balance. When carbon dioxide combines with water, H_2CO_3 is formed. Therefore, an increase in the acid carbon dioxide lowers the pH of blood, creating an acidotic state; a decrease in the carbon dioxide level increases the pH, causing the blood to become more alkaline. After H_2CO_3 is formed, it dissociates into carbon dioxide and water. The carbon dioxide is transferred to the lungs, where it diffuses into the alveoli and is eliminated through exhalation. Therefore, the rate of respiration affects the hydrogen ion concentration. An increase in respiratory rate causes carbon dioxide to be blown off by the lungs, resulting in an increase in pH. Conversely, a decrease in respiratory rate causes retention of carbon dioxide and thus a decrease in pH. This means that the lungs can either hold the hydrogen ions until the deficit is corrected or inactivate the hydrogen ions into water molecules to be exhaled with the carbon dioxide as vapor, thereby correcting the excess. It takes from 10 to 30 minutes for the lungs to inactivate the hydrogen molecules by converting them to water molecules (Lee, 1996).

RENAL REGULATION

The kidneys regulate the hydrogen ion concentration by increasing or decreasing the HCO_3 ion concentration in the body fluid by a series of complex chemical reactions that occur in the renal tubules. The regulation of acid–base balance by the kidneys occurs chiefly by increasing or decreasing the HCO_3 ion concentration in body fluids. Hydrogen is secreted into the tubules of the kidney, where it is eliminated in the urine. At the same time, sodium is reabsorbed from the tubular fluid into the ECF in exchange for hydrogen and combines with HCO_3 ions to form the buffer, $NaHCO_3$.

The kidneys help to regulate the extracellular concentration of HCO_3. Two buffer systems help the kidney to eliminate excess hydrogen in the urine: the phosphate buffer system and the ammonia buffer system. With each of these, an excess of hydrogen is secreted and HCO_3 ions are formed; sodium is reabsorbed, thus forming $NaHCO_3$. The time it takes for a change to occur in the acid–base balance can range from a fraction of a second to more than 24 hours. Although the kidneys are the most powerful regulating mechanism, they are slow to make major changes in the acid–base balance (Metheny, 2000).

MAJOR ACID–BASE IMBALANCES

There are two types of acid–base imbalances: (1) metabolic (base bicarbonate deficit and excess) **acidosis** and **alkalosis** and (2) respiratory (carbonic acid deficit and excess) acidosis and alkalosis. The balanced pH of the arterial blood is 7.4, and only small variations of up to 0.05 can exist without causing ill effects. Deviations of more than five times the normal concentration of H^+ in the ECF are potentially fatal (Horne & Derrico, 1999).

METABOLIC ACID–BASE IMBALANCE

NORMAL REFERENCE VALUE: 22 TO 26 mEq/L

METABOLIC ACIDOSIS: BASE BICARBONATE DEFICIT

Metabolic acidosis (HCO_3 deficit) is a clinical disturbance characterized by a low pH and low plasma HCO_3 level. This condition can occur by a gain of hydrogen (H^+) ion or a loss of HCO_3.

Pathophysiology and Etiology

Metabolic acidosis occurs with loss of HCO_3 from diarrhea, draining fistulas, and administration of TPN. Diabetes mellitus, alcoholism, and starvation cause ketoacidosis. Respiratory or circulatory failure, ingestion of certain drugs or toxins (e.g., salicylates, ethylene glycol, or methyl alcohol), some hereditary disorders, and septic shock cause lactic acidosis. It can also result when renal failure results in excessive retention of hydrogen ions.

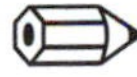 **NOTE:** Hyperkalemia is usually present in clinical cases of acidosis (Metheny, 2000).

Signs and Symptoms

Patients with metabolic acidosis may experience CNS-related symptoms such as headache, confusion, drowsiness, increased respiratory rate, and Kussmaul respirations. Other symptoms include nausea, vomiting, decreased cardiac output, and bradycardia (when serum pH is <7.0).

Diagnostic Tests

- ABG values: pH <7.35, HCO_3 less than 22 mEq/L
- $Paco_2$: <38 mm Hg
- Serum HCO_3: <22 mEq/L
- Serum electrolytes: Elevated potassium possible, because of exchange of intracellular potassium for hydrogen ions in the body's attempt to normalize acid–base environment
- ECG: Dysrhythmias caused by hyperkalemia (Horne & Swearingen, 1993)

Treatment and Management

Patients with metabolic acidosis are treated by (1) reversing the underlying cause (e.g., diabetic ketoacidosis, alcoholism related to ketoacidosis, diarrhea, acute renal failure, renal tubular acidosis, poisoning, or lactic acidosis); (2) eliminating the source (if the cause is caused by excessive administration of sodium chloride); and (3) administering $NaHCO_3$ (7.5% 44.4 mEq/50 mL or 8.4% 50 mEq/50 mL I.V. when pH is equal to or less than 7.2). Concentration depends on severity of acidosis and presence of any serum sodium disorders.

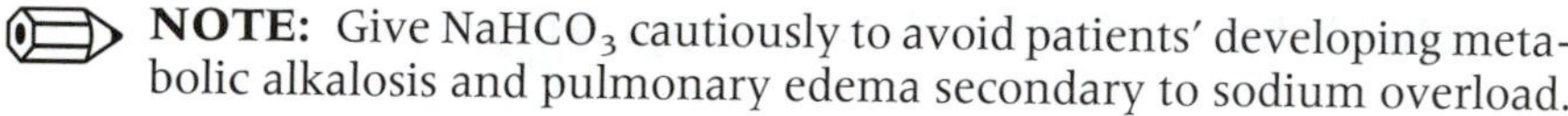

NOTE: Give $NaHCO_3$ cautiously to avoid patients' developing metabolic alkalosis and pulmonary edema secondary to sodium overload.

Potassium replacement: hyperkalemia is usually present, but potassium deficit can occur. If a deficit of less than 3.5 mEq/L is present, the potassium deficit must be corrected before $NaHCO_3$ is administered because the potassium shifts back into the ICF when the acidosis is correct.

Nursing Management

Nursing assessment includes:

1. Obtain a patient history of health problems that relate to metabolic acidosis such as diabetes or renal disease.
2. Obtain baseline vital signs with focus on the respiration and cardiac functioning.
3. Assess for symptoms of metabolic acidosis.
4. Obtain baseline values for ABGs and laboratory tests, note the serum electrolytes, serum CO_2 content, HCO_3 and blood sugar level.

Key nursing interventions include:

1. Providing safety precautions when a patient is confused
2. Monitoring the patient's dietary and fluid intake and output record.

3. Monitoring laboratory results for changes.
4. Monitoring the patient for changes in vital signs, especially changes in respiration, cardiac function, and CNS signs.

METABOLIC ALKALOSIS: BASE BICARBONATE EXCESS

Metabolic alkalosis (i.e., HCO_3 excess) is a clinical disturbance characterized by a high pH and a high plasma HCO_3 concentration and can be produced by a gain of HCO_3 or a loss of hydrogen ion.

Pathophysiology and Etiology

Metabolic alkalosis occurs with GI loss of hydrogen ions from gastric suctioning and vomiting. Renal loss of hydrogen ions occurs from potassium-losing diuretics, excess of mineralocorticoid, hypercalcemia, and hypoparathyroidism. In patients with hypokalemia and carbohydrate refeeding after starvation, hydrogen ions shift from ECF into the cells, depleting serum levels. This also occurs when excessive ingestion of alkalis (e.g., antacids such as Alka-Seltzer), parenteral administration of $NaHCO_3$ during cardiopulmonary resuscitation, and massive blood transfusions increase serum levels of HCO_3.

Signs and Symptoms

Patients with metabolic alkaloses may experience dizziness and depressed respirations in addition to impaired mentation, tingling of fingers and toes, circumoral paresthesia, and hypertonic reflexes. Other symptoms include hypotension, cardiac dysrhythmias, hyperventilation, hypokalemia, and decreased ionized calcium (i.e., carpopedal spasm).

Diagnostic Tests

- ABG values: pH >7.45; HCO_3 >26 mEq/L
- $Paco_2$: >42 mm Hg
- Serum HCO_3: >26 mEq/L
- Serum electrolytes: Low serum potassium (<4 mEq/L) and low serum chloride
- ECG: Assess for dysrhythmias (Horne & Swearingen, 1993)

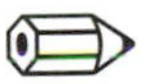 **NOTE:** Hypokalemia is often present in patients with alkalosis.

Treatment and Management

Patients with metabolic alkalosis are treated by (1) reversing the underlying cause; (2) administering sufficient chloride for the kidney to excrete the excess HCO_3; and (3) replacing potassium if a chloride deficit is also present (Horne & Swearingen, 1993).

Nursing Management

Nursing assessment includes:

1. Obtain history of health problems related to metabolic alkalosis (e.g., peptic ulcer, vomiting, adrenocortical hormone abnormalities).
2. Obtain baseline vitals signs.
3. Assess for signs and symptoms of metabolic alkalosis.
4. Obtain baseline values for ABGs and serum electrolyte, serum CO_2 content, and HCO_3.

Key nursing interventions include:

1. Providing safety precautions for hyperexcitability states
2. Monitoring the patient's fluid intake and output
3. Monitoring laboratory results for changes
4. Monitoring the patient for changes in vital signs,with particular attention to respirations and CNS
5. Monitoring for changes in cardiac rhythm, especially in patients taking cardiac glycosides

RESPIRATORY ACID-BASE IMBALANCE

NORMAL REFERENCE VALUE: PARTIAL PRESSURE OF CARBON DIOXIDE ($Paco_2$): 38 TO 42 mm Hg.

RESPIRATORY ACIDOSIS: CARBONIC ACID EXCESS

Respiratory acidosis is caused by inadequate excretion of carbon dioxide and inadequate ventilation, resulting in an increase of serum levels or carbon dioxide and H_2CO_3. Acute respiratory acidosis is usually associated with emergency situations.

Pathophysiology and Etiology

Acute respiratory acidosis can result from pulmonary, neurologic, and cardiac causes, such as pulmonary edema; aspiration of a foreign body; pneumothorax; severe pneumonia; severe, prolonged exacerbation of acute asthma; overdose of sedatives; cardiac arrest; and massive pulmonary embolism.

Chronic respiratory acidosis results from emphysema, bronchial asthma, bronchiectasis, postoperative pain, obesity, and tight abdominal binders.

Signs and Symptoms

Acute signs and symptoms include tachypnea, dyspnea, dizziness, seizures, warm, flushed skin, and ventricular fibrillation. Chronic signs and symptoms occur if $PaCO_2$ exceeds the body's ability to compensate, which include respiratory symptoms.

Diagnostic Tests

- ABG values: *Acute:* pH <7.35, $Paco_2$ >42 mm Hg, HCO_3 >26 mEq/L. *Chronic:* pH <7.35, $Paco_2$ >42 mm Hg, HCO_3 normal or slight increase
- Serum HCO_3: Reflects acid–base balance; initial values normal unless mixed disorder is present
- Serum electrolytes: Usually not altered
- Chest radiography: Determines the presence of underlying pulmonary disease
- Drug screen: Determines the quantity of drug if patient is suspected of taking an overdose

Treatment and Management

Respiratory acidosis is treated by carrying out the following:

1. Improve ventilation.
2. Administer bronchodilators or antibiotics for respiratory infections as indicated.
3. Administer oxygen as indicated.
4. Administer adequate fluids (2 to 3 L/d) to keep mucous membranes moist and help remove secretions.

Nursing Management

Nursing assessment includes:

1. Obtain history of pneumonia, chronic obstructive pulmonary disease (COPD), narcotic use, or emphysema.
2. Obtain baseline vital signs.
3. Assess for signs and symptoms of respiratory acidosis.
4. Obtain baseline values for laboratory tests, especially $Paco_2$.

Key nursing interventions include:

1. Providing safety precautions when a patient is confused
2. Monitoring laboratory results for changes, especially pH and $Paco_2$
3. Monitoring for changes in vital signs
4. Monitoring oxygen and mechanical ventilator when in use
5. Elevating the head of the patient's bed
6. Encouraging the patient to perform deep-breathing exercise
7. Performing chest percussions to break up mucus when appropriate

RESPIRATORY ALKALOSIS: CARBONIC ACID DEFICIT

Respiratory alkalosis is usually caused by hyperventilation, which causes "blowing off" of carbon dioxide and a decrease in H_2CO_3 content. Respiratory alkalosis can be acute or chronic.

Pathophysiology and Etiology

Acute respiratory acidosis results from pulmonary disorders that produce hypoxemia or stimulation of the respiratory centers. Underlying causes of hypoxemia include high fever, pneumonia, congestive heart failure, pulmonary emboli, hypotension, asthma, and inhalation of irritants. Causes of stimulation of respiratory centers include anxiety (most common), excessive mechanical ventilation, CNS lesions involving the respiratory center, and salicylate overdose (an early sign).

Signs and Symptoms

Respiratory alkalosis causes light-headedness, the inability to concentrate, numbness and tingling of the extremities (circumoral paresthesia), tinnitus, palpitations, epigastic pain, blurred vision, precordial pain (tightness), sweating, dry mouth, tremulousness, seizures, and loss of consciousness.

Diagnostic Tests

- ABG values: pH >7.45, Pa_{CO_2} <38 mm Hg, HCO_3 <22 mEq/L
- Serum electrolytes: Presence of metabolic acid–base disorders
- Serum phosphate: May fall to less than 0.5 mg/dL
- ECG: Determines cardiac dysrhythmias

Treatment and Management

Treatment of patients with respiratory alkalosis consists of (1) treating the source of anxiety (instruct patient to breathe slowly into a paper bag); (2) administering a sedative as indicated; and (3) treating the underlying cause (Metheny, 2000).

Nursing Management

Nursing assessment includes:

1. Obtaining a patient history of hysteria, fever, or severe infection.
2. Checking for signs and symptoms of respiratory alkalosis.
3. Obtaining baseline vital signs.
4. Obtaining ABG values.

Key nursing interventions include:

1. Encouraging the patient who is hyperventilating to breathe slowly

2. Have the patient rebreathe expired air by breathing into a paper bag
3. Administering a sedative as directed
4. Listening to the patient who is in emotional distress

Table 4–6 presents a summary of acute acid–base imbalances.

TABLE 4–6

SUMMARY OF ACUTE ACID–BASE IMBALANCES

Acid–Base Imbalance	pH	$Paco_2$	HCO_3	Signs and Symptoms	Causes
Acute metabolic acidosis	↓	↓	↓*	Tachypnea; Kussmaul respirations; hypotension; cold, clammy skin; coma; dysrhythmias	Shock, arrest, ketoacidosis, starvation, acute renal failure, ingestion of acids, diarrhea
Metabolic alkalosis	↑	↑	↑*	Muscular weakness, hyporeflexia, dysrhythmias, apathy, confusion, stupor	Volume depletion, gastric drainage, vomiting, diuretic use, aldosteronism, severe potassium depletion, excessive alkali intake
Respiratory acidosis	↓	↑	No change	Tachycardia, tachypnea, diaphoresis, headache, restlessness, coma, cyanosis, dysrhythmias, hypotension	Acute respiratory failure, drug overdose, chest wall trauma, asphyxiation, CNS trauma, cardiopulmonary disorders, impaired muscle of respiration
Respiratory alkalosis	↑	↓	No change	Paresthesia (fingers), dizziness, lethargy, confusion	Hyperventilation, slixylate poison, hypoxia with pneumonia, pulmonary edema, gram-negative sepsis, CNS lesion, inappropriate mechanical ventilation

*Compensatory response.

NURSING PLAN OF CARE

ELECTROLYTE IMBALANCE

Focus Assessment

Subjective

- History of precipitating illness or disorder
- Complaints of weakness, lethargy, and fatigue
- Use of drugs that may cause problem

Objective

- Serum laboratory values consistent with specific electrolyte imbalance
- Urine specific gravity, pH, and osmolarity consistent with specific electrolyte imbalance
- Neuromuscular, cardiovascular, and neurologic assessment findings consistent with specific electrolyte imbalance

Patient Outcome Criteria

Patient Will:

- Be mobile without evidence of weakness, pain, or fractures.
- Have an adequate cardiac output, blood pressure with normal range, absence of clinical signs of heart failure and cardiac dysrhythmias.
- Exhibit voiding pattern and urine characteristics with normal range.
- Have no injury caused by neuromuscular or sensory alterations.
- Have an effective breathing pattern with normal depth and rate.

Nursing Diagnoses

- Sensory perceptual alterations secondary to hyponatremia
- Altered health maintenance related to poor dietary habits or perceptual or cognitive impairment
- Constipation related to weakened peristalsis
- Fluid volume deficit related to failure of the regulatory mechanism
- Impaired physical mobility related to activity intolerance, decreased strength and endurance, pain, discomfort, neuromuscular impairment, or musculoskeletal impairment related to electrolyte imbalance
- Ineffective breathing pattern related to biochemical imbalances
- Altered comfort related to injuring agent (e.g., stones associated with excessive calcium)
- Risk for injury related to confusion, altered thought processes resulting from: (1) electrolyte imbalance, tetany, and seizures; (2) severe hypocalcemia or sensory changes; (3) hypercalcemia; or (4) severe hypokalemia, hypocalcemia, or hypophosphatemia

(continued)

(continued)

- Impaired gas exchange related to altered oxygen resulting from laryngeal spasm in patients with severe hypokalemia, hyperkalemia, hypocalcemia, or hypophosphatemia
- Altered urinary elimination pattern related to changes in renal function resulting from hypercalcemia
- Risk for impaired verbal communication related to confusion, lethargy, or electrolyte imbalance

Nursing Management

1. Consult with physician if the signs and symptoms of fluid or electrolyte imbalance persist or clinically worsen.
2. Monitor for abnormalities in serum electrolytes as indicated.
3. Monitor ECG for dysrhythmias.
4. Monitor patient response to electrolyte replacement therapy.
5. Administer supplemental electrolytes as indicated.
6. Monitor for loss of electrolyte-rich body fluids, such as nasogastric suctioning, ileostomy drainage, diarrhea, wound drainage, or diaphoresis.
7. Closely monitor serum potassium levels in patients taking diuretics with digoxin.
8. Monitor for side effects of prescribed electrolyte supplements.
9. Obtain ordered specimens for laboratory analysis of serum and urine electrolytes and ABGs as indicated.
10. Maintain I.V. solution containing electrolytes at a constant flow rate.
11. Provide a safe environment for patients with neurologic and neuromuscular manifestations of electrolyte imbalances.
12. Maintain accurate intake and output.
13. Maintain patent I.V. line.

Source: Sparks & Taylor, 1998.

PATIENT EDUCATION

- Provide written material and verbal instructions regarding any medications.
- Review indicators of digitalis toxicity, if appropriate.
- Provide information on dietary sources of electrolytes in deficit situations when appropriate.
- Educate regarding salt substitutes, potassium-sparing diuretics, and other predisposing drugs.
- Provide information on over-the-counter medications (e.g., magnesium and aluminum hydroxide, antacids and phosphorus-binding antacids, laxatives, multivitamin and mineral supplements) when appropriate.
- Educate the patient with cancer about symptoms of hypercalcemia.
- Educate the patient about appropriate use of laxatives if deficit is caused by abuse.
- Educate the patient on the high phosphorus content of processed foods, carbonated beverages, and over-the-counter medications when appropriate.

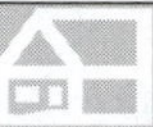

HOME CARE ISSUES

Patients disease states that might require home electrolyte replacement therapy include:

- Cardiopulmonary disorders: potassium relplacement.
- Gastrointestinal disorder: intractable diarrhea, hyperemesis gravidarum
- Patients receiving chemotherapy
- Electrolyte replacement therapies usually last from 1 to 7 days. The electrolytes are provided through a peripheral indwelling venous access device unless a long-term access device is available.
- Assess patients taking oral electrolyte supplements for compliance.

KEY POINTS

✓ The seven major electrolytes and their symbols are:

CATIONS:

- Sodium: Na^+
- Potassium: K^+
- Calcium: Ca^{++}
- Magnesium: Mg^{++}

ANIONS:

- Chloride: Cl^-
- Phosphate: HPO_4^-
- Bicarbonate: HCO_3^-
- The prefix hypo: deficit in an electrolyte
- The prefix hyper: excess in an electrolyte

✓ Key nursing interventions for electrolyte imbalances:

- Monitor laboratory values
- Frequent assessments of neurologic, cardiovascular respiratory, GI, integumentary status; special senses; body weight; and vital signs
- Monitor ECG
- Monitor for phlebitis
- Monitor for symptoms of fluid overload
- Accurate intake and output
- Safety precautions when the patient is confused
- Patients taking digitalis need to be monitored carefully for digoxin toxicity
- Monitor arterial blood gases when appropriate

✓ Key laboratory values that the nurse must recognize:

- Potassium K^+ 3.5 to 5.5 mEq/L
- Calcium: Na^+ 135 to 145 mEq/L
- Magnesium (Mg^{++}) 1.5 to 2.5 mEq/L
- Phosphate (HPO_4^-) 3.0 to 4.5 mg/dL
- Chloride (Cl^-) 95 to 108 mEq/L

✓ Critical guidelines for infusion potassium include:

- Never give potassium I.V. push.
- Concentrations of potassium greater than 60 mEq should not be given in a peripheral vein.
- Concentrations greater than 8 mEq/100 mL can cause pain and irritation of peripheral veins, leading to phlebitis.
- Do not add potassium to a hanging container.
- Administer potassium at a rate not exceeding 10 mEq/h through peripheral veins.
- Calcium and phosphate have a reciprocal relationship: when one is elevated, the other is decreased.
- Patients with calcium imbalances may need seizure precautions.
- Monitor for calcemia in patients receiving massive transfusions of citrated blood.
- Trousseau's sign and Chvostek's sign are specific for calcium deficit.
- Patients with calcium excess (i.e., hypercalcemia) need to be treated with saline diuresis and may need hemodialysis.
- The most dangerous symptom of hypocalcemia is laryngospasm.
- The four major acid–base imbalances in the body are respiratory acidosis (carbonic acid excess), respiratory alkalosis (carbonic acid deficit), metabolic acidosis (base bicarbonate deficit), and metabolic alkalosis (bicarbonate excess).
- Acid–base balance is maintained through three major reaction-specific buffer systems that regulate hydrogen ion concentration: the carbonic acid-bicarbonate system, the phosphate buffer system, and the protein buffer system.

CHAPTER ACTIVITIES

COMPETENCY CRITERIA: Patient Assessment of Electrolyte Balance
COMPETENCY STATEMENT: Competent I.V. therapy nurses will be able to monitor patients for signs and symptoms of electrolyte imbalances.
Note: The cognitive (knowledge) information that is embedded within this performance-based competency includes assessment of fluid balance, principles of fluid balance, movement of electrolytes between extracellular and intracellular compartments, function of electrolytes, treatment of electrolyte imbalance, and interpretation of laboratory data.
This competency *links* to the competencies assessment of fluid balance and delivery of parenteral fluids.

Performance	Skilled	Needs Education
Critical Action Statements		
1. Performs physical assessment directed at identifying electrolyte abnormalities A. Sodium Skin turgor Mentation B. Potassium Recognize abnormalities in ECG tracing Deep tendon reflexes C. Calcium Trousseau's sign Chvostek's sign Deep tendon reflexes Mentation D. Magnesium Chvostek's sign Trousseau's sign Circulation, motion, and sensation of extremities Mentation E. Phosphorus Mentation Deep tendon reflex F. Chloride Deep tendon reflexes Respirations		
2. Demonstrates recording of data on appropriate documentation form Physical assessment Graphics		

EVALUATION CRITERIA

1. Validation of assessment skills performed at bedside with preceptor or in simulation laboratory on partner.
2. Observation and review of documentation.
3. Implementation of appropriate nursing interventions (i.e., seizure precautions, fall precautions, notification of physician) when applicable.

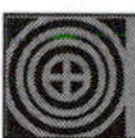

CRITICAL THINKING ACTIVITY

1. Identify the patients in your work environment who are potentially at risk for hypokalemia.

2. Review the chemistry laboratory report on one patient. Write down the patient's values and compare these values with normal laboratory values. Did you identify any electrolyte imbalances?

3. Discuss in a group why patients who have nasogastric tubes to suction are at risk for metabolic alkalosis. Develop a care plan for the patient.

4. A 50-year-old woman with chronic glomerulonephritis took Maalox to alleviate gastric discomfort. She is admitted to your unit with lethargy and difficulty in breathing. Her serum magnesium level was found to be 7.8 mEq/L. Hemodialysis was initiated. Magnesium-containing medications are contraindicated in patients with acute or chronic renal disease. What other medications should be discussed in patient education to prevent this complication?

POST-TEST

Match the signs and symptoms in Column I to the clinical manifestation in Column II.

COLUMN I	COLUMN II
1. CNS depression, drowsiness, lethargy	**a.** Hypomagnesemia
2. Hyperirritability, tremors, increased tendon reflexes	**b.** Hypermagnesemia
3. Carpopedal spasm, laryngeal spasm, convulsions	**c.** Hypocalcemia
4. Bone tumors, prolonged immobilization, increased PTH secretion	**d.** Hypercalcemia
5. Fatigue, headache, apprehension, serum Na^+ 115	**e.** Hypernatremia
6. Serum Na^+ 150, urine Na^+ <40 mEq/L, urine specific gravity >1.125	**f.** Hyponatremia
7. ECG with flat or inverted T wave, depressed ST segment	**g.** Hypokalemia
8. ECG with peaked, narrow T wave, shortened QT interval, prolonged PR interval followed by disappearance of P wave	**h.** Hyperkalemia

9. Treatment for a patient with metabolic alkalosis includes:
- **a.** Removal of underlying cause
- **b.** I.V. fluid administration with NaCl
- **c.** Replacement of potassium deficit
- **d.** All of the above

10. To correct metabolic acidosis, the parenteral fluid of choice is:
- **a.** $NaHCO_3$
- **b.** NaCl
- **c.** Albumin
- **d.** 5 percent dextrose in water

11. The pH range of arterial blood is:
- **a.** 7.25–7.35
- **b.** 7.35–7.45
- **c.** 7.45–7.55
- **d.** 7.56–8.05

12. A nursing diagnosis that would be appropriate for the patient with calcium deficit would be:
- **a.** Ineffective breathing pattern related to biochemical imbalances
- **b.** Altered comfort related to injuring agent
- **c.** Risk for injury related to electrolyte imbalance, tetany, and seizures
- **d.** Altered urinary elimination pattern related to changes in renal function

REFERENCES

Horne, C., & Derrico, D. (1999). Mastering ABGs. *American Journal of Nursing*, 99(8),26–33.

Lee, C.A., Barrett, C.A., & Ignatavicius, D. (1996). *Fluids and Electrolytes* (4th ed.). Philadelphia: F.A. Davis Co.

Metheny, N.M. (2000). Fluids and Electrolyte Balance. In *Nursing Considerations* (4th ed.). Philadelphia: Lippincott-Williams & Wilkins.

National Student Nurses'Association (1997). Specific electrolyte imbalances. In McEntee, M.A., & Gil, G.M. (eds.): *Fluids and Electrolytes*. Albany, NY: Delmar Publishers, pp. 36–70.

Phillips, L.D., & Kuhn, M. (1999). *Manual of IV Medications* (2nd ed.). Philadelphia: J.B. Lippincott.

Sparks, S.M., & Taylor, C.M. (1998). *Nursing Diagnosis Reference Manual* (4th ed.). Springhouse, PA: Springhouse Corporation.

Weldy, N.J. (1996). *Body Fluids and Electrolytes. A Programmed Presentation* (7th ed.). St. Louis: Mosby, pp. 83–119, 127.

ANSWERS TO CHAPTER 4

Pre-Test

1. b, **2.** c, **3.** c, **4.** d, **5.** b, **6.** a, **7.** b, **8.** a, **9.** a, **10.** b

Post-Test

1. b, **2.** a, **3.** c, **4.** d, **5.** f, **6.** e, **7.** g, **8.** h, **9.** d, **10.** a, **11.** b, **12.** c

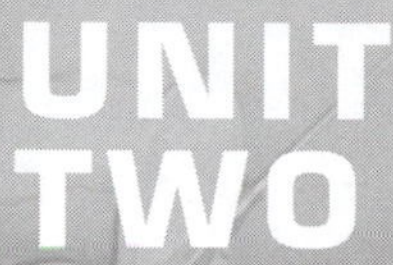

Basic Infusion Practice

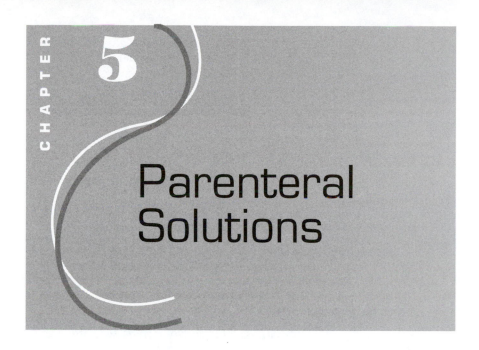

CHAPTER 5

Parenteral Solutions

Let the patient's taste decide. You will say that, in cases of great thirst, the patient's craving decides that it will drink a great deal of tea, and that you cannot help it. But in these cases be sure that the patient requires diluents for quite other purposes than quenching the thirst; he wants a great deal of some drink, not only of tea, and the doctor will order what he is to have, barley water or lemonade, or soda water and milk, as the case may be.

Florence Nightingale, 1859

CHAPTER CONTENTS

LEARNING OBJECTIVES

Upon completion of this chapter, the reader will be able to:

1. Define terminology related to parenteral solutions.
2. Identify the three objectives of parenteral therapy.
3. List the key elements in intravenous (I.V.) solutions.
4. List the uses of maintenance fluids.
5. List the four functions of glucose as a necessary nutrient when administered parenterally.
6. Explain the roles of vitamin C and vitamin B complex in maintenance therapy.
7. Describe the uses of hypotonic, isotonic, and hypertonic fluids.
8. Identify the major groupings of I.V. solutions.
9. Compare the advantages and disadvantages of dextrose, sodium chloride, hydrating fluids, and multiple electrolyte fluids.
10. Identify the main role of hydrating fluids.
11. Compare the properties of a crystalloid with those of a colloid solution.
12. Identify the use of alkalinizing and acidifying fluids.
13. State the most commonly used hypotonic multiple electrolyte solution.
14. State the most commonly used isotonic multiple electrolyte fluid.
15. State the use of albumin, hetastarch, and dextran.

GLOSSARY

Balanced solution Parenteral solution that contains portions of electrolytes similar to plasma; also contains bicarbonate or acetate ion

Catabolism The breakdown of chemical compounds by the body; an energy-producing metabolic process

Colloid A substance (e.g., blood, plasma, albumin, dextran) that does not dissolve into a true solution and is not capable of passing through a semipermeable membrane

Crystalloid A substance that forms a true solution and is capable of passing through a semipermeable membrane (e.g., lactated Ringer's solution, isotonic saline)

Dehydration A deficit of body water; can involve one fluid compartment or all three

Hydrating fluid A solution of water, carbohydrate, sodium, and chloride used to determine adequacy of renal function

Hypotonic solution A solution with an osmolarity lower than that of plasma

Hypertonic solution A solution with an osmolarity higher than that of the plasma

Isotonic solution A solution with the same osmolarity of plasma

Maintenance therapy Fluids that provide all nutrients necessary to meet daily patient requirements

Normal saline Solution of salt (0.9% sodium chloride)

Plasma substitute A solution of a synthetic substance, such as dextran, used as a substitute for plasma

Replacement therapy Replenishment of losses when maintenance cannot be met and when patient is in a deficit state

Restoration therapy Reconstruction of fluid and electrolyte needs on a continuing basis until homeostasis returns

PRE-TEST

1. Hypotonic solutions are used to:
   a. Hydrate cells
   b. Increase vascular space
   c. Supply sodium and chloride in deficit states
2. The expected outcome of administering a hypertonic solution is to:
   a. Shift ECF from intracellular space to plasma
   b. Hydrate cells
   c. Supply free water to vascular space
3. What is(are) the function(s) of parenteral glucose?
   a. Improve hepatic function
   b. Supply necessary calories for energy
   c. Spare body protein
   d. Minimize ketosis
   e. All of the above
4. What is the role of vitamin C in parenteral therapy?
   a. Increase the tensile strength of collagen
   b. Protect cells against oxidation
   c. Promote wound healing
   d. Help with metabolism of carbohydrates
5. What is the main role of a hydrating solution?
   a. Check kidney function
   b. Expand the ECF compartment
   c. Hydrate the cells
   d. Supply sodium and chloride in deficit states
6. What is the most commonly used multiple electrolyte solution?
   a. 5% dextrose in water
   b. 0.9% sodium chloride
   c. Lactated Ringer's solution
   d. 5% dextrose and sodium chloride
7. What is the most common complication of dextran administration?
   a. Fluid overload
   b. Hypersensitivity reactions
   c. Hyponatremia
   d. Hyperkalemia
8. What is the purpose of a colloid solution?
   a. Expand the interstitial compartment
   b. Replace electrolytes
   c. Expand the intravascular compartment
   d. Correct acidosis
9. How many grams of dextrose are in 1000 mL of 5% dextrose in water?
   a. 25
   b. 50
   c. 75
   d. 100

10. Dextrose and hypotonic sodium chloride solutions are considered hydrating fluids because:

a. They provide more water than is required for excretion of sodium.
b. The water they provide equals that needed for excretion of sodium.
c. They maximize retention of potassium in the cell.
d. They maximize the retention of sodium.

● ● ●

In the mid-1950s fewer than 20 percent of hospital patients received I.V. therapy. At that time, I.V. solutions were used primarily during surgery and for the treatment of patients with dehydration. Solutions for surgical patients were infused over 3- to 4-hour periods and discontinued at night. The only solutions available were 5 percent dextrose in water and 5 percent dextrose and 0.9 percent sodium chloride. Today, more than 90 percent of hospitalized patients receive I.V. therapy with more than 200 different types of parenteral solutions.

RATIONALES AND OBJECTIVES OF PARENTERAL THERAPY

To understand the use of parenteral solutions the nurse must understand two important concepts: (1) the rationale for the physician's order of I.V. therapy and (2) the type of solution ordered and the composition and clinical use of that solution.

Objectives or rationales for administration of I.V. therapy fall into three broad categories:

1. Maintenance therapy for daily body fluid requirements
2. Replacement therapy for present losses
3. Restoration therapy for concurrent or continuing losses.

These three objectives differ in the time necessary to complete the therapy, the purpose of the I.V. fluid, and the type of patient who is to receive the I.V. solution. Factors affecting the choice of objective in prescribing parenteral fluid and the rate of administration by the physician are the patient's renal function, daily maintenance requirements, existing fluid and electrolyte imbalance, clinical status, and disturbances in homeostasis as a result of parenteral therapy (Metheny, 2000).

MAINTENANCE THERAPY

Water has the priority in maintenance therapy. The body needs water to replace insensible loss, which can occur as perspiration from the skin and moisture from respirations. The average adult loses 500 to 1000 mL of water over 24 hours through insensible loss. Water is also an important dilutor for waste products excreted by the kidneys. Approximately 30 mL of fluid is needed per kilogram of body weight (i.e., 15 mL/kg) for maintenance needs (Metheny, 2000). In addition, an individual's fluid requirements are based on age, height, weight, and amount of body fat.

Maintenance therapy provides nutrients that meet the daily needs of a patient for water, electrolytes, and dextrose. Water has priority. The typical patient profile for maintenance therapy is one who is allowed nothing by mouth (NPO) or has restricted oral intake for any reason

(O'Shea, 1993). Remember that insensible loss is approximately 500 to 1000 mL every 24 hour. Maintenance therapy should be 1500 mL per square meter (m^2) of body surface over 24 hours (Metheny, 2000). For example, a man weighing 85 kg (187 lb) has a body surface area of 2 (m^2); 1500 times 2 equal 3000; therefore, he needs 3000 mL of fluids for maintenance therapy.

Balanced solutions for maintenance therapy include water, daily needs of sodium and potassium, and glucose. Glucose, a necessary component in maintenance therapy, is converted to glycogen by the liver. It has four main uses in parenteral therapy:

1. Improves hepatic function.
2. Supplies necessary calories for energy
3. Spares body protein
4. Minimizes ketosis

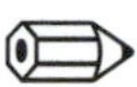

NOTE: The basic caloric requirement for an adult is 1600 calories/d for a 70-kg adult at rest. Approximately 100 to 150 g of carbohydrates are needed daily to minimize protein catabolism and prevent starvation. In 1 L of 5 percent dextrose in water, there are 50 g of dextrose (Metheny, 2000).

Hospitalized patients receiving additional saline or glucose infusions are prone to developing potassium deficiency. Hospitalized patients are usually under stress. Excretion of potassium in their urine can increase to 60 to 120 mEq/d even with limited intake. Tissue injury significantly increases the loss of potassium. Normal dietary intake of potassium is 80 to 200 mEq/d.

Vitamins are necessary for utilization of other nutrients. Vitamin C and vitamin B complex are used frequently in parenteral therapy, especially in postoperative patients. Vitamin C promotes wound healing, and vitamin B complex has a role in metabolism of carbohydrates and maintenance of gastrointestinal (GI) function (Weinstein, 1997).

REPLACEMENT THERAPY

Replacement therapy is necessary to meet the fluid, electrolyte, or blood product deficits of patients in acute distress; this type of therapy is supplied over a 48-hour period. Examples of conditions of patients needing replacement infusion therapy (and their replacement requirements) are:

- Hemorrhage (for replacement of cells and plasma)
- Low platelet count (for replacement of clotting factors)
- Vomiting and diarrhea (for replacement of losses of electrolytes and water)
- Starvation (for replacement of losses of water and electrolytes)
- When the maintenance of body requirements cannot be met, the physician should institute replacement therapy. The physician

must figure the losses and calculate replacement over a 48-hour period. Kidney function is the first thing that should be checked before replacement therapy is begun. Patients requiring replacement therapy, except those in shock, require potassium. Patients under stress from tissue injury, wound infection, or gastric or bowel surgery also require potassium. Potassium 20 mEq/L achieves adequate replacement (Metheny, 2000).

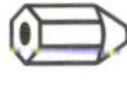

NOTE: Because it can create a life-threatening situation, never give more than 120 mEq of potassium in 24 hours unless cardiac status is monitored continuously.

Carefully monitor balanced solutions with potassium for the following patients:

1. Those with dysfunction of the:
   - Renal system
   - Cardiovascular system
   - Adrenal glands
   - Pituitary gland
   - Parathyroid gland
2. Those with deficits of:
   - Sodium
   - Calcium
   - Base bicarbonate
   - Blood volume (hypovolemic)
3. Those with excess of:
   - Base bicarbonate
   - Extracellular potassium
   - Extracellular calcium

NOTE: Key nursing assessment: Check kidney function before administering potassium in replacement therapy.

RESTORATION THERAPY

Restoration therapy for concurrent losses is achieved on an ongoing daily basis. Critical evaluation of concurrent losses of fluid and electrolyte therapy is done at least every 24 hours. Accurate documentation of intake and output is extremely important in this type of management of fluid and electrolyte therapy. Restoration of homeostasis depends on the nursing assessment of intake of I.V. fluids as well as on the documentation of all body fluid losses. The types of clinical patients who require 24-hour evaluation are those with draining fistulas, abscesses, nasogastric tubes, burns, and abdominal wounds.

The fluid and electrolyte management of these patients cannot be completed in 48 hours. Therefore, maintenance therapy and replacement therapy do not meet these patients' needs. A day-by-day restoration of vital fluids and electrolytes is necessary. With these types of patients, you will see frequent changes in the types of solutions ordered, in the amount of electrolytes ordered based on laboratory values ordered, and in the rate of infusion.

The type of restoration fluid ordered depends on the type of fluid that is being lost. For example, excessive loss of gastric fluid must be replaced by solutions resembling that fluid; with nasogastric suctioning, chloride, potassium, and sodium are lost continually. Restoration of electrolyte imbalance is imperative for proper homeostatic management therapy. Rather than waiting to make daily rounds to evaluate the 24-hour totals and change infusion orders, physicians are ordering multiple electrolyte solutions to be used as a replacement solution through the main infusion system on an ongoing basis. This replacement need is reevaluated every 1 to 8 hours. Table 5–1 presents an example of how restoration fluids are ordered and administered. Restoration of fluids and electrolytes is challenging for nurses. One must be on time and accurate so as not to overload.

TABLE 5–1

ADMINISTRATION OF RESTORATION FLUIDS

The physician orders 1000 mL of 5 percent dextrose/0.45 percent sodium chloride every 8 hours as a primary solution. A multiple electrolyte solution, such as lactated Ringer's solution, is ordered in addition to the primary solution to replace nasogastric output milliliter for milliliter over 4 hours. The primary I.V. solution is continuously infused at 125 mL/h. If the nasogastric suction container is emptied of 400 mL of gastric secretions, the nurse will need to infuse 400 mL of lactated Ringer's solution over the next 4 hours, or 100 mL/h. (See sample schedule below.) The primary solution (5 percent dextrose/0.5 percent sodium chloride) will infuse at 125 mL, and the lactated Ringer's solution will infuse at 100 mL/h for a total of 225 mL/h. The nurse will then empty the nasogastric suction container 4 hours later and recalculate the replacement solution.

Time	8 AM	9 AM	10 AM	11 AM	12 noon	1 PM
Gastric suction, mL	400				300	
Primary fluids, mL	125	125	125	125	125	125
Restoration fluids (lactated Ringer's solution), mL	100	100	100	100	75	75
Total, mL	225	225	225	250	200	200

KEY ELEMENTS IN PARENTERAL SOLUTIONS

The key elements that make up parenteral fluids include water, carbohydrates (glucose), protein, vitamins, electrolytes, and pH.

WATER

Normal daily maintenance requirements for water in an adult are roughly 1000 mL/d. These water needs are increased in patients with sensible water losses such as respiratory rate above 20, fever, diaphoresis, and in low humidity; in patients with decreased renal concentration ability; and in elderly people. The average adult loses 500 to 1000 mL in the form of insensible water every 24 hours. Water must be provided for adequate kidney function.

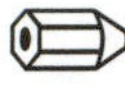 **NOTE:** High humidity, such as that in an incubator, minimizes insensible water loss (Metheny, 2000).

CARBOHYDRATES (GLUCOSE)

Glucose, a nutrient included in maintenance, restoration, and replacement therapies, is converted into glycogen by the liver, which improves hepatic function. By supplying calories for energy, it spares body protein. Sources of carbohydrates include dextrose (glucose) and fructose. When glucose is supplied by infusion, all the parenteral glucose is bioavailable.

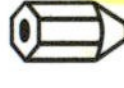 **NOTE:** The addition of 100 g of glucose per day minimizes starvation. Every 2 L of 5 percent dextrose in water contains 100 g of glucose (Weinstein, 1997).

AMINO ACIDS

Amino acids (protein) are the body-building nutrients whose major function is contributing to tissue growth and repair, replacing body cells, healing wounds, and synthesizing vitamins and enzymes. Amino acids are the basic units of protein. Current parenteral proteins are elemental, provided as synthetic crystalline amino acids. These proteins are available in concentrations of 3.5 to 15 percent and are used in total parenteral nutrition (TPN) centrally or peripherally. When administered by infusion, protein bypasses the GI and portal circulation (Metheny, 2000).

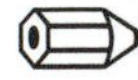 **NOTE:** The usual daily requirement is 1 g protein/kg of body weight. For example, a 54-kg woman needs 54 g of protein per day.

VITAMINS

Vitamins are added to restorative and replacement therapies. Certain vitamins (i.e., the fat-soluble A, D, E, and K and water-soluble B and C vitamins) are necessary for growth and act as catalysts for metabolic processes. Some disease conditions alter vitamin requirements (Metheny, 1996). Vitamins B and C are the most frequently used in parenteral therapy. Vitamin B complex is important in the metabolism of carbohydrates and the maintenance of GI function, which is especially important in postoperative patients. Vitamin C promotes wound healing.

ELECTROLYTES

Electrolytes are the major additives to replacement and restorative therapies. The correction of electrolyte imbalances is important in the prevention of serious complications associated with excess or deficit of electrolytes. There are seven major electrolytes contained in normal body fluids and seven major elements supplied in manufactured I.V. solutions. (Chapter 4 reviews these electrolyte functions.) The electrolytes of major importance in parenteral therapy are potassium, sodium, chloride, magnesium, phosphorus, calcium, and bicarbonate or acetate ion (important for acid–base balance).

pH

The pH reflects the degree of acidity or alkalinity of a solution. Blood pH is not a significant problem for routine parenteral therapy. Normal kidneys can achieve an acid–base balance as long as enough water is supplied. The USP standards require that solution pH must be slightly acidic (between a pH of 3.5 and 6.2). Many solutions have a pH of 5. The acidity of solutions allows them to have a longer shelf life (Weinstein, 1997).

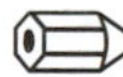

NOTE: As the acidity of a solution increases, the solution's ability to irritate vein walls increases.

OSMOLARITY OF PARENTERAL SOLUTIONS

The choice of I.V. solution depends on the amount of solutes in the solution and the osmolarity of the infusate. The effect of I.V. fluid on the body fluid compartments depends on how its osmolarity compares with the patient's serum osmolarity. I.V. fluids can change the fluid compartment in one of three ways:

1. Expand the intravascular compartment

2. Expand the intravascular compartment and deplete the intracellular and interstitial compartments
3. Expand the intracellular compartment and deplete the intravascular compartment

I.V. fluids are hypotonic, isotonic, or hypertonic, depending on the amount of solutes in the solution.

HYPOTONIC FLUIDS

Hypotonic fluids have an osmolarity below 250 mOsm/L. By lowering serum osmolarity, the body fluids shift out of blood vessels into cells and interstitial spaces. **Hypotonic solutions** hydrate cells and can deplete the circulatory system. Water moves from the vascular space to the intracellular space when hypotonic fluids are infused.

Examples: 0.45 percent sodium chloride, mOsm/L = 154
Use: To hydrate cells and lower serum sodium levels
Caution: Hypotonic fluids cause depletion of the circulatory system

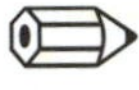

NOTE: Do not give hypotonic solutions to patients with low blood pressure because it will further a hypotensive state.

ISOTONIC FLUIDS

Isotonic solutions have an osmolarity of 250 to 375 mOsm/L. They are used to expand the extracellular fluid (ECF) compartment. Many isotonic solutions are available.

Examples: 0.9 percent sodium chloride, 5 percent dextrose in water, lactated Ringer's solution
Use: To expand the intravascular compartment
Caution: The danger with the use of isotonic solutions is circulatory overload. These solutions do not cause fluid shifts into other compartments.
The problem with overexpanding the vascular compartment is that the fluid dilutes the concentration of hemoglobin and lowers hematocrit levels.

HYPERTONIC FLUIDS

Hypertonic fluids have an osmolarity of 375 mOsm/L or higher. These fluids are used to replace electrolytes. When hypertonic dextrose solutions are used alone, they also are used to shift ECF from the interstitial fluid to the plasma.

Examples: Five percent dextrose and 0.9 percent sodium chloride, 5 percent dextrose and lactated Ringer's solution, 10 percent dextrose in water, 20 percent dextrose in water

Use: To replace electrolytes and to shift fluid from interstitial space to plasma
Caution: **Hypertonic solutions** are irritating to vein walls and may cause hypertonic circulatory overload

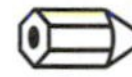

NOTE: Give hypertonic solutions slowly to prevent circulatory overload (Kuhn, 1999).

TYPES OF PARENTERAL SOLUTIONS

CRYSTALLOID SOLUTIONS

Crystalloids are materials capable of crystallization (i.e., have the ability to form crystals). Crystalloids are solutes that, when placed in a solution, mix with and dissolve into a solution and cannot be distinguished from the resultant solution. Because of this, crystalloid solutions are considered true solutions that are capable of diffusing through membranes (Josephson, 1999). The vascular fluid is 25 percent of the ECF, and 25 percent of any crystalloid administered remains in the vascular space. Crystalloids must be given in three to four times the volume to expand the vascular space equal to a **colloid** solution. Types of crystalloid solutions include dextrose solutions, sodium chloride solutions, multiple electrolyte solutions, and alkalizing and acidifying solutions.

Dextrose Solutions

Dextrose in water. Carbohydrates can be administered by the parenteral route as dextrose, fructose, or invert sugar. Dextrose is the most commonly administered carbohydrate. The percentage solutions express the number of grams of solute per 100 g of solvent. A 5 percent dextrose in water (D5W) infusion contains 5 g of dextrose in 100 mL of water (Josephson, 1999).

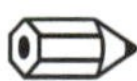

NOTE: One mL of water weighs 1 g, and 1 mL is 1 percent of 100 mL. Milliliters, grams, and percentages can be used interchangeably when calculating solution strength. Thus, 5 percent dextrose in water equals 5 g dextrose in 100 mL, and 1 L of 5 percent dextrose in water contains 50 g of dextrose (Weinstein, 1997). Example: 250 mL of a 20 percent dextrose in water solution contains 50 g of dextrose.

Approximately 1600 calories are needed daily for an adult at bed rest; this is a basal figure and does not allow for fever or other causes of increased metabolism (Metheny, 1996). When carbohydrate needs are inadequate, the body will use its own fat to supply calories. Dextrose fluids are used to provide calories for energy, reduce catabolism of protein, and reduce protein breakdown of glucose to help prevent a negative nitrogen balance (Weinstein, 1997).

The monohydrate form of dextrose used in parenteral solutions provides 3.4 kcal/g. It is difficult to administer enough calories by I.V.

infusion, especially with 5 percent dextrose in water, which provides only 170 calories per liter. One would have to administer 9 L to meet calorie requirements, and most patients cannot tolerate 9000 mL of fluid in 24 hours. Concentrated solutions of carbohydrates in 20 to 70 percent dextrose are useful for supplying calories. These solutions containing high percentages of dextrose must be administered slowly for adequate absorption and utilization by the cells (Metheny, 2000).

Dextrose is a nonelectrolyte, and the total number of particles in a dextrose solution does not depend on ionization. Dextrose is thought to be the closest to the ideal carbohydrate available because it is well metabolized by all tissues. The tonicity of dextrose solutions depends on the particles of sugar in the solution. Dextrose 5 percent is rapidly metabolized and has no osmotically active particle after it is in the plasma. The osmolarity of a dextrose solution is determined differently from that of an electrolyte solution. Dextrose is distributed inside and outside the cells, with 8 percent remaining in the circulation to increase blood volume. The USP pH requirements for dextrose is 3.5 to 6.5 (Weinstein, 1997).

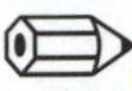 **NOTE:** Hypotonic dextrose solutions hydrate the intracellular compartment more than they hydrate the intravascular space.

The other two types of carbohydrates used for infusions, fructose and invert sugar, have their own specific uses. Fructose is similar to glucose but is less irritating to veins. The important point about fructose is that it can be metabolized by adipose tissue independent of insulin. However, fructose cannot be used if the patient is in acidosis. Invert sugar contains the same equimolar quantities of glucose and fructose, but less invert sugar is lost in the urine (Metheny, 2000).

Advantages

- Acts as a vehicle for administration of medications
- Provides nutrition
- Can be used as treatment for hyperkalemia (using high concentrations of dextrose)
- Can be used in treatment of patients with dehydration
- Provides free water

Disadvantages

- If solutions of 20 to 70 percent dextrose are infused rapidly, they act as an osmotic diuretic and pull interstitial fluid into plasma, causing severe cellular **dehydration.** Any solution of dextrose infused rapidly can place the patient at risk for dehydration. To prevent this adverse reaction, infuse the dextrose solution at the prescribed rate.
- If 20 to 70 percent dextrose is infused too rapidly, it can irritate the vein wall. Rapid infusion of 20 to 70 percent dextrose can also

lead to transient hyperinsulin reaction, in which the pancreas secretes extra insulin to metabolize the infused dextrose. Sudden discontinuation of any hypertonic dextrose solution may leave a temporary excess of insulin.

To prevent hyperinsulinism, infuse an isotonic dextrose solution (5 to 10%) to wean the patient off hypertonic dextrose. The infusion rate should be gradually decreased over 48 hours. When administering dextrose solutions, remember that they do not provide any electrolytes. Dextrose solutions cannot replace or correct electrolyte deficits, and continuous infusion of 5 percent dextrose in water places patients at risk for deficits in sodium, potassium, and chloride. In addition, dextrose cannot be mixed with blood components because it causes hemolysis (i.e., agglomeration) of the cells.

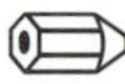

NOTE: Before any medication is added to a dextrose solution, compatibility information should be checked. Dextrose may also affect the stability of admixtures (e.g., ampicillin sodium) (Terry & Hedrick, 1995).

Do not play "catch up" if the solution infusion is behind schedule. Make sure the I.V. solution does not "run away" and infuse rapidly into the patient.

All dextrose solutions are acidic (pH 3.5 to 5.0) and may cause thrombophlebitis. Assess the I.V. site frequently.

Table 5–2 presents the types and contents of available dextrose solutions.

Sodium Chloride Solutions

Sodium Chloride. Sodium chloride injection (0.9%) is an isotonic solution. It is isotonic owing to the higher than normal sodium (Na^+)and chloride (Cl^-) ions. Sodium chloride 0.9 percent solution has 154 mEq of both sodium and chloride or about 9 percent higher than normal plasma levels of sodium and chloride ions without other plasma electrolytes. See Table 5–2 for the types of available sodium chloride solutions.

Advantages

- Provides ECF replacement when chloride loss is greater than or equal to sodium losses (e.g., a patient undergoing nasogastric suctioning)
- Treats patients with metabolic alkalosis in the presence of fluid loss (the 154 mEq of chloride helps compensate for the increase in bicarbonate ions)
- Treats patients with sodium depletion
- Initiates or terminates a blood transfusion (the saline solutions are the only solutions to be used with any blood product)

TABLE 5–2

CONTENTS OF AVAILABLE INTRAVENOUS FLUIDS

Solution	Osmolarity	Dextrose, g/100 mL	pH	Cal/100 mL	Na	Cl	K	Ca	Mg	Acetate	Lactate
			Dextrose in Water (D/W)								
2.5%D/W	Hypotonic	2.5	4.5	8							
5%D/W	Isotonic	5	4.8	17							
10%D/W	Hypertonic	10	4.7	34							
20%D/W	Hypertonic	20	4.8	68							
50%D/W	Hypertonic	50	4.6	170							
70%D/W	Hypertonic	70	4.6	237							
			Sodium Chloride (NaCl)								
0.2%NaCl (1/4 strength)	Hypotonic		4.5		34	34					
0.45% NaCl (1/2 strength)	Hypotonic		5.6		77	77					
0.9% NaCl (full strength)	Isotonic		6.0		154	154					
3% NaCl	Hypertonic		6.0		513	513					
5% NaCl	Hypertonic		6.0		855	855					

			Dextrose and Sodium Chloride (D/NaCl)								
0.2% D and 0.9% NaCl	Isotonic	2.5	4.5	8	154	154					
5% D and 0.2% NaCl	Isotonic	5	4.6	17	34	34					
5% D and 0.45 NaCl	Hypertonic	5	4.6	17	77	77					
5% D and 0.9% NaCl	Hypertonic	5	4.4	17	154	154					
			Multiple Electrolyte Solutions								
Lactated Ringer's solution	Isotonic	6.5			130	109	4	3			28
Ringer's injection	Isotonic	5.5			147	156	4	4			
Normosol-R	Isotonic	6.4		18	140	98	5		3	27	
Plasmalyte-A	Isotonic	5.5			140	98	5		3	27	
Isolyte E	Isotonic	6.0			140	103	10		3	49	

(Continued)

TABLE 5–2

CONTENTS OF AVAILABLE INTRAVENOUS FLUIDS ***(Continued)***

Solution	Osmolarity	Dextrose, g/100 mL	pH	Cal/100 mL	Na	Cl	K	Ca	Mg	Acetate	Lactate
Specialty Solutions											
1/6M sodium lactate	Isotonic (335)	6.5			167						167
10% Mannitol	Hypertonic	5.7									
20% Mannitol	Hypertonic	5.7									
NaHCO3	Isotonic (333)	8.0			595						595
6% Dextran and 0.9% NaCl	Isotonic	5.0			154	154					
10% Dextran and 0.9% NaCl	Isotonic	5.0			154	154					

Ca = Calcium
Cal = Calories
Cl = Chloride
K = Potassium
Mg = Magnesium
Na = Sodium

Disadvantages

- Provides more sodium and chloride than patients need, causing hypernatremia. The adult dietary sodium requirements are 90 to 250 mEq daily. [Three liters of sodium chloride (0.9%) provides a patient with 462 mEq of sodium, a level that exceeds normal tolerance.] To prevent this overload of electrolytes, assess for signs and symptoms of sodium retention.
- Can cause acidosis in patients receiving continuous infusions of 0.9 percent sodium chloride because sodium chloride provides one third more chloride than is present in ECF. The excess chloride leads to loss of bicarbonate ions, leading to an imbalance of acid.
- May cause low potassium levels (i.e., hypokalemia) because of the lack of the other important electrolytes over a period of time.
- Can lead to circulatory overload. Isotonic fluids expand the ECF compartment, which can lead to overload of the cardiovascular compartments.

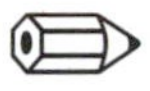

NOTE: During stress, the body retains sodium, adding to hypernatremia.

Hypotonic saline (0.45%) can be used to supply normal daily salt and water requirements safely. Hypertonic saline solution (3 to 5%) is used only to correct severe sodium depletion and water overload (Keithley & Fraulini, 1982).

Hyperosmolar saline (3 or 5% NaCl) can be dangerous when administered incorrectly. Nurses should follow these steps to ensure safe administration of hyperosmolar saline:

- Check serum sodium level before and during administration.
- Administer only in intensive care settings.
- Monitor aggressively for signs of pulmonary edema.
- Only small volumes of hyperosmolar fluids are usually administered.
- Use a volume-controlled devices or electronic infusion pump (NSNA, 1997).

AGE-RELATED CONSIDERATIONS

Be aware of the increased dangers in administering saline solutions to elderly patients, patients with severe dehydration, and patients with chronic glomerulonephritis.

Dextrose Combined with Sodium Chloride

When sodium chloride is infused, the addition of 100 g dextrose prevents formation of ketone bodies. Dextrose prevents **catabolism,** which is the breakdown of chemical compounds by the body. Consequently, there is a loss of potassium and intracellular water (Weinstein, 1997).

Carbohydrates and sodium chloride fluid combinations are best used when there has been an excessive loss of fluid through sweating, vomiting, or gastric suctioning (Kuhn, 1999). See Table 5–2 for types of available dextrose and sodium chloride solutions.

Advantages

- Temporarily treats patients with circulatory insufficiency and shock caused by hypovolemia in the immediate absence of a plasma expander
- Provides early treatment of burns, along with plasma or albumin
- Replaces nutrients and electrolytes
- Acts as a **hydrating solution** to assist in checking kidney function before replacement of potassium

Disadvantages

- Same as for sodium chloride solutions (see earlier section): hypernatremia, acidosis, and circulatory overload.

Hydrating Fluids (Combinations of Dextrose and Hypotonic Sodium Chloride)

Solutions that contain dextrose and hypotonic saline provide more water than is required for excretion of salt and useful as hydrating fluids. Hydrating fluids are used to assess the status of the kidneys. The administration of a hydrating solution at a rate of 8 mL/m^2 of body surface per minute for 45 minutes is called a fluid challenge. When urinary flow is established, it indicates that the kidneys have begun to function; the hydrating solution may then be replaced with a specific electrolyte solution. If the urinary flow is not restored after 45 minutes, the rate of infusion should be reduced and monitoring of the patient should continue without electrolyte additives (especially potassium; Metheny, 1996). Carbohydrates in hydrating solutions reduce the depletion of nitrogen and liver glycogen and are also useful in rehydrating cells.

Hydrating solutions are potassium free. Potassium is essential to the body but can be toxic if the kidneys are not functioning effectively and are therefore unable to excrete the extra potassium (Kuhn, 1999). See Table 5–2 for types of hydrating fluids.

Advantages

- Helps assess the status of the kidneys before replacement therapy is started
- Hydrates patients in dehydrated states
- Promotes diuresis in dehydrated patients (Weinstein, 1997)

Disadvantage

- Requires cautious administration in edematous patients (e.g., patients with cardiac, renal, or liver disease)

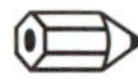

NOTE: Do not give potassium to any patient unless kidney function has been established. Use hydrating fluid to check kidney function.

Multiple Electrolyte Fluids

A variety of balanced electrolyte fluids are available commercially. Balanced fluids are available as hypotonic or isotonic maintenance and replacement solutions. Maintenance fluids approximate normal body electrolyte needs; replacement fluids contain one or more electrolytes in amounts over those found in normal body fluids. Balanced fluids also may contain lactate or acetate (yielding bicarbonate), which helps to combat acidosis and provide a truly "balanced solution." See Table 5–2 for types of multiple electrolyte solution.

Multiple electrolyte fluids are recommended for use in patients with trauma, alimentary tract fluid losses, dehydration, sodium depletion, acidosis, and burns.

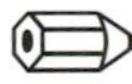

NOTE: Dextrose (5%) is usually added to balanced multiple electrolyte solutions.

Balanced Hypotonic Fluids (Maintenance Fluids)

Hypotonic balanced multiple electrolyte fluids are used for maintaining body homeostasis. These solutions contain 5 percent dextrose for its protein-sparing effect. Dextrose increases the tonicity of these solutions. The balancing of hypotonic electrolytes (lower than within normal body levels) is ideal for maintaining body homeostasis. Balanced solutions contain sodium, potassium, calcium, magnesium, chloride, and lactate. Potassium is usually not added to maintenance multiple electrolyte fluids.

Hypotonic multiple electrolyte fluids are used for (1) routine maintenance;(2) conditions that increase fluid losses through urine, stool, or expired air; and (3) stress leading to inappropriate release of antidiuretic hormone.

Advantage

- Useful for maintaining water. Water maintenance equals 1600 mL/m^2 body surface area per day (Drug and Therapeutic Information, 1970). Because of the hypotonicity of these multiple electrolyte fluids, water should be provided for urinary and metabolic needs to take advantage of the body's homeostatic mechanisms (Weinstein, 1997).

Disadvantages

- Can cause hyperkalemia
- Can cause water intoxication

Balanced Isotonic and Hypertonic Fluids (Replacement Fluids)

Many types of replacement fluids are available. Special fluids are available by each manufacturer for gastric replacement, which provide the typical electrolytes lost by vomiting or gastric suction. These isotonic fluids usually contain ammonium ions, which are metabolized in the liver to hydrogen ions and urea, replacing hydrogen ions lost in gastric juices. Lactated Ringer's injection is considered an isotonic multiple electrolyte solution.

Hypertonic multiple electrolyte solutions are also used as replacement fluids and usually have the addition of 5 percent dextrose, which raises the osmolarity of the solution.

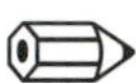 **NOTE:** Do not use gastric replacement fluid in patients with hepatic insufficiency or renal failure.

Advantage

- Isotonic multiple electrolyte solutions are balanced and have an ionic composition similar to that of plasma

Disadvantage

- May cause hypernatremia (3 L of isotonic multiple electrolyte fluid can provide up to 390 mEq of sodium)

Lactate Fluids

The Ringer's solutions (i.e., Ringer's injection and lactated Ringer's injection) are classified as balanced or isotonic solutions because their fluid and electrolyte content are similar to those of plasma. They are used to replace electrolytes at physiologic levels in the ECF compartment.

Ringer's Solution (Injection)

Ringer's injection is a fluid and electrolyte replenisher, which is used over 0.9 percent sodium chloride for treating patients with dehydration after reduced water intake or water loss. Ringer's solution (injection) is similar to **normal saline** (i.e., 0.9% sodium chloride) with the substitution of potassium and calcium for some of the sodium ions in concentrations equal to the plasma. Ringer's injection, however, is superior to 0.9 percent sodium chloride as a fluid and electrolyte replenisher and it is preferred to normal saline treating patients with dehydration after drastically reduced water intake or water loss (e.g., with vomiting, diarrhea, or fistula drainage). This solution has some incompatibilities with medications, so it is necessary to check drug compatibility literature for guidelines.

Ringer's injection does not contain enough potassium or calcium to be used as a maintenance fluid or to correct a deficit of these electrolytes.

Ringer's injection is used for the following:

- Treatment of any type of dehydration
- Restoration of fluid balance before and after surgery
- Replacement of fluids resulting from dehydration, GI losses, and fistula drainage

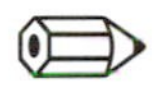

NOTE: Use this solution instead of lactated Ringer's when the patient has liver disease and is unable to metabolize lactate.

Advantages

- Tolerated well in patients who have liver disease
- May be used as blood replacement for a short period of time

Disadvantages

- Provides no calories
- May exacerbate sodium retention, congestive heart failure, and renal insufficiency
- Contraindicated in renal failure

Lactated Ringer's Solution

This solution is also called Hartmann's solution. Lactated Ringer's is the most commonly prescribed solution. This solution has an electrolyte concentration closely resembling that of the ECF compartment. This solution is commonly used to replace fluid loss from burns, bile, and diarrhea. Lactated Ringer's is used for the following:

- Rehydration in all types of dehydration
- Restoration of fluid volume deficits
- Replacement of fluid lost as a result of burns
- Treatment of mild metabolic acidosis
- Treatment of salicylate overdose

This solution has some incompatibilities with medications, so it is necessary to check drug compatibility literature for guidelines.

Advantages

- Contains the bicarbonate precursor to assist in acidosis
- Most similar to body's extracellular electrolyte content

Disadvantages

- Three liters of lactated Ringer's solution contains about 390 mEq of sodium, which can quickly elevate the sodium level in a patient who does not have a sodium deficit (Weinstein, 1997).
- Lactated Ringer's solution should not be used in patients with impaired lactate metabolism, such as those with liver disease, Addison's disease, severe metabolic acidosis or alkalosis, profound hypovolemia, or profound shock or cardiac failure.

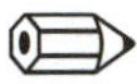

NOTE: In the above conditions, serum lactate levels may already be elevated (Griffith, 1986).

Alkalizing and Acidifying Infusions Fluids

Alkalizing Fluids

Metabolic acidosis can occur in clinical situations in which dehydration, shock, liver disease, starvation, or diabetes causes retention of chlorides, ketone bodies, or organic salts or when excessive bicarbonate is lost. Treatment consists of infusion of an alkalizing fluid. Two I.V. fluids are available when excessive bicarbonate is lost and metabolic acidosis occurs: 1/6 molar isotonic sodium lactate and 5 percent sodium bicarbonate injection. The lactate ion must be oxidized in the body to carbon dioxide before it can affect the acid–base balance. Sodium lactate to bicarbonate requires 1 to 2 hours. Oxygen is needed to increase bicarbonate concentrations. The isotonic solution sodium bicarbonate injection provides bicarbonate ions in clinical situations in which excessive bicarbonate is lost.

Alkalizing fluids are used for vomiting, starvation, uncontrolled diabetes mellitus, acute infections, renal failure, and severe acidosis with severe hyperpnea (sodium bicarbonate injection).

The 1/6 molar sodium lactate solution is useful whenever acidosis has resulted from sodium deficiency; however, it is contraindicated in patients suffering from lack of oxygen and in those with liver disease. Patients receiving this fluid should be watched for signs of hypocalcemic tetany (Weinstein, 1997).

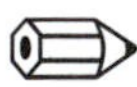

NOTE: Sodium bicarbonate injection is used to relieve dyspnea and hyperpnea; the bicarbonate ion is released in the form of carbon dioxide through the lungs, leaving behind an excess of sodium.

Acidifying Fluids

Metabolic alkalosis is a condition associated with an excess of bicarbonate and deficit of chloride. Isotonic sodium chloride (0.9%) provides conservative treatment of metabolic alkalosis. Ammonium chloride is the solution used to treat metabolic alkalosis. Acidifying fluids are used for severe metabolic alkalosis caused by a loss of gastric secretions or pyloric stenosis.

An advantage is that the ammonium ion is converted by the liver to hydrogen ion and to ammonia, which is excreted as urea. However, a disadvantage is that ammonium chloride must be infused at a slow rate to enable the liver to metabolize the ammonium ion. In fact, rapid infusion can result in toxicity, causing irregular breathing and bradycardia.

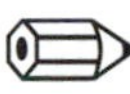
NOTE: Ammonium chloride must be used with caution in patients with severe hepatic disease or renal failure and is contraindicated in any condition with a high ammonium level.

Potassium Chloride Solutions

Several premixed solutions of potassium chloride (KCl) are available from the manufacturer. Potassium 20 or 40 mEq is added to 5 percent dextrose in water or 5 percent dextrose and 0.45 percent sodium chloride. Follow special nursing considerations in administration of I.V. potassium chloride. Chapter 4 provides more information about potassium chloride, including the critical guidelines for the administration of potassium chloride fluids.

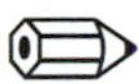
NOTE: As packaged from the manufacturer, potassium has a clear red label to distinguish it from I.V. solutions without additives.

COLLOID SOLUTIONS

Patients with fluid and electrolyte disturbances occasionally require treatment with colloids. Colloid solutions contain protein or starch molecules that remain distributed in the extracellular space and do not form a "true" solution. When colloid molecules are administered, they remain in the vascular space for several days in patients with normal capillary endothelia. These fluids increase the osmotic pressure within the plasma space, drawing fluid to increase intravascular volume.

Colloid solutions do not dissolve and do not flow freely between fluid compartments. Infusion of a colloid solution increases intravascular colloid osmotic pressure (pressure of plasma proteins).

Dextran

Dextran fluids are polysaccharides that behave as colloids. They are available as low molecular weight dextran (dextran 40) and high molecular weight dextran (dextran 70). Dextran 70 is more effective than dextran 40 as a substitute for plasma expansion. It is important to monitor the patient's pulse, blood pressure, and urine output every 5 to 15 minutes for the first hour of administration of dextran and then every hour after that. Dextran should be administered at a rate of 20 mL/kg of body weight over 24 hours to prevent hypersensitivity reactions and decrease the risk of bleeding (Phillips & Kuhn, 1999).

Dextran fluids are used for **plasma substitution** or expansion. An advantage of dextran use is that the intravascular space is expanded in excess of the volume infused. Disadvantages are the possibility of hypersensitivity reactions (i.e., anaphylaxis) and an increased risk of bleeding.

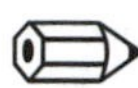

NOTE: Dextran is contraindicated in patients with severe bleeding disorders, congestive heart failure, and renal failure. It is important to draw blood for typing and cross-matching before administering dextran.

Albumin

Albumin is a natural plasma protein prepared from donor plasma. This colloid is available as a 5 or 25 percent solution. Five percent albumin is osmotically and oncotically equivalent to plasma. The 25 percent solution is equivalent to 500 mL of plasma or two units of whole blood (Phillips & Kuhn, 1996).

Albumin is used for maintenance of blood volume, emergency treatment of shock caused by acute blood loss, hypovolemic shock caused by plasma rather than whole blood loss, hypoproteinemic conditions, and treatment of erythroblastosis fetalis (25% solution).

Advantage

- These products are subject to an extended heating period during preparation and therefore do not transmit viral disease

Disadvantages

- May precipitate allergic reactions (e.g., urticaria, flushing, chills, fever, or headache)
- May cause circulatory overload (greatest risk with 25% albumin)
- May cause pulmonary edema
- May alter laboratory findings

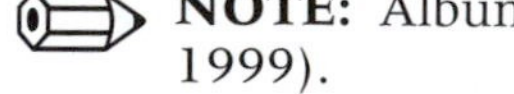

NOTE: Albumin is not a source of nutrition (Phillips & Kuhn, 1999).

Mannitol

Mannitol is a sugar alcohol substance that is available in concentrations from 5 to 25 percent. It is used to promote diuresis in patients with oliguric acute renal failure, promote excretion of toxic substances in the body, reduce excess cerebrospinal fluid (CSP), reduce intraocular pressure, and treat intracranial pressure and cerebral edema.

Advantage

- May reduce excess CSP within 15 minutes

Disadvantages

- May cause fluid and electrolyte imbalances
- May cause cell dehydration or fluid overload by drawing fluid from cells into the vascular system
- Requires cautious use for patients with impaired cardiac or renal system
- May lead to skin irritation and tissue necrosis because of extravasation of mannitol (Terry & Hedrick, 1995)

Hetastarch

Hetastarch (hydroxyethyl glucose) is a synthetic colloid made from starch. It is available under the name Hespan as a 6 or 10 percent solution, diluted in isotonic sodium chloride in a 500-mL container. These starches are not derived from donor plasma and are therefore less toxic and less expensive. Hetastarch is equal in plasma volume expansion properties to 5 percent human albumin.

Advantage

- Hetastarch does not interfere with blood typing and cross-matching, as do other colloidal solutions

Disadvantage

- Possibility of allergic reaction

Hetastarch may alter the coagulation mechanism (i.e., with transient prolongation of the prothrombin, partial thromboplastin, and clotting times). Thus, this solution is contraindicated in patients with severe bleeding disorders, severe congestive heart failure, and anuric renal failure (Terry & Hedrick, 1995).

NOTE: Use cautiously in patients whose conditions predispose them to fluid retention.

Table 5–3 presents a summary of common I.V. fluids.

TABLE 5–3

QUICK-GLANCE CHART OF COMMON I.V. FLUIDS

Solutions	Indications	Precautions
	Dextrose Solutions	
5% Dextrose 10% Dextrose 20% Dextrose 50% Dextrose 70% Dextrose	Spares body protein Provides nutrition Provides calories Provides free water Acts as a diluent for I.V. drugs Treats dehydration Treats hyperkalemia	Possible compromise of glucose tolerance by stress, sepsis, hepatic and renal failure, corticosteroids, and diuretics Does not provide any electrolytes May cause vein irritation, water intoxication, and possible agglomeration Use cautiously in the early postoperative period to prevent water intoxication; ADH secretions as a stress response to surgery Hypertonic fluids may cause hyperglycemia, osmotic diuresis, hyperosmolar coma, or hyperinsulinism
	Sodium Chloride (NaCl) Solutions	
0.2% NaCl 0.45% NaCl 0.9% NaCl 3% NaCl 5% NaCl	Replaces ECF and electrolytes Replaces sodium and chloride Treats hyperosmolar diabetes Acts as diluent for I.V. drug administration Used for initiation and discontinuation of blood products Replaces severe sodium and chloride deficit Helps to correct water overload Acts as an irrigant for intravascular devices	Hyponatremia (excessive use of 0.25 or 0.45% NaCl); calorie depletion; hypernatremia or hyperchloremia; circulatory overload; deficit of other electrolytes Can induce hyperchloremic acidosis because of a loss of bicarbonate ions Does not provide free water or calories Use with caution in older adults

Combination Dextrose and Sodium Chloride Solutions		
5% Dextrose/0.2% NaCl (hydration solution) 5% Dextrose/0.45 NaCl (hydration solution) 5% Dextrose/0.9% NaCl	Assesses kidney function Hydrates cells Promotes diuresis For temporary treatment of circulatory insufficiency hydrating fluids Replaces nutrients and electrolytes Supplies some calories Reduces nitrogen depletion Used in place of plasma expanders	Use with caution in patients with edema and those with cardiac, renal, or liver disease Do not use in patients in diabetic coma Do not use in patients who are allergic to corn
Multiple Electrolyte Solutions		
A. Maintenance solutions	Provide free water, calories, and electrolytes	
Plasma-Lyte M (Baxter) (an electrolyte solution and 5% dextrose)	Provides routine maintenance Relieves physiologic stress leading to inappropriate release of ADH	Water intoxication May cause increased potassium levels
B. Replacement solutions	Provide calories and electrolytes	
Plasma-Lyte R (Baxter) injection Plasma-Lyte 148 and 5% dextrose	Provides fluid and electrolyte replacement	Hypernatremia Fluid overload
5% Dextrose in Ringer's injection	Provides calories Spares protein Replaces ECF losses and electrolytes	Contraindicated in patients with renal failure Use with caution in patients with CHF Composition similar to plasma Tolerated well in patients with liver disease

(Continued)

TABLE 5–3

QUICK-GLANCE CHART OF COMMON I.V. FLUIDS ***(Continued)***

Solutions	Indications	Precautions
5% Dextrose and lactated Ringer's solutions	Treats mild metabolic acidosis Replaces fluid losses from burns and trauma Replaces fluid losses from alimentary tract Rehydrates in all types of dehydration	Contraindicated in patients with lactic acidosis Circulatory overload May cause metabolic acidosis Ionic composition similar to plasma Contains bicarbonate precursor
	Specialty Fluids	
A. Alkalizing	Treats metabolic acidosis Relieves dyspnea and hyperpnea	
Sodium bicarbonate 1/6 Molar sodium lactate	Corrects metabolic acidosis Reduces severe hyperkalemia Treats uncontrolled diabetes mellitus, acute infections, and renal failure	1/6 Molar contraindicated in patients suffering from the lack of oxygen or in those with liver disease, hypocalcemia (tetany), or hypernatremia
B. Plasma expanders		
Dextran 70 (6%) and 0.9% NaCl Dextran 40 (10%) and 0.9% NaCl	Provides plasma expansion Treats perioperative shock Counteracts shock or anticipated shock related to trauma, surgery, burns, or hemorrhage Prevents venous thrombosis and pulmonary embolism during surgery	Hypersensitivity reactions Increased risk of bleeding Pre-existing hypervolemic conditions should be considered (e.g., renal or cardiac disease) Do not add any medications to dextran solutions

10% Mannitol 20% Mannitol	Reduces intraocular pressure Decreases intracranial pressure, reducing cerebral edema Promotes diuresis and excretion of toxic substances Increases granulocyte yield during leukapheresis	Hypervolemia Extravasation Skin irritation Tissue necrosis Interferes with laboratory testing Pre-existing conditions should be considered with caution owing to possible crystal formation
5% Albumin 25% Albumin	Restores circulatory dynamics Counteracts shock or impending shock caused by hypovolemia Provides protein (for hypoproteinemia) Treats hyperbilirubinemia and erythroblastosis fetalis	Allergic reactions Circulatory overload Alteration of laboratory tests Extensive heating period during preparation prevents transmission of viral disease
6% Hetastarch in 0.9% NaCl 10% Hetastarch in 0.9% NaCl	Provides fluid replacement Restores circulatory dynamics Provides volume expansion	May alter coagulation mechanism Allergic reactions Hypervolemia Do not use with severe bleeding disorder Does not interfere with blood typing and cross-matching

NURSING PLAN OF CARE

ADMINISTRATION OF PARENTERAL FLUIDS

Focus Assessment

Subjective

- History of present illness of fluid loss

Objectives

- Observe ability to ingest and retain fluids
- Monitor vital signs
- Monitor weight
- Assess symptoms of fluid disturbance
- Assess for complications associated with infusion therapy (phlebitis, erratic flow rates, infiltration)

Patient Outcome Criteria

The Patient Will:

- Demonstrate improved fluid balance as evidenced by urine output of 30 mL/h with normal specific gravity, stable vital signs, moist mucous membranes, good skin turgor, and capillary refill of less than 3 seconds.
- Verbalize understanding of condition and treatment.

Nursing Diagnoses

- Anxiety (mild, moderate, severe) related to threat to or change in health status; misconceptions regarding therapy
- Altered nutrition less than body requirements related to inability to ingest or digest food or absorb nutrients; inadequate nutrient replacement
- Decreased cardiac output related to reaction to parenteral solution, contamination
- Fluid volume excess related to infusion of I.V. fluid
- Knowledge deficit related to new procedure and maintaining I.V. therapy
- Fluid volume deficit related to deviations affecting intake and absorption of fluids; factors influencing fluid needs (e.g., hypermetabolism state)
- Impaired tissue integrity related to irritating fluids
- Risk for infection related to broken skin or traumatized tissue
- Risk for sleep pattern disturbance related to external sensory stimuli (e.g., I.V. fluid and tubing)

(continued)

(continued)

Nursing Management

1. Administer I.V. fluids at room temperature.
2. Administer I.V. medications at prescribed rate and monitor for results.
3. Monitor I.V. site during infusion.
4. Monitor for fluid overload and physical reactions.
5. Monitor for I.V. patency before administering I.V. medications.
6. Replace I.V. cannula and apparatus every 48 to 72 hours.
7. Replace fluid containers at least every 24 hours.
8. Flush I.V. lines between administration of incompatible solutions.
9. Record intake and output.
10. Monitor urine output and specific gravity.
11. Provide information outlining current I.V. therapy.
12. Maintain standard precautions.

PATIENT EDUCATION

- Instruct on reason for therapy (e.g., replacement fluid, vitamins, nutrition, volume replacement)
- Instruct to report signs and symptoms of complications (e.g., burning at infusion site, redness, any discomfort).

Most infusion therapies in the home are used for delivery of specific treatment such as antibiotics, chemotherapy, total parenteral nutrition, growth hormones, blood products, and hydration therapy.

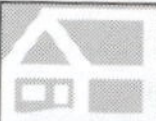

HOME CARE ISSUES

Home care for hydration therapy is used for dehydration and fluid and electrolyte imbalance resulting from:

- Cardiopulmonary disorders
- Fistulas
- Hyperemesis gravidarum
- Intractable diarrhea
- Chemotherapy (before and after)
- Radiation enteritis
- Short bowel syndrome

Short-term therapy lasts from 1 to 7 days and is usually administered via a peripheral lock or long-term access device.

Educate patients about the need for therapy, aseptic technique, set up and administration of specific solution, and possible complications.

Monitor the patient's weight, hydration status, and laboratory tests.

KEY POINTS

PARENTERAL SOLUTIONS

Three main objectives of I.V. therapy are to:

1. Maintain daily requirements
2. Replace previous losses
3. Restore concurrent losses

Solutions have an osmolarity of hypotonic, isotonic, or hypertonic:

- Hypotonic is 250 mOsm/L or below.
- Isotonic ranges from 250 to 375 mOsm/L.
- Hypertonic is above 375 mOsm/L.

Give hypertonic solutions slowly to prevent circulatory overload.

As the acidity of the solution increases, irritation to the vein wall increases.

Do not play "catch-up" with I.V. solutions that are behind schedule; recalculate the infusion.

Always check compatibility before adding medication to dextrose solutions.

Do not give potassium solutions to any patient unless kidney function has been established.

Infusates are categorized as:

- Crystalloids: Solutions that are considered true solutions and whose solutes, when placed in a solvent, mix, dissolve, and cannot be distinguished from the resultant solutions. Crystalloids are able to move through membranes. Examples are dextrose and sodium chloride solutions and lactated Ringer's solution.
- Colloids: Substances whose particles, when submerged in a solvent, cannot form a true solution because their molecules cannot dissolve, but remain suspended and distributed in the fluid. Examples are dextran, albumin, mannitol, blood products, and hetastarch.

CHAPTER ACTIVITIES

COMPETENCY CRITERIA: Administration of Peripheral Parenteral Fluids
COMPETENCY STATEMENT: Competent nurses will be able to administer peripheral parenteral solutions safely following policy and standardized procedures.
Note: The cognitive (knowledge) that is embedded within this performance-based competency includes aseptic techniques, composition of parenteral fluids, and fluid and electrolytes.
This competency *links* to steps in initiating peripheral I.V. therapy.

Performance	Skilled	Needs Education
Critical Action Statements		
1. Verifies written order for appropriate solution, rate, and volume A. Inspects fluids for abnormalities (cracks, punctures, expiration date, clarity)		
2. Chooses appropriate administration set A. Primary or Y set B. Vented or nonvented		
3. Documents solution, rate, time		
4. Documents education provided to patient and family		

EVALUATION CRITERIA

1. Validation of spiking, priming, and administration of solution with preceptor
2. Review of charting
3. Validation of correct I.V. solution compared with physician's order with preceptor

CRITICAL THINKING ACTIVITY

1. Describe a situation in which you observed a solution administered too rapidly.

2. Become familiar with the solutions available in your work environment. Are they primarily solutions without additives? If they are multiple electrolyte solutions, are they arranged on the shelf so as not to be mistaken for each other?

3. The solutions with red lettering on top are usually solutions with additives such as lidocaine and aminophylline. How are these solutions dispensed at your facility? Are they in such a place that they could be "grabbed" by mistake and hung in an emergency?

4. You discover that a solution has been rapidly infused into a patient. Can this potentially harm the patient? What would you do to remedy this situation?

POST-TEST

Match the term in column I with the definition in column II.

COLUMN I	COLUMN II
1. Crystalloid	**a.** Substance that does not dissolve and does not pass through a semipermeable membrane
2. Hydrating solution	**b.** Ability to restore equilibrium
3. Homeostasis	**c.** Solution of water, carbohydrate, and sodium chloride used to check kidney function
4. Colloid	**d.** Breakdown of chemical compounds by the body's energy, producing metabolic process
5. Catabolism	**e.** A substance that forms a true solution

6. The three objectives of I.V. therapy are:
- **a.** Maintenance, peristaltic, and replacement therapy.
- **b.** Replacement, expansion, and restoration therapy.
- **c.** Maintenance, replacement, and restoration therapy.
- **d.** Restoration, hydration, and dehydration therapy.

7. The functions of glucose in parenteral therapy include all of the following **EXCEPT:**
- **a.** Provides calories for energy
- **b.** Helps to prevent negative nitrogen balance
- **c.** Reduces catabolism of protein
- **d.** Serves as vehicle for blood transfusions

8. Maintenance solutions are used for patients who are:
- **a.** Ingesting nothing by mouth for a short period of time
- **b.** Experiencing hemorrhage
- **c.** Dehydrated from GI losses
- **d.** Experiencing draining fistulas

9. An example of a true solution is:
   a. Lactated Ringer's solution
   b. Hetastarch
   c. Mannitol
10. How many grams of dextrose are in 250 mL of 10% dextrose in water?
   a. 25
   b. 50
   c. 75
   d. 100

REFERENCES

Grace, L.A., & Tomaselli, B.J. (1995). Intravenous therapy in the home. In Terry, J., Baranowski, L., Lonsway, R., & Hedrick, C. (eds.): *Intravenous Therapy: Clinical Principles and Practice.* Philadelphia: W.B. Saunders, p. 513.

Josephson, D.L. (1999). *Intravenous Infusion Therapy for Nurses: Principles and Practice.* Albany, NY: Delmar Publishers, pp. 110–127.

Kuhn, M. (1999). *Pharmacotherapeutics: A Nursing Process Approach* (4th ed.). Philadelphia: F.A. Davis, pp. 173–193.

Metheny, N.M. (2000). Fluid and Electrolyte Balance. In *Nursing Considerations* (4th ed.). Philadelphia: Lippincott-Williams & Wilkins, pp. 169–171.

National Student Nurses Association (1997). Specific electrolyte imbalances. In McEntee, M.A., & Gill, G.M. (eds.): *Fluids and Electrolytes.* Albany, NY: Delmar Publishers, pp. 36–70.

Phillips, L.D., & Kuhn, M. (1999). *Manual of I.V. Drugs* (2nd ed.). Philadelphia: J.B. Lippincott.

Terry, J., & Hedrick, C. (1995). Parenteral fluids. In Terry, J., Baranowski, L., Lonsway, R., & Hedrick, C. (eds.): *Intravenous Therapy: Clinical Principles and Practices.* Philadelphia, W.B. Saunders, pp. 151–164.

Weinstein, S. (1997). *Principles and Practices of I.V. Therapy* (5th ed.). Boston: Little, Brown, p. 304.

ANSWERS TO CHAPTER 5

Pre-Test

1. a, **2.** a, **3.** e, **4.** c, **5.** a, **6.** c, **7.** b, **8.** c, **9.** b, **10.** a

Post-Test

1. e, **2.** c, **3.** b, **4.** a, **5.** d, **6.** c, **7.** d, **8.** a, **9.** a, **10.** a

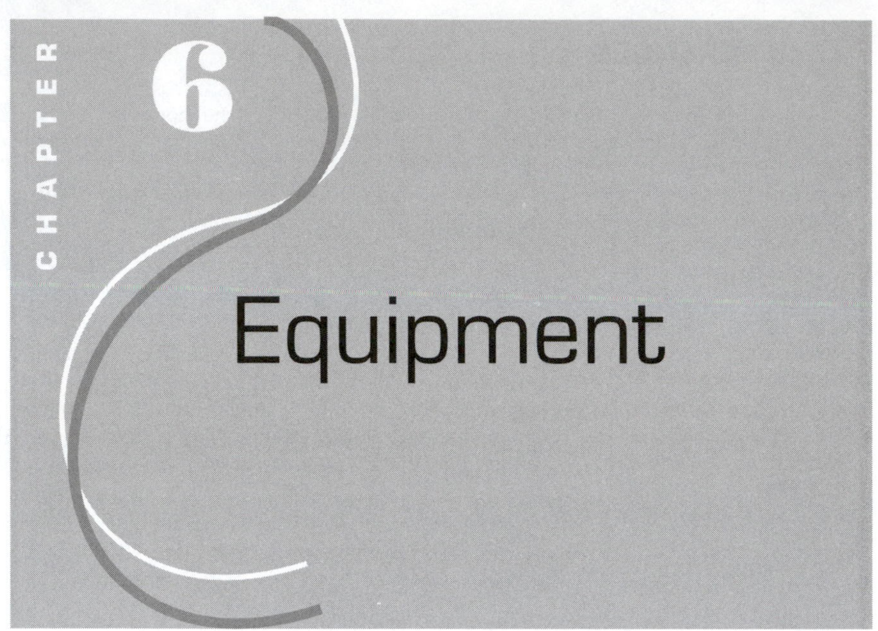

Equipment

All rituals and ceremonials which our modern worship of efficiency may devise, and all our elaborate scientific equipment will not save us if the intellectual and spiritual elements in our art are subordinated to the mechanical, and if the means come to be regarded as more important than ends.

Isabel M. Stewart, 1929

CHAPTER CONTENTS

LEARNING OBJECTIVES

Upon completion of this chapter, the reader will be able to:

1. Define the terminology related to I.V. equipment.
2. Identify the types and characteristics of three infusate containers.
3. Identify the use of vented and nonvented administration sets with the appropriate solution containers.
4. Identify the types and characteristics of peripheral and central infusion devices.
5. State the major advantages and disadvantages associated with over-the-needle catheters and scalp vein needles.
6. Identify the characteristics and uses of electronic infusion devices.
7. Describe the use of filters in the infusion of solutions and blood products.
8. Describe the use of miscellaneous adjuncts to aid in the administration of safe infusions.
9. Identify the Intravenous Nurses Society (INS) and the Centers for Disease Control and Prevention (CDC) recommendations for standards of practice related to equipment safety and use

GLOSSARY

Cannula A tube or sheath used for infusing fluids
Check valve A device that functions to prevent retrograde solution flow; also called a backcheck valve
Coring Visible, as well as microscopic, particles of rubber bung displaced by the spike during piercing of the glass container or needle during access of implanted vascular access devices
Drip chamber Area of the I.V. tubing usually found under the spike where the solution drips and collects before running through the I.V. tubing
Drop factor The number of drops needed to deliver 1 mL of fluid
Filter A special porous device used to prevent the passage of undesired substances
Gauge Size of cannula opening
Hub Female connection point of an I.V. cannula where the tubing or other equipment attaches
Implanted port A catheter surgically placed into a vessel or body cavity and attached to a reservoir; the reservoir is placed under the skin
Infusate I.V. solution
Lumen The space within an artery, vein, or catheter
Macrodrip Drop factor of 10 to 20 drops equivalent to 1 mL based on manufacturer's specifications
Microaggregate Microscopic collection of particles, such as platelets, leukocytes, and fibrin that can exist in stored blood
Microdrip Drop factor of 60 drops/mL
Midclavicular catheter Long (24 to 24 in) I.V. access device made of a soft flexible material inserted into one of the superficial veins of the peripheral vascular system and advanced to proximal axillary or subclavian veins
Midline Peripherally inserted catheter with the tip terminating in the proximal portion of the extremity, usually 6 inches in length
PCA Patient-controlled analgesia
PICC Peripherally inserted central catheter. Long (20 to 24 in) I.V. access device made of a soft flexible material inserted into one of the superficial veins of the peripheral vascular system and advanced to the superior vena cava
Port Point of entry
PRN (pro re na'ta) According to circumstances. Used to describe devices used for intermittent infusions.
psi pounds per square inch; a measurement of pressure: 1 psi equals 50 mm Hg or 68 cm H_2O
Radiopaque Material used in I.V. catheter that can be identified by radiographic examination
Rubber bung Stopper of glass container composed of numerous substances including rubber, chemical particles, and cellulose fibers
Stylet Needle or guide that is found inside a catheter used for vein penetration
Tunneled catheter A catheter designed to have a portion lie within a subcutaneous passage before exiting the body

PRE-TEST

1. When using a closed-glass system, the administration set should be:
   a. Vented
   b. Nonvented
2. Inline filters are useful for:
   a. Filtering nonviable contaminants such as particles of metal, lint, and glass
   b. Filtering viable contaminants such as bacteria and fungi
   c. Filtering air from the administration set
   d. All of the above
3. A disadvantage of Teflon over-the-needle catheters for peripheral infusion is:
   a. The risk of phlebitis
   b. The risk of infiltration
   c. They can be used for only 24 hours
   d. The risk of septicemia
4. The infusate solution containers should be inspected for:
   a. Clarity, expiration date, and air vents
   b. Clarity, expiration date, punctures, and cracks
   c. Punctures, cracks, presence of ports, and clarity
5. Volumetric pumps require:
   a. A 170-micron filter
   b. A 0.22-micron filter
   c. Special cassette (cartridge) tubing
   d. Microdrip tubing
6. Advantages of over-the-needle catheters include all of the following **EXCEPT:**
   a. They are patent longer than scalp vein needle.
   b. They are radiopaque.
   c. They have decreased infiltration risks.
   d. They have low incidence of mechanical phlebitis.
7. Locking devices must be monitored every 4 hours and kept patent with:
   a. Saline flushes
   b. Heparin flushes
   c. Medication
   d. Saline or heparin based on hospital policy and physician preference
8. Y-type infusate administration sets are used:
   a. With collapsible infusion containers
   b. For administration of I.V. solutions
   c. For administration of lipids
   d. For administration of blood products
9. Needleless systems are now being marketed to:
   a. Decrease the risk of needlestick injuries
   b. Protect the I.V. line's integrity
   c. Decrease tubing changes
   d. Enable quicker blood draws

10. An EID with a controller mode functions:

a. As an electronic eye that watches the drops flow, according to a preset rate through a drop sensor

b. By providing a driving force to overcome resistance to pressure in order to propel the infusate

c. As a piston-driven force

d. By flow restriction (rubber band infusion)

● ● ●

INFUSION DELIVERY SYSTEMS

Two infusion systems are available for delivery of I.V. fluids: the glass system and the plastic system (Fig. 6–1). Sterile evacuated glass containers became available in 1929. The rigid glass containers contain a standard mix of materials, glass, metal, and rubber. The combination of materials is a disadvantage because of incompatibilities with other fluids and additives and the breakdown of the materials during heat sterilization. In 1950, plastic containers became accessible for the storage and delivery of blood products. Today, the plastic system is used 90 to 95 percent of the time for administering solutions and blood products.

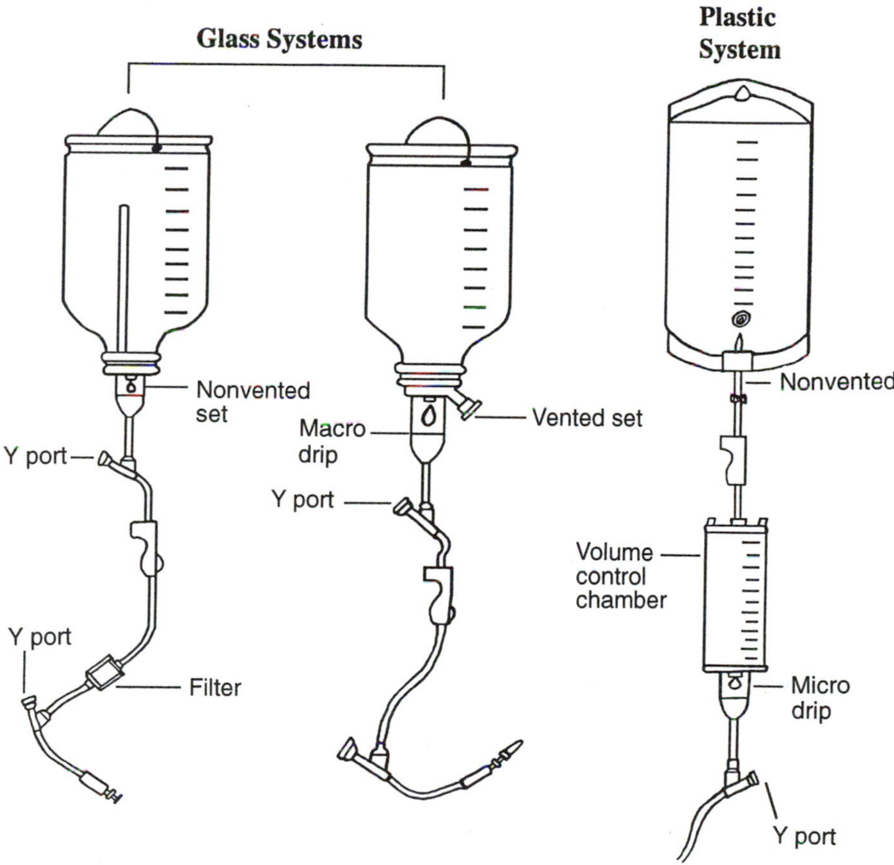

FIG. 6–1. Comparison of glass and plastic infusion delivery systems. (Drawings by Timothy D. Mitas.)

THE GLASS SYSTEM

The glass system has a partial vacuum and requires air vents (unlike the plastic system). In the open-glass system, air enters through a plastic tube in the container and collects in the air space in the bottle, allowing for displacement of the solution. In the closed-glass system, air is filtered into the container via vented tubing. The closed-glass system must use vented tubing to allow air into the container.

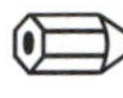

NOTE: In the open-glass system, the straw must extend above the fluid level to prevent bubbling of the air through the infusate (I.V. solution). Bubbling increases the risk of contamination. This system has been replaced by the use of closed-glass and plastic systems.

The glass system has a stopper, also called the **rubber bung.** During insertion of the administration set, **coring** can occur, which results in the introduction of fragments of the rubber core into the solution. Twisting the spike through the rubber bung can displace visible and microscopic particles of the rubber bung. Because of the combination of materials in the glass system, there have been some disadvantages to this system during heat sterilization procedures. Openings between the external environment and the internal container occur at peak heating and early cooling phases of sterilization. Recalls of endogenously contaminated fluids in the United States were caused by the expansion of metal, rubber, and glass during the sterilization procedure.

Checking the Glass System for Clarity

To ensure safety in the administration of solutions, the nurse must check the solution's clarity and expiration date before connecting it to the administration set. To check the glass system, hold the glass bottle up to the light and check for flashes of light, floating particles, or discoloration. The glass system should be crystal clear; if it is not, mark the container as contaminated and return it to the central supply. Check the expiration date on the label.

Advantages

- Crystal clear; allows good visualization of contents
- Fluid level easy to read
- Inert; has no plasticizers

Disadvantages

- Breakage and shattering of glass
- Storage
- Coring (because of the rubber bung)
- Cumbersome disposal

- Rigidity
- Container constructed of mixed materials

THE PLASTIC SYSTEM

Most I.V. fluids are packaged in plastic containers that are flexible or semi-rigid (Fig. 6–2)

The flexible plastic container has several unique features. The entire structure that comes in contact with the fluid, including the closure, is made of the same material; it is all polyvinyl chloride (PVC) or other suitable material. There is no combination of metal, rubber, or glass as in the rigid glass system. The plastic system is a truly closed system.

Plastic containers are commonly made of PVC, which is a polymeric material. The introduction of PVC plastic solution containers has been accompanied by concerns of compatibility, specifically with the plasticizer diethylhexylphthalate (DEHP). DEHP is a plasticizer added to PVC that allows PVC to become flexible (Table 6–1).

The plastic system does not contain a vacuum; therefore, the containers must be flexible and collapsible. The plastic system does not need air to replace fluid flowing from the container. Either a vented or nonvented administration set is acceptable for delivery of the infusate. A membrane seals both the medication and the administration ports of the container, and there is no entry of air into this system. Because there is no rubber

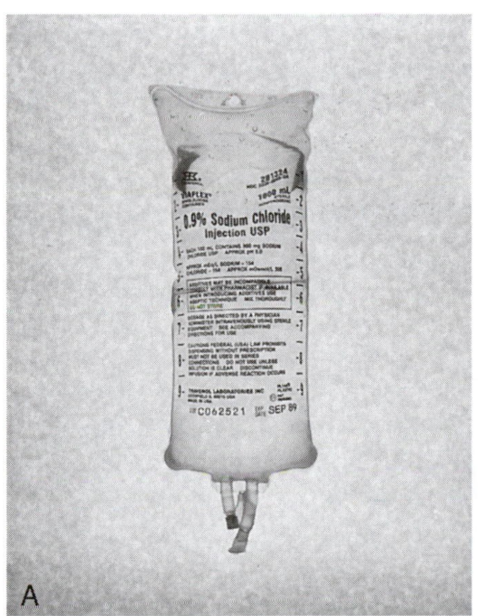

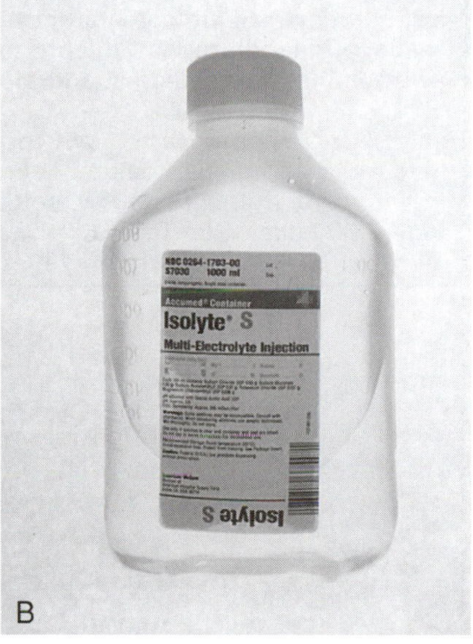

FIG. 6–2. Plastic infusion system. I.V. solutions are available in both (*A*) a flexible plastic container and (*B*) a more rigid type of container. (Courtesy of D. Anderson, Chico, California.)

TABLE 6–1

CONCERNS OVER POLYVINYL CHLORIDE AND DEHP

Polyvinyl chloride is a commonly used plastic found in many consumer, industrial, and medical products. A phthalate (DEHP) is a plasticizer that is added to PVC that allows PVC to become flexible. In 1972, potential hazards of transfusing blood that contained DEHP derived from blood bags and tubing were identified. In 1986, California Proposition 65 listed DEHP as a chemical that is known to cause cancer. In 1988, the Environmental Protection Agency (EPA) identified DEHP as a probable human carcinogen.

When incinerated, PVC releases hydrogen chloride gas (identified as a toxic air pollutant and cause of acid rain) and possible dioxin. When PVC products are incinerated, they produce HCl, a corrosive gas that has been identified a toxic air pollutant. PVC materials are also not biodegradable, and DEHP may leach into the soil.

There are two reasons why the use of PVC I.V. containers is contraindicated in many I.V. therapies:

1. Absorption
2. Leaching

DEHP is not chemically bound to the polymer and can leach out during use. This extraction occurs either by DEHP's directly leaching out of the PVC product or when an extracting material (blood or I.V. fluids) diffuses into the PVC matrix, dissolves the plasticizer and then the two diffuse out together. The most important factors in DEHP's leaching from medical devices are temperature, concentration of the phthalate, agitation, storage time, and surrounding media. DEHP is leached from PVC blood bags, I.V. bags, and tubing into blood, blood products, and medical solutions (Healthcare without Harm, 1999). Certain drugs (e.g., Taxol, cyclosporine, diazepam, miconazole, nitroglycerine, warfarin, sodium carmustin), fat emulsions, and blood products enhance the leaching of DEHP (B. Braun, 1999).

Health Care Without Harm (www.noharm.org/DEHP) initiated a collaborative international campaign advocating environmentally responsible health care. In the 1980s, I.V. solutions were provided by B. Braun in non-PVC bags. (See Table 6-2, page 247, for a list of PVC alternatives.) (Health Care Without Harm, 1999).

---

bung on the plastic system, spiking the system can be accomplished by means of a simple twisting motion (Fig. 6–3). Because the plastic can be easily perforated during use, careful attention should be paid to the integrity of this container during preparation and infusion delivery.

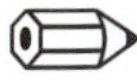

NOTE: Never write directly on a flexible plastic bag with a ballpoint or indelible marker; the pen may puncture the bag and the marker ink may absorb into the plastic.

The advantages of the semirigid, hard plastic unit are that it is made of polyolefin, contains no plasticizers, and the fluid level marks are easier to

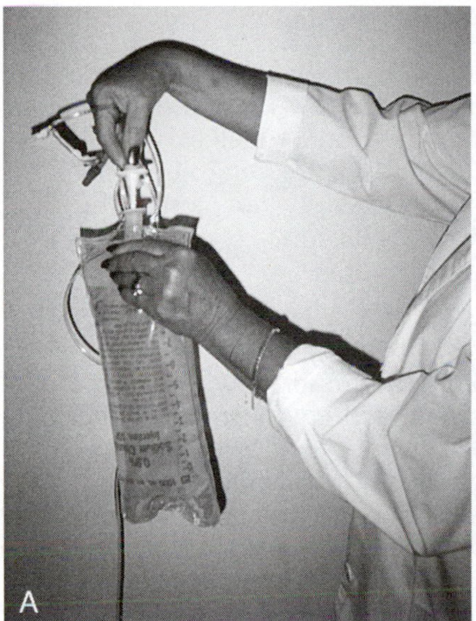

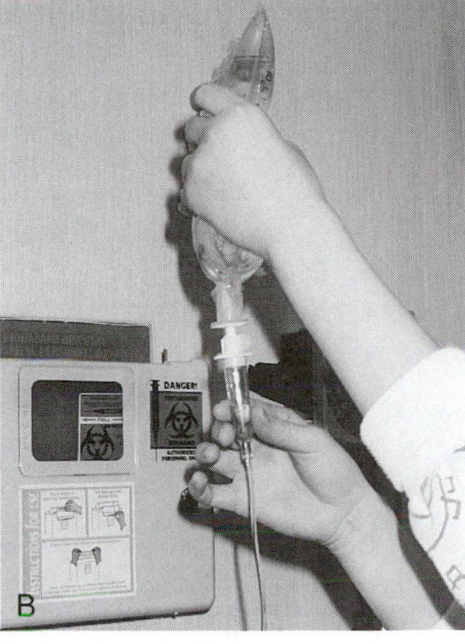

FIG. 6–3. Spiking the plastic container. (*A*) To spike the plastic container, insert the piercing pin of the I.V. tubing into the outlet port of the infusion bag using a twisting motion to ensure that the seal is pierced completely open. (*B*) Invert the container and squeeze drip chamber to fill.

read. This system is also impermeable to moisture. A disadvantage is that it does not completely collapse; therefore, the last 50 mL of the solution may be difficult to infuse.

The flexible and semirigid plastic systems, when used in a series with other similar containers, may promote movement of residual air into the I.V. line.

Advantages

- Closed system
- Flexible
- Lightweight
- Container composed of one substance
- Better storage

Disadvantages

- Punctures easily
- Fluid level difficult to determine
- Composed of plasticizers
- Not completely inert (potential for leaching)
- Environmentally unsafe

Checking the Plastic System for Clarity

The plastic container should be held up to the light and checked for clarity. If the plastic system is not crystal clear, any discoloration or floating particles in the solution should be identified and labeled contaminated. The plastic system must be squeezed to check for pinholes. Check the expiration date on the label to ensure patient safety and be sure the outer wrap of the plastic system is free of pooled solution.

USE-ACTIVATED CONTAINERS

Use-activated containers are compartmentalized with premeasured ingredients that form an admixture when mixed. The containers are useful for high-use infusions that have a short shelf life after admixture. These systems are useful in the emergency department because they enable ease of use in acute situations (such as in an ambulance), in field use, and during transport. The ambulatory and home care settings also benefit from use-activated systems (Fig. 6–4).

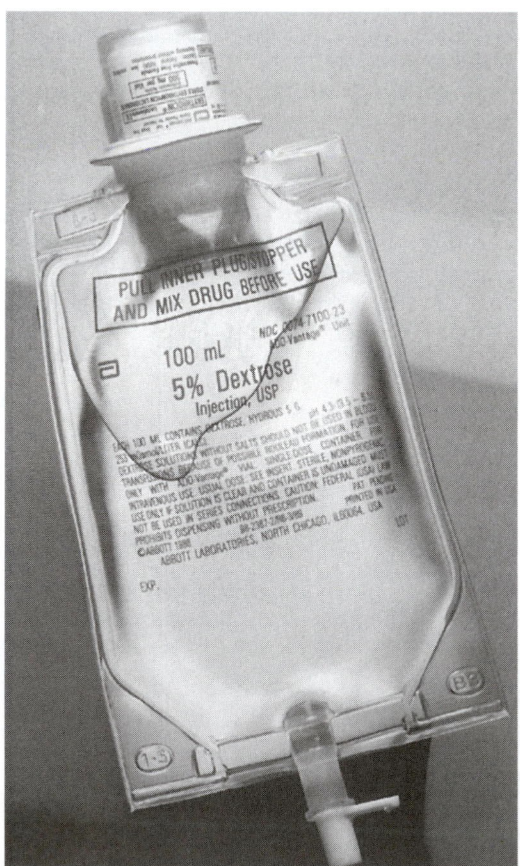

FIG. 6–4. Use-activated system. This Abbott ADD-Vantage system allows drugs to be reconstituted quickly and safely in an appropriate amount of diluent immediately before use. (Courtesy of Abbott Laboratories, North Chicago, Illinois. Used with permission.)

ADMINISTRATION SETS

The most frequently used administration sets include:

- Single-line sets, which include primary (standard) sets, secondary sets (also called "piggyback" sets), and volume-controlled sets.
- Primary Y sets.
- Administration sets, which vary among manufacturers and drop factor, all have the basic components (Fig. 6–5).

BASIC COMPONENTS OF ADMINISTRATION SETS

The basic components of administration sets include:

1. *Spike/piercing pin:* The spike/piercing pin is a sharply tipped plastic tube designed to be inserted into the infusate container. It is connected to the flange, drop orifice, and drip chamber.
2. *Flange:* The flange is a plastic guard that helps prevent touch contamination during insertion of the spike.
3. *Drop orifice:* The drop orifice is an opening that determines the size and shape of the fluid drop. The size of this drop orifice determines the **drop factor.**
4. *Drip chamber:* The drip chamber is a pliable, enlarged clear plastic tube that contains the drop orifice. It is connected to the tubing.
5. *Tubing:* The plastic tubing connects to the drip chamber. Depending on the manufacturer, the tubing may have a variety of clamps, ports, connectors, or filters built into the system. The average length of primary tubing is 66 to 100 inches. The length of secondary administration sets averages from 32 to 42 inches.
6. *Clamp:* The flow clamp control device operates on the principle of compression of the tubing wall. Each manufacturer supplies a clamp (roller, screw, or slide), and all operate on the principle of compression. The roller and screw clamps are equally reliable. The slide clamp is viewed as less reliable in controlling flow.
7. *Injection ports:* Injection ports serve as an access into the tubing and are located at various points along the administration set. Usually the ports are used for administration of medication. Small needles should be used to access these ports (21- to 25-gauge) to ensure resealing.
8. *Backcheck valve:* The valve allows the primary solution to resume after the piggyback is completed.
9. *Hub:* The adaptor to connect the administration set to the I.V. catheter or a needleless system is also called the male Luer-Lok.
10. *Final filter:* The final filter removes foreign particles from the infusate. It can be purchased as part of the administration set tubing, or filters can be added on.

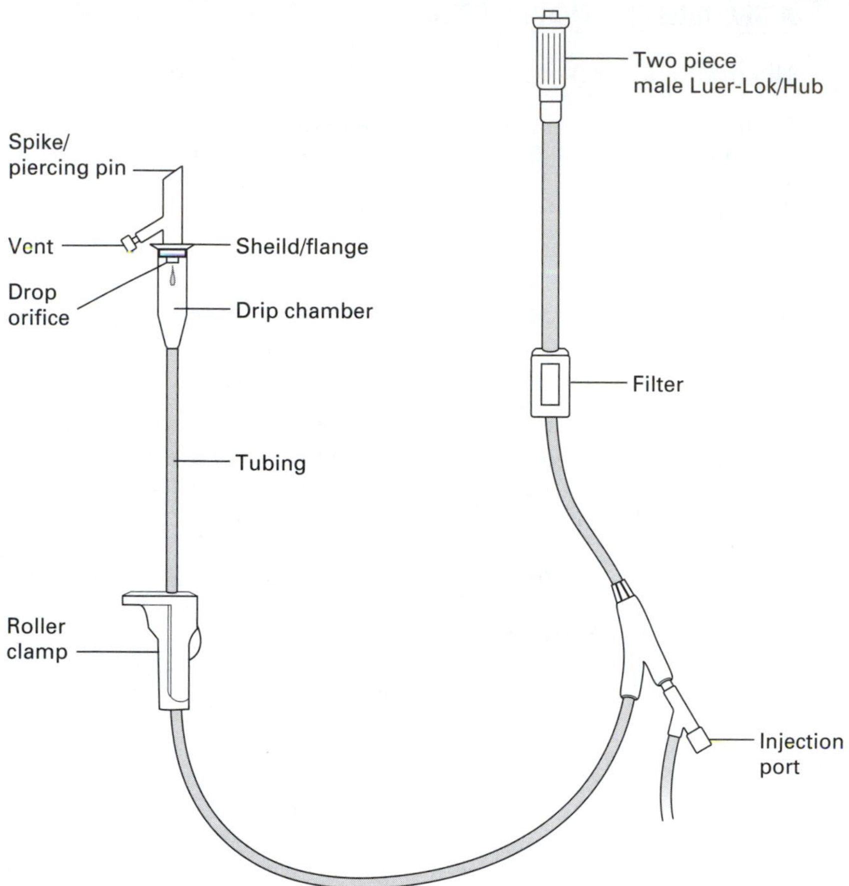

FIG. 6–5. Basic administration system.

SINGLE-LINE ADMINISTRATION SETS

Single-line sets have only one spike that extends proximally from the drip chamber. Only one main bag of infusate is used with this system. The tubing distal to the **drip chamber** terminates in one male-adapter end that connects to the **hub** of a vascular access device.

Primary Sets

Primary sets are referred to as standard sets and are available as vented or nonvented. Vented sets have an air filter attached to the spike pin that allows air to enter the container. Vented sets must be used on the closed-glass system. Nonvented sets have a straight spike pin without an air vent device. Nonvented sets can be used on any open-glass or plastic system. Primary sets are available in **macrodrip** form (10 to 20 drops/mL) or in **microdrip** form (60 drops/mL). The calibration is clearly specified on the box of each administration set, as well as in the accompanying literature. The microdrip set, also called a minidrip or pediatric set, is used when small amounts of fluid are required (Fig. 6–6).

A **check valve** (also called backcheck valve) is a device that functions to prevent retrograde flow of the solution. Check valves are in-line components of many primary administration sets. The check valve is an important feature when secondary I.V. lines are in place for intermittent infusions. The check valve inhibits the backflow of secondary **infusate** into the primary infusate.

Check valves function when the:

- Primary infusate is infusing at the prescribed rate by gravity.
- Secondary infusate, of a lesser volume, is piggybacked into the primary line.
- Level of the secondary infusate is higher than the primary container.
- Clamp on the tubing of the secondary container is opened, activating the backcheck valve because of the pressure exerted by the piggyback solution.
- Secondary infusate container empties and its fluid descends into its tubing; the decreased pressure in the line causes the backcheck valve to release, thus activating flow in the primary line (Fig. 6–7).

INS STANDARDS Primary and secondary continuous administration sets shall be changed every 72 hours and immediately upon suspected contamination or when the integrity of the product or system has been compromised. (INS, 2000, 54)

An organization that exhibits an increased rate of catheter-related blood-stream infection with the practice of 72-hour administration set changes should return to a 48-hour administration set change. (INS, 2000, 24)

Secondary Administration Sets

Two types of secondary administration sets are available: the piggyback set and the volume-controlled set.

Piggyback Set

The piggyback set has short tubing (30 to 36 in) with a standard drop factor of 10 to 20 drops/mL. It is used to deliver 50 to 100 mL of infusate. These sets are widely used because of the administration of multiple drug therapies to patients. They are connected with a needleless adapter into an **injection port** immediately distal to the backcheck valve of the primary tubing (Josephson, 1999). In setting up the piggyback set, the primary infusion container is positioned lower than the secondary container, using the extension hook provided in the secondary line box.

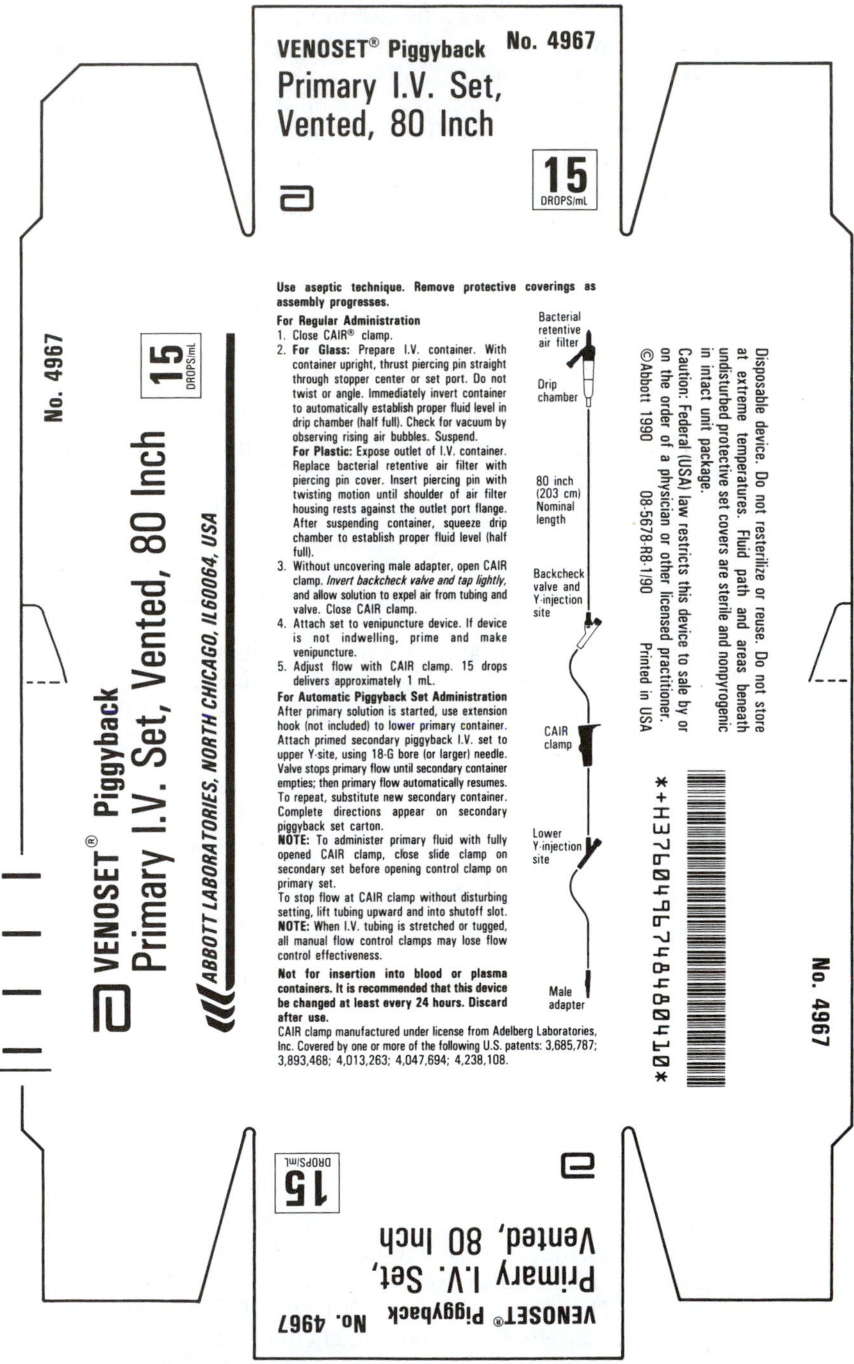

VENOSET® Piggyback No. 4967
Primary I.V. Set, Vented, 80 Inch
15 DROPS/mL
No. 4967
VENOSET® Piggyback
Primary I.V. Set, Vented, 80 Inch
15 DROPS/mL
ABBOTT LABORATORIES, NORTH CHICAGO, IL60064, USA
Use aseptic technique. Remove protective coverings as assembly progresses.
For Regular Administration
1. Close CAIR® clamp.
2. For Glass: Prepare I.V. container. With container upright, thrust piercing pin straight through stopper center or set port. Do not twist or angle. Immediately invert container to automatically establish proper fluid level in drip chamber (half full). Check for vacuum by observing rising air bubbles. Suspend.
For Plastic: Expose outlet of I.V. container. Replace bacterial retentive air filter with piercing pin cover. Insert piercing pin with twisting motion until shoulder of air filter housing rests against the outlet port flange. After suspending container, squeeze drip chamber to establish proper fluid level (half full).
3. Without uncovering male adapter, open CAIR clamp. Invert backcheck valve and tap lightly, and allow solution to expel air from tubing and valve. Close CAIR clamp.
4. Attach set to venipuncture device. If device is not indwelling, prime and make venipuncture.
5. Adjust flow with CAIR clamp. 15 drops delivers approximately 1 mL.
For Automatic Piggyback Set Administration
After primary solution is started, use extension hook (not included) to lower primary container. Attach primed secondary piggyback I.V. set to upper Y-site, using 18-G bore (or larger) needle. Valve stops primary flow until secondary container empties; then primary flow automatically resumes. To repeat, substitute new secondary container. Complete directions appear on secondary piggyback set carton.
NOTE: To administer primary fluid with fully opened CAIR clamp, close slide clamp on secondary set before opening control clamp on primary set.
To stop flow at CAIR clamp without disturbing setting, lift tubing upward and into shutoff slot.
NOTE: When I.V. tubing is stretched or tugged, all manual flow control clamps may lose flow control effectiveness.
Not for insertion into blood or plasma containers. It is recommended that this device be changed at least every 24 hours. Discard after use.
CAIR clamp manufactured under license from Adelberg Laboratories, Inc. Covered by one or more of the following U.S. patents: 3,685,787; 3,893,468; 4,013,263; 4,047,694; 4,238,108.
Bacterial retentive air filter
Drip chamber
80 inch (203 cm) Nominal length
Backcheck valve and Y-injection site
CAIR clamp
Lower Y-injection site
Male adapter
Disposable device. Do not resterilize or reuse. Do not store at extreme temperatures. Fluid path and areas beneath undisturbed protective set covers are sterile and nonpyrogenic in intact unit package.
Caution: Federal (USA) law restricts this device to sale by or on the order of a physician or other licensed practitioner.
©Abbott 1990 08-5678-R8-1/90 Printed in USA
+H3760496748480410
No. 4967
VENOSET® Piggyback No. 4967
Primary I.V. Set,
Vented, 80 Inch
15 DROPS/mL

FIG. 6–6. Primary administration set package. (Courtesy of Abbott Laboratories, Hospital Products Division, North Chicago, Illinois.)

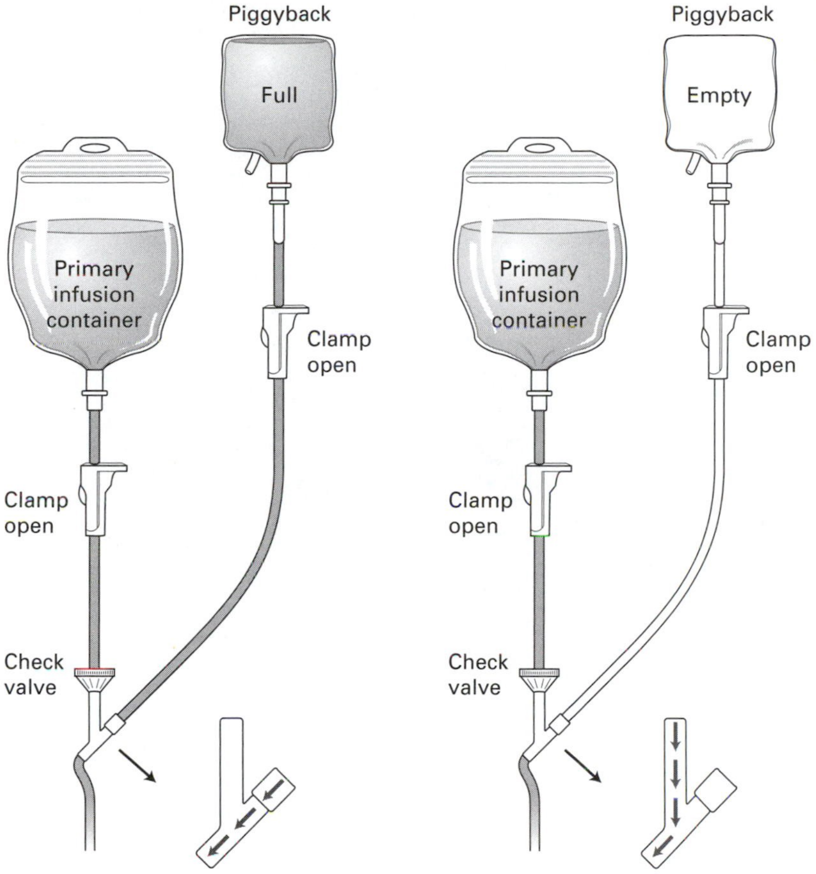

FIG. 6–7. Check valve (also called backcheck valve) acts to prevent retrograde solution flow.

Volume-Controlled Set

The volume-controlled set, also called metered-volume chamber set, is designed for intermittent administration of measured volumes of fluid with a calibrated chamber. These sets are calibrated in much smaller increments than other infusion devices, thus limiting the amount of solution available to the patient (usually for reasons of safety). Most chambers hold 100 to 150 mL of solution, but neonatal chambers may hold only 10 to 50 mL. The volume-controlled set is most frequently used for pediatric patients and critically ill patients when small, well-controlled delivery of medication or solution is needed (Fig. 6–8).

INS STANDARDS Primary intermittent administration sets shall be changed every 24 hours and immediately upon suspected contamination or when the integrity of the product or system has been compromised. (INS, 2000, 54)

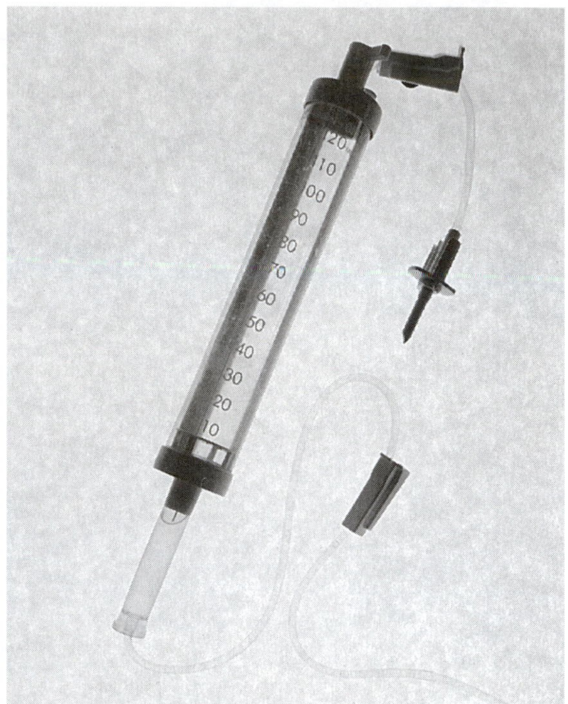

FIG. 6-8. Volume chamber control set for intermittent infusion. (Courtesy of D. Anderson, Chico, California.)

PRIMARY Y ADMINISTRATION SETS

The primary Y administration set is used for rapid infusion or for administration of more than one solution at a time. Each leg of the Y set is capable of being the primary set. The Y set has two separate spikes with a separate drip chamber and short length of tubing with individual clamps. Primary Y sets are made up of large-bore tubing because this tubing is meant to infuse large amounts of fluid in acute situations. Blood components can be administered through primary Y sets. A Y set allows for priming of the administration set before the blood is administered. Most blood administration Y sets contain inline filters with a pore size of 170 microns and have a drop factor of 10 to allow for the safe infusion of blood cells.

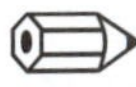 **NOTE:** Primary Y sets are not provided as vented sets, so caution applies to bottles with venting straws or a venting apparatus added to the bottle. Collapsible containers should be used with Y sets. Any

air emboli associated with tubing of this inner lumen size are considered significant (Jensen, 1995).

INS STANDARDS Administration sets that are used to accommodate blood or blood components shall be changed after each unit or at the end of 4 hours. (INS, 2000, S4)

PUMP-SPECIFIC ADMINISTRATION SETS

Pump-specific administration sets are made specifically for use with electronic infusion devices (EIDs). These sets also come in a number of configurations, with each set specific for respective electronic delivery systems. For specifics on each pump administration set, see the literature that accompanies each EID.

LIPID ADMINISTRATION SETS

Lipids or fat emulsions are supplied in glass containers and require special vented tubing that is supplied by the manufacturer. Lipid-containing infusates have been known to leach phthalates from the bags and tubing of PVC. Fat emulsions are supplied in glass containers with non-PVC infusion sets.

ACCESSORY DEVICES FOR ADMINISTRATION SETS

Accessory, or add-on, devices for administration sets include:

- Filters
- Extension tubings
- Adapters and connectors
- Stopcocks
- Injection access ports
- Needleless systems

When an add-on device is used, it should be of a Luer-Lok configuration. Aseptic technique and infection control measures must be followed for all add-on device changes. Adding accessories to an existing administration set is referred to as breaching the infusion line. Whenever an infusion line is breached, the possibility for the introduction of contaminates exists.

INS STANDARDS When add-on devices are used, they should be changed with each catheter or administration set replacement, or whenever the integrity of either product is compromised. (INS, 2000, 35)

FILTERS

Inline I.V. Solution Filters

Inline, or "final," **filters** are used in the delivery of I.V. therapy to filter microorganisms, which, if alive, will multiply in the bloodstream or, if dead, will enter the tissue and cause a sterile abscess. There are two groups of particulate matter: (1) nonviable contaminants such as particles of metal, lint, asbestos, rubber, cotton, dust, and glass; and (2) viable contaminants, consisting of bacteria and fungi. Inline filters remove undissolved drug powders or crystals and precipitates from incompatible admixtures.

Inline filters are available in a variety of forms, sizes, and materials:

- 5- to 1.2-micron filters remove most particulate matter but do not remove fungi or bacteria.
- 0.45-micron filters remove fungi or bacteria.
- 0.22-micron filters remove all fungi and bacteria but reduce flow rates.

The Food and Drug Administration (FDA, 1994) recommends the use of inline filter devices for removal of bacteria, fungi, particulate, air, and some endotoxins from I.V.-delivered fluids. The National Coordinating Committee on Large Volume Parenteral (NCCLVP) has established priorities for the use of filters and recommends the use of filters with tissue plasminogen activator (TPN) admixtures; for immunodeficient or immunocompromised patients; and for I.V. infusions containing additives, especially those that are heavily precipitated (Sevick, 1995).

INS STANDARDS A 0.2-micron filter is considered a bacterial/particulate retentive, air-eliminating filter and is recommended for use to decrease the potential of air emboli. To achieve final filtration, the filter should be located as close to the **cannula** site as possible. The filter should be an integral part of the administration set. (INS, 2000, 38)

Two commonly used filters are the depth filter and the membrane filter.

Depth Filter

The depth filter is composed of fibers or fragmented material that has been pressed or bonded to form a maze; the pore size is nonuniform. Fluid flows through a random path that absorbs and traps the particles. These filters can clog when large amounts of particles are retained. Depth filters prime easily and are capable of air elimination.

Membrane Filter

Membrane filters are screen filters with uniformly sized pores. A 5-micron screen will retain on the flat portion of the membrane all particles larger than 5 microns. Filters of 0.2 microns are for bacteria, fungus, and air retention. The 0.22-micron air-venting filters automatically vent air through a nonwettable (hydrophobic) membrane and permit uniform high-gravity flow through large wettable (hydrophilic) membrane (Weinstein, 1997).

To be effective, an infusion membrane filter must have the ability to:

- Maintain high flow rates
- Automatically vent air
- Retain bacteria, fungi, particulate matter, and endotoxins
- Tolerate pressures generated by infusion pumps
- Act in a nonbinding fashion to drugs (Weinstein, 1997)

Membrane filters are used when:

1. An additive has been combined with the solution.
2. The injection port on the tubing is used.
3. The patient is susceptible to infusion phlebitis.
4. The infusion is given centrally.
5. The solution is a three-in-one TPN solution.

Filters range in size from 5 microns (largest) to 0.22 micron (smallest). They allow liquids but not particles to pass through them. The finer the membrane, the more fully it will filter the liquid.

Prescribed therapies in which a 0.2-micron filter is contraindicated include administration of blood or blood components, lipid emulsions, and low-dose (<5 micron/mL) solutions. Other contraindications include the administration of low-volume medications (total amount <5 mg over 24 hours), I.V. push medications, medications in which pharmacologic properties are altered by the filter membrane, and medications that adhere to the filter membrane.

All filters have a certain pressure value at which they will allow the passage of air from one side of a wetted hydrophilic membrane to the other. This pressure valve is called the bubble point.

Filters are also rated according the pounds per square inch (**psi**) of pressure they can withstand. The filter should withstand the psi exerted by the infusion pump or rupture may occur. If the psi rating of the housing is less than that of the membrane, excess force will break the housing (Weinstein, 1997).

INS STANDARDS When using a positive pressure EID, consideration should be given to the psi rating of a filter. The psi exerted by the device should never exceed the psi capacity of the filter. (INS, 2000, 38)

Filters for Parenteral Therapy

An air-eliminating 0.2-micron filter set designed for 96-hour bacteria and endotoxin retention is indicated for use with I.V. administration sets for the removal of inadvertent particulate debris, microbial contaminates and their associated endotoxin, and entrained air that may be found in solutions intended for I.V. administration (Pall, 2000) (Fig. 6–9).

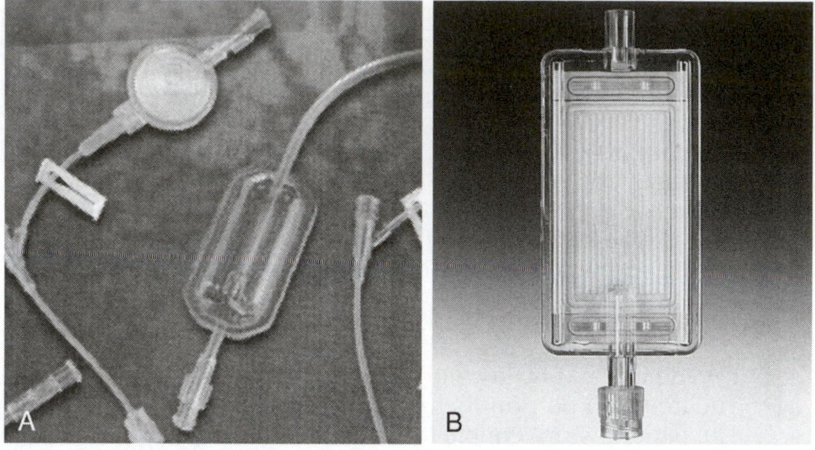

FIG. 6–9. (*A*) Inline 0.22-micron filter: Filterflow. (Courtesy of B. Braun Medical Inc., Bethlehem, Pennsylvania.) (*B*) Intravenous 0.2-micron filter. (Courtesy of Pall Corporation, Port Washington, New York.) Filter, for use with any I.V. administration set, eliminates air and removes inadvertent particulate debris, microbial contamination and associated endotoxins, and any entrained air that may be in the solutions.

A filter set for total nutritional admixture administration has a 1.2-micron air-eliminating filter. This filter set is indicated for use with any nutritional I.V. administration containing lipids for the removal of inadvertent particulate debris, fungal contaminants, and entrained air (Pall, 2000; Fig. 6–10).

When lipid emulsions are administered, a 0.45-micron filter is available for the removal of inadvertent particulate debris; air; and microbial contaminates such as *Candida albicans, Moraxella osloensis, Staphylococcus auras,* and *Klebsiella pneumoniae* (Fig. 6–11).

Blood Filters

The American Association of Blood Banks states that blood must be transfused through a sterile, pirogue-free transfusion set that has a filter capable of retaining particles that are potentially harmful to the recipient (Vengelen-Tyler, 1996). Commercially available filters include the standard clot filter, the microaggregate filter, and the leukocyte depletion filter. For further details on blood filters, see Chapter 12.

INS STANDARDS Blood filters are used to remove particulate matter from blood and its components. Nurses should be knowledgeable regarding filters and filter requirements of various blood components. (INS, 2000, 38)

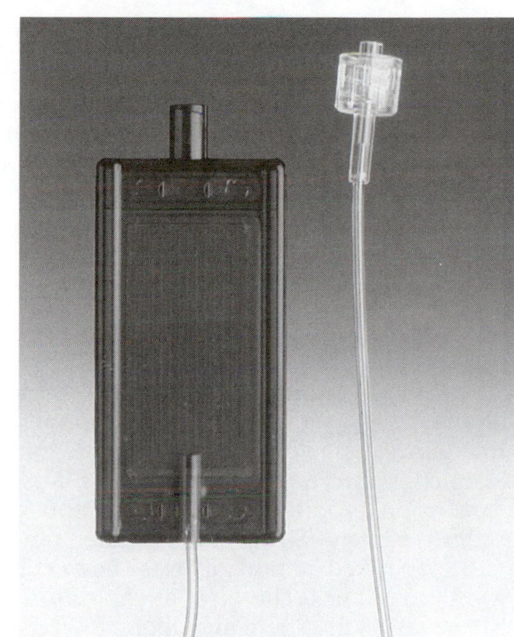

FIG. 6–10. Air-eliminating filter set designed for total nutrient admixture solutions. This filter has a 1.2-micron nylon membrane that provides an effective barrier for patient from inadvertent particulate contamination, uncontrollable precipitate contamination, and entrained air. (Courtesy of Pall Corporation, Port Washington, New York.)

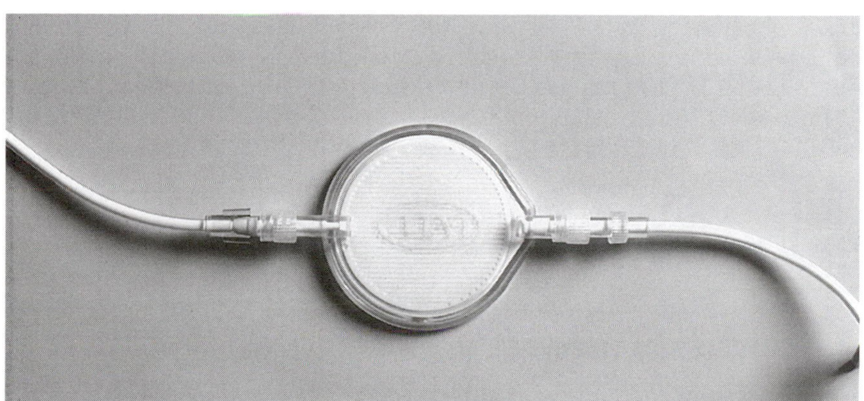

FIG. 6–11. Lipipor emulsive filter contains a 0.45-micron filter used for removal of inadvertent particulate debris, entrained air, and microbial contamination of drug lipid emulsions. (Courtesy of Pall Corporation, Port Washington, New York.)

Standard Clot Filters

Blood administration sets have a standard clot filter of 170 to 220 microns. They are intended to remove coagulated products, microclots, and debris resulting from collection and storage. These filters allow passage of smaller particles called microaggregates, which are composed of nonviable leukocytes, primarily granulocytes, platelets, and fibrin strands. The microaggregates can cause pulmonary dysfunction (adult respiratory distress syndrome) when large quantities of stored bank blood are infused.

Microaggregate Filters

A supplementary filter (transfusion filter) can be added to an in-use administration set, permitting infusion of blood, easy replacement of the filter (if clogging occurs), and multiple infusion of blood units. The 20- to 40-micron **microaggregate** blood filters remove most debris from the transfusion product but can slow the administration of blood to an undesirable rate. The 40-micron filter allows blood to be transfused easily in the specified period of time; however, filtration is less refined. The 80-micron filter is the filter of choice in many institutions because of its safe level of filtration and high flow rate potential (Jensen, 1995). A microaggregate filter is a free-flow, low priming volume device that provides a 40-micron rated screen filter medium for the removal of potentially harmful blood components, microaggregates, and nonblood component particulate matter (Pall, 2000) (Fig. 6–12).

Leukocyte Depletion Filters

Leukocyte depletion filters are used to remove leukocytes (including leukocyte-mediated viruses) from red blood cells and platelets. Leukocyte-poor filters are classified according to efficiency level, not micron size (Pall Biomedical Corporation, 2000). These filters can be used to remove 99.9 percent of leukocytes from red blood cells, platelets, and plasma (Pall, 2000) (Fig. 6–13).

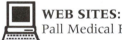

WEB SITES:
Pall Medical Filter information: *www.pall.com/medical*

EXTENSION TUBINGS

Extension tubings are add-on sets used to add I.V. line length. Commonly used with active patients, these sets, which come in various lengths, aid in tubing changes without site manipulation. Extension tubing is also frequently used as primary tubing for syringe pumps and ambulatory pumps. Disadvantages are an added cost and an additional site for bacteria to enter the system.

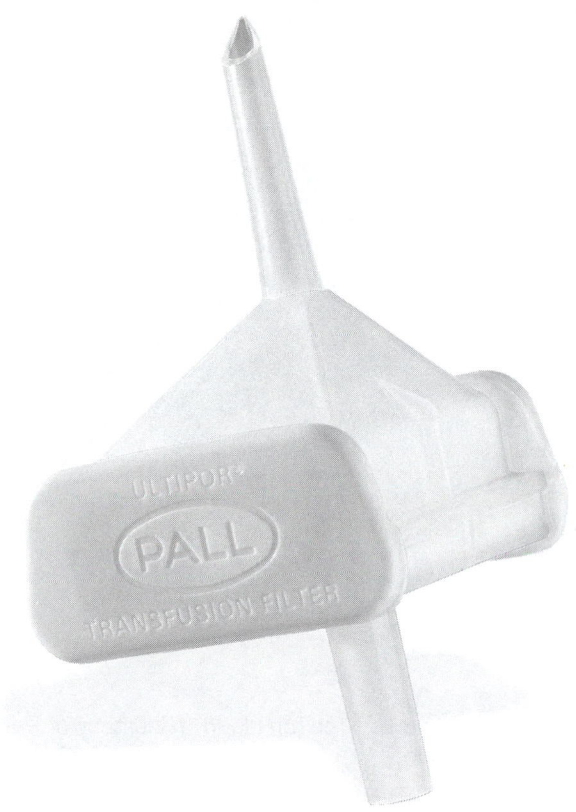

FIG. 6–12. Microaggregate blood transfusion filter. (Courtesy of Pall Corporation, Port Washington, New York.)

ADAPTERS AND CONNECTORS (LOOPS)

J-, U-, or T-shaped adapters and connectors may be used at the injection site. The T port is a common add-on device that is usually about 4 to 6 inches long and is made of standard or microbore tubing with a hard plastic T-shaped connector on one end. One leg of the T connector attaches to the I.V. device with the other a resealable latex port.

The J loop or U connector has the same purpose as the T connector. Their rigid shape is maintained when connected to an I.V. site.

Disadvantages of I.V. adapter and connector loops are increased cost and increased potential for infection because of the increased opportunity for manipulation and risk of separation. Their use should be limited (Fig. 6–14).

INS STANDARDS All add-on devices should be of Luer-Lok design. Tape should not be used as a means of junction securement. (INS, 2000, 35)

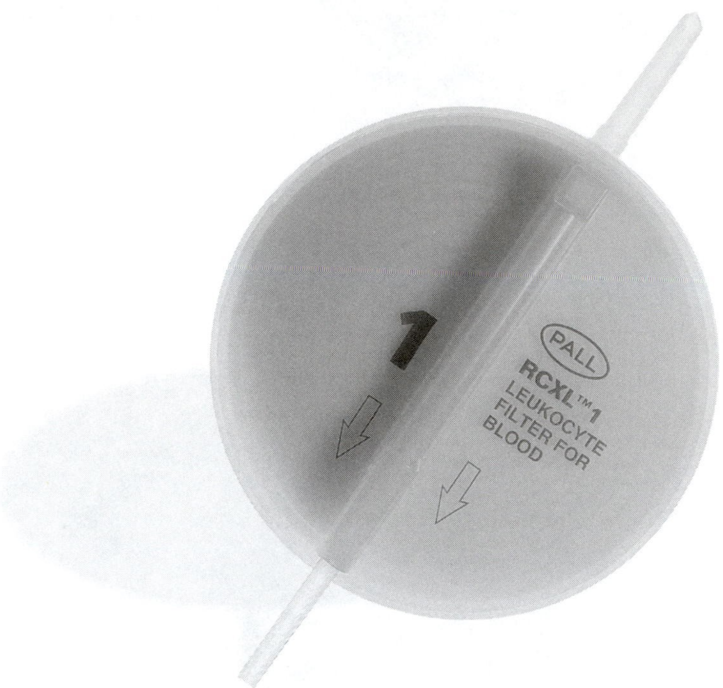

FIG. 6–13. RCXL 1 leukocyte filter for blood. (Courtesy of Pall Corporation, Port Washington, New York.)

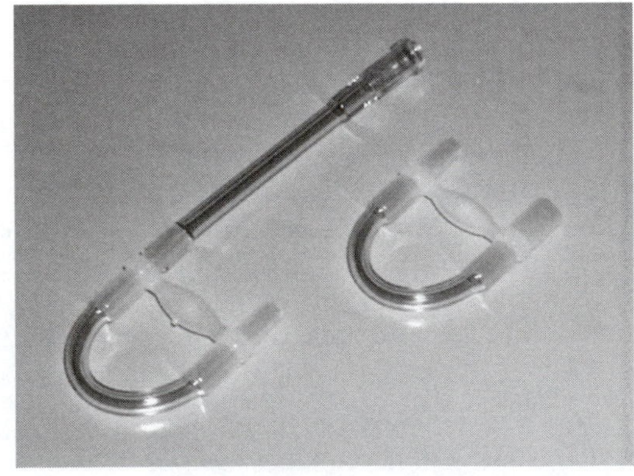

FIG. 6–14. J- and U-shaped add-on devices. (Courtesy of Becton Dickinson, Franklin Lakes, New Jersey.)

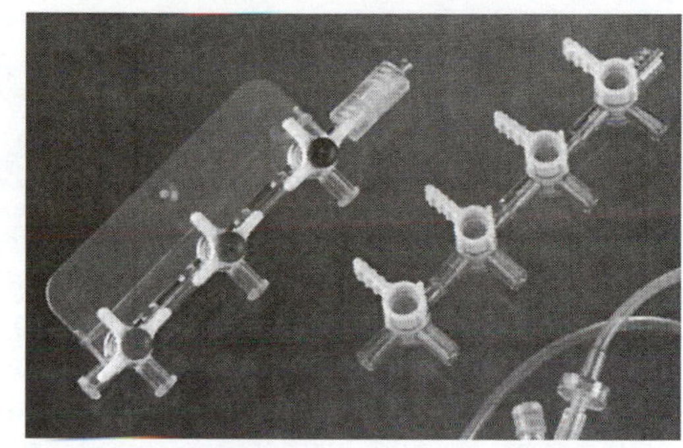

FIG. 6–15. Stopcocks: (Courtesy of B. Braun Medical Inc., Bethlehem, Pennsylvania.)

STOPCOCKS

A stopcock is a device that controls the direction of flow of an infusate through manual manipulation of a direction-regulating valve (Fig. 6–15). A stopcock is usually a three- or four-way device. A three-way stopcock connects two lines of fluid to a patient and provides a mechanism for either one to run to the patient (similar to a faucet). With a four-way stopcock, the valve can be manipulated so that one or both lines can run to the patient, alone, or in combination (Josephson, 1999).

The general use of stopcocks is strongly discouraged because of the issue of contamination. When the stopcock portals are uncapped, they are vulnerable to touch contamination. The stopcock itself is small and requires handling in such a way that sterility can easily be compromised. Syringes are frequently attached to I.V. push administration, and the portal is poorly protected after use (Jensen, 1995).

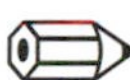 **NOTE:** Caution should be used when using a stopcock because of the risk of contamination of the I.V. system or accidental disconnection if a Luer-Lok connection is not used or if the stopcock is accidentally turned. Also, the infusion may be interrupted or administered incorrectly.

INJECTION ACCESS PORTS

Injection access ports or caps are locking devices also known as resealable **PRN** devices. A **locking device** is a capped resealable diaphragm that may have a Luer-Lok or Luer slip connection. The diaphragms may be made of latex, but many manufacturers are now making latex-free diaphragms because of increased sensitivities to latex. This type of device can convert continuous I.V. infusion to an intermittent device when a resealable plug is inserted into the cannula hub. The resealable lock is used for saline or heparin flush (Fig. 6–16).

A disadvantage of the resealable lock is that it can separate at the hub or plug junction, allowing bacteria to enter the system because of inadequate

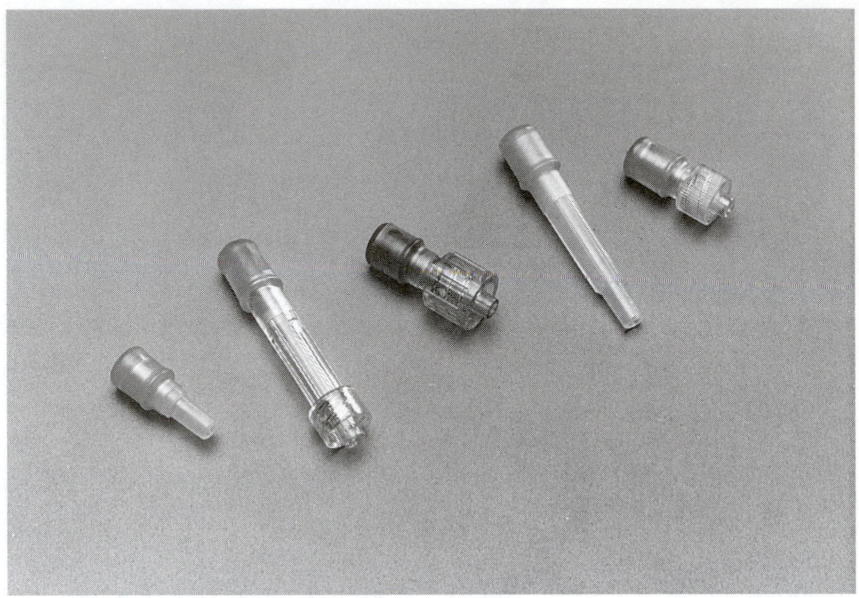

FIG. 6–16. Injection access ports (PRN adapters). (Courtesy of Becton-Dickinson.)

flushing of blood cells from under the latex rubber. In addition, an occlusion or blood clot can occur within the locking device.

INS STANDARDS Injection access ports should be aseptically cleansed with an approved antimicrobial solution immediately before use. (INS, 2000, 41)

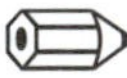

NOTE: Large-bore needles or frequent needle punctures may remove a plug of rubber from the **port,** resulting in coring. The risk of coring is difficult to predict; therefore, injection caps should be routinely changed according to institutional protocol.

NEEDLELESS SYSTEMS

Needleless systems and needle safety systems are the state-of-the-art technology of needle systems and are used to connect I.V. devices, administer infusates and medications, and sample blood.

Needlestick injuries among healthcare workers occur at an estimated 1 million per year (Goodman, 1997). Nurses and other healthcare workers are at risk of occupation exposure to HIV, hepatitis B and C virus (HBV and HCV), and other bloodborne pathogens. Chapters 1 and 2 provide detailed information on risks associated with infusion therapy.

The current cost for a single percutaneous injury is estimated at between $500 and $1000, with more than $500 million being spent annually for needlestick injuries.

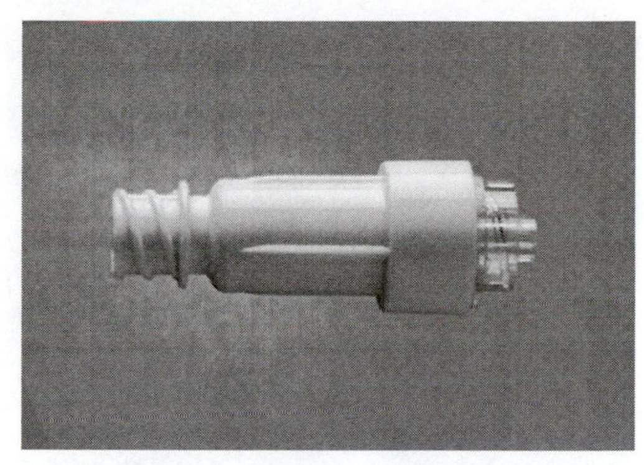

FIG. 6–17. ULTRASITE needle-free valve. (Courtesy of B. Braun Medical Inc., Bethlehem, Pennsylvania.)

The use of protected needles or needleless equipment significantly decreases the risk of needlestick injuries (Chiarello, Nagin, & Laufer, 1992). Two types of devices are available: (1) I.V. delivery systems that are needleless and (2) shielded needles. Needleless systems were introduced in March of 1992 when the United States Occupational Safety and Health Administration (OSHA, 1992) mandated that healthcare facilities "look for engineering controls that make the environment healthier and safer for workers" (Horner, 1998).

The needleless system consists of a blunt-tipped plastic insertion device and an injection port that opens and immediately reseals (Figs. 6–17 and 6–18).

The shielded needle design provides FDA guidelines that require that the device be designed to require the worker's hands to remain behind the needle as it is covered (FDA, 1995). The shielded needle provides protection for the practitioner after the stylet is withdrawn from the catheter during insertion into a vein. The needle is usually locked within a needle guard (Fig. 6–19).

To purchase a report on needlestick prevention devices, contact the Emergency Care Research Institute (ECRI) which is an independent, nonprofit agency evaluating medical devices.

ECRI
5200 Butler Pike
Plymouth Meeting, PA 19462
610-825-6000 ext. 5888

WEB SITES:

Emergency Care Research Institute (ECRI): *www.ECRI.com*
Johnson & Johnson Vanishpoint: *www.vanishpoint.com*
Service Employees International Union (SEIU): *www.serv.org/new*
International Health Care Worker Safety Center: *hsc.virginia.edw/epinet*

Table 6–2 presents a list of I.V. safety products and devices.

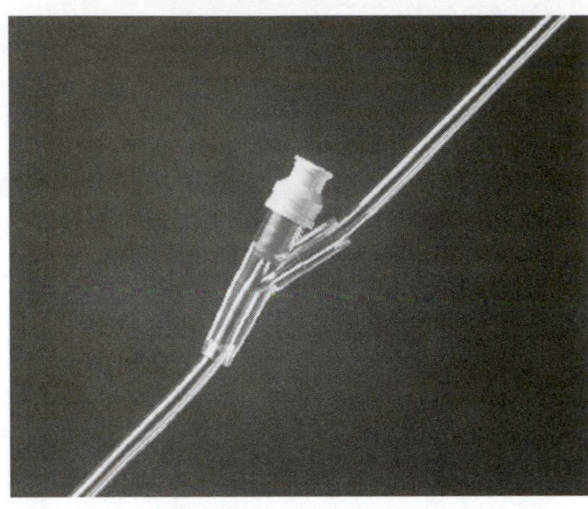

FIG. 6–18. SmartSite needle-free system. (Courtesy of Alaris Medical Systems, San Diego, California.)

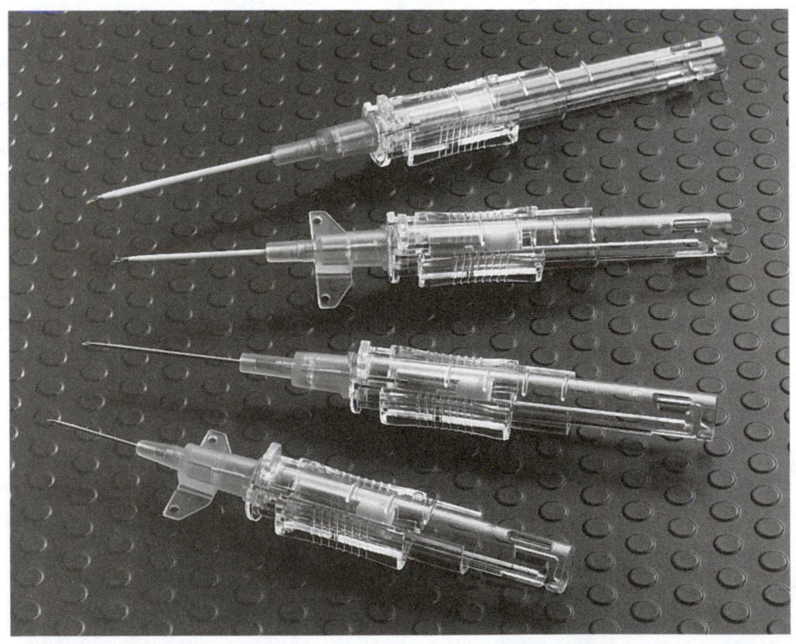

FIG. 6–19. Shielded needle system PROTECTIV catheters. (Courtesy of Johnson & Johnson, Arlington, Texas.)

TABLE 6–2

SAFETY PRODUCTS AND DEVICES

Retractable needles
- NMT Safety Syringe: New Medical Technology, Inc.
- Vanish Point Syringe: Retractable Technologies Safety 1st R Safety Syringe: Safety 1st Medical Inc.

Recessed or protected needle
- LifeShield Connector: Abbott Laboratories
- Needle Lock Device: Baxter/Becton Dickinson
- Versa-Lok and Pro-Lok: Beech Medical
- Click Lock and Piggy Lock: ICU Medical
- Protected Needle System: B.Braun
- Centurion Uni-Guard Piggy Back Connector: Tri-State Hospital Supply

Needle-free valve
- Safsite System: B.Braun
- Clave connector: ICU Medical
- AVI Checkvalve: 3M Health Care

I.V. insertion equipment
- Shielded or retracting peripheral I.V. catheters
  - Insyte Auto Guard shielded I.V. catheter: Becton Dickinson
  - Saf-T-Intima I.V. catheter safety system: Becton Dickinson
  - ProtectIV and ProtectIV Plus I.V. catheter safety system: Johnson & Johnson Medical, Inc
- Midline I.V. catheters
  - Biovue PICC/Midline catheter with Protective Safety Introducer: Johnson & Johnson Medical, Inc.

I.V. medication delivery systems
- Needle-free I.V. access-blunted cannulas
  - Life Shield System: Abbott Laboratories
  - Interlink I.V. Access System: Baxter/Becton Dickinson
  - POSIFLOW valve: Becton Dickinson

PVC alternatives
- I.V. bags
  - B.Braun, CharterMed
- Film for I.V. bags
  - Dow Plastics, Cryovac North America, Huntsman Polymer Corp., Montell Polyolefins, Eastman Chemical Co.
- Tubing
  - Huntsman Polymer Corp, 3M Co., Exxon Chemical, Dupont Dow Elastomers, Norton Performance Plastics Corp.
- Plasma collection bags
  - Medsep Corp.
- 3-in-1 mixing containers
  - B.Braun
- Gloves
  - Coast Scientific

PERIPHERAL INFUSION DEVICES

Several types of peripheral infusion devices are commercially available: scalp vein needles, over-the-needle catheters, through-the-needle catheters, midline catheters, and dual **lumen** catheters. The catheter-type devices usually have **radiopaque** material or stripping added to ensure radiographic visibility. Radiopacity aids in the identification of a catheter embolus, a rare complication. The hub of a cannula is plastic and color coded to indicate the length and **gauge.**

The most common catheter materials include polytetrafluoroethylene (Teflon) which is less thrombogenic and less inflammatory than polyurethane or PVC, and Vialon a newer material that is nonhemolytic and free of plasticizers. Vialon is slick when wetted and softens after insertion, minimizing venous trauma and clot induction. For a comparison of the types of peripheral infusion devices, see Table 6–3.

INS STANDARDS The cannula selected shall be of the smallest gauge and the shortest length to accommodate the prescribed therapy. Catheters shall be radiopaque. A short peripheral catheter is defined as one that is smaller than 3 inches in length. The term "cannula" refers to a stainless steel needle or the catheter. (INS, 2000, 44)

SCALP VEIN NEEDLES

The wing-tipped or butterfly needles are types of scalp vein needles. Scalp vein needles are made of stainless steel with odd-numbered gauges (i.e., 17, 19, 21, 23, 25) and lengths of 0.5 to 1.0 inch. The wings attached to the shaft are made of rubber or plastic, and the flexible tubing extending behind the wings varies from 3 to 12 inches long (Fig. 6–20).

These needles are most frequently used for short-term therapy, usually in patients with expected indwelling catheter times of less than 24 hours, such as with single-dose therapy, I.V. push medications, or blood sample retrieval (Jensen, 1995). Steel needles are biocompatible, and low rates of inflammation or phlebitis have been documented. Steel cannulas do not flex or yield with resistance; therefore, the steel tip can easily puncture the vasculature after placement, increasing the risk of infiltration.

INS STANDARDS Because stainless steel needles tend to dislodge and infiltrate more frequently than catheters, their use should be limited to short-term or single-dose administration. (INS, 2000, 44)

OVER-THE-NEEDLE CATHETERS

The over-the-needle catheter (ONC) consists of a needle with a catheter sheath (Fig. 6–21). The point of the needle extends beyond the tip of the catheter. After venipuncture, the needle (**stylet**) is withdrawn and discarded, leaving a flexible catheter within the vein. The cannula consists of a catheter with a length of 0.5 to 2.0 inches and gauges of even numbers

TABLE 6–3

COMPARISON OF PERIPHERAL INFUSION DEVICES

Cannula	Advantages	Disadvantages	Uses
Scalp vein needle	Excellent for one-time I.V. medication, blood withdrawal, in patients allergic to nylon or Teflon Wings allow ease of insertions and secure taping Attached extension permits easy tubing change	Needle increases the risk of infiltration Not recommended for use in flexor areas Needle not flexible Repuncture by contaminated needle possible	Infants and children Elderly and other adults with small veins Adults receiving short-term therapy
Over-the-needle	Easy to insert Stays patent longer Catheter tip tapered to prevent peelback Radiopaque feature makes radiographic detection easy Infiltration rare Winged cannula easy to tape Stable; allows for greater patient mobility	Depending on the hub, sometimes difficult to secure with tape Long inflexible stylet increases the risk of accidental puncture; pressure marks from hub Some catheters drag through the skin on insertion Increased risk of phlebitis	Long-term therapy Delivery of viscous liquids: blood and total parenteral nutrition Arterial monitoring
Through-the-needle	Permits insertion of catheter into the SVC Less likely to damage veins Stable	Needle remains secured outside the skin; risk of catheter embolus Plastic catheter may support infection or trigger phlebitis in central veins	Long-term therapy Delivery of viscous liquid Delivery of drugs Central venous pressure monitoring

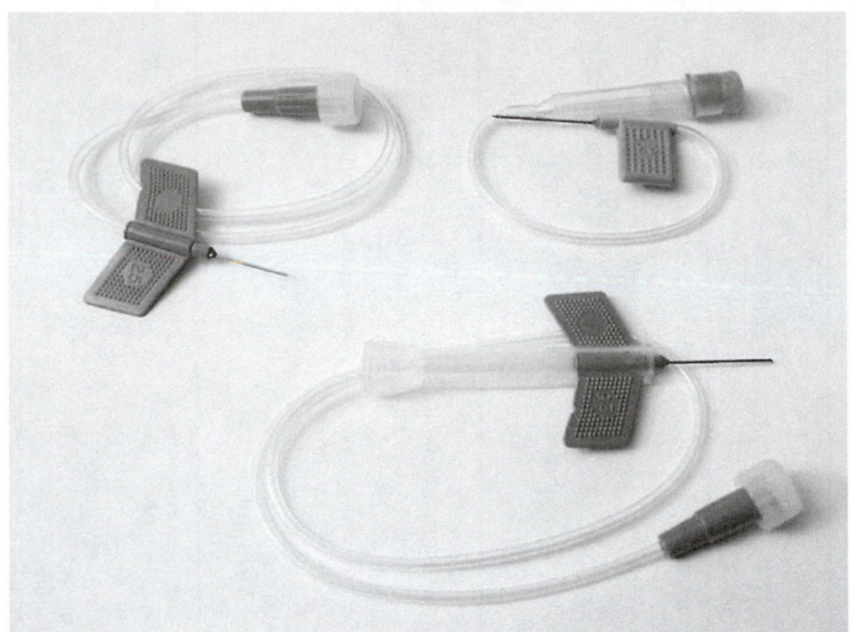

FIG. 6–20. Types of scalp vein needles. (Courtesy of Becton Dickinson, Franklin Lakes, New Jersey.)

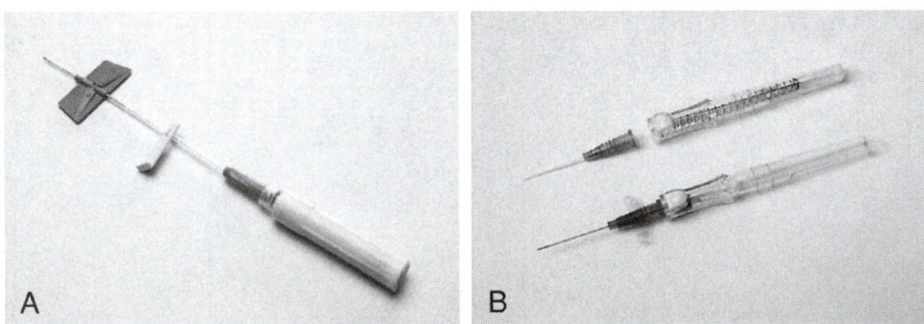

FIG. 6–21. Over-the-needle catheters: (*A*) Integrated I.V. catheter with safety shield SAF-T-INTIMA. (*B*) Insyte with safety shield. (Courtesy of Becton Dickinson, Franklin Lakes, New Jersey.)

ranging from 12 to 24. Use the following as a guide regarding when to use the different gauge catheters:

- 14 to 16 gauge: Multiple trauma, heart surgery, transplantation procedures
- 18 gauge: Major trauma or surgery, blood administration
- 20 gauge: Minor trauma or surgery, blood administration
- 22 gauge: Pediatric use, person with small veins, administration of platelets or plasma (avoid using 22-gauge catheters when administering packed red blood cells, whole blood, and antibiotic therapy)

Catheters are made of various biocompatible materials such as Teflon and Vialon (Becton Dickinson). Teflon, a polyurethane material, has been shown to provide low cost, low rates of infiltration, and comparatively low rates of phlebitis. Teflon is a plastic-coated catheter material that is less thrombogenic and less inflammatory than simple PVC or polyurethane (Altavela, Haas, & Nowak, 1993). Teflon over-the-needle catheters tend to increase the risk of infusion-related phlebitis with small peripheral venous catheters (Maki & Ringer, 1991).

Vialon, an elastomer of polyurethane, is a high-strength material that provides a smooth-surfaced catheter for easy insertion. After it is inside a vein, Vialon becomes soft and pliable, permitting the catheter to float in the vein rather than against the intima of the vein wall. Vialon is also designed to minimize local reactions under conditions of extended use (McKee et al., 1989).

INS STANDARDS Radiopaque over-the-needle catheters are recommended for routine infusion therapy. (INS, 2000, 44)

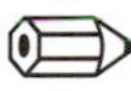

NOTE: With any catheter use, the shortest length and the smallest gauge to deliver the ordered therapy. Also, use a vein large enough to sustain sufficient blood flow because this will decrease irritation to the vein wall.

THROUGH-THE-NEEDLE CATHETERS

A through-the-needle catheter (TNC) consists of a catheter between 14 and 19 gauges in diameter lying inside a needle. The needle may be from 1 to 2 inches long, and the catheter may be 8 to 36 inches long. The newer type of through-the-needle catheters, mainly seen in peripherally inserted central venous access devices, have a steel or plastic encasement that can be removed after the catheter is advanced into the vein. After the catheter is placed, the needle is withdrawn and secured outside the skin. Because the catheter is radiopaque, confirmation by radiographic examination can be done before administration of viscous solutions.

DUAL-LUMEN PERIPHERAL CATHETERS

The dual-lumen peripheral catheter is available in a range of catheter gauges with corresponding lumen sizes. Two totally separate infusion channels exist, making it possible to infuse two solutions simultaneously. They are available as 16-gauge catheters with 18- and 20-gauge lumens or as 18-gauge catheters with 22- and 20-gauge lumens. Dual-lumen catheters are also available as midlines.

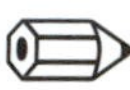 **NOTE:** Controversy still exists regarding simultaneous infusions of known incompatible solutions or medications through a dual-lumen peripheral catheter because of the limited hemodilution achievable in any peripheral vessel (Collins & Lutz, 1991).

MIDLINE AND MIDCLAVICULAR CATHETERS

Numerous controversial issues and practice inconsistencies surround the use and application of peripherally placed non–central venous catheters with tip location in the upper arm and axillary–subclavian vein areas. Other terms for the midline or midclavicular catheters include "long line," "halfway," "midline," "PIC," and "extended peripheral" (INS, 1997).

Any catheter placed between the antecubital area and the head of the clavicle is called a midline catheter. **Midline catheters** are designed for intermediate-term therapies of up to 28 days of isotonic or near isotonic therapy. The catheters are 6 inches long and are made of elastomeric hydrogel. Approximately 2 hours after insertion, this type of catheter becomes 50 times softer, allowing it to increase 2 gauges in size and 2.5 cm in length (Meares, 1992). It is placed midline in the antecubital region in the basilic, cephalic, or median antecubital site and is then advanced into the larger vessels of the upper arm for greater hemodilution (Fig. 6–22).

Radiologic confirmation of the tip location is recommended in the following clinical situations:

- Difficulty with catheter advancement
- Pain or discomfort after catheter advancement
- Inability to obtain free-flowing blood return
- Inability to flush the catheter easily
- When the guidewire is difficult to remove or is bent after removal

Midclavicular catheters are peripherally inserted with the tip location in the proximal axillary or subclavian vein. If a line intended for the superior vena cava (SVC) location falls short and ends up in the brachiocephalic (innominate) vein, it should be considered midclavicular. The tip location in this anatomic area is not considered a "midline" or a **peripherally inserted central catheter (PICC)**. The intended tip location is the proximal axillary or subclavian vein.

Midclavicular catheters may be the appropriate choice for I.V. fluid, electrolytes, and other medications commonly administered through peripheral veins and administration of isotonic solutions. This type of

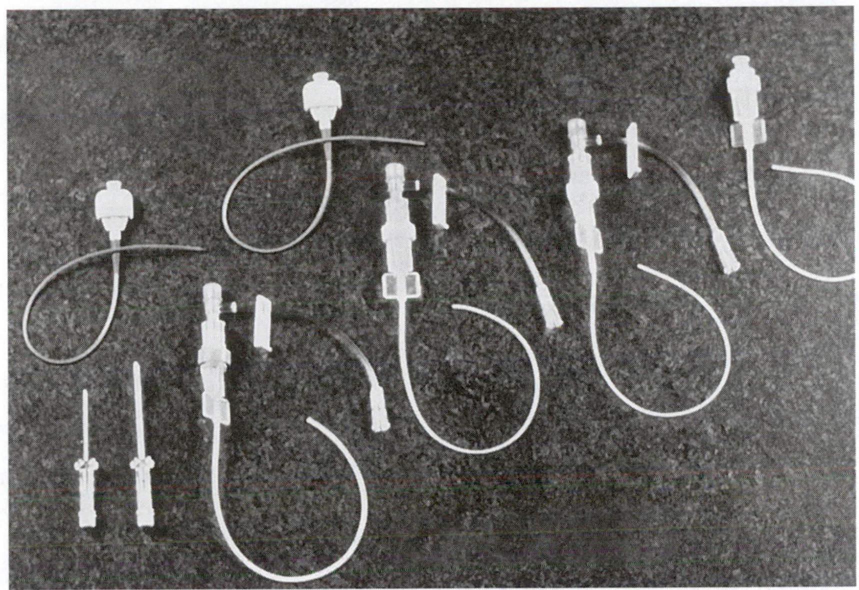

FIG. 6-22. Examples of midline catheters. (Courtesy of BARD Access Systems, Salt Lake City, Utah.)

catheter may be most appropriate if disease-produced or surgically created anomalies prevent tip location in SVC. Radiologic confirmation of the tip location is recommended for midclavicular catheters and is the same as for midline catheters with the addition of pain, discomfort, feelings of fullness or coldness, or hearing gurgling sounds during flushing (INS, 1997).

INS STANDARDS The choice of catheter and appropriate nursing care for midline catheters should be established in organizational policy and procedure. (INS, 2000, 44)

Guidelines for PICC, midline, and midclavicular catheters are presented in Chapter 11.

CENTRAL INFUSION DEVICES

Long-term I.V. therapy may require venous access over weeks, months, or even years. Special central venous catheters have been designed specifically for long-term access, patient comfort, and decreased complications associated with multiple therapies. There are three general types of placement of central venous lines: centrally placed percutaneous catheters and central venous tunneled catheters, both of which must be inserted by a physician, and PICCs, which can be inserted by a nurse specifically trained in their insertions.

Central catheters are made of soft, medical grade silicone elastomers, thermoplastic polyurethane, or PVC and are commercially available in many designs. Polyurethane catheters are the most commonly used catheters because of the material's versatility, malleability (tensile strength and elongation characteristics), and biocompatibility (Brown, 1995).

Central lines include:

- Percutaneous catheters
- Central venous tunneled catheters
- Implantable venous access ports
- PICCs

Various types of central line catheters in use today are discussed in detail in Chapter 11.

PERCUTANEOUS CATHETERS

In 1961, the first I.V. catheter for accessing the central circulation was introduced (Stewart & Sanislow, 1961). The percutaneous catheter is placed by an infraclavicular approach through the subclavian vein (or the jugular or femoral vein) and secured by suturing. The final tip location should be in the SVC. The catheter may remain in place for a few days to several weeks. This type of catheter provides access to larger venous circulation for the delivery of hypertonic solutions.

CENTRAL VENOUS TUNNELED CATHETERS

Central venous **tunneled catheters** (CVTCs) are made of soft, medical grade silicone elastomers. CVTs have a Dacron cuff near the subcutaneous exit site of the catheter that anchors it in place, acts as a securing device, and serves as a microbial barrier. CVTCs are surgically inserted through percutaneous cutdown under local or general anesthesia. The distal catheter tip is advanced into the vessel and is placed in the SVC. The proximal end is subcutaneously tunneled to an incisional exit site on the anterior or posterior trunk of the body. The usual exit sites for CVTCs are the mid- to lower thoracic or upper abdominal regions. The Broviac, Hickman, and Groshong were prototypes of many of the more recently developed CVTCs. These catheters are 20 to 30 inches long and have a 22- to 17-gauge internal lumen diameter. The thickness of the silicone wall varies by manufacturer. Silicone catheters can be single, dual, triple, or quadruple lumen (Fig. 6–23).

IMPLANTABLE VENOUS ACCESS PORTS

The implantable venous access port is a completely closed system consisting of an implanted device with a drug reservoir, or port, with a self-sealing system connected to an outlet catheter. The device is surgically implanted into a convenient body site in a subcutaneous pocket. The

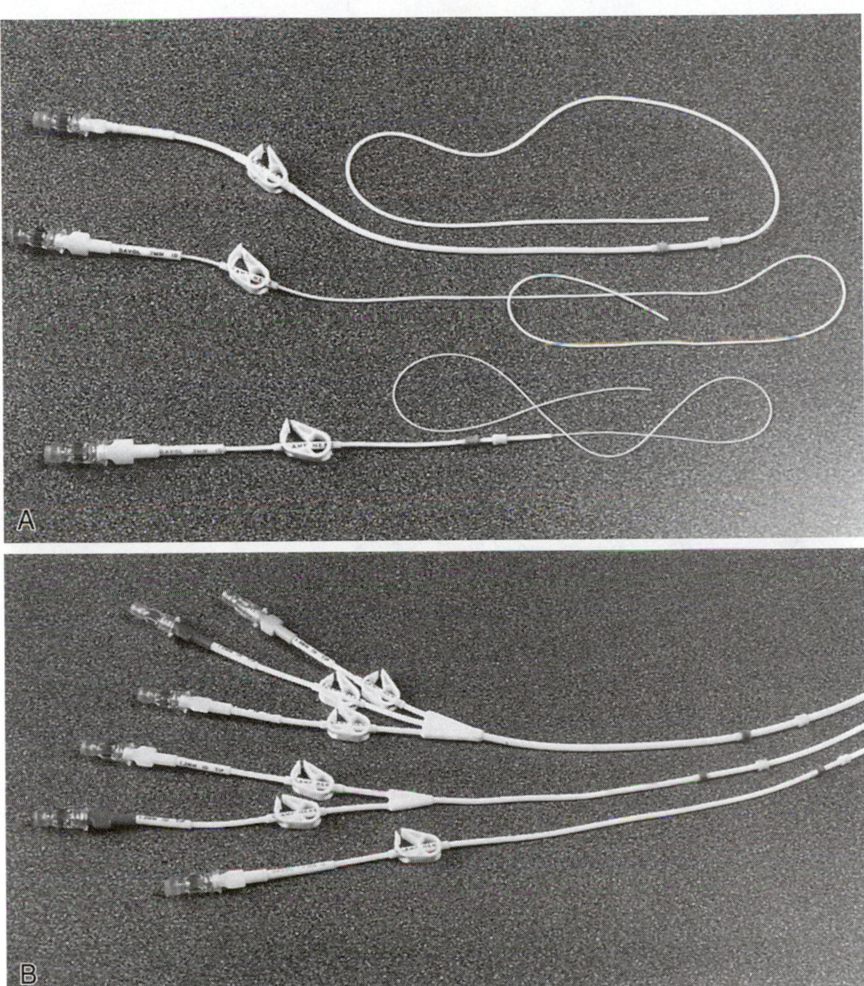

FIG. 6–23. (*A*) Hickman (top) and Broviac (bottom two) catheters. (*B*) Triple-lumen (top), double-lumen (middle), and single-lumen (bottom) central venous tunneled catheters.

self-sealing septum can withstand up to 2000 needle punctures. This device provides venous access for blood withdrawal, I.V. solution infusion, blood transfusion, and chemotherapy. The **implanted port** must be accessed with a Huber needle (noncoring) for safe and proper penetration of the septum of the port. Because these are noncoring needles, they contribute to the long lifetime of the port. The needles are sized from 19 to 24 gauge and range from 1 to 2 inches in length. The needles are available in 90-degree or straight-needle designs (Fig. 6–24).

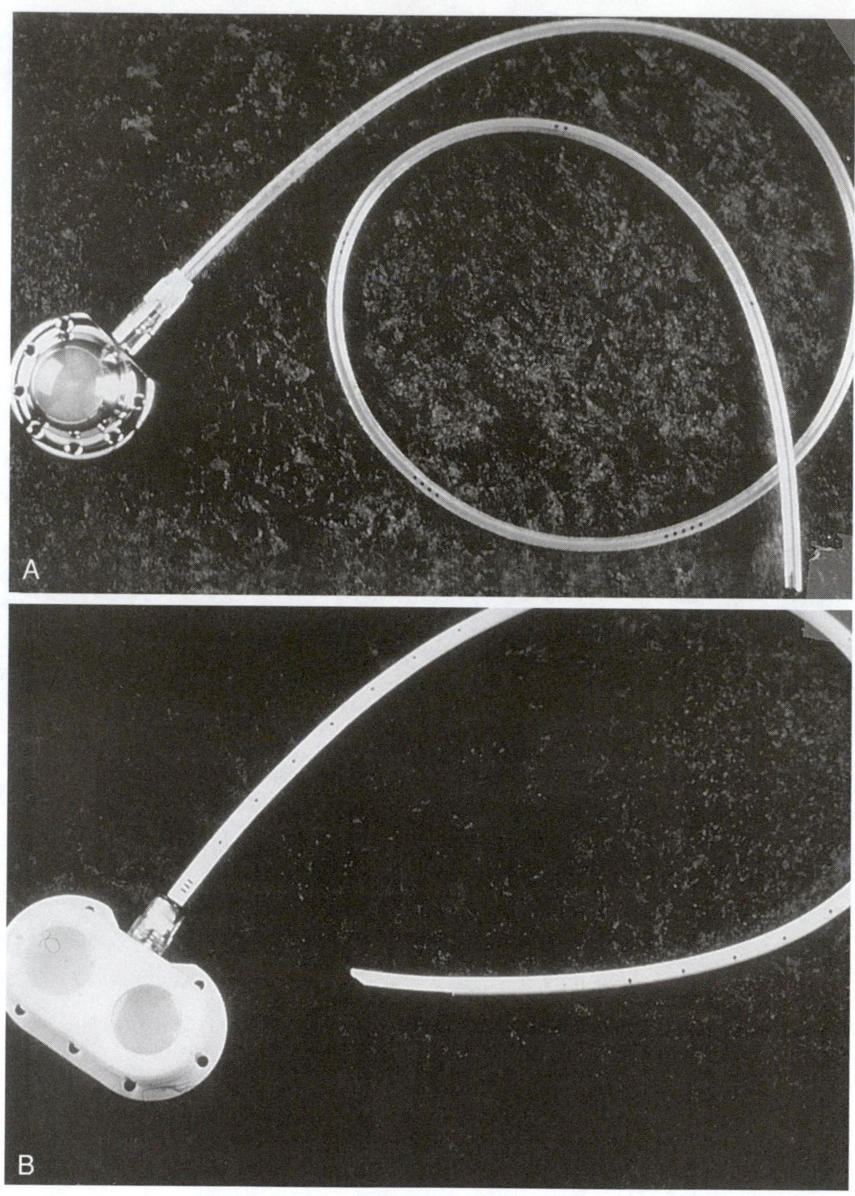

FIG. 6–24. (*A*) Dome port with Groshong valve. (*B*) MRI dual port. (Courtesy of BARD Access Systems, Salt Lake City, Utah.)

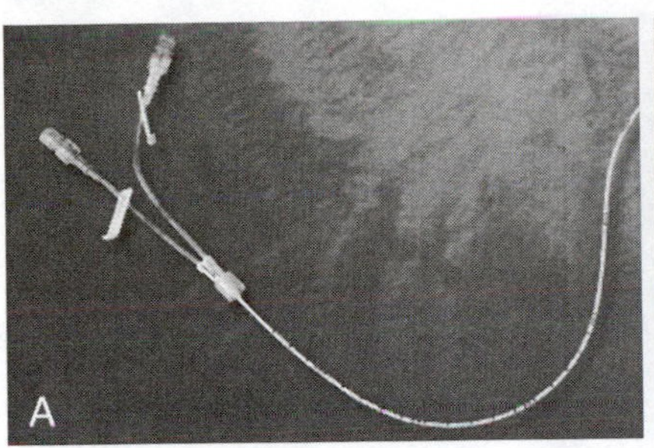

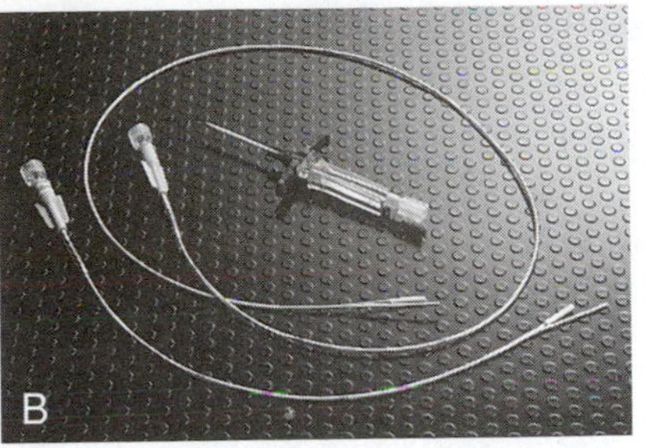

FIG. 6–25. Peripherally inserted central venous catheters (PICC) (*A*) ACCUGUIDE PICC catheter. (Courtesy of B. Braun Medical, Bethlehem, Pennsylvania.) (*B*) BIOVUE PICC/midline catheter with PROTECTIV safety introducer. (Courtesy of Johnson & Johnson, Arlington, Texas.)

PERIPHERALLY INSERTED CENTRAL VENOUS CATHETERS

A PICC is placed with tip location in the SVC. This catheter usually ranges from 16 to 26 gauges and from 20 to 24 inches in length. The peripheral catheter is inserted into a peripheral site and advanced into the SVC. To reach the SVC in the average adult, a catheter at least 20 inches long is required. The catheter is made of silicone, which has proven reliability and biocompatibility over the years in central venous catheter application as well as a variety of implant uses. Silicone elastomer is soft, flexible, nonthrombogenic, and biocompatible (Fig. 6–25).

A PICC may be used to deliver all types of therapy. It is the appropriate choice for parenteral nutrition with dextrose content greater than 10 percent, continuous infusion of vesicant medications or medications with the ability to cause necrosis if they infiltrate, therapies with extreme variations in tonicity of pH, or anticipated extended I.V. therapy.

INS STANDARDS The catheter selected for a PICC shall be a radiopaque catheter designed for central placement by peripheral access. The length of the catheter should be such that the tip resides in the SVC. (INS, 2000, 44)

INFUSION REGULATION DEVICES

Historically, infusion systems were regulated with a roller clamp, which the nurse adjusted manually with the roller or screw clamp on the administration set. Today there are numerous mechanical and electronic devices available to assist nurses in maintaining an accurate infusion rate.

INS STANDARDS A flow-control device is used to assist in regulating a prescribed administration rate. (INS, 2000, 39)

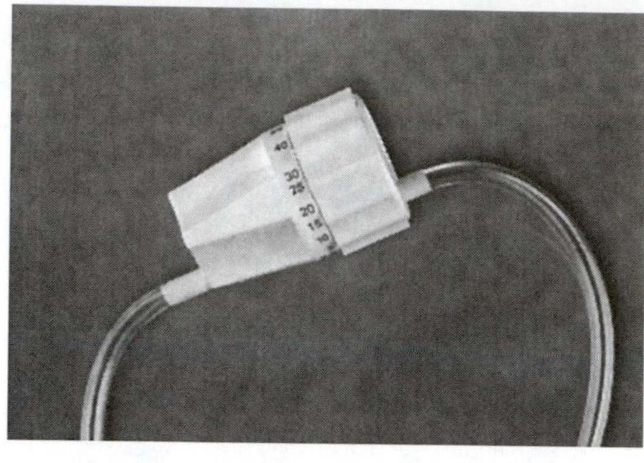

FIG. 6–26. Mechanical controller: Rate flow regulator. (Courtesy of B. Braun Medical Inc., Bethlehem, Pennsylvania.)

MECHANICAL GRAVITY DEVICES

Flow-regulating mechanisms that attach to the primary infusion administration sets are called mechanical gravity control devices (or mechanical controllers). They are manually set to deliver specified volumes of fluid per hour. They are available as dials, with clocklike faces, or a barrel-shaped device with cylindrical controls. Flow markings on the dials help to approximate the drops per minute, based on the set drop factor, but should be verified by counting the drops (Fig. 6–26).

INS STANDARDS Manual flow-control devices should achieve accurate delivery of prescribed therapy with minimal deviation and are an adjunct to nursing care and are not intended to alleviate the nurses responsibility for monitoring the flow rate of the therapy. (INS, 2000, 39)

ELECTRONIC INFUSION DEVICES

The use of EIDs (or flow-control devices) should be guided by the patient's age and condition, setting, and prescribed therapy. These devices provide an accurate flow rate, are easy to use, and have alarms that signal problems with the infusion. However, hourly assessment, responsibility, and accountability for safe infusion still lie with the professional nurse. To use these devices effectively, the nurse should know: (1) indications for their use, (2) their mechanical operation, (3) how to troubleshoot, (4) their psi rating, and (5) safe usage guidelines (Weinstein, 1997).

Infusion control devices have come a long way since their introduction in 1958. The very early models had serious accuracy and safety problems: air embolisms, fluid containers that ran dry, and clogged catheters were common. The pumps were large, hard to troubleshoot, and limited in their reliability and usability.

IVAC Corporation introduced the concept of the rate controller in 1972; today there are many models and types on the market, including:

- Controllers
- Positive pressure infusion pumps

- Volumetric pumps
- Peristaltic pumps
- Syringe pumps
- Patient-controlled analgesia (PCA) systems
- Multichannel and dual channel
- Ambulatory pumps
- Disposable pumps (Elastomere balloon pumps)

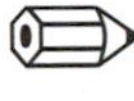

NOTE: Because of the many controllers and volumetric and peristaltic pumps on the market, refer to the manufacturer's recommendations for guidelines for set up and trouble shooting of each EID.

INS STANDARDS EIDs shall be used when warranted by the patient's age, condition, setting, and prescribed therapy. The nurse is responsible and accountable for the use of the EID. (INS, 2000, 39)

Controllers

Controllers operate strictly on gravity flow and do not exert positive pressure greater than the head height of the infusion bag, which is usually 2 psi. Some controllers can reach a psi of 5, but this pressure is uncommon. The maximum flow rate is affected by how high the I.V. container is hung above the I.V. site. Controllers cannot detect infiltrations. After the I.V. catheter leaves the vein and infiltrates into the tissues, the pressure drops. Because the infusion device is "looking" for pressure to signal an infiltration, it may be a long time with significant fluid accumulation before the infuser actually detects infiltration. It is always best to recommend that the nurse monitor the infusion visually and not rely on the infusion device to detect infiltrations.

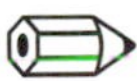

NOTE: One psi and 50 mm Hg exert the same amount of pressure.

A drop sensor and electric feedback mechanism regulate the gravity flow of the fluid. Controllers reduce the potential for rapid infusion of large amounts of solution (runaways) and empty bottles. Controllers assist the nurse in detecting infiltrations and maintaining accurate flow rates. It is estimated that 80 percent of I.V. fluid and drug administration can safely be regulated by the use of a controller.

The I.V. bag is usually hung 36 inches above a patient's head for adequate gravity pressure. When there is resistance to the flow, the controller's alarm will sound, signaling that it cannot maintain the preset rate. Resistance can occur when the patient is restless and frequently changing positions, if the catheter tip is at a flexion point, or if the patient lies on the tubing. Many of the newer controllers can deliver blood components safely (Fig. 6–27).

Positive Pressure Infusion Pumps

Positive pressure infusion pumps average 10 psi, with up to 15 psi considered to be safe, although newer technology has the psi set as low as

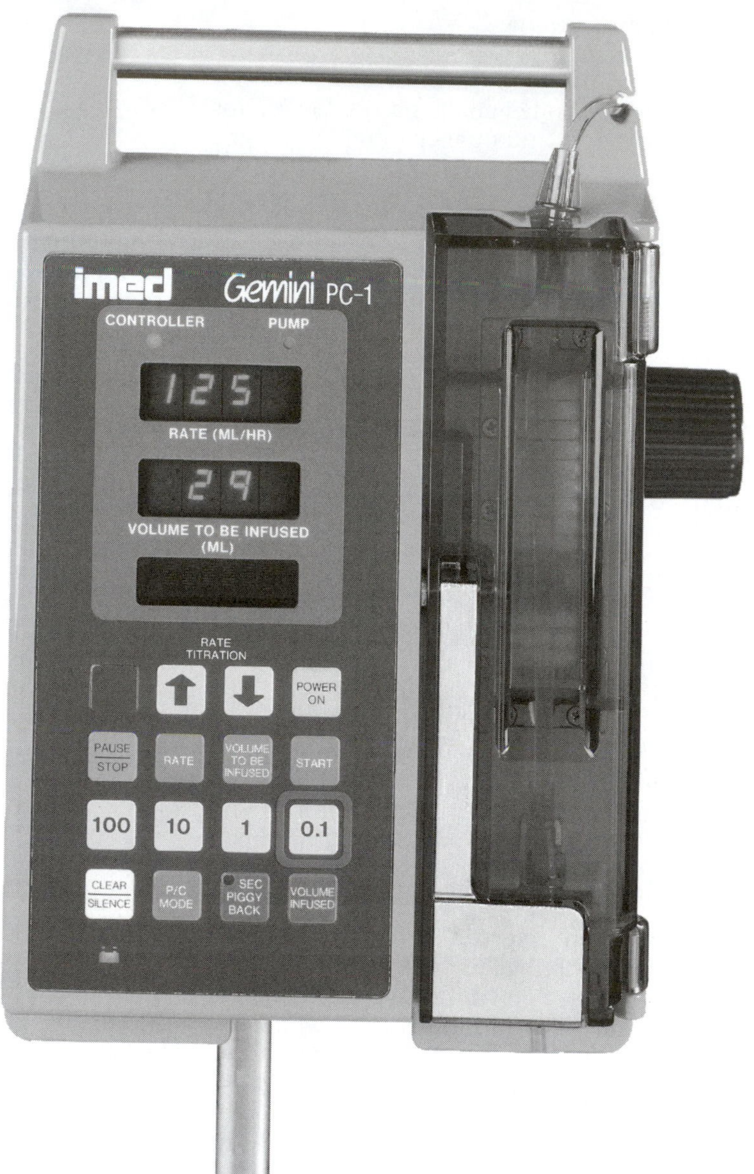

FIG. 6–27. Controller: IMED Gemini PC-1. (Courtesy of Alaris Medical Systems, San Diego, California.)

0.1 psi. Older pumps still in use may pump at dangerous pressures of 16 to 22 psi. Pressures greater than 15 to 20 psi should be used with extreme caution.

Positive pressure infusion pumps are used for delivering high volumes and complex therapies in high-acuity situations. The pumps are more precise than controllers; accurately deliver the fluid as programmed; and have many features, such as the ability to keep track of fluid amounts and to sound alarms for various malfunctions. These pumps totally control the flow rate.

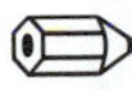

NOTE: All positive pressure pumps should have an "anti–free-flow" alarm to prevent inadvertent free-flowing solution.

Volumetric Pumps

Volumetric pumps calculate the volume delivered by measuring the volume displaced in a reservoir that is part of the disposable administration set. The pump calculates every fill and empty cycle of the reservoir. The reservoir is manipulated internally by a specific action of the pump. The industry standard for the accuracy of electronic volumetric infusion pumps is plus or minus 5 percent (Jensen, 1995).

Pressure terminology includes the terms "fixed" and "variable." With fixed infusion pressure, the pump is set internally to infuse up to a certain psi but not more (occlusion limit). Variable pressure pumps allow individual judgment about the psi needed to safely deliver therapy. Nurses can adjust a variable pressure pump through programming. Variable pressure devices have a conservative upper limit (usually 10 psi) and a lower limit of 2 psi similar to that of a controller. A psi setting of 4 to 8 is common.

Volumetric pumps have proved invaluable in neonatal, pediatric, and adult intensive care units, where critical infusions of small volumes of fluid or doses of high-potency drugs are indicated. A cartridge pumps the solution to be delivered; therefore, blood and red blood cells can be administered without damage to the blood cells.

Many pumps use microprocessor technology for a more compact unit and for easier troubleshooting. All volumetric pumps require special tubing (Fig. 6–28).

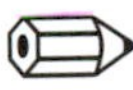

NOTE: To ensure safe, efficient operation, review the literature that accompanies the pump to become familiar with the operation of the pump. Observe all precautions.

Peristaltic Pumps

Peristaltic refers to the controlling mechanisms: a peristaltic device moves fluid by intermittently squeezing the I.V. tubing. The device may be rotary or linear. In a rotary peristaltic pump, a rotating disk or series of rollers compresses the tubing along a curved or semicircular chamber, propelling the fluid when pressure is released. In a linear device, one or more projections intermittently press the I.V. tubing. Peristaltic pumps are primarily used for the infusion of enteral feedings.

Syringe Pumps

Syringe pumps are piston-driven infusion pumps that provide precise infusion by controlling the rate by drive speed and syringe size,

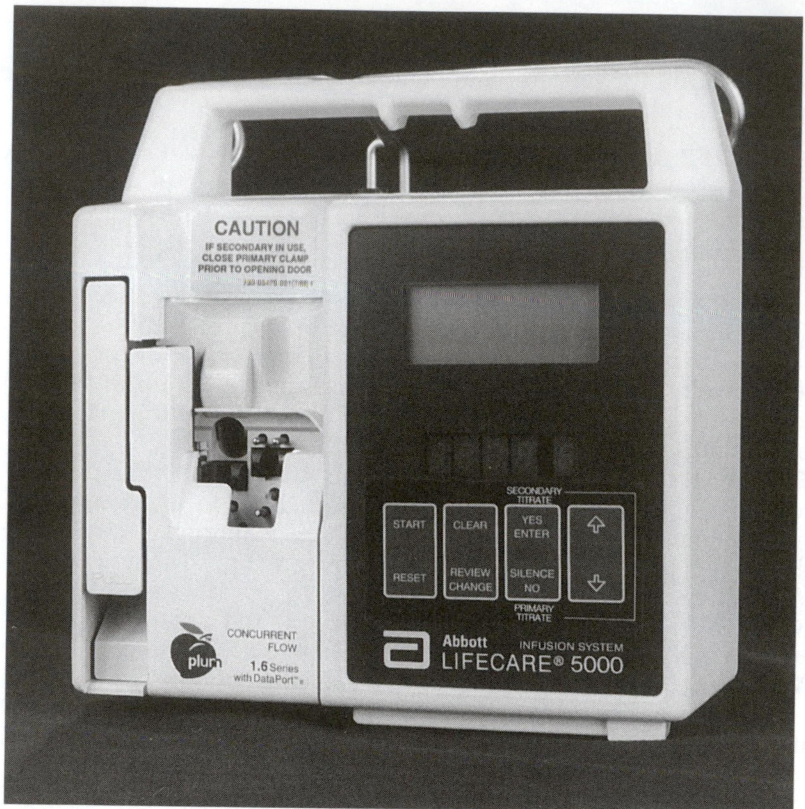

FIG. 6–28. Infusion pump: LIFECARE 5000. (Courtesy of Abbott Laboratories Hospital Products Division, North Chicago, Illinois.)

thus eliminating the variables of the drop rate. Syringe pumps are valuable for critical infusions of small doses of high-potency drugs. A lead, screw motor-driven system pushes the plunger to deliver fluid or medication at a rate of 0.01 to 99.9 mL/h. It is a precisely accurate delivery system that can be used to administer very small volumes. Some models have program modes capable of administration in meg/kg/min, mcg/min, and mL/h. The syringe is usually filled in the pharmacy and stored until used.

These pumps are used most frequently for delivery of antibiotics and small-volume parenteral therapy. Syringe pump technology was applied to PCA infusion devices. Syringe pumps are used frequently in the areas of anesthesia, oncology, and obstetrics.

The volume of the syringe pump is limited to the size of the syringe; a 60-mL syringe is usually used. However, the syringe can be as small as 5 mL. The tubing usually is a single, uninterrupted length of kink-resistant tubing with a notable lack of Y injection ports. Syringe pumps can use

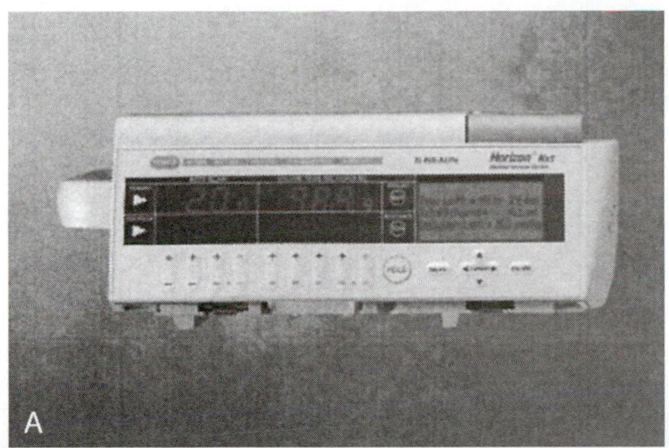

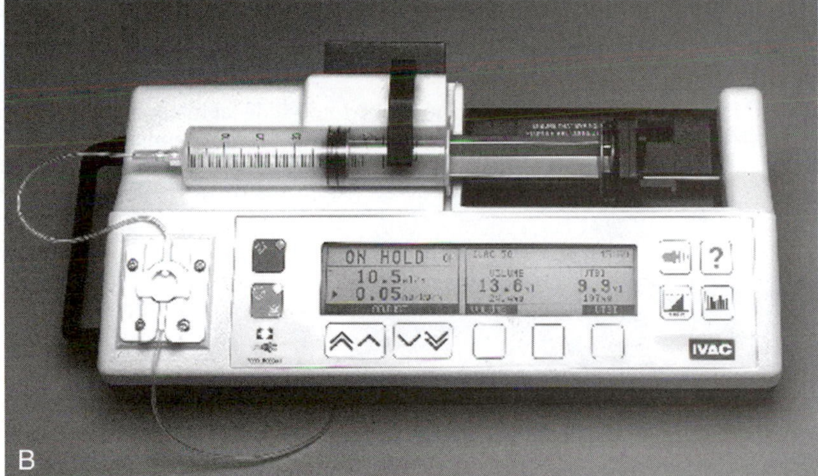

FIG. 6–29. Syringe pumps: (*A*) Horizon Nxt modular infusion system. (Courtesy of B. Braun Medical Inc., Bethlehem, Pennsylvania.) (*B*) IVAC Signature Edition. (Courtesy of Alaris Medical Systems. San Diego, California.)

primary or secondary sets, depending on the intended use (Jensen, 1995) (Fig. 6–29).

Patient-Controlled Analgesia Pumps

Patient-controlled analgesia (PCA) pumps have been developed to assist patients in controlling their pain at home or in the hospital. PCA pumps can be used to deliver medication through I.V., epidural, or subcutaneous routes. These pumps are different from other infusion devices in that they have a remote bolus control in which the patient or nurse can deliver a bolus of medication at set intervals. PCA pumps are available in ambulatory or pole-mounted models.

There are three types of PCA pumps: basal, continuous, and demand. All three afford some type of pain control with varying degrees of patient interaction.

- The basal mode is designed to achieve pain relief with minimal medication with intermittent dosing, thus allowing the patient to remain alert and active without sedation.
- The continuous mode of therapy is designed for patients who need maximum pain relief; it usually does not fluctuate from hour to hour and should completely relieve pain or achieve a constant effect.
- The demand mode dose is delivered by intermittent infusion when a button attached to the pump is pushed. The demand dose can be used alone or with the basal type of infusion (Fig. 6–30).

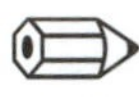

NOTE: PCA pumps must be programmed with parameters to prevent overmedication. These pumps are designed with a special key or locking device for security of the medications.

INS STANDARDS Nurses should be knowledgeable about the preparation and use of the PCA devices, including programming the device to deliver prescribed therapy, administration and maintenance procedures, and the use of lock-out devices. Additionally, nurses should have

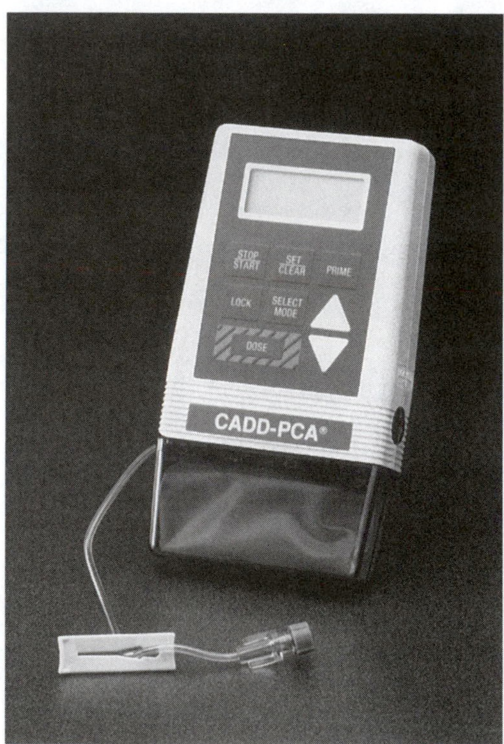

FIG. 6–30. Ambulatory patient-controlled analgesia (PCA) pump: CADD-PCA. (Courtesy of SIMS Deltec, St. Paul, Minnesota.)

knowledge of the pharmacologic implications of the medication, monitor the patient for therapeutic response, recognize untoward responses, implement nursing interventions as required, and document in the medical record. (INS, 2000, 72)

Multichannel and Dual-Channel Pumps

Multiple-drug delivery systems are computer generated, and many use computer-generated technology. Multichannel and dual-channel pumps can deliver several medications and fluids simultaneously or intermittently from bags, bottles, or syringes (Weinstein, 1997). Multichannel pumps (usually with three or four channels) require manifold-type sets to set up all channels, whether or not they are in use; each channel must be programmed independently. Programming a multichannel pump can be challenging (Fig. 6–31).

Dual-channel pumps offer a two-pump mechanism assembly, with a common control and programming panel. This type of pump uses one administration set for each channel (Fig. 6–32).

Ambulatory Pumps

Ambulatory pumps are lightweight, compact infusion pumps. These have made a significant breakthrough in long-term care. This device allows the patient freedom to resume a normal life. Ambulatory pumps range in size and weight; most weigh less than 6 lb and are capable of delivering most infusion therapies. Features include medication delivery, delivery of several different dose sizes at different intervals, memory of programs, and safety alarms. The main disadvantage of ambulatory pumps is limited power supply; they function on a battery system that requires frequent recharging (Fig. 6–33).

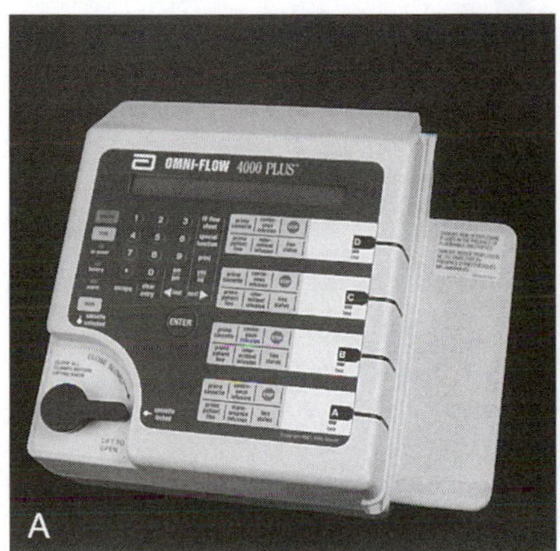

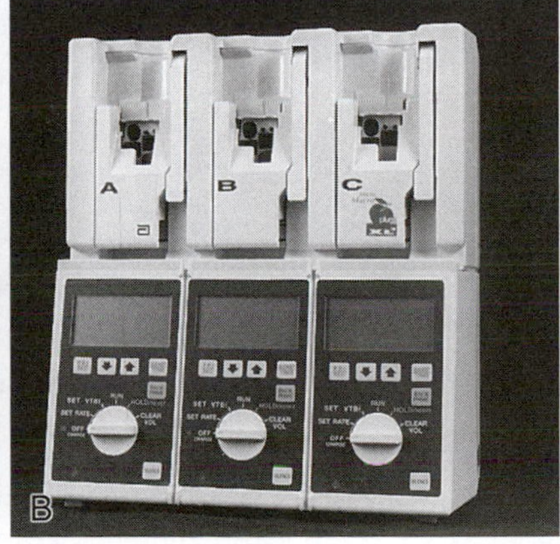

FIG. 6–31. Multiple-channel pump: (*A*) OMNI-FLOW 4000 Plus. (*B*) Plum XL-3. (Courtesy of Abbott Laboratories, North Chicago, Illinois.)

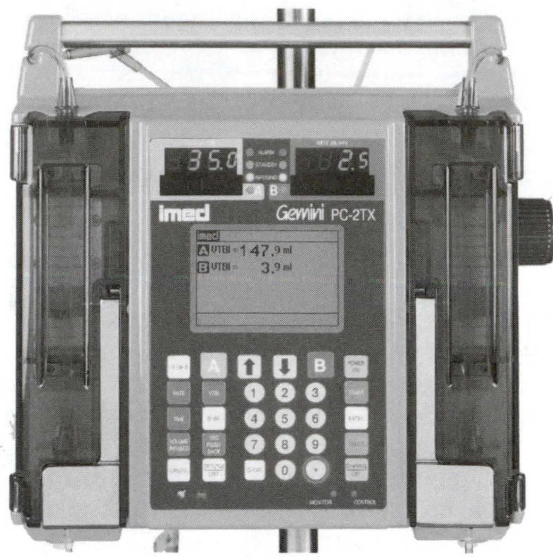

FIG. 6–32. Multiple-channel pump: IMED Gemini PC 2tx. (Courtesy of Alaris Medical Systems, San Diego, California.)

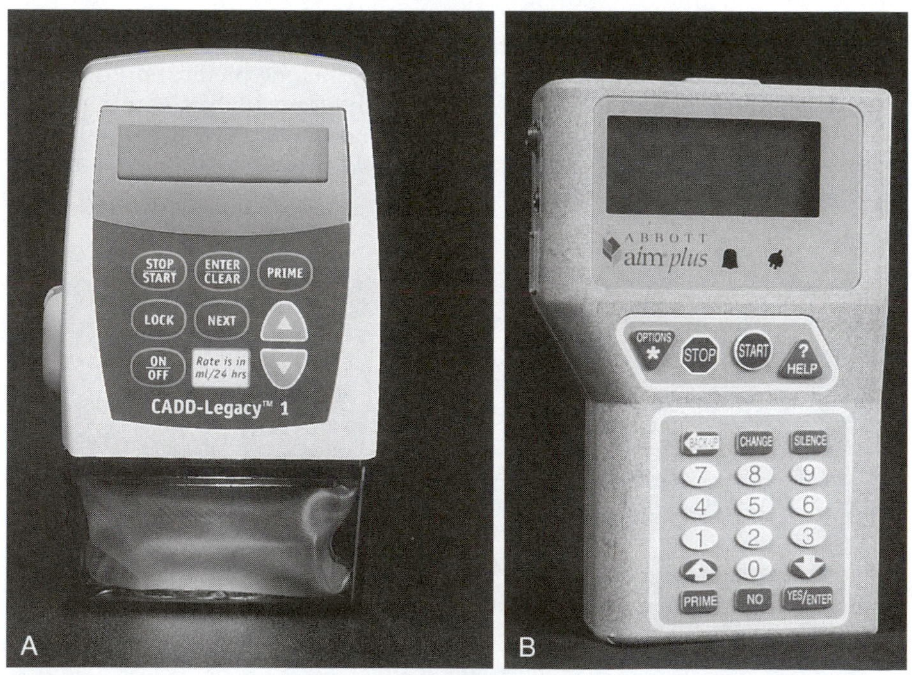

FIG. 6–33. Ambulatory pumps: (*A*) CADD-Legacy 1. (Courtesy of SIMS-Deltec, St. Paul, Minnesota.) (*B*) a*i*m *plus*. (Courtesy of Abbott Laboratories, North Chicago, Illinois.)

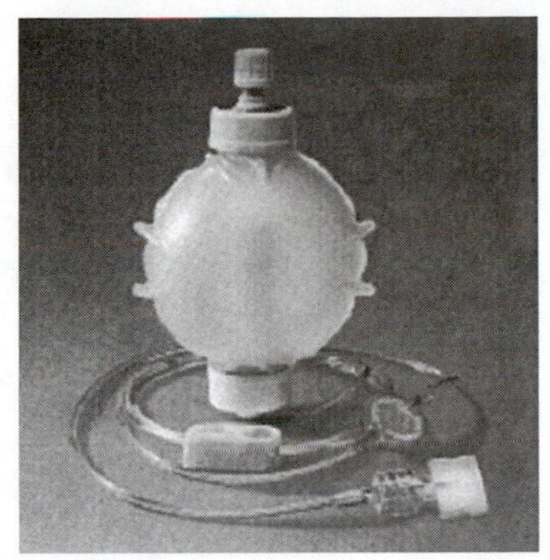

FIG. 6-34. Elastomere balloon pump: Eclipse elastomeric pump. (Courtesy of B. Braun Medical Inc., Bethlehem, Pennsylvania.)

Disposable Pumps

The elastomere balloon pump system is a portable device with an elastomeric reservoir, or balloon, that works on flow restrictions. The balloon, which is made of a soft rubberized material capable of being inflated to a predetermined volume, is safely encapsulated inside a rigid, transparent container. When the reservoir is filled, the balloon exerts positive pressure to administer the medication with an integrated flow restrictor that controls the flow rate. This system requires no batteries or electronic programming and is not reusable (Figs. 6–34 and 6–35).

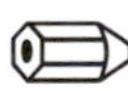 **NOTE:** Elastomere balloon devices are used primarily for the delivery of antibiotics. The typical volume for these devices is 50 to 100 mL, but these balloons are available in sizes up to 250 mL.

PROGRAMMING ELECTRONIC INFUSION DEVICES

To be able to program any type EID, one needs to be familiar with the terminology for delivering infusion and the device enhancements, including alarms.

Infusion Terminology

- *Rate:* Amount of time over which a specific volume of fluid is delivered. Infusion pumps deliver in increments of mL/h. The most common rate parameters for regular infusion pumps are 1 to 999 mL/h. Many newer pumps are capable of setting rates that offer parameters of 0.1 mL in increments of 0.1 to 99.9 mL, then in 1-mL increments up to 999 mL.
- *Volume infused:* Measurement that tells how much of a given solution has been infused. This measurement is used to monitor the amount of fluid infused in a shift. It can also be used in home health to monitor the infusion periodically during the day or over

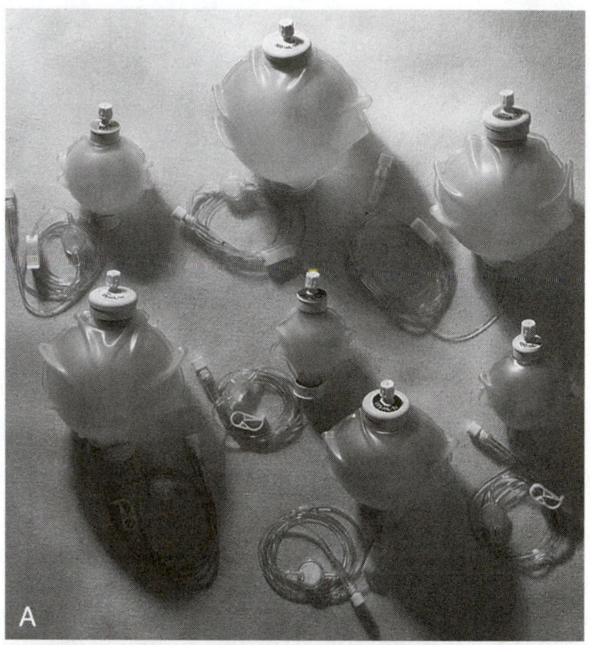

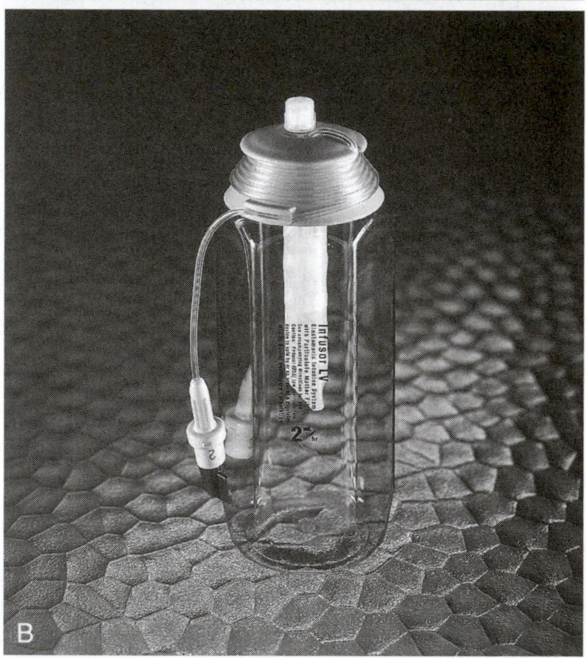

FIG. 6–35. Small-volume infusion pumps. (*A*) Eclipse elastomeric pumps come in a variety of sizes ranging in volume from 50 to 500 mL. (Courtesy of B. Braun Medical Inc., Bethlehem, Pennsylvania.) (*B*) Infusor LV system. (Courtesy of Baxter Healthcare Corporation, Round Lake, Illinois.)

several days. The "counter" must be returned to 0 at the beginning of each shift.

- *Volume to be infused:* Usually the amount of solution hanging in the solution container. A pump is designed to sound an alarm when the volume to be infused is reached.

Enhancement Terminology

- *Drop sensors:* Used with a controller to confirm the presence or absence of flow. The drop sensor is attached to the drop chamber of the administration set or can be located internally on the controller as the flow passes through a chamber.

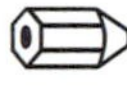

NOTE: The drop chamber must remain still to ensure that the counter senses or detects each drop as it falls. Splashing or multiple drops result in sudden rate changes.

Alarm Terminology

- *Air-in-line:* Designed to detect only visible bubbles or microscopic bubbles. This alarm is necessary for all positive pressure pumps and infusion controllers. Volumetric pumps are usually equipped with air-in-line detectors.
- *Occlusion:* Standard alarm for infusion devices. Controllers may be able to indicate only "no flow." With an occlusion alarm, controllers are able to indicate upstream (between pump and container) or downstream (between patient and pump) occlusion by absence of flow. Many newer pumps are able to differentiate between upstream (or proximal) and downstream (or distal) occlusions. This is often detected by changes in pressure

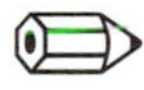

NOTE: In a number of EIDs, the pressure is "user" selectable from 0.10 to 10 psi. Occlusion alarms at low psi settings are common because the pumps are sensitive to even slight changes in pressure and very small I.V. catheter or patient movement. Many of the current EIDs infuse fluids using very low infusion pressures, often lower than the pressure of a gravity delivery. These devices are not, however, designed to detect infiltrations. When an infiltration occurs, the in-line pressure may actually drop; therefore, the EID will not detect the infiltration. Visual monitoring of the I.V. site by a professional nurse is mandatory for patients with EIDs.

- *Infusion complete:* Alarm triggered by a preset volume limit ("infusion complete"). These alarms are helpful in preventing the fluid container from running dry because they can be set to sound before the entire solution container is infused.
- *Low battery or low power:* Gives the user ample warning of the pump's impending inability to function. A low-battery alarm means that the batteries need to be replaced or external power source needs to be connected. As a protective measure, when

low-battery and low-power alarms are continued over a preset number of minutes, the pumps usually convert to a keep-vein-open (KVO) rate. The preset KVO rate is usually between 0.1 and 5 mL.

- *Nonfunctional or malfunctional:* Alarm that means the pump is operating outside parameters and the problem cannot be resolved. When this alarm sounds, the pump should be disconnected from the patient and returned to biomedical engineering or to the manufacturer for evaluation. The alert signifying a nonfunctional alarm may be worded in many ways, depending on the manufacturer.
- *Not infusing:* Indicates that all of the pump infusion parameters are not set. This feature prevents tampering or setting changes from happening accidentally. The pump must be programmed or changed and then told to "start."
- *Parameters or timed-out:* Reminds the programmer that all settings have not been completed.
- *Tubing:* Used generally with controllers. Ensures that the correct tubing has been loaded into the pump. If tubing is incorrectly loaded, this alarm will also sound.
- *Door:* Indicates that the door that secures the tubing is not closed. Cassette pumps may give a "cassette" alarm if the cassette is unable to infuse within device operating parameters.
- *Free flow:* Detects the rapid infusion of fluid, which can occur when the set is removed from the pump. Disengaging the tubing from the pump requires a deliberate act. Most newer devices have free-flow protection, meaning that when the door is opened accidentally, there should be no fluid flow to the patient without nurse intervention.

ADDITIONAL ELECTRONIC INFUSION DEVICE ENHANCEMENTS

Many other functions have been added to newer pumps. These include:

- Preprogrammed drug compatibility
- Retrievable patient history data
- Infiltration or thrombus detection alarm
- Central venous pressure monitor
- Positive pressure fill stroke
- Modular self-diagnosing capability
- Printer read-out
- Nurse call system
- Remote site programming
- Syringe use for secondary infusion
- Adjustable occlusion pressures
- Opaque infusions (for blood, fat emulsions, iron dextran)

- Secondary rate settings
- Lock level for security

(See Appendix D for a Summary of Recommendations from the CDC [1995] on Procedures for Maintenance of Intravascular Catheters, Administration Sets, and Parenteral Fluids.)

NURSING PLAN OF CARE

PATIENTS RECEIVING PERIPHERAL I.V. THERAPY

Focus Assessment

Subjective

- Knowledge of therapies and equipment used to deliver therapy

Objective

- Suitable vascular access device for length and type of therapy
- Adequate level of consciousness and compliance

Patient Outcome Criteria

The patient will be:

- Free of complications associated with I.V. therapy
- Free of injury

Nursing Diagnoses

- Risk for injury related to environmental conditions, lack of knowledge regarding equipment
- Knowledge deficit related to new procedure and maintaining I.V. therapy
- Impaired physical mobility related to placement and maintenance of I.V. cannula
- Anxiety (mild, moderate, or severe) related to new equipment technology

Nursing Management

1. Follow the manufacturer's guidelines on the setup and maintenance of specific EIDs.
2. Select and prepare infusion pumps as indicated.
3. Correct any malfunctioning equipment.
4. Plug equipment into electrical outlets connected to an emergency power source.
5. Have equipment periodically checked by bioengineers as appropriate.
6. Set alarm limits on equipment as appropriate.
7. Respond to equipment alarms appropriately.
8. Consult with other healthcare team members and recommend equipment and devices for patient use.

(continued)

(continued)

9. Compare machine-derived data with nurse's perception of patient's condition.
10. Explain potential risks and benefits of using equipment technology.
11. Follow INS Standards of Practice in rotation of I.V. sites, administration set changes, and dressing management to maintain integrity of site.
12. Use filters when appropriate.
13. Use appropriate administration set (vented or nonvented) with the appropriate fluid container.
14. Inspect fluid containers, administration sets, and cannulas for integrity before use.

PATIENT EDUCATION

- Instruct the patient by demonstrating the preparation and administration of therapy.
- Teach the patient and family how to operate equipment, as appropriate.
- Advise the patient regarding pump alarms and advise him or her to contact the nurse if the alarm is triggered.
- Instruct the patient and family on the use of PCA pumps for pain control.
- Teach the patient and family the expected patient outcomes and side effects associated with using the equipment.
- Document the patient's and family's understanding of the education provided to them.

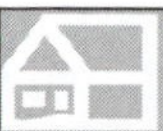

HOME CARE ISSUES

Reimbursement is a challenge in the home care setting. Before any equipment is acquired, the reimbursement status of the clientele served and the anticipated need should be thoroughly explored (Jensen, 1995).

Home care infusion devices are designed to allow the patient maximum portability and freedom of movement. The aim is for small, quiet, lightweight infusion pumps with pouches to enclose the infusion container. Equipment used at home must offer safety features because the caregiver in most situations is the patient or family.

Equipment used frequently in home care management include:

- Medical teaching dolls (Legacy Products): Facilitate visual, hands-on approach to educate patients of all ages and families about vascular access site, equipment, and procedures
- Vascular access devices: Easy to administer medication by home healthcare professional, patient, or family
- Tubing, connectors, and filters: Include needleless systems for use in home to prevent needlestick injuries
- EIDs: Syringe pumps, elastomeric infusers, ambulatory pumps
- Premixed medications
- Transport storage pouch

KEY POINTS

EQUIPMENT

- Types of infusion delivery systems include glass and plastic (rigid and flexible).
- Check all solutions for clarity and expiration date. Squeeze to check for leaks, floating particles, and clarity.
- Concerns over PVC and DEHP: Plasticizer phthalate (DEHP) added to many I.V. products for flexibility. EPA warning that PVC leaches into I.V. solutions and toxic absorption can occur. Many new products on market without DEHP.
- Administration sets

  Single-line sets: Most frequently used; follow INS standards for frequency of set changes. Available in vented and nonvented sets.

  Primary (standard) set, volume-controlled sets

  Primary Y sets: Most often used with blood components

  Pump-specific sets: Used with EIDs

  Lipid administration sets: Used with fat emulsion, which are supplied in glass containers with special vented tubing
- Filters

  Inline I.V. solution filters

  Depth: Filters in which pore size is not uniform

  Membrane (screen): Air-venting, bacteria-retentive, 0.22-micron filter

  Blood filters

  Standard clot: 170 to 220 microns; used on blood administration sets to remove coagulated products, microclots, and debris

(continued)

KEY POINTS *(continued)*

- Filters *(continued)*
  - Microaggregate: 20, 40, and 80 microns; can be added to an in-use blood administration set, permitting infusion of blood, and easy replacement of the filter for delivery of multiple units
  - Leukocyte depletion: Used to remove 95 to 99.9 percent of leukocytes from red blood cells
- Adaptors and connectors
  - J-, U-, or T-shaped ports that are used at the injection side. Add-on devices add length for manipulation. Add-on devices are used only when an integral system is not available to deliver the prescribed therapy.
- Stopcocks
  - Control the direction of flow of an infusate through manual manipulation of a direction regulation valve
- Resealable locks (PRN device)
  - Attach to hub of catheter and convert the cannula into an intermittent device
- Needleless systems
  - State-of-the-art technology to replace needles to connect I.V. devices and administer infusates
- Peripheral infusion devices
  - Scalp vein needles: For short-term therapy; odd-numbered gauges
  - Over-the-needle catheters: For peripheral therapy, made from Teflon, Vialon; even-numbered gauges
  - Through-the-needle catheters: Example is a PICC
  - Midline catheters: 6 inches long; indwelling time, 28 days
- Central infusion devices
  - Percutaneous catheters
  - Central venous tunneled catheters (CVTCs)
  - Implantable ports: Closed system composed of implanted device with reservoir, port, and self-sealing system; require the use of a noncoring needle to access port
  - Peripherally inserted central catheters (PICCs): Inserted peripherally and threaded to the SVC; can be placed by physicians, nurses, or nurse practitioners
- Infusion Regulation Devices
  - EIDs
  - Controller: Used in 80 percent of situations requiring rate control device; gravity-dependent; many are nonvolumetric; some volumetric controllers available with peristaltic action
  - Pumps
    - Volumetric: Calibrated in mL/h; require special cassette or cartridge to be used with the machine, very accurate, and used in delivery of high-potency drugs or when accuracy is imperative
    - Peristaltic: Calibrated in mL/h; used primarily for delivery of enteral feedings; have a rotary disk or rollers to compress tubing
    - Syringe: Piston-driven pump that controls rate of infusion by drive speed and syringe size
    - Patient-controlled analgesia (PCA): Can be used at home or in hospital to deliver pain medication
    - Ambulatory infusion: Lightweight, compact infusion pumps
    - Elastomere balloons: Portable device designed with an elastomeric reservoir for delivery of medication

CHAPTER ACTIVITIES

COMPETENCY CRITERIA: Equipment Management
COMPETENCY STATEMENT: Competent I.V. nurses will be able to demonstrate use of technical equipment and devices to deliver I.V. therapy.
Note: The cognitive (knowledge) information that is embedded within this performance-based competency includes aseptic technique and vein anatomy.
This competency *links* to the competency of infection control and initiation of peripheral I.V therapy.

Performance	Skilled	Needs Education
Critical Action Statements		
1. Chooses appropriate gauge and length of cannula for peripheral I.V. therapy A. Pediatric B. Adult C. Geriatric		
2. Chooses administration set for use with therapy being provided A. Straight set B. Vented C. Nonvented D. Y-set E. Volume-control set		
3. Checks I.V. solution container for: A. Clarity B. Expiration date C. Cracks or leaks		
4. Demonstrates use of EIDs A. Pump B. Syringe pump C. Elastomeric pump D. PCA		
5. Demonstrates use of inline filters A. 0.22 micron B. 70 micron C. Leukocyte D. Microaggregate		
6. Demonstrates appropriate use of adjunct equipment A. J, U, or T connectors B. Fluid warmers		

(continued)

(continued)

Performance	Skilled	Needs Education
Critical Action Statements		
7. Demonstrates connection of PRN device (resealable lock) to cannula		
8. Demonstrates spiking and priming I.V. container		

EVALUATION CRITERIA

1. Validation of spiking and priming I.V. setup.
2. Validation of setup and troubleshooting of EIDs.
3. Validation of use of PRN device.

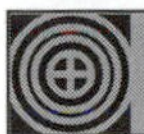

CRITICAL THINKING ACTIVITY

1. You are asked to set up an I.V. piggyback of 150 mL of 5 percent dextrose in water with 20 mEq of potassium chloride added. What type of rate regulation device would you use?

2. In setting up the regulation infusion device for a potassium piggyback, you find that the facility in which you are working uses a regulation pump that you have never used. What are your options for solving this problem?

3. You are asked to add an inline filter (0. 22 micron) to an I.V. line that is connected to an infusion pump. What do you have to do before adding the filter?

POST-TEST

In 1 through 5, match the term in Column I with the definition in Column II.

COLUMN I	COLUMN II
1. Cannula	**a.** A female connection point of an I.V. cannula where the tubing or other equipment attaches
2. Drip chamber	**b.** Point of entry
3. Lumen	**c.** Area of the I.V. tubing usually found under the spike where the solution drips and collects
4. Hub	**d.** Space within an artery, vein, or catheter
5. Port	**e.** A tube or sheath used for infusing fluids

6. When using a flexible plastic system, what type of administration set could you choose?
   - **a.** Vented
   - **b.** Nonvented
   - **c.** Vented or nonvented; both work with this system

7. A 0.22-micron filter should be used when:
   - **a.** An additive has been combined with the solution
   - **b.** The patient is susceptible to infusion phlebitis
   - **c.** The infusion is delivered by the central route
   - **d.** All of the above

8. The standard blood administration set has a clot filter of how many microns?
   - **a.** 170
   - **b.** 40
   - **c.** 20
   - **d.** 10

9. Microaggregate filters are used for:
   - **a.** Administration of protein solutions
   - **b.** Administration of whole blood and packed cells stored more than 5 days
   - **c.** Removal of bacteria for infusion
   - **d.** Filtering air from the set

10. A disadvantage of the glass system is that it:
   - **a.** Is breakable and difficult to store
   - **b.** Reacts with some solutions and medications
   - **c.** May be difficult to read fluid levels
   - **d.** May develop leaks

REFERENCES

Altavela, J.L., Haas, C.E., & Nowak, D.R. (1993). Comparison of polyethylene and polyvinyl chloride sets for the administration of intravenous nitroglycerin to treat ischemic heart disease (abstract). Presented at the American College of Clinical Pharmacists Annual Meeting, Reno, NV.

Centers for Disease Control and Prevention. (1995). Guideline for prevention of intravenous therapy-related infections. U.S. Department of Health and Human Services, Atlanta, GA.

B. Braun Medical Inc. (1999). Is the IV container as important as the solution being infused? Intravenous Nurses Society Annual Conference. Charlotte, North Carolina, May 3–5.

Brown, S.L., Morrison, A.E., Parmentier, C.M., et al. (1997). Infusion pump adverse events: Experience from medical device reports. *Journal of Intravenous Nursing,* 20(1), 41–49.

Brown, J.M. (1995). Polyurethane and silicone: Myths and misconceptions. *Journal of Intravenous Nursing,* 18(3), 120–122.

Chiarello, L.A., Nagin, D., & Laufer, F. (1992). *Pilot Study of Needle Stick Prevention Devices.* Albany: New York State Department of Health.

Collins, J.L., & Lutz, R.J. (1991). In vitro study of simultaneous infusion of incompatible drugs in multilumen catheters. *Heart Lung,* 20, 271–277.

Food and Drug Administration (1994). Safety alert: Hazards of precipitation associated with parenteral nutrition. *American Journal of Hospital Pharmacy,* 51, 1427–1428.

Goodman, E. (1997). Safe workplace: New technology sharpens workplace safety by removing the fear of needle sticks. Internet. Available: http://www.vanishpoint.com/article-Goodwin.htm.

HealthCare Without Harm (1999). Citizen petition for a food and drug administration regulation or guideline to label medical devices that leach phthalate plasticizers and to establish a program to promote alternative. Internet. Available June 14, 1999.

Horner, K.A. (1998). Technology assessment of two needleless systems. *Journal of Intravenous Nursing,* 21(40), 203–208.

Intravenous Nursing Society (1997). Position paper: Midline and midclavicular catheters. *Journal of Intravenous Nursing,* 20(4), 175–178.

Intravenous Nursing Society. (2000). Intravenous Nursing Standards of Practice. *Journal of Intravenous Nursing,* 21, S35–44, 72.

Jensen, B.L. (1995). Intravenous therapy equipment. In J. Terry, L. Baranowski, R. Lonsway, & C. Hedrick (eds.): *Intravenous Therapy: Clinical Principles and Practice.* Philadelphia: W.B. Saunders, pp. 303–338.

Josephson, D.L. (1999). *Intravenous Infusion Therapy for Nurses: Principles and Practice.* Albany: Delmar Publishers, pp. 146–180.

Maki, D.G., & Ringer, M. (1991). Risk factors for infusion-related phlebitis with small peripheral venous catheters: A randomized controlled study. *Annals of Internal Medicine,* 114, 945.

McKee, J.M., Shell, J.A., Warren, T.A., & Campbell, V.P. (1989). Complications of intravenous therapy: A randomized perspective study: Vialon vs Teflon. *Journal of Intravenous Therapy,* 12(5), 288.

Meares, C. (1992). P.I.C.C. & M.L.C. lines options worth exploring. *Nursing 92,* (10), 52–56.

Millam, D.A. (1990). Controlling the flow: Electronic infusion devices. *Nursing 90,* 65–68.

Pall Biomedial Corporation (2000). New York: Pall Biomedical Products Corporation.

Salahuddin-Mobashi, G. (1999). Sharps injury prevention program: A step by step guide. American Hospital Association.

Sevick, S. (1995). Intravenous in-line filtration: choice or necessity? *Technical Report Gelman Sciences,* 1–3.

Vengelen-Tyler, V. (1996). American Association of Blood Banks Technical Manual. Bethesda, MD, American Association of Blood Banks.

Weinstein, S. (1997). *Plumer's Principles and Practices of Intravenous Therapy* (6th ed.) Philadelphia: J.B. Lippincott.

Widman, F.K. (1991). *Standards for Blood Banks and Transfusion Services* (14th ed.) Arlington, VA: American Association of Blood Banks, pp. 39.

RESOURCES: EQUIPMENT MANUFACTURERS AND SUPPLIERS

Alaris Medical Systems: *www.alarismed.com*
B. Braun: *www.bbraunusa.com*
Bard Access Systems: *www.bardaccess.com*
Becton Dickinson/Baxter: *www.bd.com*
Johnson & Johnson: *www.jnjmedical.com*
SIMS Deltec, Inc.: *www.deltec.com*

ANSWERS TO CHAPTER 6

Pre-Test

1. a, **2.** d, **3.** a, **4.** b, **5.** c, **6.** d, **7.** d, **8.** d, **9.** a, **10.** a

Post-Test

1. e, **2.** c, **3.** d, **4.** a, **5.** b, **6.** c, **7.** d, **8.** a, **9.** b, **10.** a

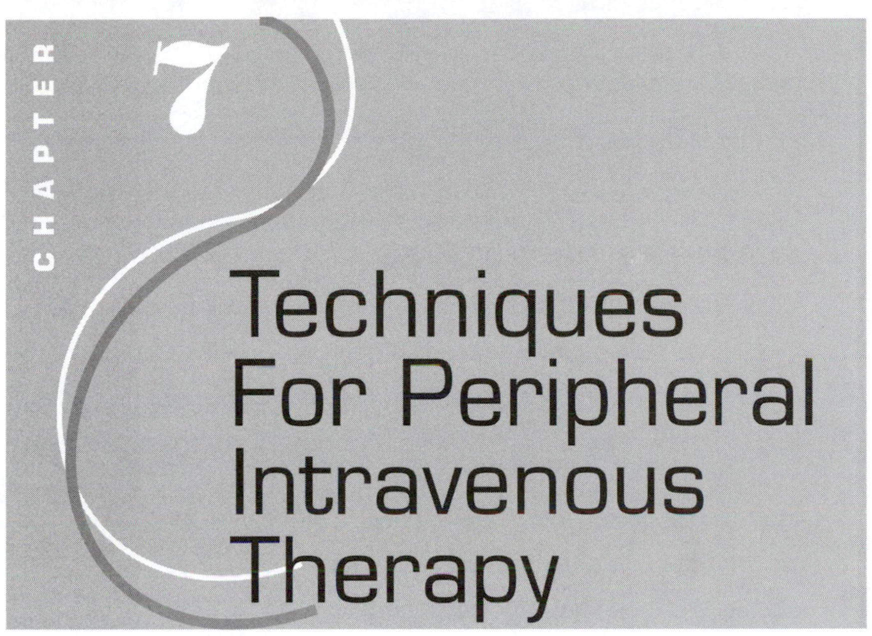

CHAPTER 7 Techniques For Peripheral Intravenous Therapy

Challenges make you discover things about yourself that you really never knew. They're what make the instrument stretch—what make you go beyond the norm.

Cicely Tyson, American Actress

CHAPTER CONTENTS

Worksheet 7–3: Math Calculation Worksheet 2 and Answers
POST-TEST
REFERENCES
ANSWERS TO CHAPTER 7

LEARNING OBJECTIVES

Upon completion of this chapter, the reader will be able to:

1. Define the terminology related to peripheral veins.
2. Recall the anatomy and physiology related to the venous system.
3. Identify the five tissue structures that therapists must penetrate for a successful venipuncture.
4. Identify the peripheral veins appropriate for venipuncture.
5. List the factors affecting site selection.
6. Document the initiation of I.V. therapy.
7. Demonstrate Phillips' 15-step approach for initiating I.V. therapy.
8. List the sites appropriate for labeling.
9. State the Intravenous Nursing Standards of Practice for peripheral infusions.
10. Recall the steps in performing a saline lock flush.
11. Describe the advantages and disadvantages of resealable locking devices.
12. Contrast the advantages and disadvantages of saline lock flush versus heparin lock flush.
13. Identify the uses of lidocaine and topical creams in the initiation of I.V. therapy.
14. Calculate drops per minute using varied drop-factor tubing.
15. Use the nursing process in techniques for initiation of I.V. therapy.

GLOSSARY

Antimicrobial An agent that destroys or prevents the development of microorganisms

Bevel Slanted edge on opening of a needle or cannula device

Cannula A hollow plastic tube used for accessing the vascular system

Dermis The corium layer of the skin composed of connective tissue, blood vessels, nerves, muscles, lymphatics, hair follicles, sebaceous and sudoriferous glands

Distal Farther from the heart; farthest from point of attachment (below the previous site of cannulation)

Drop factor The number of drops needed to deliver 1 mL of fluid

Endothelial lining A thin layer of cells lining the blood vessels and heart

Epidermis The outermost layer of skin covering the body that is composed of epithelial cells and is devoid of blood vessels

Gauge Size of a cannula (catheter) opening; gradual measurements of the outside diameter of a cannula

Macrodrip Drop factor of 10 to 20 drops equivalent to 1 mL based on manufacturer

Microabrasion Superficial break in skin integrity that may predispose the patient to infection

Microdrip Drop factor of 60 drops/mL

Palpation Examination by touch

Prime To fill the administration set with infusate for the first time

Proximal Nearest to the heart; closest point to attachment (above the previous site of cannulation)

Spike To insert the administration set into the infusate container

PRE-TEST

1. The three layers of a vein are the:
   a. Tunica center, tunica media, and facia
   b. Tunica intima, tunica media, and tunica adventitia
   c. Tunica intima, epidermis, and dermis
2. A physician's verbal order must be validated by a written order within how many hours?
   a. 12
   b. 24
   c. 48
   d. 72
3. The first step in heparin flush of an intermittent infusion device is to:
   a. Flush with sodium chloride
   b. Check for patency of the catheter
   c. Flush with heparin
   d. Administer medication
4. According to the Intravenous Nurses Standards of Practice, I.V. sites should be rotated every:
   a. 24 to 48 hours
   b. 36 to 48 hours
   c. 48 to 72 hours
   d. 72 to 96 hours
5. Which peripheral vein is appropriate for antibiotic therapy?
   a. Cephalic vein
   b. Dorsal metacarpal vein
   c. Digital vein
   d. Median antecubital vein
6. The calculation of the drop rate depends on the:
   a. Tubing length
   b. Filter size
   c. Drop factor of the tubing
   d. mL/h
7. Labels should be applied to the:
   a. Catheter site
   b. Tubing
   c. Solution container
   d. All of the above
8. What factor(s) affect site selection?
   a. Type of solution
   b. Condition of vein
   c. Duration of therapy
   d. Presence of disease, shunts, or grafts in the extremity
   e. All of the above

9. The purpose of intermittent infusion devices is to:
   a. Prevent phlebitis
   b. Provide access to the vascular system without administration of solutions
   c. Administer solutions at a more rapid rate
   d. Prevent infiltration
10. If a patient who is on anticoagulant therapy needs to have an I.V. initiated, which of the following would be appropriate?
   a. Avoid use of a tourniquet if possible or apply loosely
   b. Avoid excess pressure when cleansing the skin
   c. Use alcohol or adhesive remover when removing adhesive dressing
   d. All of the above
11. The order is for 1000 mL of 5 percent dextrose in water at 100 mL/h. Calculate the drip rate using 15-gtt factor tubing.

● ● ●

ANATOMY AND PHYSIOLOGY RELATED TO I.V. PRACTICE

To accurately perform I.V. therapy, nurses must know the anatomy and physiology of the skin and venous system and be familiar with the physiologic response of veins to heat, cold, and stress. It is also important to become familiar with the skin thickness and consistency at various sites.

SKIN

The skin consists of two main layers, the **epidermis** and **dermis,** which overlies the superficial fascia. The epidermis, composed of squamous cells that are less sensitive than underlying structures, is the first line of defense against infections. The epidermis is the thickest on the palms of the hands and soles of the feet and is thinnest on the inner surfaces of the extremities. Thickness varies with age and exposure to the elements, such as wind and sun.

The dermis, a much thicker layer, is located directly below the epidermis. The dermis consists of blood vessels, hair follicles, sweat glands, sebaceous glands, small muscles, and nerves. As with the epidermis, the thickness of the dermis varies with age and physical condition. The skin is a special-sense touch organ, and the dermis reacts quickly to painful stimuli, temperature changes, and pressure sensation. This is the most painful layer during venipuncture because of the large amount of blood vessels and the many nerves contained in this sheath.

The hypodermis, or fascia, lies below the epidermis and dermis and provides a covering for the blood vessels. This connective tissue layer varies in thickness and is found over the entire body surface. Because any infection in the fascia, called superficial cellulitis, spreads easily throughout the body, it is essential to use strict aseptic technique when inserting infusion devices. This superficial tissue layer connects with deeper fascia (Fig. 7–1.)

SENSORY RECEPTORS

There are five types of sensory receptors, four of which affect parenteral therapy. The sensory receptors transmit along afferent fibers. Many types of stimulation, such as heat, light, cold, pressure, and sound, are processed along the sensory receptors (Guyton, 1991). Sensory receptors related to parenteral therapy include:

1. Mechanoreceptors, which process skin tactile sensations and deep tissue sensation (**palpation** of veins)
2. Thermoreceptors, which process cold, warmth, and pain (application of heat or cold)
3. Nociceptors, which process pain (puncture of vein for insertion of the **cannula**)

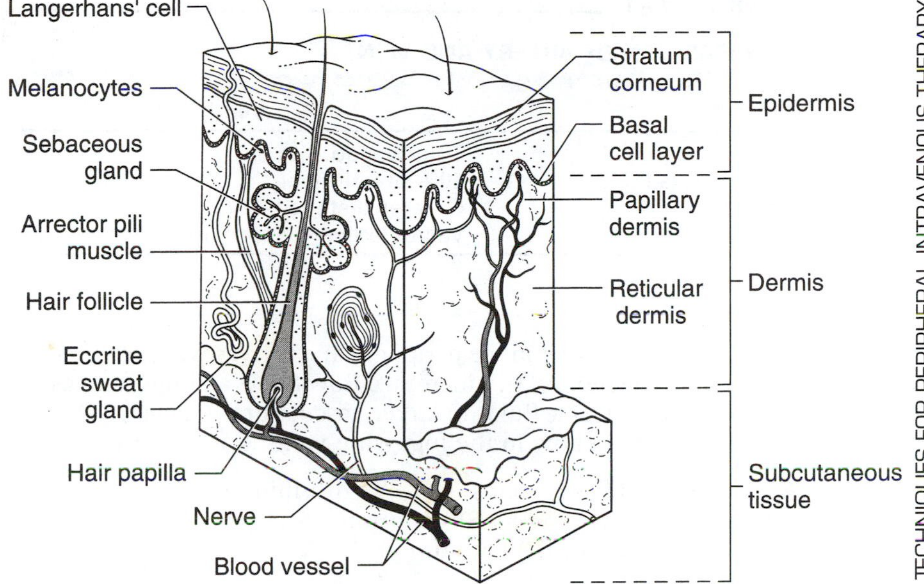

FIG. 7–1. Anatomy of skin.

4. Chemoreceptors, which process osmotic changes in blood and decreased arterial pressure (decreased circulating blood volume)

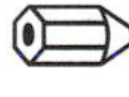 **NOTE:** To decrease the patient's pain during venipuncture, keep the skin taut by applying traction to it and move quickly through the skin layers and past the pain receptors.

VENOUS SYSTEM

The body transport mechanism, the circulatory system, has two main subdivisions—the cardiopulmonary and the systemic systems. The systemic circulation, particularly the peripheral veins, is used in I.V. therapy. Veins function similarly to arteries but are thinner and less muscular (Table 7–1.)

The wall of a vein is only 10 percent of the total diameter of the vessel, compared with 25 percent in the artery. Because the vein is thin and less muscular, it can distend easily, allowing for storage of large volumes of blood under low pressure. Approximately 75 percent of the total blood volume is contained in the veins.

Some veins have valves, particularly those that transport blood against gravity, as in the lower extremities. Valves, made up of endothelial leaflets, help prevent the **distal** reflux of blood. Valves occur at points of branching, producing a noticeable bulge in the vessel (Smeltzer & Bare, 1999). Arteries and veins have three layers of tissue that form the wall, the tunica intima, tunica adventitia, and tunica media (Fig. 7–2.)

TABLE 7–1

COMPARISON OF ARTERY AND VEIN

Artery*	Vein*
Thick-walled	Thin-walled
25% of arterial wall	10% of vein wall
Lacks valves	Greater distensibility
Pulsates	Valves present approximately every 3 in

*Has three tissue layers.

Venous blood flows slower in the periphery and increases in turbulence in the larger veins of the thorax. This increased flow rate is an important aspect in administering hypertonic fluids in larger vasculatures (Fabian, 1998).

The amount of blood flow in the following veins is as follows:

- Cephalic and basilic veins: 45 to 95 mL/min
- Subclavian vein: 150 to 300 mL/min
- Superior vena cava: 2000 mL/min

Tunica Adventitia

The outermost layer, called the tunica adventitia, consists of connective tissue that surrounds and supports a vessel. The blood supply of this layer, called the vasa vasorum, nourishes both the adventitia and media layers. Sometimes during venipuncture, you can feel a "pop" as you enter the tunica adventitia.

Tunica Media

The middle layer, called the tunica media, is composed of muscular and elastic tissue with nerve fibers for vasoconstriction and vasodilation. The tunica media in a vein is not as strong and rigid as it is in an artery, so

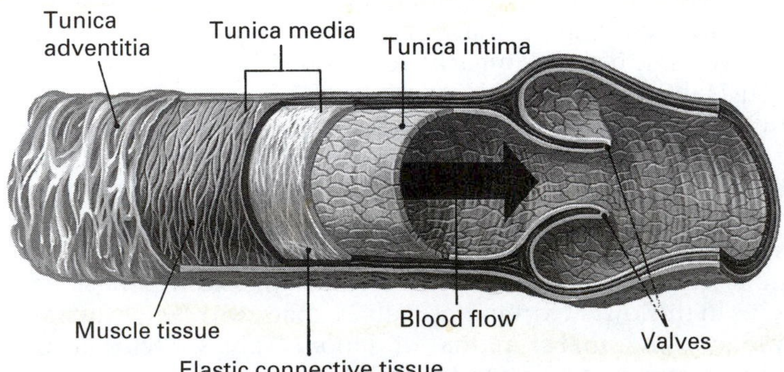

FIG. 7–2. Anatomy of a vein. (Source: Medical Economics Publishing, Montvale, New Jersey, with permission.)

it tends to collapse or distend as pressure decreases or increases. Stimulation by change in temperature or mechanical or chemical irritation can produce a response in this layer. For instance, cold blood or infusates can produce spasms that impede blood flow and cause pain. Application of heat promotes dilatation, which can relieve a spasm or improve blood flow (Weinstein, 1997).

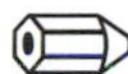

NOTE: During venipuncture, if the tip of the catheter has nicked the tunica adventitia or is placed in the tunica media layer, a small amount of blood will appear in the catheter; however, the catheter will not thread because it is trapped between layers. If you cannot get a steady backflow of blood, the needle might be in this layer, so advance the stylet of the cannula slightly before advancing the catheter.

Tunica Intima

The innermost layer, called the tunica intima, has one thin layer of cells, referred to as the **endothelial lining.** The surface is smooth, allowing blood to flow through vessels easily. Any roughening of this bed of cells during venipuncture while the catheter is in place, or on discontinuing the system, fosters the process of thrombosis formation (see Chapter 8).

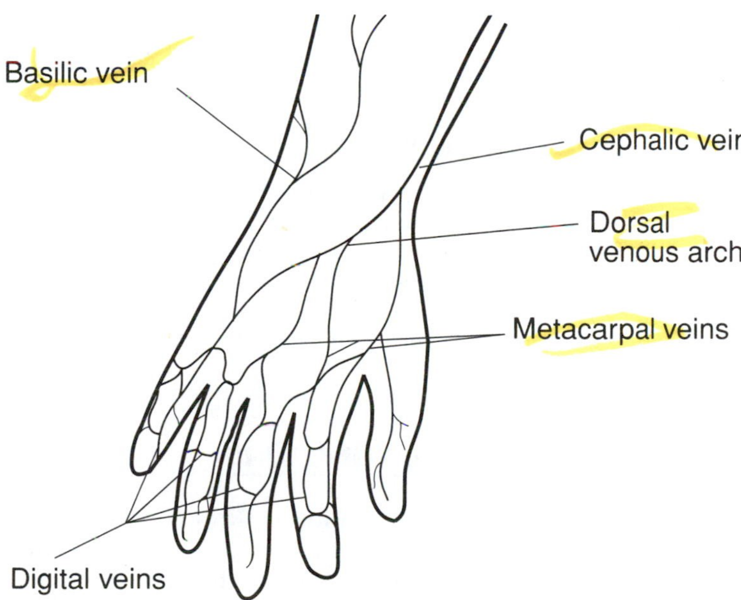

FIG. 7–3. Superficial veins of the dorsum of the hand. (Courtesy of Becton Dickinson, Sandy, Utah.)

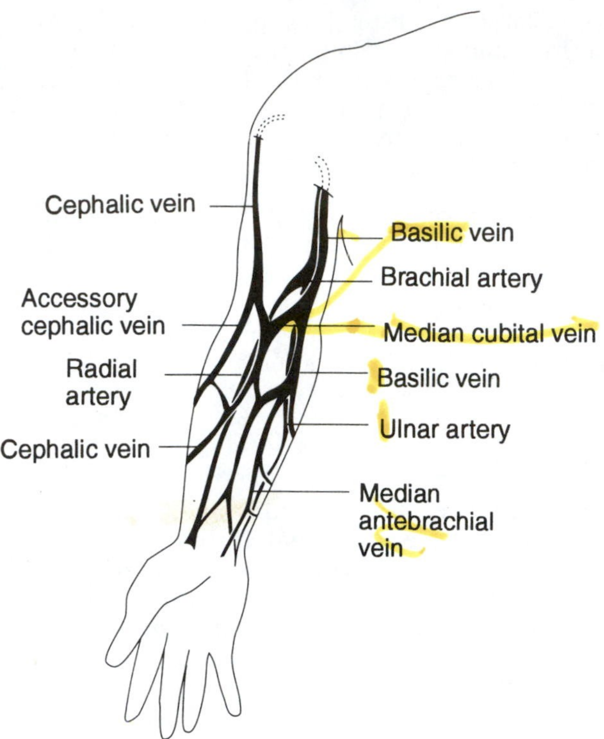

FIG. 7–4. Superficial veins of the forearm. (Courtesy of Becton Dickinson, Sandy, Utah.)

Veins of the Hands and Arms

Several veins can be used to infuse I.V. fluids, but the veins of the hands or arms are most commonly used (Figs. 7–3 and 7–4).

When selecting the best site, many factors must be considered, such as ease of insertion and access, type of needle or catheter that can be used, and comfort and safety for the patient. Table 7–2 provides information on identifying and selecting the most effective I.V. site for the clinical situation of the patient.

APPROACHES TO VENIPUNCTURE

Performing a successful venipuncture requires mastery and knowledge of infusion therapy as well as psychomotor clinical skill. Many aseptic approaches to venipuncture techniques provide safe parenteral therapy. The Phillips 15-step venipuncture method, outlined in Table 7–3 and explained in detail in this chapter, is an easy-to-remember step approach for beginning practitioners.

TABLE 7–2

SELECTING AN INSERTION SITE FOR THE SUPERFICIAL VEINS OF THE DORSUM OF THE HAND AND THE ARM

Vein and Location	Insertion Device	Considerations
Digital Lateral and dorsal portions of the fingers	Small-gauge cannula 20- to 22-gauge catheter 21- to 25-gauge steel needle	Use a padded tongue blade to splint the cannula. Use only solutions that are isotonic without additives because of the risk of infiltration.
Metacarpal Dorsum of the hand formed by union of digital veins between the knuckles	20- to 22-gauge to ¾–1 in length over the needle catheter 21- to 25-gauge steel needle (short-term)	Good site to begin therapy Usually easily visualized Avoid if infusing antibiotics, potassium chloride, or chemotherapeutic agents
Cephalic Radial portion of the lower arm along the radial bone of the forearm	18- to 22-gauge cannulas, usually over-the-needle catheter	Large vein, easy to access First use most distal section and work upward for long-term therapy Useful for infusing blood and chemically irritating medications
Basilic Ulnar aspect of the lower arm and runs up the ulnar bone	18- to 22-gauge, usually over-the-needle catheter	Difficult area to access Large vein, easily palpated, but moves easily; stabilize with traction during venipuncture Often available after other sites have been exhausted
Accessory cephalic Branches off the cephalic vein along the radial bone	18- to 22-gauge, usually over-the-needle catheter	Medium to large size and easy to stabilize May be difficult to palpate in persons with large amounts of adipose tissue Valves at cephalic junction may prohibit cannula advancement Short length may prohibit cannula use

(Continued)

TABLE 7–2

SELECTING AN INSERTION SITE FOR THE SUPERFICIAL VEINS OF THE DORSUM OF THE HAND AND THE ARM *(Continued)*

Vein and Location	Insertion Device	Considerations
Upper cephalic Radial aspect of upper arm above the elbow	16- to 20-gauge, usually over-the-needle catheter	Difficult to visualize Excellent site for confused patients (who tend to pull at their I.V. line)
Median antebrachial Extends up the front of the forearm from the median antecubital veins	18- to 22-gauge, usually over-the-needle catheter	Area has many nerve endings and should be avoided Infiltration occurs easily.
Median basilic Ulnar portion of the forearm	18- to 22-gauge, usually over-the-needle catheter	Good site for I.V. therapy
Median cubital Radial side of forearm; crosses in front of the brachial artery at the antecubital space	18- to 22-gauge, usually over-the-needle catheter	Good site for I.V. therapy
Antecubital In the bend of the elbow	All sizes especially 16- to 18-gauge; used for midline catheters and peripherally inserted central catheters	Should be reserved for blood draws for laboratory analysis only, unless in an emergency Uncomfortable placement site, owing to the arm extending in an unnatural position Area difficult to splint with armboard If used in an emergency situation, change site within 24 hours

PRECANNULATION

Before initiating cannulation, you must follow steps 1 through 5: checking the physician's order, handwashing, preparing the equipment, assessing and preparing the patient, and selecting the vein and the site of insertion.

TABLE 7-3

PHILLIPS 15-STEP VENIPUNCTURE METHOD

Precannulation
1. Checking physician's order
2. Handwashing procedure
3. Equipment preparation
4. Patient assessment and psychological preparation
5. Site selection and vein dilation

Cannulation
6. Needle selection
7. Gloving
8. Site preparation
9. Vein entry, direct versus indirect
10. Catheter stabilization and dressing management

Postcannulation
11. Labeling
12. Equipment disposal
13. Patient education
14. Rate calculations
15. Documentation

Step 1: Checking the Physician's Order

A physician's order is necessary to initiate I.V. therapy. The physician's order should be clear, concise, legible, and complete. All I.V. solutions should be checked against the physician's order. The physician's order should include:

- Date and time of the day
- Infusate name
- Route of administration
- Dosage of administration
- Volume to be infused
- Rate of infusion
- Duration of infusion
- Physician's signature (Josephson, 1999)

INS STANDARDS Verbal orders written by a nurse in the medical record in a hospital setting should be signed by the prescriber within an appropriate time frame.

Verbal orders taken in a home setting must be sent to the prescriber for signature. (INS, 2000, 10)

Step 2: Handwashing Procedure

Handwashing has been shown to significantly decrease the risk of contamination and cross-contamination. Touch contamination is a common cause of transfer of pathogens. Soap and water are adequate for handwashing before the insertion of cannula; however, an antiseptic solution such as chlorhexidine may be used. Wash hands for 15 to 20 seconds before equipment preparation and before insertion of a catheter. Do not apply hand lotion after handwashing (CDC, 1995). The agent that you use for washing has an effect on efficiency. Bar, powdered, leaflet, or liquid soaps that do not contain an antibacterial agent are unacceptable for surgical scrubs. Agents recommended for handwashing are antiseptic soaps containing chemicals of iodine or chlorhexidine. Avoid wearing false fingernails, which can increase the number of hand-carried microorganisms (NITA, 1985).

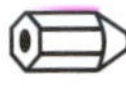

NOTE: Touch contamination is a common cause of transmission of pathogens. The risk of cross-contamination is reduced by handwashing, length of time, place, and method of handwashing (INS, 1998, 16).

INS STANDARDS Handwashing shall be performed before and immediately after all clinical procedures and after removal of gloves. (INS, 1998, 16)

Step 3: Equipment Preparation

Inspect the infusate container at the nurses' station, in the clean utility, or in the medication room. In modern practice, two systems are available—glass system (open or closed) and plastic system (rigid or soft).

To check the glass system, hold the container up to the light to inspect for cracks as evidenced by flashes of light. Glass systems are crystal clear. Rotate the container and look for particulate contamination and cloudiness. Inspect the seal and check the expiration date.

To check a plastic system, squeeze the soft plastic infusate container to check for breaks in the integrity of the plastic; squeeze the system to detect pinholes. Observe for any particulate contamination and check the expiration date. The plastic systems are not crystal clear. The outer wrap of the soft plastic systems should be dry.

Select either a vented or nonvented primary tubing set or a secondary set, depending on the rationale for infusion. It is wise to "**spike**" the solution container and "**prime**" the administration set at the nurses' station to detect defective equipment. Choose the correct tubing to match the solution container. For closed glass use vented only; for plastic, use vented or nonvented. (See Chapter 6 for more detailed information on I.V. equipment.)

Step 4: Patient Assessment and Psychological Preparation

First, provide privacy for the patient. Explain the procedure to decrease his or her anxiety and instruct the patient regarding the purpose of the I.V. therapy, the procedure, what the physician has ordered in the infusate and why, and the limitations.

Evaluate the patient's psychological preparedness for the I.V. procedure by talking with the patient before assessing the vein. The therapist should consider aspects such as autonomy and independence, along with invasion of personal space when I.V. placement is necessary. Often the patient has a fear of pain associated with venipuncture because of the lack of understanding related to necessity of the therapy.

Questions to ask the patient:

- What is your primary medical diagnosis?
- Do you have a chronic disease that places you at risk of complications?
- Do you have epilepsy?
- Do you have a history of vasovagal reactions during venipuncture or when you see blood?
- Do you have fragile peripheral veins?
- Have you had previous vascular access devices?
- Will you be in one setting for the course of therapy or will you be transferred to another setting?
- If you will be going home with the access device, are you (or a caregiver) capable of managing the device at home? (Hadaway, 1999a)

Step 5: Site Selection and Vein Dilatation

Site selection is based on INS standards.

INS STANDARDS Vein selection shall include assessment of the patient's condition, age, and diagnosis; vein condition size and location; and type and duration of therapy. The vein shall accommodate the gauge and length of the cannula required by the prescribed therapy. (INS, 1998, S49)

Vein Dilatation

Several factors should be considered before a venipuncture is attempted. These factors help therapists make competent choices of location for the infusion.

1. *Type of solution:* Fluids that are hypertonic (i.e., more than 375 mOsm), such as antibiotics and potassium chloride, are irritating to vein walls. Select a large vein in the forearm to initiate this therapy. Start at the best, lowest vein.
2. *Condition of vein:* A soft, straight vein is the ideal choice for venipuncture. Palpate the vein by moving the tips of the fingers down the vein to observe how it refills. The dorsal metacarpal veins in elderly patients are a poor choice because blood extravasation (i.e., hematoma) occurs more readily in small, thin veins. When a patient is hypovolemic, peripheral veins

CULTURAL AND ETHNIC CONSIDERATIONS: PERFORMING I.V. THERAPY

Transcultural nursing is becoming a specialty field; however, every nurse must use transcultural knowledge to facilitate culturally appropriate care. Practitioners performing I.V. therapy must make every effort to deliver culturally sensitive care that is free of inherent biases based on gender, race, and religion.

Culturally diverse nursing care must take into account six cultural phenomena that vary with application and use yet are evident in all cultural groups: (1) communication, (2) space, (3) social organization, (4) time, (5) environmental control, and (6) biologic variations.

In preparing to perform I.V. therapy–related procedures on patients from different cultures, is important to remember some key guidelines.

- Plan care based on the communicated needs and cultural background.
- Learn as much as possible about the patient's cultural customs and beliefs.
- Encourage the patient to reveal cultural interpretations of health, illness, and health care.
- Be sensitive to the uniqueness of the patient.
- Identify sources of discrepancy between patient's and your own concepts of health and illness.
- Communicate at the patient's personal level of functioning.
- Modify communication approaches to meet cultural needs.
- Understand that respect for the patient and his or her communication needs is central to the therapeutic relationship.
- Communicate in a nonthreatening manner.
- Follow acceptable social and cultural amenities.
- Adopt special approaches when the patient speaks a different language.
- Use a caring tone of voice and facial expression.
    - Speak slowly and distinctly but not loudly.
    - Use gestures, pictures, and play acting to help the patient understand.
    - Repeat the message in different way.
    - Be alert to words the patient seems to understand and use them frequently.
    - Keep messages simple and repeat them.
    - Avoid using medical terms and abbreviations.
    - If available, use an appropriate language dictionary.
    - Use interpreters to improve communication (Giger & Davidhizar, 1999).

collapse more quickly than larger veins (Weinstein, 1997). Avoid:
- Bruised veins
- Red, swollen veins
- Veins near previously infected areas
- Sites near a previously discontinued site

3. *Duration of therapy:* Choose a vein that supports I.V. therapy for at least 72 hours. Start at the best, lowest vein. Use the hand only if a nonirritating solution is being infused. Long courses of infusion therapy make preservation of veins essential. Perform venipuncture distally with each subsequent puncture **proximal** to previous puncture and alternate arms. Avoid:
   - A joint flexion
   - A vein too small for cannula size
4. *Cannula size:* Hemodilution is important. The **gauge** of the cannula should be as small as possible. When performing transfusion therapy, an 18-gauge catheter is preferred so the cellular portion of blood will not be damaged during infusion.
5. *Patient age:* Infants do not have the accessible sites that older children and adults have owing to infants' increased body fat. Veins in the hands, feet, and antecubital region may be the only accessible sites. Veins in elderly persons are usually fragile; approach venipuncture gently and evaluate the need for a tourniquet (Fabian, 1995).

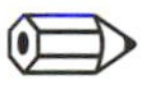

NOTE: Fragile veins can be penetrated with less extravasation of blood if a tourniquet is not used and an indirect (2-step) method is used.

6. *Patient preference:* Consider the patient's personal feelings when determining the catheter placement site. Evaluate the extremities, taking into account the dominant hand.
7. *Patient activity:* Ambulatory patients using crutches or a walker will need cannula placement above the wrist so the hand can still be used.
8. *Presence of disease or previous surgery:* Patients with vascular disease or dehydration may have limited venous access. Avoid phlebitis-infiltrated sites or a site of infection. If a patient has a condition with poor vascular venous return, the affected side **must be avoided.** Examples are cerebrovascular accident, mastectomy, amputation, orthopedic surgery of the hand or arm, and plastic surgery of the hand or arm.

INS STANDARDS A physician's order is required for vein selection in the arm of a patient who has undergone mastectomy or axillary node dissection. (INS, 2000, 43)

9. *Presence of shunt or graft:* Do not use a patient's arm or hand that has a patent graft or shunt for dialysis.

10. *Patients receiving anticoagulation therapy:* Patients receiving anticoagulant therapy have a propensity to bleed. Local ecchymoses and major hemorrhagic complications can be avoided if the nurse is aware that the patient is taking anticoagulant therapy. Precautions can be taken when initiating I.V. therapy. Venous distention can be accomplished with minimal tourniquet pressure. Use the smallest cannula that will accommodate the vein and deliver the ordered infusate. Dressing must be removed gently using alcohol or adhesive remover.
11. *Patient with allergies:* Determine whether a patient has allergies. Allergies to iodine need to be identified because iodine is contained in products used to prep the skin before venipuncture. Question the patient regarding allergies to shellfish. If there is a doubt, use 70 percent isopropyl alcohol to prep the skin and cleanse the ports. Other allergies of concern to delivery of safe patient care include allergies to medications, foods, animals, and environmental substances.

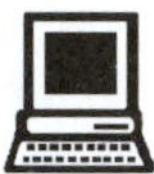

WEB SITES: *www.allergy.mcg.edu*
Other:______________________________________

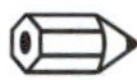

NOTE: Always question the patient regarding allergies before administering medication, especially those given parenterally.

Cannulation of the lower extremities in adults should be avoided, because this increases the risk of thrombophlebitis and embolism. (INS, 1998, 49)

There are many ways to increase the flow of blood in the upper extremities. Factors affecting the capacity for dilatation are blood pressure, presence of valves, sclerotic veins, and multiple previous I.V. sites.

Ways to dilate veins are:

1. *Gravity:* Position the extremity lower than the heart for several minutes.
2. *Fist clenching:* Instruct the patient to open and close his or her fist. Squeezing a rubber ball or rolled washcloth works well.
3. *Tapping:* Using thumb and the second finger, flick the vein; this releases histamines beneath the skin and causes dilatation.
4. *Warm compresses:* Apply warm towels to the extremity for 10 minutes. Do not use a microwave to heat towels; the temperature can become too hot and cause a burn.
5. *Blood pressure cuff:* This is an excellent choice for vein dilatation. Pump the cuff up slightly (e.g., about 30 mm Hg). This method prevents constriction of the arterial system.

NOTE: Care must be used when using a blood pressure cuff not to start the I.V. too close to the cuff owing to excessive back pressure.

6. *Tourniquet:* Apply the tourniquet 6 to 8 inches above the venipuncture site if the blood pressure is within normal range. If the patient is hypertensive, the tourniquet should be placed high on

the extremity; occasionally, the tourniquet is not needed with severely hypertensive patients. With hypotensive patients, move the tourniquet as close as possible to the venipuncture site without contamination of prepped area. (See Chapter 9 for multiple tourniquet techniques.)

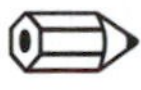

NOTES: Use the tourniquet only once. Using the same tourniquet on more than one patient can result in cross-contamination.

Tourniquets may be sources of latex exposure (INS, 1998, 51).

Use a nonlatex tourniquet (Becton Dickinson [1-800-237–2762] or Baumgarten's Plastiband [1-800-247–5547]) or place clothing or a stockinette over the latex tourniquet.

INS STANDARDS Site selection should be routinely initiated in the distal areas of the upper extremities, and subsequent cannulation should be made proximal to the previously cannulated site. Avoid using veins at areas of flexion unless the area is immobilized. Veins in the antecubital fossa should be reserved for peripheral central line and midline access and for drawing blood samples. (INS, 2000, 43)

7. *Multiple tourniquets:* Applying additional tourniquets to increase the oncotic pressure and bring deep veins into view is discussed in detail in Chapter 9.
8. *Transillumination:* Use of a penlight or Venoscope to illuminate veins in patients with dark skin is discussed in detail in Chapter 9.

CANNULATION

Cannulation involves steps 6 through 10: selecting the needle, gloving, preparing the site, direct or indirect entry into the vein, and stabilizing the catheter and managing the dressing.

Nursing goals for choosing an appropriate site include the following:

- The site must tolerate the rate of flow.
- The site must be capable of delivering the medications ordered.
- The site must tolerate the gauge of cannula needed.
- The patient must be comfortable with the site chosen.
- The site must not impede the patient's activities of daily living (Fabian, 1998).

Table 7–4 presents tips for selecting veins.

Step 6: Needle Selection

Infusions may be delivered with a plastic or steel cannula. (See Chapter 6 for needle choice and sizes.) The choice of catheter depends on the purpose of the infusion and the condition and availability of the veins. Steel needles are generally avoided, except for bolus injections or infusions lasting only a few hours. Inflexible steel needles greatly increase the risk of vein injury and infiltration.

TABLE 7–4

TIPS FOR SELECTING VEINS

- A suitable vein should feel relatively smooth, pliable with valves well spaced.
- Veins will be difficult to stabilize in a patient who has recently lost weight.
- Debilitated patients and those taking corticosteroids have fragile veins that bruise easily.
- Sclerotic veins are common among narcotic addicts.
- Sclerotic veins are common among the elderly population.
- Dialysis patients usually know which veins are good for venipuncture.
- Start with distal veins and work proximally.
- Veins that feel bumpy like running your finger over a cat's tail are usually thrombosed or extremely valvular.

Catheters made of radiopaque material are the best quality. Most hospitals, clinics, and home care agencies have policies and procedures for the selection of catheters. Recommended gauges are:

- 18 to 20 gauge for infusion of hypertonic or isotonic solutions with additives
- 18 to 20 gauge for blood administration
- 22 to 24 gauge for pediatric patients
- 22 gauge for fragile veins in elderly persons if unable to place a 20-gauge catheter

The tip of the catheter should be inspected for integrity before venipuncture to note the presence of burrs on the needle, peeling of catheter material, or other abnormalities.

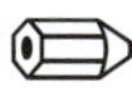

NOTE: Only two attempts at venipuncture are recommended because multiple unsuccessful attempts cause unnecessary trauma to the patient and limit vascular access. When aseptic technique is compromised (i.e., in an emergency situation), the cannula is also considered compromised and a new catheter should be placed within 24 hours.

INS STANDARDS The cannula selected shall be the smallest gauge and shortest length to accommodate the prescribed therapy. Catheters shall be radiopaque. (INS, 2000, 44)

INS STANDARDS A peripheral short catheter shall be removed every 72 hours and immediately upon suspected contamination, complication, or therapy discontinuation. An organization that fails to maintain an ongoing phlebitis rate of 5% or less with the practice of 72 hour catheter site rotation should return to a 48-hour site rotation interval. (INS, 2000, 55)

Step 7: Gloving

The CDC (1995) recommends following standard precautions whenever exposure to blood or body fluids is likely. Latex and vinyl gloves protect wearers from contact with blood and body fluids. However, latex, a natural material, is more flexible than vinyl and molds to the wearer's hand, allowing freedom of movement. Its lattice-type structure allows tiny punctures to reseal automatically.

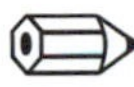
NOTE: Latex and the powder used in the gloves are associated with potentially severe allergic reactions in susceptible persons. Avoid using this material if you have experienced any reactions to their use. (For more information on latex allergy, see Chapter 1.)

Gloves made of polyvinyl chloride, the synthetic rubber known as vinyl, do not reseal, are less flexible and less durable, and are of limited usefulness in high-risk, heavy-usage situations (Korniewicz, Kirwin, & Larson, 1991).

Step 8: Site Preparation

Hair should only be removed with scissors or clippers. Shaving is not recommended because of the potential for **microabrasions,** which increase the risk of infection. The use of depilatories is not recommended because of the potential for allergic reactions. Electric hair removal devices are not used unless they are effective and meet the criteria for preservation of skin integrity (INS, 1998, 52).

Cleansing the insertion site reduces the potential for infection. The following **antimicrobial** solutions may be used to prepare the cannula site:

- Tincture of iodine 2 percent
- Iodophor (povidone-iodine)
- 70 percent isopropyl alcohol
- Chlorhexidine

Aqueous benzalkonium-like compounds and hexachlorophene should not be used as preparatory solutions before venipuncture (INS, 1998, 54).

In preparing the site, use a vigorous circular motion working from the center outward to a diameter of 2 to 3 inches for 20 seconds. The solutions should be allowed to air dry. Use 70 percent alcohol as a defatting agent before application of the povidone-iodine. If the patient is allergic to iodine, use 70 percent alcohol with friction for at least 30 seconds.

INS STANDARDS Do not apply 70 percent isopropyl alcohol after a povidone-iodine prep because alcohol negates the effect of the povidone-iodine. (INS, 2000, 47)

Step 9: Vein Entry

Gloves should be in place before venipuncture and kept on until after the cannula is stabilized. Gloves should be removed only *after* the risk of exposure to body fluids has been eliminated. Venipuncture can be performed using with a *direct* (1-step) or *indirect* (2-step) method. The direct method is appropriate for small-gauge needles, fragile hand veins, or rolling veins and carries an increased risk of causing a hematoma. The indirect method can be used for all venipunctures. (Procedure 7–1: Venipuncture describes the steps to use.)

PROCEDURE 7–1: VENIPUNCTURE

Step 1: Pull skin below puncture site to stabilize the skin and prevent the rolling of the vein.

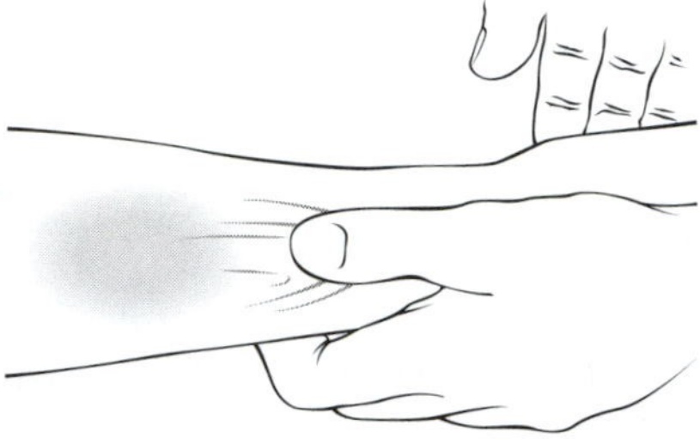

Step 2: Grasp the flashback chamber.

Step 3: Insert the needle of choice **bevel** up at a 30- to 45-degree angle, depending on the vein location and catheter, while applying traction on the vein to keep skin taut.

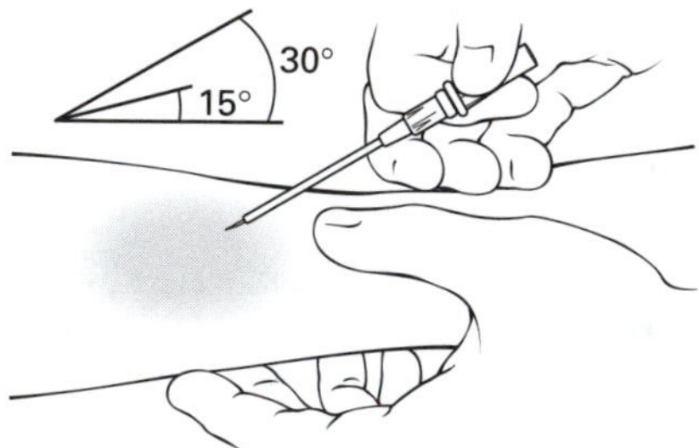

Step 4: Insert the catheter by direct or indirect method with a steady motion.

For the Direct (One-Step) Method:

A. Insert the cannula directly over the vein at a 30- to 45-degree angle.
B. Penetrate all layers of the vein with one motion.

For the Indirect (Two-Step) Method:

A. Insert the cannula at a 30- to 45-degree angle to the skin alongside the vein; gently insert the cannula distal to the point at which the needle will enter the vein.

B. Maintain parallel alignment and advance through the subcutaneous tissue.
C. Relocate the vein and decrease the angle as the cannula enters the vein.

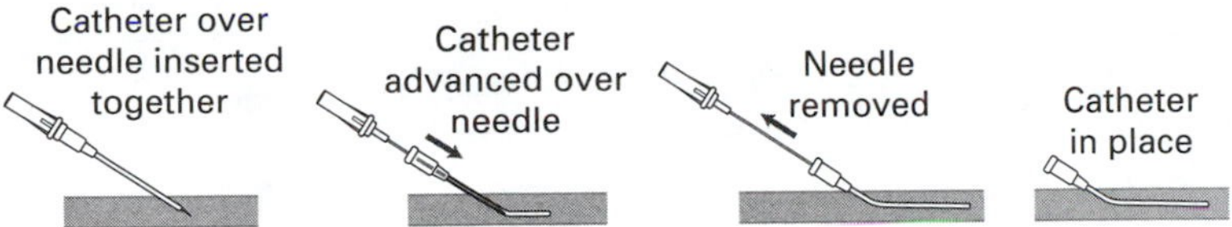

Jabbing, stabbing, or quick thrusting should be avoided because such actions may cause rupture of delicate veins (Enrich, 1991). For performing a venipuncture on difficult veins, follow these guidelines:

- For paper-thin transparent skin or delicate veins: Use the smallest catheter possible (preferably 22 gauge); use direct entry; decrease angle of entry to 15 degrees; apply minimal tourniquet pressure.
- For an obese patient or if you are unable to palpate or see veins: Create a visual image of venous anatomy and select a longer catheter (preferably 2 in).
- If the veins roll when venipuncture is attempted: Apply traction to the vein with thumb during venipuncture, keeping skin taut; leave tourniquet on to promote venous distention; use a blood pressure cuff for better filling of the vein; use 16- or 18-gauge catheter.

Step 5: After the bevel enters the vein and blood flashback occurs, lower the angle of the catheter and stylet (needle) as one unit and advance into the vein. After the catheter tip and bevel are in the vein, advance the catheter forward off the stylet and into the vein. A steady backflow of blood indicates a successful entry. If the catheter is shorter than the needle, backflow may occur before the catheter tip is fully in the vein.

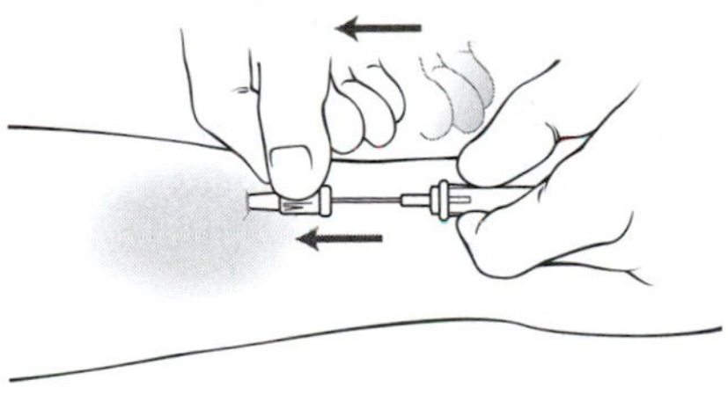

Step 6: After the vein is entered, cautiously advance the cannula into the vein lumen. Hold the catheter hub with your thumb and middle finger and use your index finger to advance the catheter, maintaining skin traction. A one-handed technique is recommended to advance the catheter off the stylet so that the opposite hand can maintain proper traction on the skin and maintain vein alignment (Weinstein, 1997). (A two-handed technique

(continued)

(continued)

can be used, but this increases the risk of vessel rupture during threading of a rigid cannula in a nonstabilized vein.)

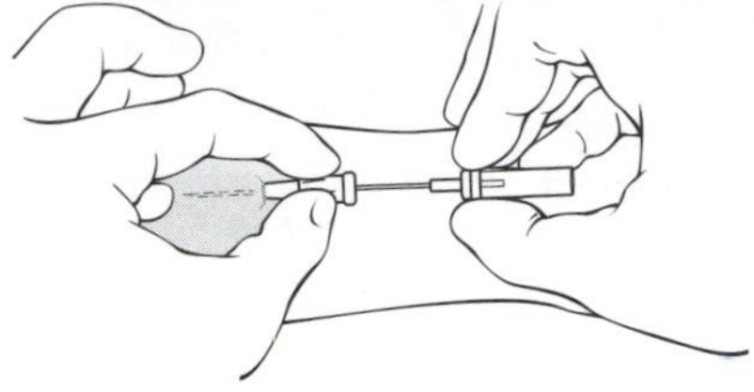

Step 7: While the stylet is still partially inside the catheter, release the tourniquet.
Step 8: Remove the stylet.
Step 9: Connect the adaptor on the administration set to the hub of the catheter.
(Figures Courtesy of Critikon, a Johnson & Johnson Company.)

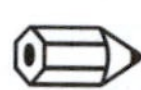 **NOTES:** Blood may ooze from the catheter, depending on the brand of needle used. If there is no blood, the catheter may not be placed correctly or may have penetrated the vein wall. If this is the case, remove the catheter and restart with a sterile cannula.

If the vein has sustained a through-and-through puncture and a hematoma develops, immediately remove the catheter and apply direct pressure to the site. Do not reapply a tourniquet to an extremity immediately after a venipuncture because a hematoma will form (Weinstein, 1997).

Step 10: Catheter Stabilization and Dressing Management

Catheter Stabilization

The catheter should be stabilized in a manner that does not interfere with visualization and evaluation of the site. Stabilization reduces the risk of complications related to I.V. therapy such as phlebitis, infiltration, sepsis, and cannula migration.

There are three methods appropriate for stabilization of the catheter hub: the U method, the H method, and the chevron method (Table 7–5).

When tape is used, it should only be applied to the cannula hub or wings and should not be applied directly to the skin–cannula junction site (INS, 1998, S56).

Using an armboard to stabilize the catheter site is not usually necessary with over-the-needle catheters. If it is necessary because of an erratic flow rate caused by the patient's frequent change of position, use a disposable lightweight armboard. To absorb perspiration, cover the armboard with a washcloth or a paper cover (usually provided with armboards). Secure the

TABLE 7–5

STABILIZING THE CATHETER*

U Method	H Method	Chevron Method
U Method 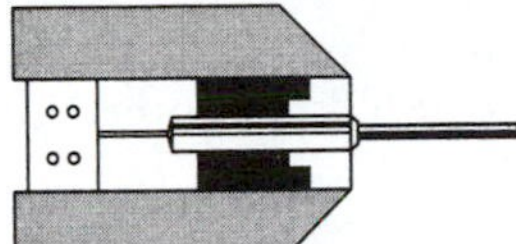 Use for Winged Set	H Method 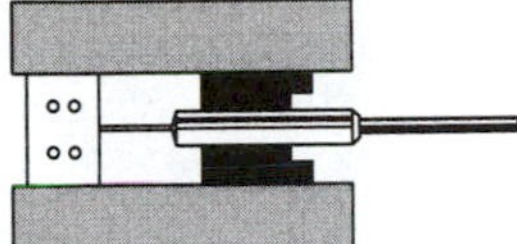 Use for Winged Set	Chevron Method 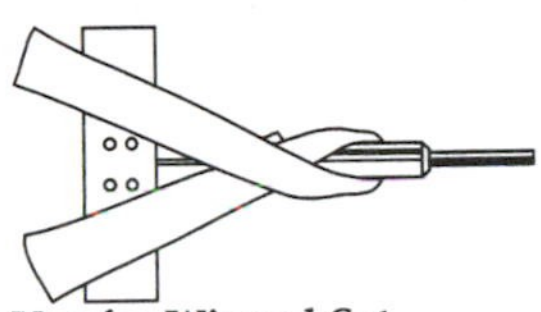 Use for Winged Set
Use for Winged Set	**Use for Winged Set**	**Use for Winged Set**
1. Cut three strips of ½-in tape. With sticky side up, place one strip under tubing. 2. Bring each side of the tape up, folding it over the wings of the needle. Press it down, parallel with the tubing. 3. Loop the tubing and secure it with a piece of 1-in tape.	1. Cut three strips of 1-in tape. 2. Place one strip of tape over each wing, keeping the tape parallel with the needle. 3. Place another strip of tape perpendicular to the first two. Place over the wings to stabilize wings and hub.	1. Cover the venipuncture with transparent dressing or 2 × 2 gauze dressing. 2. Cut a long 5- to 6-in strip of ½-in tape. Place one strip of tape, sticky side under hub, parallel with the dressing. 3. Cross the end of the tape over the opposite side of the needle so that the tape sticks to the patient's skin. 4. Apply a piece of 1-in tape across the wings of the chevron. Loop the tubing and secure it with another piece of 1-in tape.

*For all methods, include on the last piece of tape the date, time of insertion, size of gauge, length of needle or catheter, and your initials.

armboard with two or three pieces of double-backed tape to protect the patient's skin. Do not tape over the site but do leave the patient's fingers free for movement.

INS STANDARDS Cannulas need to be stabilized in a manner that does not interfere with assessment and monitoring of the infusion site or impede delivery of the prescribed therapy. (INS, 2000, 49)

Junction Securement

The use of junction securement minimizes the risk of complications related to infusion therapy. A method of securement should always be used at junction points of I.V. tubing and add-on devices. Examples of junction securement are Luer locks, clasping devices, and threaded devices. The use of tape is not recommended because of the potential risks of air embolism and hemorrhage that may lead to a life-threatening situation caused by separation of the I.V. system and risk of infection (INS, 1998, 57).

Dressing Management

There are two methods for dressing management: (1) a gauze dressing secured with tape and (2) a transparent semipermeable membrane dressing (TSM). A sterile gauze dressing can be applied aseptically with edges secured with tape.

INS STANDARDS Gauze dressings should be changed every **48 hours** on peripheral sites or when the integrity of the dressing is compromised. (INS, 2000, 50)

To apply the gauze dressing:

1. Cleanse the area of excess moisture after venipuncture.
2. Secure the cannula hub.
3. Apply the dressing.

INS STANDARDS The use of a nonocclusive type adhesive bandage strip in place of a gauze dressing is not recommended. (INS, 2000, 50)

Transparent semipermeable membrane dressings should be applied aseptically and changed every 48 to 72 hours, depending on the standard of practice within the institution. The dressing and catheter should be replaced together, unless the integrity of the dressing is impaired; then removal of the dressing with replacement of a new sterile TSM is required. Do not use ointment of any kind under a TSM dressing. Adhesive-coated semipermeable film is available from many manufacturers. The TSM dressing should be applied only to the cannula hub and wings.

To apply a TSM:

1. Cleanse the area of excess moisture after venipuncture.
2. Center the transparent dressing over cannula site and partially over the hub.
3. Press down on the dressing, sealing the catheter site.
4. Apply tape to secure administration set. (See Procedure 7–2: Applying a Dressing.)

PROCEDURE 7–2: APPLYING A DRESSING

Step 1: Cover the insertion site and catheter hub with the transparent dressing.

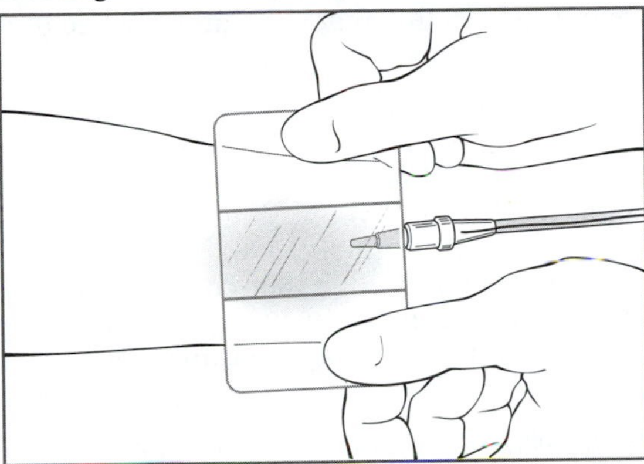

Step 2: Pinch the transparent dressing around the catheter hub to secure the hub.

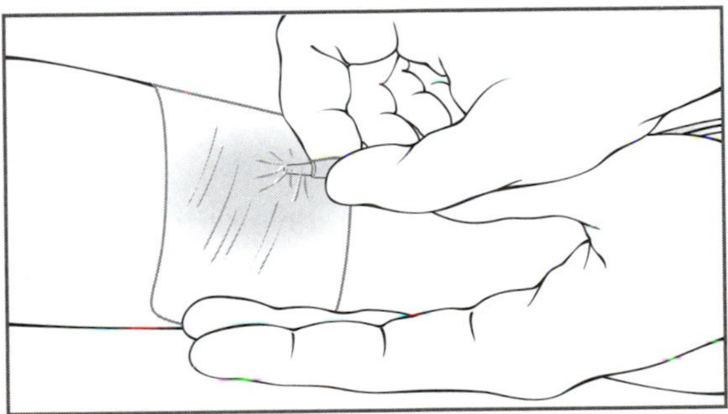

Step 3: Label the insertion site, noting the catheter gauge, date and time of insertion, and initials of the person who performed the venipuncture.

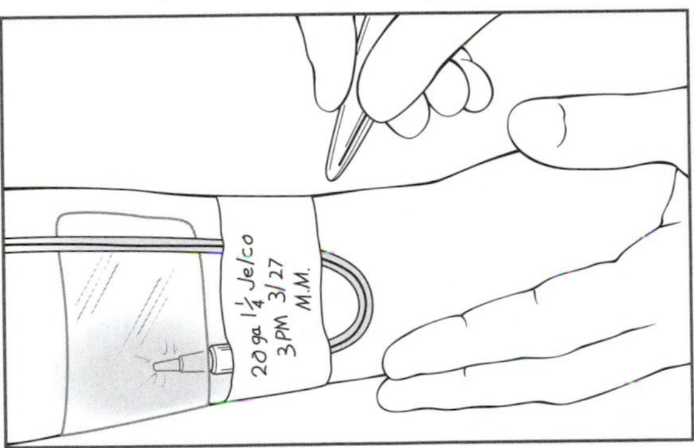

(Figures Courtesy of Critikon, a Johnson & Johnson Company.)

INS STANDARDS TSM dressings should be changed on peripheral short catheters at the time of site rotation or sooner if the integrity has been compromised. (INS, 2000, 50)

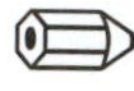

NOTE: Do not put tape over the transparent film because it is difficult to remove the transparent film when the dressing needs to be changed.

Advantages of TSM dressings include that they allow continuous inspection of the site, are more comfortable than gauze and tape, and permit patients to bathe and shower without saturating the dressing (Maki & Mermel, 1998). A disadvantage of TSM dressings is that they are more costly than gauze and tape (Maki & Mermel, 1998).

Ongoing clinical trials based on the knowledge that cutaneous occlusions with tape or impervious plastic films result in an explosive increase in cutaneous microflora, with overgrowth of gram-negative bacilli and yeasts (Prager, 1984).

NOTE: Polyurethane dressing are semipermeable. That is, they are impervious to extrinsic microbial contaminates and liquid-phase moisture and variably permeable to oxygen, carbon dioxide, and water vapor. Other studies in healthy volunteers have shown little effect of these dressing on the cutaneous flora (Hoffmann, 1992).

Step 11: Labeling

The I.V. setup should be labeled in three spots: the insertion site, the tubing, and the solution container, which should be time stripped.

INS STANDARDS Distinctive legible labeling shall provide pertinent and easily identified information relative to the cannula, dressing, solution, medication, and administration set. (INS, 2000, 17)

1. The venipuncture site should be labeled on the side of the transparent dressing or across the hub. Do not place the label over the site because this obstructs visualization of the site. Include on the label:
   - Date and time
   - The type and length of the catheter (e.g., 20-gauge, 1 in)
   - The nurse's initials
2. Label the tubing according to agency policy and procedure so that practitioners on subsequent shifts will be aware of when the tubing must be changed.
3. Place a time strip on all parenteral solutions with the name of the solution and additives, initials of the nurse, and the time the solution was started.

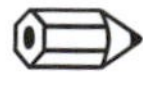

NOTE: Time strips are helpful for assessing whether the solution is on schedule.

Step 12: Equipment Disposal

Recapping needles increases the risk of needlestick injuries to the practitioner. Needles and stylets should be disposed of in nonpermeable tamper-proof containers. Needles and stylets should not be recapped, broken, or bent in accordance with the Occupational Safety and Health Administration (OSHA) and the Joint Commission on Accreditation of Healthcare Organizations (JCAHO, 1995; CDC, 1995). After venipuncture is complete, dispose of all paper and plastic equipment in a container suitable for burning.

INS STANDARDS Needles and stylets (sharps) shall be disposed of in nonpermeable, tamper-proof containers. (INS, 2000, 31)

Step 13: Patient Education

Patients have the right to receive information on all aspects of their care in a manner they can understand, as well as the right to accept or refuse treatment (INS, 1998, S22).

After the catheter is stabilized, the dressing applied and the labeling complete:

- Inform the patient of any limitations on movement or mobility.
- Explain all alarms if an electronic control device is used.
- Instruct the patient to call for assistance if the venipuncture site becomes tender or sore or if redness or swelling develops.
- Advise the patient that the venipuncture site will be checked by the nurse.

INS STANDARDS When a patient requires continued care in his or her home, the nurse shall provide comprehensive education to the patient and caregiver that includes the behavioral domains of cognitive affective and psychomotor, along with a written set of instructions on all pertinent aspects of treatment. (INS, 2000, 12)

Step 14: Rate Calculations

Many clinical environments require delivery of I.V. medications, unusual infusion rates, and administration of primary and secondary infusions, so I.V. therapists must be capable of accurate calculations. Calculating the proper I.V. rate for medication and solution delivery can be time intensive. All I.V. infusions should be monitored frequently for accurate flow rates and complications associated with infusion therapy.

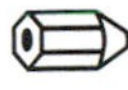

NOTE: Refer to the section on math calculations for further guidance on rate calculations.

Step 15: Monitoring and Documentation

Monitoring of the patient should include cannula, exit site, and surrounding area; flow rate; clinical data; patient response; and compliance to the prescribed therapy. The frequency of monitoring provides for patient protection and is an integral part of quality and risk management. Information that is obtained by monitoring should be communicated to other healthcare professionals responsible for the patient's care by documentation (INS, 1998, S23).

Documentation of I.V. therapy procedures generally includes:

- Date and time of insertion
- Manufacturer's brand name and style of device
- The gauge and length of the device
- Specific name and location of the accessed vein
- The infused solution and rate of flow
- Infusing by gravity or pump
- The number attempts for a successful I.V. start
- The patient's specific comments related to the procedure
- Signature (Masoorli, 1995)

Documentation should be legible, accessible to healthcare professionals, and readily retrievable.

INS STANDARDS Documentation in the patient's medical record should contain sufficient information to identify infusion procedures, prescribed treatments, complications, nursing interventions, and patient outcomes. (INS, 2000, 17)

Patient education is lacking in most audits of charts; therefore, documentation of patient response to the procedure needs to be included in the charting format. This needs to be addressed in narrative charting or in a check-off format, which includes the status of the patient, the reason for restart, the procedure used, and comments.

Table 7–6 summarizes the steps of starting a peripheral infusion.

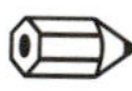

NOTE: Refer to Appendix D for CDC (1995) recommendations for the use of peripheral venous catheters.

DISCONTINUATION OF THE I.V. CANNULA

I.V. therapy should be discontinued if the integrity of the cannula is compromised or the physician orders the discontinuation of therapy. To discontinue the I.V. cannula:

1. Put on gloves.
2. Obtain a dry 2-in by 2-in gauze pad. Avoid one with alcohol because it causes stinging and promotes bleeding.
3. Loosen the tape and apply the gauze pad loosely over the site.
4. Remove the cannula and transparent dressing as one unit, without pressure over the site.

TABLE 7–6

SUMMARY OF STEPS IN INITIATING I.V. THERAPY

Precannula Insertion

1. Check physician order; confirm all parts of the order for accuracy.
2. Wash hands for 15 to 20 seconds using bactericidal soap. Prepare equipment: Check for breaks in integrity and check expiration date; spike and prime the infusion system.
3. Provide privacy. Explain procedure to the patient. Evaluate the patient's psychological preparation for I.V. therapy.
4. Make assessment of site and vein dilatation.
5. Assess both arms keeping the factors for vein selection in mind. Make a choice whether to use blood pressure cuff or tourniquet for dilatation. Use other methods for venous distension, such as warm packs, gravity, or tapping, if necessary.

Cannula Insertion

6. Choose the appropriate catheter for duration of infusion and type of infusate based on facility policy and procedure. Rewash hands.
7. Use gloves, following universal precautions for exposure to blood or body fluids.
8. Prepare site by using 70 percent alcohol to cleanse the site followed by a 20-second scrub with povidone-iodine or chlorhexidine. Let the povidone-iodine or chlorhexidine air dry. Do not remove. If the patient is allergic to iodine, use alcohol for a 30-second vigorous scrub as a substitute. Do not retouch. Put on gloves before venipuncture.
9. Insert the over-the-needle catheter with the direct or indirect method. Thread the catheter while removing the stylet needle. Connect the catheter hub to I.V. tubing or insert a locking device (PRN device).
10. Stabilize the catheter hub with the chevron taping method or use transparent dressing directly over the hub and site. There are two methods of dressing management: (1) 2-in × 2-in gauze with all edges taped; change every 48 hours or (2) transparent film (TSM) applied with aseptic technique and changed every 48 to 72 hours or if the integrity of the dressing is compromised.

Postcannula Insertion

11. Label the insertion site with cannula size, date, time, and initials; label the tubing with the date and time; strip the solution.
12. To facilitate equipment disposal, use OSHA and JCAHO standards for disposal of the needle.
13. Explain to the patient the limitations, provide information on the equipment being used, and give instructions for observation of the site.
14. Remember when doing rate calculations that if a roller clamp or electronic controller is used, the drops per minute should be calculated based on the drop factor.
15. Monitor the patient for response to prescribed therapies. Document the procedure performed, how the patient tolerated the venipuncture, and what instructions were given to the patient.

5. After the catheter is removed, apply direct pressure with the sterile gauze pad over the site.
6. An adhesive bandage may be applied to the venipuncture site after bleeding is controlled.
7. Document the site appearance, how the patient tolerated the procedure, and the intactness of the cannula.

INTERMITTENT INFUSION DEVICES

Intermittent infusion devices or resealable locks, also called PRN devices, intermittent I.V. lock devices, and saline or heparin locks have been a standard of practice in most hospitals for over a decade. Maintaining these devices is typically accomplished by flushing with dilute heparinized saline at the end of an infusion and between injections. Controversies have arisen regarding standardization of heparin flushing protocols and the use of saline flushes for maintaining patency of peripheral lines (Fry, 1992).

Resealable locks consist of a cap that fits over the proximal end of the I.V. catheter with a resealable diaphragm. A number of sets are available commercially. Heparin locks were originally used for pediatric and geriatric patients.

Advantages:

- Provide access to the vascular system, allowing for more flexibility than hanging I.V. fluids
- Allow or reduced volume of fluid administered, which can be important for cardiac patients
- Can be used to collect blood samples for glucose tolerance tests, eliminating multiple puncture sites
- Provide access for delivery of emergency medications

Disadvantages

- Occlusion or blood clotting within the lock
- Possibility of speed shock and damage from drug being rapidly introduced into the circulation

INTERMITTENT INFUSION MAINTENANCE

The CDC (1995) recommends that heparin only be used when intermittent infusion devices are used for blood sampling. This is a change based on studies that suggest that 0.9 percent sodium chloride is just as effective as heparin in maintaining catheter patency and reducing phlebitis. How devices are kept patent is determined by institution policy.

Currently, the INS recommends using sodium chloride injection for flushing peripheral I.V. cannulas.

INS STANDARDS Flushing with 0.9 percent sodium chloride injection solution to ensure and maintain patency of an intermittent peripheral I.V. cannula should be performed at intervals. (INS, 2000, 56)

Sodium Chloride Lock Flush

Cost-effectiveness is a driving factor influencing the choices of practice in today's healthcare field. Use of 0.9 percent sodium chloride rather than heparin to maintain heparin locks has been investigated as a way of reducing cost.

Advantages:

- Fewer steps
- Lower cost
- Takes 2 minutes for a nurse to administer and document a flush (eliminating two thirds of the flushes per year saves nursing time)

Disadvantages:

- Loss of patency
- Phlebitis
- Increased patient stress caused by catheter starts (Cyganski, Donohue, & Heaton, 1987)

Heparin Lock Flush

Heparin inhibits reactions that lead to blood coagulation and the formation of fibrin clots in vitro and in vivo. The anticoagulant effect of heparin is almost immediate. Heparin acts indirectly by means of a plasma cofactor, thereby neutralizing several activated clotting factors. Because of these properties, it can be used therapeutically as a flushing agent.

Heparin is injected into the diaphragm (hub) of the device after each use or every 8 hours if not in use (Fry, 1992). A study by Andersen and Holland (1992) found that 10 U/mL heparin was as effective as 100 U/mL heparin in maintaining the patency of peripherally inserted central catheters.

The use of heparinized saline has been successful for many years and is a recognized standard of practice in the medical community. It is recommended that the lowest possible concentration of heparin be used.

Advantages:

- Reduced risk of phlebitis
- Low incidence of side effects when properly used
- Low risk of tort liability with heparin flushing practices
- One dose of heparin solution will maintain anticoagulation within the lumen of the device for up to 4 hours

Despite pressures to reduce costs by eliminating the flush, hospitals legally and ethically can support only policies that benefit or at least have no adverse effect on the patient.

Disadvantages:

- Must be used with caution in patients with known hypersensitivity to pork and beef
- Local and systemic allergic-type reactions with the use of multidose vial preparations are thought to be associated with a preservative hypersensitivity
- Has one extra step
- Increased cost to patients
- Complications, including hypersensitivity reactions, transient increases in activated partial thromboplastin time, and delayed fibrinolysis with platelet aggregation and thrombocytopenia (Baldwin, 1989; Chang, 1987)
- Has bioincompatibilities (Nelson, Young, & Lammin, 1987)

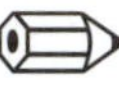

NOTES: Do not use the heparin sequence in flushing a peripheral I.V. unless backed by institutional policy or specifically ordered by a physician (Josephson, 1999).

When flushing the device, positive pressure within the lumen of the catheter must be maintained during and after administration of the flush solution to prevent reflux of blood into the cannula lumen.

INS STANDARDS The amount of heparin and the frequency of the flush should be such that the patient's clotting factors are not altered. (INS, 2000, 56)

Table 7–7 presents a comparison of the heparin and saline lock flush procedures.

TABLE 7–7

COMPARISON OF PROCEDURE FOR HEPARIN LOCK FLUSH AND SALINE LOCK FLUSH

Heparin Lock Flush*	Saline Lock Flush
1. Check patency of lock.	1. Check patency of the lock.
2. Flush lock with 1 mL saline to clear lock of any bioincompatibility.	2. Flush with 1 mL of 0.9% sodium chloride.
3. Administer medication.	3. Administer medication.
4. Flush with saline again to clear lock of any bioincompatibility.	4. Flush with 1 mL of 0.9% sodium chloride.
5. Heparinize with 10 to 100 units of heparin in 1 mL saline to reseal the lock.	

*This is the SASH method: saline = administration = saline = heparin.

CONTROVERSIAL PRACTICES

Controversy exists in the administration of anesthetics either on or in the skin before venipuncture. These include the use of lidocaine (xylocaine hydrochloride) intradermal injection as well as transdermal application of xylocaine (EMLA cream) and topical nitroglycerin.

LIDOCAINE

Lidocaine has been used in clinical practice since 1948 and is one of the safest anesthetics. Lidocaine is an amide that works by stopping impulses at the neural membrane. The anesthetized site is numb to pain, but the patient perceives touch and pressure and has control of his or her muscles. The anesthetic becomes effective within 15 to 30 seconds and lasts 30 to 45 minutes. The nurse must have knowledge of the actions and side effects associated with lidocaine. A history of previous allergies precludes the administration of lidocaine.

The use of lidocaine is a simple process:

1. Check for patient allergy and lidocaine sensitivity.
2. Select appropriate arm, apply the tourniquet, and select a suitable vein.
3. Draw up 0.1 cc of 1 percent lidocaine (plain) in a TB syringe. More than 0.1 cc increases the risk for vasospasm.
4. Put on gloves.
5. Prep site with alcohol for 30 seconds and allow it to dry.
6. Reapply the tourniquet. The vein should be fully dilated, pulled taut by stretching, and stabilized while the local anesthetic is administered.
7. Insert the needle at a 15- to 25-degree angle. Inject the lidocaine intradermally into the side of the vein next to the desired insertion site. Do not nick the vein.
8. Withdraw the needle. Allow 5 to 10 seconds for the anesthetic to take effect.
9. Continue with the steps in starting the I.V. (e.g., prep skin with Betadine).

INS STANDARDS Local anesthesia, including lidocaine, shall not be routinely used for the insertion of a cannula. (INS, 2000, 46)

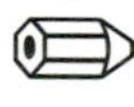

NOTE: Local anesthetics should not be injected into a vein because of the possibility of an undesirable systemic effect. The local anesthetic will not "freeze" the venipuncture site if it is injected into the vein (Fig. 7–5).

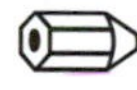

NOTE: Some clinicians believe administration of lidocaine before catheter insertion increases patient comfort and decreases anxiety. However, lidocaine may expose a patient to complications that include (but are not limited to) allergic reaction, anaphylaxis,

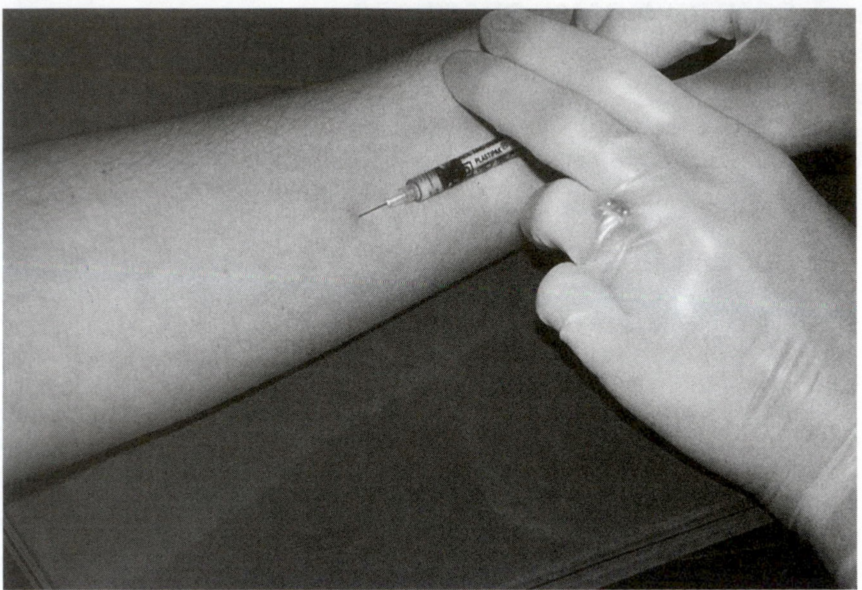

FIG. 7–5. Intradermal lidocaine administered before venipuncture using 0.1 to 0.2 mL of 1% lidocaine and a tuberculin syringe entering the skin at a 15- to 25-degree angle.

inadvertent injection of the drug into the vascular system, and obliteration of the vein.

TRANSDERMAL ANALGESIA

EMLA cream is a mixture of two local anesthetics (lidocaine 2.5% and prilocaine 2.5%). When EMLA is applied to the skin under an occlusive dressing, a release of lidocaine and prilocaine from the cream into the epidermal and dermal layers of the skin provides analgesia. The two agents stabilize neuronal membranes by inhibiting the conduction of impulses, therefore affecting local anesthetic action (Astra, 1992).

Follow these steps when applying EMLA cream:

1. Apply 2.5 g in a thick layer at the intended site of the venipuncture.
2. Place an occlusive dressing over the EMLA cream and smooth down the edges. Be sure to write down the time of application on the dressing.
3. Remove the occlusive dressing, cleanse the skin with an antiseptic, and prepare the patient for the venipuncture. (Fig. 7–6).

In a study, Cooper and coworkers (1987), found that EMLA cream reduced the pain associated with venipuncture in children when a

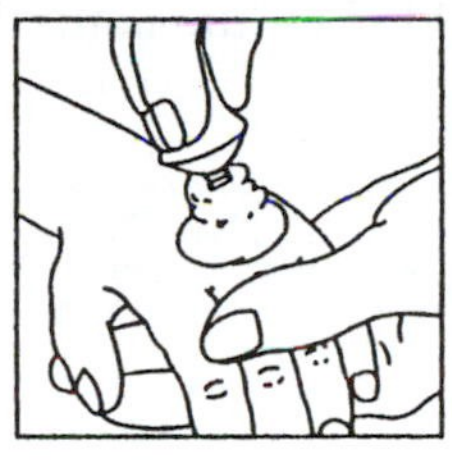

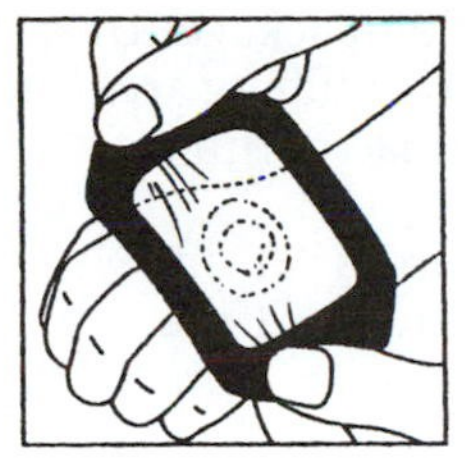

A B

FIG. 7-6. (*A*) Application of EMLA cream to the intended venipuncture site. (*B*) Placement of an occlusive dressing over the cream. (Courtesy of Astra Pharmaceutical Products, Inc., Westborough, Massachusetts.)

25-gauge needle was used. Sixty minutes are required to achieve effective analgesia.

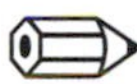

NOTE: Apply EMLA cream under occlusive dressing for one hour before venipuncture.

EMLA cream is contraindicated in patients who have known histories of sensitivity to amide-type local anesthetics.

TOPICAL NITROGLYCERIN

The use of 1 to 2 mg of nitroglycerin rubbed topically into the surrounding skin area has been studied as a method of dilating veins before venipuncture. Hecker and associates (1983) have studied this technique in Australia. In their study, which needs replication, they found that the use of topical Nitrobid distended the veins without the need for other adjuncts such as tapping, swabbing, or clenching the fist.

CALCULATING THE I.V. RATE

PRIMARY I.V. RATE CALCULATIONS

The ability to calculate I.V. rates is essential in many clinical environments. I.V. practitioners must be able to calculate accurately. For proper I.V. rate calculations for medication and solution delivery, two key components must be understood: (1) the drip rate of the I.V. administration set to be used is called the **drop factor,** and (2) the amount of solution to be infused over 1 hour.

Macrodrip Sets

To correctly calculate the drip rate, note the drop factor of the administration set. This is usually located on the side, front, or back of the administration package. Drop factors provided by the administration set for **macrodrip** tubing are as follows:

Primary (macrodrip) sets

- 10 drops = 1 mL
- 15 drops = 1 mL
- 20 drops = 1 mL

Use macrodrip sets whenever (1) a large amount of fluid is ordered to be infused over a short period of time or (2) the microdrips per minute are too many, making counting too difficult (Henke, 1999).

Microdrip Sets

Special administration sets such as pediatric (**microdrip**) sets and transfusion administration sets are also available. All manufacturers of microdrip sets are consistent in having 60 drops equaling 1 mL.

Pediatric (microdrip) sets

- 60 drops = 1 mL

Use microdrip sets whenever (1) the I.V. is to be administered over a long period of time, (2) a small amount of fluid is to be administered, or (3) the macrodrops per minute are too few (Henke, 1999).

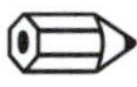

NOTE: Blood flow through veins exerts a pressure: if the I.V. is too slow, blood pressure may force blood into the administration set, where it clots. The I.V. will stop.

Blood Administration Sets

Transfusion administration need a larger drop orifice, so all manufacturers of administration sets specific for blood have 10 drop orifices.

Blood administration sets

- 10 drops = 1 mL

Table 7–8 presents a drop factor conversion chart.

DETERMINING THE AMOUNT OF SOLUTION TO BE INFUSED

The physician orders the amount of solution to be infused. Orders are written in one of two ways: (1) in the total amount over a specified length of time, such as 1000 mL over 8 hours; or (2) in the amount to be delivered per hour (e.g., 125 mL/h).

TABLE 7–8

CONVERSION CHART: RATE CALCULATION

	Drop Factors			
Order: mL/hour	**10 Drops/mL**	**15 Drops/mL**	**20 Drops/mL**	**60 Drops/mL**
10	2	3	3	10
15	3	4	5	15
20	3	5	7	20
30	5	8	10	30
50	8	13	17	50
75	13	19	25	N/A
80	13	20	27	N/A
100	17	25	33	N/A
120	20	30	40	N/A
125	21	31	42	N/A
150	25	38	50	N/A
166	27	42	55	N/A
175	29	44	58	N/A
200	33	50	67	N/A
250	42	63	83	N/A
300	50	75	100	N/A

Microdrip tubing is not appropriate for rates over 50 mL/h.

Formula for I.V. Flow Rates Using Drops per Minute

After the drop factor of the tubing and the amount of solution to be infused are known, the following formula can be used to calculate the drop rate per minute:

$$\frac{\text{mL per hour} \times \text{drops per mL (drop factor [DF])}}{\text{60 (minutes in an hour)}} = \text{drops per minute}$$

$$\text{Formula: } \frac{\text{mL/h} \times \text{DF}}{\text{minutes}} = \text{gtt/min}$$

Formula for I.V. Flow Rates Using an Electronic Rate Control Device

Calculations are particularly important when an electronic rate control device is not being used or when an electronic controller is used that does not have a mechanism to dial in milliliters per hour.

NOTES: Rule: Problems in I.V. calculations are solved in two steps.
Step 1 is used to solve problems requiring an infusion pump and to simplify the math needed for microdrip and macrodrip.
Step 2 will solve micro- and macrodrip problems (Henke, 1999).

Macrodrip Infusion

Example:
Physician orders are for 125 mL/h and the primary tubing selected has a drop factor of 15. Two steps are needed.

$$\text{Formula: } \frac{\text{mL/h} \times \text{DF}}{\text{minutes}} = \text{gtt/min}$$

$$\text{Step 1: } \frac{125 \times 15}{60} = \text{gtt/min}$$

$$\text{Step 2: } \frac{125}{4} = 31 \text{ gtt/min}$$

Microdrip Infusion

When using a microdrip (pediatric tubing) that is 60 drops/mL, the drops per minute equal the milliliters per hour, so only 1 step is needed.

Example:
The physician orders 35 mL of solution per hour for a 2-year-old girl. You would set up your rate calculation as follows, using only 1 step.

$$\text{Formula: } \frac{\text{mL/h} \times \text{DF}}{\text{minutes}} = \text{gtt/min}$$

$$\text{Step 1: } \frac{135 \times 60}{60} = \text{gtt/min} = 35 \text{ gtt/min}$$

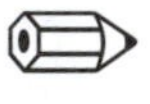

NOTES: Do the practice problems in Math Calculations Worksheet 1 at the end of this chapter to test your comprehension of rate calculation.

The conversion chart in Table 7–8 can be cut and laminated for use in your clinical practice to assist in rate calculation.

Formula for I.V. Flow Rates Using Milliliters per Hour

When using an electronic infusion device that has a setting for milliliters per hour, the amount of solution to be infused in 1 hour is dialed in on the infusion pump.

Example:
The physician orders the I.V. solution at 125 mL/h. Only one step is required. The rate for the pump would be dialed in for 125 mL/h.

ADJUSTING THE FLOW RATE

It is the responsibility of the nurse to maintain the rate of flow of I.V. fluid, especially those with additives. Many factors can interfere with the flow: kinking of the tube, movement of the client, the effect of gravity, or placement of the catheter. It is not at the discretion of the nurse to arbitrarily speed up or slow down the flow rate.

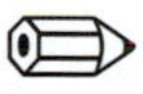

NOTE: Recalculation of flow rates must be included in hospital policy and must not vary from the original rate by more than 25 percent.

A recalculation of the flow rate is indicated when, during routine observation, the flow rate of the I.V. has either increased or decreased. Recalculate the flow rate to administer the total milliliters remaining over the number of hours remaining of the original order.

Example:

The order reads 1000 mL of 5 percent dextrose in water over 8 hours. The drop factor is 15 gtt/mL and the I.V. is correctly set at 31 gtt/min. You would expect that after 4 hours, 50 percent of the total or 500 mL of the solution would be infused. However, checking the I.V. bag the fourth hour after starting the IV, you find 600 mL remaining. You would compute a new flow rate for the 600 mL to run for the remaining 4 hours.

Step 1: Hourly volume to be infused:

$600 \times 4 \text{ hours} = 150 \text{ mL/h}$

Step 2: Know the drop factor of the tubing: 15

Calculation of example:

$$\frac{15 \times 150}{60} = 37.5 = 38 \text{ gtt/min}$$

(It is standard practice to round up if the fraction is above 0.5.)

Secondary Infusion: Solutions to Be Infused in Less Than 1 Hour

A medication may be ordered to be dissolved in a small amount of I.V. fluid (usually 50 to 100 mL) and run "piggyback" to the regular I.V. fluid (Picker, 1999).

To set the rate of the secondary infusion the formula must be changed to adjust for the time change.

Formula:

$$\frac{\text{mL per hour} \times \text{drops per mL (drop factor)}}{\text{Hourly volume varies}} = \text{drops per minute}$$

Example:

Kefzol 0.5 g in 100 mL of dextrose in water to run IVPB over 30 minutes. Administration set is 20 drop factor.

$$\frac{20 \times 100 \text{ mL}}{30 \text{ minutes}} = 2000$$

$$\frac{2000}{30} = 67 \text{ gtt/min}$$

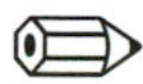

NOTE: Do the practice problems in Math Calculations Worksheet 2 at the end of this chapter to test your comprehension of recalculations and secondary infusions.

NURSING PLAN OF CARE

INITIATION OF VENIPUNCTURE

Focus Assessment

Subjective

- Interview the patient regarding previous experiences with venipunctures.
- Review the purpose of I.V. and patient diagnosis.

Objective

- Assess arms for access.
- Assess age.
- Assess condition of skin and substructures.
- Assess presence of shunts.
- Assess previous surgery that would limit site selection.
- Assess presence of tattoos.
- Assess presence of edema.
- Assess vital signs.

Patient Outcome Criteria

The patient will:

- Demonstrate improved fluid balance.
- Verbalize understanding of need for I.V. access and consent to procedure.
- Be free of complications associated with I.V. therapy.

Nursing Diagnoses

- Anxiety (mild, moderate, or severe) related to threat to or change in health status; misconceptions regarding therapy
- Fear related to insertion of cannula
- Knowledge deficit related to new procedure and maintaining I.V. therapy
- Impaired physical mobility related to pain or discomfort resulting from placement and maintenance of I.V. cannula
- Impaired skin integrity related to I.V. cannula or I.V. solution
- Pain related to physical trauma (e.g., cannula insertion)
- Risk of infection related to broken skin or traumatized tissue

Nursing Management

1. Verify the physician's order for I.V. therapy.
2. Instruct the patient about procedure.
3. Maintain universal precautions.
4. Use strict aseptic technique during insertion of the cannula.
5. Examine the solution for type, amount, expiration date, character of solution, and integrity of container.
6. Select and prepare an I.V. infusion pump as indicated.

(continued)

(continued)

8. Administer I.V. fluids at room temperature.
9. Monitor I.V. flow rate and I.V. site during infusion following protocol.
10. Monitor for I.V. therapy complications (e.g., phlebitis, infiltration, site infection).
11. Replace I.V. cannula and administration every 48 to 72 hours.
12. Maintain integrity of occlusive dressing.

PATIENT EDUCATION

- Instruct on purpose of I.V. therapy.
- Educate regarding limitations of movement.
- Instruct to notify the nurse if pump alarms.
- Instruct to report discomfort at the infusion site.

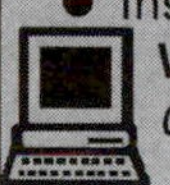

WEB SITES: Patient education: *www.patient-education.com*
Others: ____________________

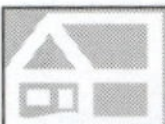

HOME CARE ISSUES

Home care issues for the initiation and maintenance of I.V. therapy revolve around technical procedures, as well as the monitoring of therapy. The technical procedures that the patient is expected to learn and perform depend on his or her cognitive ability, willingness to learn, and the specific technique being taught. Another home care issue is the number of visits that will be required to maintain the line and the proximity of the patient's home to a healthcare facility.

Many common household items contain latex. Home-bound patients who perform self-catheterization or undergo intermittent catheterization are at risk for latex-related allergic reactions. Synthetic rubber, polyethylene, silicon, or vinyl can be used effectively in the home care setting.

Territoriality (i.e., the need for space) serves four functions: security, privacy, autonomy, and self-identification. People tend to generally feel safer in their own territory because it is arranged and equipped in a familiar manner. Most people believe there is a degree of predictability associated with being in one's own personal space and that this degree of predictability is hard to achieve elsewhere (Giger & Davidhizar, 1999).

Patients or their caregivers are often expected to:

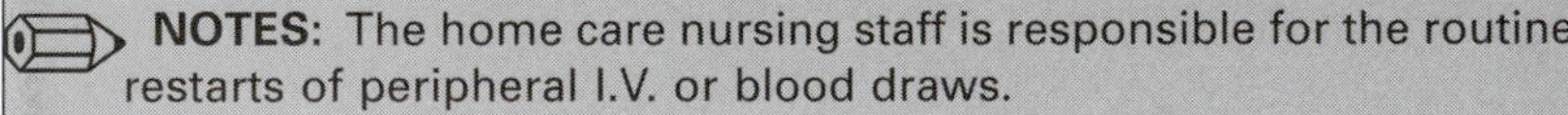

- Administer solutions or medications.
- Change dressings.
- Change administration sets.
- Set up or monitor pump equipment.
- The patient and his or her family must be taught universal precautions and aseptic technique in the home care setting.

NOTES: The home care nursing staff is responsible for the routine restarts of peripheral I.V. or blood draws.

KEY POINTS

The first step is an understanding of the anatomy and physiology of the venous system. The five layers in the approach to successful venipuncture are the epidermis, dermis, tunica adventitia, tunica media, and tunica intima.

A working knowledge of the veins in the hand and forearm is vital so the practitioner can successfully locate an acceptable vein for venipuncture and cannula placement. Keep in mind the type of solution, condition of vein, duration of therapy, patient age, patient preference, patient activity, presence of disease, previous surgery, presence of shunts or grafts, allergies, and medication history.

The steps in performing the placement of a catheter that can support I.V. therapy for 48 to 72 hours are as follows:

PRECANNULATION

- Step 1: Check physician's order.
- Step 2: Wash hands.
- Step 3: Prepare equipment.
- Step 4: Patient assessment and psychological preparedness.
- Step 5: Select site and dilate vein.

CANNULA PLACEMENT

- Step 6: Needle selection
- Step 7: Gloving
- Step 8: Site preparation
- Step 9: Vein entry
- Step 10: Catheter stabilization and dressing management

POSTCANNULATION

- Step 11: Labeling
- Step 12: Equipment disposal
- Step 13: Patient instructions
- Step 14: Rate calculation
- Step 15: Documentation

The choice of using heparin or saline to maintain latex injection ports (locks) is determined by the agency's policies and procedures and the physician's order. Check these before using the steps in heparin or saline lock flush.

- Locks must be flushed every 8 hours if not being used for medication administration.
- Use of xylocaine hydrochloride before venipuncture. Use 0.1 to 0.2 cc of 1 percent xylocaine injected intradermal. Wait 5 to 10 seconds before continuing the steps of the venipuncture.
- Use of topical transdermal analgesia cream, such as a combination of lidocaine 2.5 percent and prilocaine 2.5 percent. Apply in thick layer and cover with occlusive dressing for 1 hour.

RATE CALCULATIONS

To calculate drop rates of gravity infusions, I.V. nurses must know (1) the drop factor of the administration set and (2) the amount of solution ordered.

MACRODRIP SETS:

- 10 gtt = 1 mL
- 15 gtt = 1 mL
- 20 gtt = 1 mL

MICRODRIP SETS

- 60 gtt = 1 mL
- Transfusion administration sets: usually 10 gtt = 1 mL

CHAPTER ACTIVITIES

COMPETENCY CRITERIA: Initiation of Peripheral I.V. Therapy Based on the Phillips 15 Steps
COMPETENCY STATEMENT: Competent I.V. nurses will be able to perform venipuncture technique for support of peripheral I.V. therapy
NOTE: The cognitive (knowledge) information that is embedded within this performance-based competency includes aseptic technique, manufacturer recommendation for use of equipment, venous anatomy and physiology, fluid and electrolyte balance.
This competency *links* to the competency of infection control, management of I.V. equipment, and parenteral solutions.

Performance	**Skilled**	**Needs Education**
Critical Action Statements		
1. Verifies appropriate fluid to physician's order.		
2. Washes hands for 15 to 20 seconds.		
3. Performs inspection of I.V. equipment to ensure product integrity		
4. Informs patient of procedure, and interviews regarding previous experiences with I.V.s		
5. Examines both arms for appropriate site to support I.V. therapy		
6. Chooses appropriate size catheter		
7. Dons gloves before site preparation		
8. Performs preparation of site with povidone-iodine or alcohol A. 15- to 20- second scrub B. 30-second scrub when using alcohol		
9. Performs venipuncture technique A. Indirect or direct stick B. Angle of 30 to 45 degrees to enter skin C. Lowers angle of cannula after cannula is through skin D. Establishes blood return before threading catheter E. Connects hub of catheter to locking device or administration set		

(continued)

(continued)

Performance	**Skilled**	**Needs Education**
Critical Action Statements		
10. Performs successful venipuncture (85–95%) on initial attempt A. One attempt per I.V. device		
11. Follows Intravenous Nurses Standards of Practice for: A. Dressing management B. Gauze C. Transparent semipermeable dressing		
12. Labels site, tubing, and solution according to agency policy and procedures		
13. Provides patient education		
14. Disposes of equipment in biohazard containers		
15. Calculates rate accurately		
16. Documents initiation of peripheral I.V therapy based on institution policy and procedures A. Assessment of site B. Size and length of cannula C. Number of attempts D. Location of catheter Use of equipment (electronic infusion devices, inline filters, extension sets, resealable lock) Solution infusing and rate How patient tolerated procedure		

EVALUATION CRITERIA

1. Observation of initiation of I.V. therapy on patient or simulation on manikin.
2. Observation and review of documentation.
3. Calculation problems.

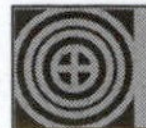

CRITICAL THINKING ACTIVITY

1. Check the policy and procedure manual at your facility to check the procedure for:
   - Flushing an intermittent infusion device
   - Recommendations for tubing changes
   - Recommendations for catheter replacement

2. Do you think checking for patency is necessary flush procedure? Why?

3. Check the I.V. setups in your agency and check for labeling practices. What did you find?

4. Identify techniques that you have observed that may contribute to contamination of an I.V. site.

WORKSHEET 7–1

SUPERFICIAL VEINS OF THE UPPER EXTREMITIES WORKSHEET AND ANSWERS

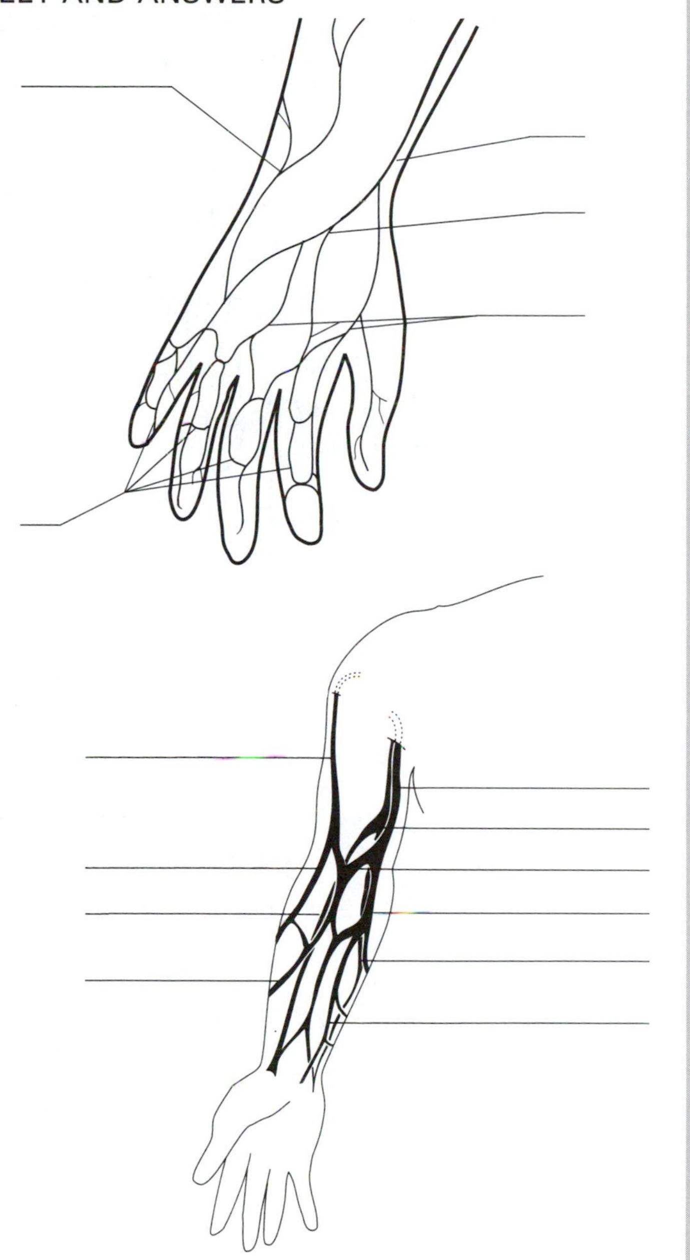

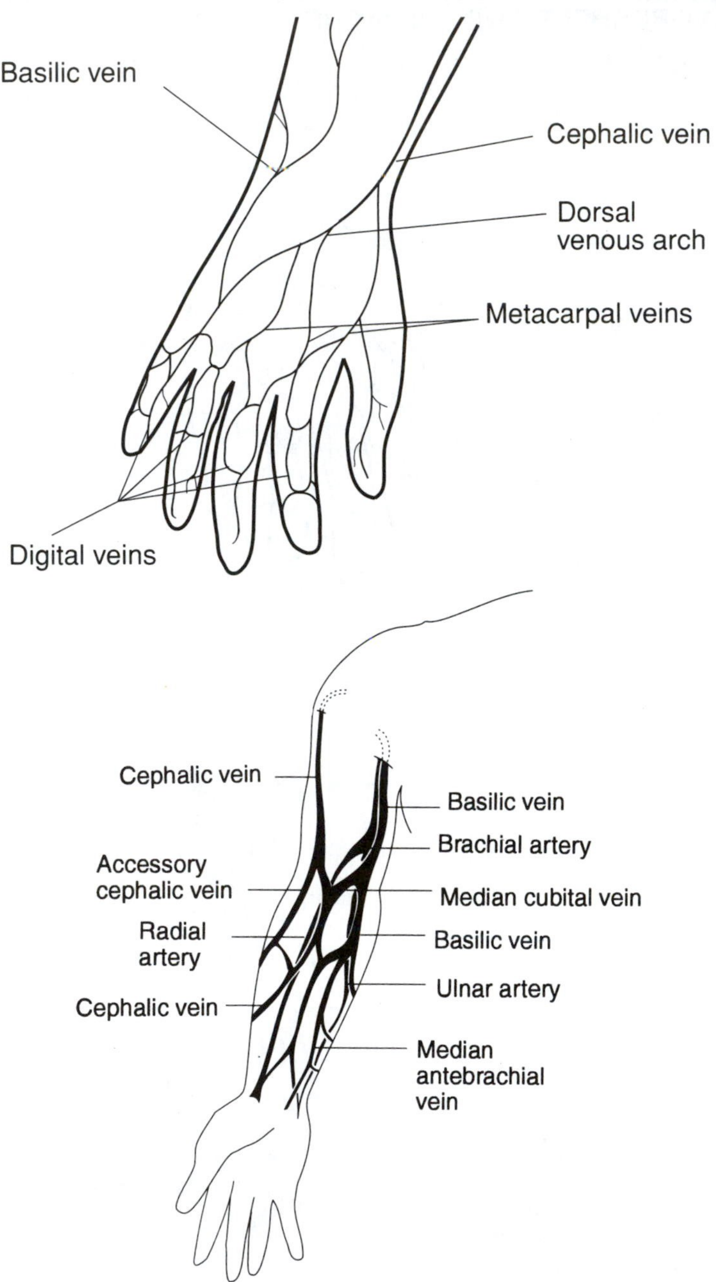
Basilic vein
Cephalic vein
Dorsal venous arch
Metacarpal veins
Digital veins
Cephalic vein
Basilic vein
Brachial artery
Accessory cephalic vein
Median cubital vein
Radial artery
Basilic vein
Cephalic vein
Ulnar artery
Median antebrachial vein

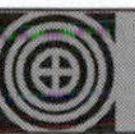

WORKSHEET 7-2

MATH CALCULATION WORKSHEET 1 AND ANSWERS

Set 1: Basic Calculation of Primary Infusions

1. The order reads 1000 mL of 5 percent dextrose in water at 125 mL/h. You have available 20 drop factor tubing. Calculate the drops per minute.

2. The order is for 1000 mL of 5 percent dextrose and 0.45 percent sodium chloride at 150 mL/h. You have available 15 drop factor tubing. Calculate the drops per minute.

3. The order is for 250 mL (1 U) of packed cells over 2 hours. Remember, blood tubing is always 10 drop factor. Calculate the drops per minute.

(continued)

4. The order is for 45 mL/h of 5 percent sodium chloride solution on an 8-month-old baby. Calculate the drops per minute if you have to use a controller that is drops per minute. (Remember, use microdrip tubing.)

5. The order reads 3000 mL of a multiple electrolyte fluid over 24 hours. You have available 20 drop factor tubing. Calculate the drops per minute

6. The order is for 250 mL of 5 percent dextrose in water to run at 25 cc/h. You will be infusing it using an infusion pump.

(continued)

WORKSHEET 7–2 *(continued)*

7. The order is for 500 mL of lactated Ringer's solution to be administered at 75 mL/h. You have available 15 drop factor tubing. Calculate the drops per minute

8. Calculate problem 7 using 20 drop factor tubing.

9. The order reads 50 mL/h of 5 percent dextrose in water to rehydrate an 85-year-old woman. You assess the patient and find her cardiovascular status compromised. What tubing do you choose, microdrip or macrodrip? Why? Calculate the drops per minute using 15 drop factor tubing and 60 drop factor tubing.

(continued)

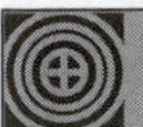

WORKSHEET 7–2 *(continued)*

10. The order is for aminophylline 500 mg in 250 mL of 5 percent dextrose in water to be infused at 50 mL/h. You will be infusing it via an infusion pump.

ANSWERS: MATH CALCULATION WORKSHEET 1

1. Formula: $\frac{\text{mL/h} \times \text{DF}}{\text{minutes}} = \text{gtt/min}$

Step 1: $\frac{125 \times 20}{60} = \text{gtt/min}$

Step 2: $\frac{125}{3} = \underline{42 \text{ gtt/min}}$

2. Formula: $\frac{\text{mL/h} \times \text{DF}}{\text{minutes}} = \text{gtt/min}$

Step 1: $\frac{150 \times 15}{60} = \text{gtt/min}$

Step 2: $\frac{150}{4} = \underline{38 \text{ gtt/min}}$

3. Formula: $\frac{\#\text{mL}}{\#\text{h}} = \text{mL/h}$

Step 1: $\frac{250}{2} = \underline{125 \text{ mL/h}}$

Formula: $\frac{\text{mL/h} \times \text{DF}}{\text{minutes}} = \text{gtt/min}$

Step 2: $\frac{125 \times 10}{60} = \text{gtt/min}$

Step 3: $\frac{125}{6} = \underline{21 \text{ gtt/min}}$

4. Formula: $\frac{\text{mL/h} \times \text{DF}}{\text{minutes}} = \text{gtt/min}$

Step 1: $\frac{45 \times 60}{60} = \underline{45 \text{ gtt/min}}$

Only one step needed for microdrop infusions.

5. Formula: $\frac{\#\text{mL}}{\#\text{h}} = \text{mL/h}$

Step 1: $\frac{3000}{8} = \underline{125 \text{ mL/h}}$

Formula: $\frac{\text{mL/h} \times \text{DF}}{\text{minutes}} = \text{gtt/min}$

Step 2: $\frac{125 \times 20}{60} = \text{gtt/min}$

Step 3: $\frac{125}{3} = \underline{42 \text{ gtt/min}}$

6. Formula: $\frac{\text{mL/h} \times \text{DF}}{\text{minutes}} = \text{gtt/min}$

Step 1: $\frac{25 \times 60}{60} = \underline{25\ \text{gtt/min}}$

Only one step needed for infusion pumps (microdrip sets).

7. Formula: $\frac{\text{mL/h} \times \text{DF}}{\text{minutes}} = \text{gtt/min}$

Step 1: $\frac{75 \times 15}{60} = \text{gtt/min}$

Step 2: $\frac{75}{4} = \underline{19\ \text{gtt/min}}$

8. Formula: $\frac{\text{mL/h} \times \text{DF}}{\text{minutes}} = \text{gtt/min}$

Step 1: $\frac{75 \times 20}{60} = \text{gtt/min}$

Step 2: $\frac{75}{3} = \underline{25\ \text{gtt/min}}$

9. Formula: $\frac{\text{mL/h} \times \text{DF}}{\text{minutes}} = \text{gtt/min}$

Microdrip:

Step 1: $\frac{50 \times 60}{60} = \underline{50\ \text{gtt/min}}$

Macrodrip:

Step 1: $\frac{50 \times 15}{60} = \text{gtt/min}$

Step 2: $\frac{50}{4} = \underline{13\ \text{gtt/min}}$

Microdrip would be a better choice because of the difficulty regulating a 13-gtt drip rate. Also, with a compromised patient, there is more flexibility if needed to adjust the rate lower with a microdrip fluid.

10. Formula: $\frac{\text{mL/h} \times \text{DF}}{\text{minutes}} = \text{gtt/min}$

Step 1: $\frac{50 \times 60}{60} = 50\ \text{gtt/min}$

Only one step needed for infusion pump.

WORKSHEET 7–3

MATH CALCULATION WORKSHEET 2 AND ANSWERS RECALCULATIONS AND SECONDARY INFUSIONS

1. The physician orders a fluid challenge of 250 mL of sodium chloride over 45 minutes. You have 20 drop factor tubing available. Calculate the drops per minute in order to accurately deliver the 250 mL over 45 minutes.

2. Administer vinblastine sulfate 50 mg diluted in 50 mL of 0.9 percent sodium chloride over 15 minutes. You have available macrodrip 15.

3. Administer 500 mg of acyclovir in 100 mL of 5 percent dextrose in water over 1 hour. You have available macrodrip 20 gtt.

(continued)

4. Administer trimethoprim-sulfamethoxazole 400 mg in 125 mL of dextrose in water over 90 minutes. You have available a microdrip set and macrodrip 15 gtt.

5. At 12 noon you discover that an infusion set to deliver 100 mL per hour from 7 AM to 5 PM has 400 mL left in the infusion bag. Recalculate the infusion using a macrodrip 10 gtt.

6. Recalculate the flow rate in drops per minute for an infusion that is scheduled for 12 hours of 1000 mL of lactated Ringer's solution. At the sixth hour, there is 850 mL remaining. It is infusing using a macrodrip 20 gtt.

7. Recalculate the flow rate in drops per minute for an infusion that is scheduled for 6 hours of 1000 mL 5 percent dextrose in water. At the end of hour 4, there is 360 mL remaining. It is infusing using a macrodrip 15 gtt.

(continued)

WORKSHEET 7-3 *(continued)*

8. Recalculate the flow rate for an infusion of 100 mL 0.9 percent sodium chloride solution to run for 4 hours. At the end of the second hour, there is 90 mL remaining. You have available a microdrip and macrodrip 15 gtt.

9. The order is for carbenicillin disodium 2 g IVPB diluted in 50 mL of 5 percent dextrose in water in infuse in 15 minutes. You have available macrodrip 20 gtt. Calculate the drip rate.

10. The order is written for vancomycin 500 mg in 100 mL of 5 percent dextrose in water over 30 minutes. You will be infusing it with an infusion pump.

ANSWERS: MATH CALCULATION WORKSHEET 2

1. Formula: $\frac{\text{mL/h} \times \text{DF}}{\text{minutes}} = \text{gtt/min}$

Step 1: $\frac{250 \times 20}{45 \text{ min}} = \text{gtt/min}$

Step 2: $\frac{250 \times 4}{9} = 1000 = \underline{111 \text{ gtt/min}}$

2. Formula: $\frac{\text{mL/h} \times \text{DF}}{\text{minutes}} = \text{gtt/min}$

Step 1: $\frac{50 \times 15}{15} = \underline{50 \text{ gtt/min}}$

3. Formula: $\frac{\text{mL/h} \times \text{DF}}{\text{minutes}} = \text{gtt/min}$

Step 1: $\frac{100 \times 20}{60} = \text{gtt/min}$

Step 2: $\frac{100}{3} = \underline{33 \text{ gtt/min}}$

4. Formula: $\frac{\text{mL/h} \times \text{DF}}{\text{minutes}} = \text{gtt/min}$

Step 1: $\frac{125 \times 15}{90 \text{ min}} = \text{gtt/min}$

Step 2: $\frac{125}{6} = 21 \text{ gtt/min}$

5. Formula: $\frac{\text{\# mL}}{\text{\# h}} = \text{mL/h}$

Step 1: $\frac{400}{5} = 80 \text{ mL/h}$

Formula: $\frac{\text{mL/h} \times \text{DF}}{\text{minutes}} = \text{gtt/min}$

Step 2: $\frac{80 \times 10}{60} = \text{gtt/min}$

Step 3: $\frac{80}{6} = \underline{13 \text{ gtt/min}}$

6. Formula: $\frac{\text{\# mL}}{\text{\# h}} = \text{mL/h}$

Step 1: $\frac{850}{6} = 142 \text{ mL/h}$

Formula: $\frac{\text{mL/h} \times \text{DF}}{\text{minutes}} = \text{gtt/min}$

Step 2: $\frac{142 \times 20}{60} = 47$ gtt/min

7. Formula: $\frac{\#\ mL}{\#\ h} = mL/h$

Step 1: $\frac{360}{2} = 180$ mL/h

Formula: $\frac{mL/h \times DF}{minutes} = gtt/min$

Step 2: $\frac{180 \times 15}{60} = gtt/min$

Step 3: $\frac{180}{4} =$ <u>45 gtt/min</u>

8. Formula: $\frac{\#\ mL}{\#\ h} = mL/h$

Step 1: $\frac{90}{2} = 45$ mL/h

Formula: $\frac{mL/h \times DF}{minutes} = gtt/min$

Step 2: $\frac{45 \times 15}{60} = 11$ gtt/min

Step 3: $\frac{30}{4} = 8$ gtt/min

9. Formula: $\frac{mL/h \times DF}{minutes} = gtt/min$

Step 1: $\frac{50 \times 20}{15} = gtt/min$

Step 2: $\frac{50 \times 4}{3} = \frac{200}{3} = 67$ gtt/min

10. Formula: $\frac{mL/h \times DF}{minutes} = gtt/min$

Step 1: $\frac{100 \times 60}{30} = gtt/min$

Step 2: $100 \times 2 = 200 =$ <u>200 gtt/min</u>

POST-TEST

In 1 through 5, match the definition in Column II to the term in Column I:

COLUMN I	COLUMN II
1. Antimicrobial	a. Peripheral vascular access device made of polyurethane
2. Cannula	b. Slanted portion of cannula device or needle
3. Bevel	c. To fill the administration set with infusate for the first time
4. Prime	d. To insert the administration set into the infusate container
5. Spike	e. An agent that destroys or prevents the development of microorganisms

6. List the four steps in maintaining patency of a saline locking device when giving a medication.
   1.
   2.
   3.
   4.
7. Before equipment setup and venipuncture, how many seconds of handwashing with an antimicrobial soap are recommended?
   a. 10 to 30
   b. 15 to 20
   c. 30 to 60
   d. 45 to 60
8. I.V. therapy labels should be on which areas?
   a. Catheter site, tubing, and solution container
   b. Tubing, solution container, and chart
   c. Solution container, catheter site, and patient's armband
9. The order reads 1000 mL of 5 percent dextrose and lactated Ringer's solution at 125 mL/h. Calculate the drip rate using 20 gtt factor tubing.

10. What is the recommended frequency in which a patient receiving infusion therapy should be monitored?
   a. Every hour or more frequently if condition warrants
   b. Every 4 hours
   c. Every shift or every 8 to 12 hours
   d. Every 24 hours

REFERENCES

Anderson, M., & Holland, J. (1992). Maintaining the patency of peripherally inserted central catheters with 10 units/cc heparin. *Journal of Intravenous Nursing,* 15(2), 84–88.

Astra Pharmaceutical Products. (1992). EMLA cream package insert. Wesborough, MA: ASTRA.

Baldwin, D.R. (1989). Heparin-induced thrombocytopenia. *Journal of Intravenous Nursing,* 12 (6), 378–382.

Byers, P.H. (1986). Comparison of application factors among three brands of transparent semipermeable films for peripheral I.V.'s *National Intravenous Therapy Association,* 8(4), 315–318.

Centers for Disease Control and Prevention. (1995). *Centers for Disease Control and Prevention intravascular device-related infections prevention; Guideline availability; notice.* Atlanta: US Department of Health and Human Services.

Cooper, C.M., Gerrish, S.P., Hardwick, M., & Kay, R. (1987). EMLA cream reduces the pain of venipuncture in children. *European Journal of Anaesthesiology,* 4, 441–448.

Cyganski, J.M., Donahue, J.M., & Heaton, J.S. (1987). The case for the heparin flush. *American Journal of Nursing,* 87, 796–797.

Delaney, C.W., & Lauer, M.L. (1988). *Intravenous Therapy: A Guide to Quality Care.* Philadelphia: J.B. Lippincott.

Enrich, M. (1991). Performing venipuncture in elderly patients. *Nursing 91,* 21.

Ellenberer, A. (1999). Starting an I.V. line. *Nursing 99,* 99(3): 56–59.

Epperson, E.L. (1984). Efficacy of 0.9% sodium chloride injection with and without heparin for maintaining indwelling intermittent injection sites. *Clinical Pharmacy,* 3, 626–629.

Fabian, B. (1995). Intravenous therapy in the older adult. In Terry, J., Baranowski, L., Lonsway, R., & Hedrick, C. (eds.). *Intravenous Therapy: Clinical Principles and Practice.* Intravenous Nurses Society. Philadelphia: W.B. Saunders, pp. 495–504.

Fabian, B. (1998). *Basic I.V. skills: Adult and pediatric.* National Academy presentation: November 1998, Phoenix, Arizona.

Fry, B. (1992). Intermittent flushing protocols: A standardization issue. *Journal of Intravenous Nursing,* 15(3), 160–163.

Giger, J.N., & Davidhizar, R.E. (1999). *Transcultural Nursing: Assessment and Intervention.* St. Louis: Mosby.

Goode, C.J., Titler, M., & Rakel, B. (1991). A meta-analysis of effects of heparin flush and saline flush: Quality and cost implications. *Nursing Research,* 40(6), 324–330.

Guyton, A.C. (1991). *Textbook of Medical Physiology* (8th ed.). Philadelphia: W.B. Saunders.

Hadaway, L. (1999). Choosing the right vascular access device, part I. *Nursing 99,* 99(2), 18.

Hadaway, L. (1999) Choosing the right vascular access device, part II. *Nursing 99,* 99(7), 28.

Hecker, J.F., Lewis, G.B., & Stanley, H. (1983). Nitroglycerine ointment as an aide to venipuncture. *Lancet,* 2, 332–333.

Henke, G. (1999). *Med-Math* (3rd ed.). Philadelphia: J.B. Lippincott, pp. 188–204.

Hoffmann, K.K., Weber, D.J., Samsa, G.P., et al. (1992). Transparent polyurethane film as an intravenous catheter dressing: a meta-analysis of the infection risks. *JAMA,* 267; 2072–2076.

Intravenous Nursing Society (2000). Revised intravenous nursing standards of practice. *Supplement Journal of Intravenous Nursing,* 21 (IS).

Josephson, D.L. (1999). *Intravenous Infusion Therapy for Nurses: Principles and Practice.* Albany: Delmar Publishers, pp. 181–205.

Korniewicz, D.M., Kirwin, M., & Larson, E. (1991). Do your gloves fit the task? *American Journal of Nursing,* 91(6), 38–39.

Maki, D.G., Botticelli, J.T., LeRoy, L.L., & Thielke, T.S. (1987). Prospective study of replacing administration sets for intravenous therapy at 48 vs 72 hour intervals. 72 Hours is safe and cost effective. *JAMA,* 258(13), 1777–1781.

Maki, D.G., Mermel, & L.A. (1998). Infection due to infusion therapy. In John Bennett and Philip Brachman (eds). *Hospital Infections* (4th ed.). Philadelphia: Lippincott-Raven, pp. 689–716.

Masoorli, S. (1995). Documentation. *Intravenous Nurses Society Newsline,* May/June, 7.

Mathewson-Kuhn, M. (1999). *Pharmacotherapeutics: A Nursing Process Approach* (4th ed.). Philadelphia: F.A. Davis, pp. 180–182.

National Intravenous Therapy Association Editorial. (1985). Infection traced to false fingernails. *Journal of Intravenous Nursing,* 6(6), 5.

Nelson, R.W., Young, R., & Lamnin, M. (1987). Visual incompatibility of dacarbazine and heparin. *American Journal of Hospital Pharmacy,* 44, 71–73.

Pauley, S. (1985). Nitro vein dilation. *National Intravenous Therapy Association,* 6(2), 5.

Perucca, R. (1995). Obtaining vascular access. In Terry, J., Baranowski, L., Lonsway, R., & Hedrick, C. (Eds.). *Intravenous Therapy: Clinical Principles and Practice.* Intravenous Nurses Society. Philadelphia: W.B. Saunders, pp. 370–399.

Peterson, F.Y., & Kirchhoff, K.T. (1991). Heparinized versus nonheparinized intravenous lines. *Heart & Lung,* 20(6), 631–637.

Prager, R.L., & Silva, J. (1984). Colonization of central venous catheters. *Southern Medical Journal,* 77: 458–461.

Smeltzer, S.C., & Bare, B.G. (1999). *Brunner and Suddarth's Textbook of Medical-Surgical Nursing* (8th ed.). Philadelphia: J.B. Lippincott.

Weinstein, S. (1997). *Plumers' Principles and Practice of Intravenous Therapy* (6th ed.). Philadelphia: J.B. Lippincott.

ANSWERS TO CHAPTER 7

Pre-Test

1. b, **2.** b, **3.** b, **4.** c, **5.** a, **6.** c, **7.** d, **8.** e, **9.** b, **10.** d, **11.** 25 gtt/min

Post-Test

1. e, **2.** a, **3.** b, **4.** c, **5.** d, **6.** Check patency; flush with 1 mL of sodium chloride; administer medication; flush with 1 mL of sodium chloride using positive pressure, **7.** b, **8.** a, **9.** 42 gtt/min, **10.** a

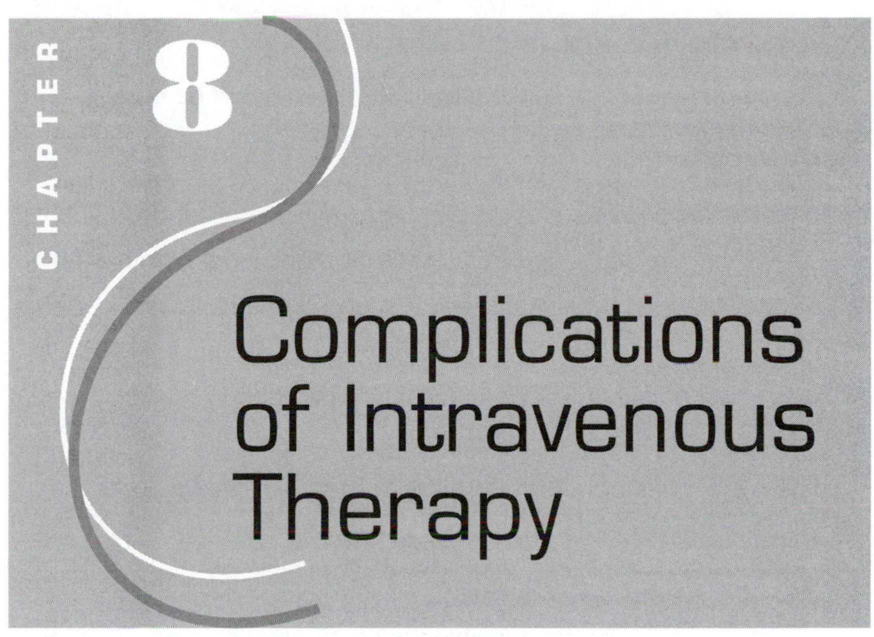

CHAPTER 8 Complications of Intravenous Therapy

The most important practical lesson that can be given to nurses is to teach them what to observe—how to observe—what symptoms indicate improvement—what the reverse—which are of importance—which are of none—which are the evidence of neglect—and of what kind of neglect.

Florence Nightingale, 1859

CHAPTER CONTENTS

LEARNING OBJECTIVES

Upon completion of this chapter, the reader will be able to:

1 Define terms related to the hazards associated with I.V. therapy.

2 Differentiate between local and systemic complications.

3 Describe the signs and symptoms of eight local complications.

4 Identify prompt treatment for local and systemic complications.

5 Document assessment of each local and systemic complication.

6 Identify the most hazardous local complication.

7 List three risk factors for phlebitis.

8 Use the phlebitis chart for identifying and rating postinfusion phlebitis.

9 Identify erratic flow rates as they relate to the hazards associated with I.V. therapy.

10 Identify organisms responsible for septicemia related to infusion therapy.

11 Identify prevention techniques for the six systemic complications.

12 State the recommendations for prevention of complications involving intravascular devices.

GLOSSARY

Ecchymosis A bruise; a "black and blue spot" on the skin caused by escape of blood from injured vessels

Embolism A sudden obstruction of a blood vessel by a clot or foreign material formed or introduced elsewhere in the circulatory system and carried to the point of obstruction by the bloodstream

Extravasation Escape of fluid from a vessel into the surrounding tissue

Hematoma A localized mass of blood outside of the blood vessel usually found in a partially clotted state

Infiltration Process of seepage or diffusion into tissue of I.V. infusate

Phlebitis Inflammation of the intima of a vein associated with chemical irritation (i.e., chemical phlebitis), mechanical irritation (i.e., mechanical phlebitis), or bacterial infection (i.e., bacterial phlebitis); postinfusion inflammation of the intima of a vein within 48 to 96 hours after cannula removal

Septicemia Systemic disease caused by the presence of pathogenic microorganisms in the body

Speed shock Systemic reaction that occurs when a substance foreign to the body is rapidly introduced into the circulation

Suppurative Formation or discharge of pus

Thrombosis Formation or presence of a blood clot; venous arrest of circulation in the vein by a blood clot; also called phlebemphraxis

Vasospasm Contraction of the muscular coats of the blood vessels; also called angiospasm

Vesicant Any agent that produces blisters

PRE-TEST

In 1 through 5, match the type of complication (local or systemic) in column II to the complication in column I.

COLUMN I	COLUMN II
1. Thrombosis	**a.** Local
2. Septicemia	**b.** Systemic
3. Speed shock	
4. Phlebitis	
5. Vasospasm	

6. The recommended treatment of phlebitis stage 2+ is to:
- **a.** Discontinue the cannula and apply heat to site.
- **b.** Watch the site and document observations.
- **c.** Leave the cannula in place and apply heat to the site.
- **d.** Flush the cannula with 0.9% sodium chloride.

7. The first symptom of venous vasospasm is:
- **a.** Sharp pain extending from the site of infusion.
- **b.** Redness along the vein.
- **c.** Increased temperature.
- **d.** Cold feeling in the extremity.

8. The organism responsible for most cases of septicemia related to infusion is
- **a.** *Proteus* spp.
- **b.** *Escherichia coli*
- **c.** Coagulase-negative staphylococci.
- **d.** *Pseudomonas* spp.

9. The risk of phlebitis is increased in which of the following patients?
- **a.** Patients receiving total parenteral nutrition
- **b.** Immunosuppressed patients
- **c.** Patients with burns
- **d.** Patients who have multiple I.V. manipulations
- **e.** All of the above

10. What complication is suspected if the patient has fever, chills, malaise, tachycardia, tachypnea, hypotension, and altered mental status?
- **a.** Local infection
- **b.** Septicemia
- **c.** Inflammatory response syndrome
- **d.** Thrombophlebitis

11. Signs and symptoms of an air embolus include:
- **a.** Dyspnea, tachypnea, cough, and diaphoresis
- **b.** Cardiac dysrhythmia, hypotension, anxiety, and substernal pressure
- **c.** Localized decreased breath sounds, chest pain with inhalation and exhalation, pleural friction rub, and a cog wheel murmur
- **d.** All of the above

COMPLICATIONS OF I.V. THERAPY

Because the nursing profession assumed the role of I.V. care in the 1940s, a large body of knowledge has been gathered about I.V. therapy. Complications such as **embolism,** catheter dislodgement or perforation, metabolic imbalance, hypervolemia, and nosocomial infections have been documented. The fact that 90 percent of hospitalized patients receive I.V. fluids and medications puts patients at risk for developing complications associated with this form of therapy.

LOCAL COMPLICATIONS

Local complications of I.V. therapy occur as adverse reactions or trauma to the surrounding venipuncture site. These complications can be recognized early by objective assessment. Assessing and monitoring are the key components in early intervention. Good venipuncture technique is the main factor related to the prevention of most local complications associated with I.V. therapy.

Local complications include hematoma, thrombosis, phlebitis, postinfusion phlebitis, thrombophlebitis, infiltration, extravasation, local infection, venous spasm, and hypersensitivity reactions.

HEMATOMA

The formation of a **hematoma** at the venipuncture site is usually related to nursing venipuncture technique. Patients who bruise easily can develop a hematoma when large cannulae are used to initiate I.V. therapy, owing to trauma to the vein during insertion (Fig. 8–1).

Hematomas are most often related to:

- Nicking the vein during an unsuccessful venipuncture attempt
- Discontinuing the I.V. cannula or needle without pressure held over the site after removal of the cannula or needle
- Applying a tourniquet too tightly above a previously attempted venipuncture site

Signs and Symptoms

Signs and symptoms of hematoma include:

- Discoloration of the skin (i.e., **ecchymoses**) surrounding the venipuncture (immediate or slow)
- Site swelling and discomfort
- Inability to advance the cannula all the way into the vein during insertion
- Resistance to positive pressure during the lock flushing procedure

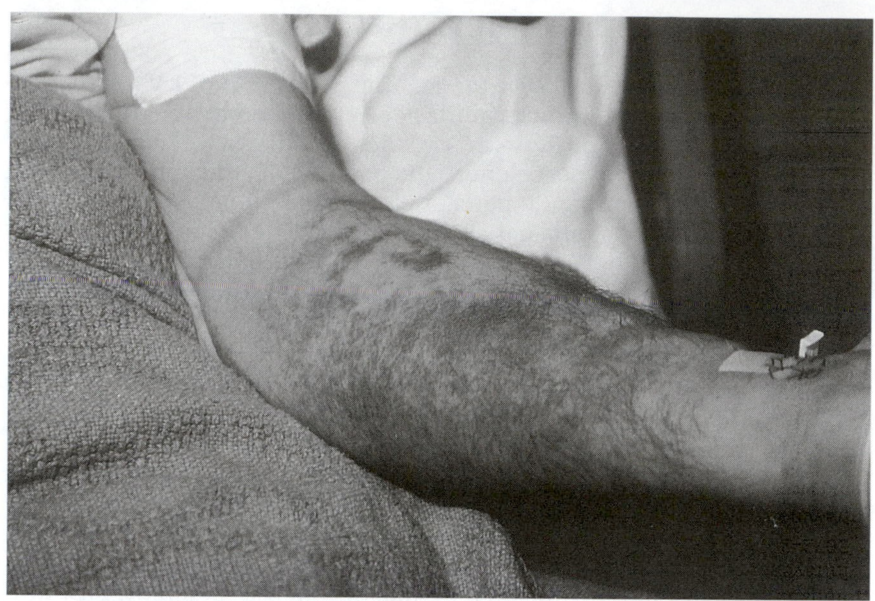

FIG. 8–1. Hematoma. (Courtesy of Beth Fabian, CRNI.)

AGE-RELATED COMPLICATIONS: HEMATOMA

Hematomas and ecchymoses are frequently seen in elderly persons. Fragile veins are easily injured.

Prevention

Techniques for prevention of hematoma formation include:

1. Use an indirect method for starting an I.V. until your technique is perfected for direct sticks. This decreases the chance of piercing through the vein and therefore causing seepage of blood into the subcutaneous tissue. (See Chapter 7 for techniques for venipuncture.)
2. Apply the tourniquet just before venipuncture.
3. For elderly patients, patients taking corticosteroids, or patients with paper-thin skin, use a small needle or catheter, preferably 20 or 22 gauge. Use a blood pressure cuff rather than a rubber tourniquet to fill the vein so you have better control of the pressure exerted on the vein.
4. Be very gentle when performing venipuncture.

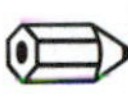 **NOTE:** The presence of both ecchymosis and hematomas limits veins from future use (Perdue, 1995).

Treatment

1. Apply direct pressure using a sterile 2 × 2 gauze pad over the site after catheter or needle is removed.
2. Have the patient elevate the extremity over his or her head or on a pillow to maximize venous return.

Documentation

Document observable ecchymotic areas. Be sure to document the nursing interventions you used for care of the site.

THROMBOSIS

Trauma to the endothelial cells of the venous wall cause platelets to adhere to the vein wall, which may lead to the formation of a clot. The **thrombosis** usually occludes the circulation of blood. Thrombus formation is manifested by the flow of the I.V. solution: the drip rate slows, or the line does not flush easily and resistance is felt, especially in a lock device. The I.V. site may appear healthy. There are two areas of great concern in assessing for a thrombosis. First, do not propel the clot into the bloodstream with pressure from a syringe, and second, keep in mind that a thrombus within a vein can trap bacteria.

Thrombosis formation is most often related to:

- Blood's backing up in the system of a hypertensive patient
- A low flow rate, which limits fluid movement to maintain patency
- The location of the I.V. cannula (e.g., a catheter placed in a flexor area may occlude when the position is changed
- Obstruction of flow rate caused by the patient's compressing the I.V. line for an extended period of time
- Trauma to the wall of the vein by the cannula

Thrombosis, along with thrombophlebitis, can lead to a systemic embolism.

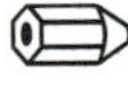 **NOTE:** Therapists must avoid injuring the vein wall, performing multiple punctures, and performing through-and-through punctures.

Signs and Symptoms

Signs and symptoms of a thrombosis include:

- Fever and malaise
- Slowed or stopped infusion rate
- Inability to flush locking device

Prevention

Techniques for the prevention of a thrombosis include:

1. Use pumps and controllers for managing rate control. Rate control devices prevent blood from backing up in the tubing and produce an alarm when the I.V. line is dry.
2. Choose microdrip tubing (60 drops/mL) when I.V. gravity flow rates are below 50 mL/h. Remember, more drops mean more movement.
3. Avoid placing I.V. cannulae in areas of flexion.
4. Use filters.
5. Avoid cannulation of lower extremities.

Treatment

1. Discontinue the cannula and restart the I.V. infusion with a new catheter in a different site.
2. Apply cold compresses to the site to decrease the flow of blood and increase platelet adherence to the clot that has already formed (Perdue, 1995).
3. Notify the physician and assess the site for circulatory impairment (Table 8–1.)

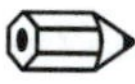

NOTES: If an occlusion occurs, do not irrigate. Irrigation of an occluded line with saline can propel the clot into the circulatory system, causing an embolism.

If there is any resistance when gentle pressure is exerted on the syringe plunger when you are attempting to flush an I.V. catheter, STOP! The application of force could dislodge the clot.

Never use a syringe with a barrel size of 2 or 3 mL to flush or aspirate clots in an I.V. line. A small syringe creates excess pressure that can damage the intima of the vein (Josephson, 1999).

Documentation

Document the change of infusion rate, the steps taken to solve the problem, and the end result. Be sure to chart the new I.V. site, its patency, and the size of the catheter used to restart the infusion. Also document the appearance of the occluded site.

PHLEBITIS

Phlebitis is a commonly reported complication of I.V. therapy. The fact that 27 to 70 percent of patients receiving I.V. therapy develop some stage of phlebitis makes this local complication one of the most common hazards associated with over-the-needle catheters in today's practice (Maki & Ringer, 1991).

TABLE 8–1

STEPS FOR CHECKING SLOWED INFUSION

Check tubing for kinks → Yes → Unkink and check flow rate → Ok → Stop
↓
No
↓
Check catheter: Is it taped too tightly? → Yes → Retape and milk tubing to restart flow rate → Ok → Stop
↓
No
↓
Suspect Clot
Milk the tubing using the side of pen or pencil OR
Strip tubing (*above lowest medicinal entry*) toward the patient with fingers.
NOTE: Stripping the tubing moves the catheter from the vein wall with minimal pressure.

↓ No	↓ Yes
Use 3-mL syringe filled with 2 mL of saline to attempt to aspirate clot (never use a 1-mL syringe because it generates too much pressure)	Blood return Flush with saline → OK

↓
No
Discontinue the I.V. and restart

Phlebitis is an inflammation of the vein in which the endothelial cells of the venous wall become irritated and cells roughen, allowing platelets to adhere and predispose the vein to inflammation-induced phlebitis. The site is tender to touch and can be very painful. At the first sign of redness or complaint of tenderness, the I.V. site should be checked. Phlebitis can prolong hospitalization unless treated early.

The process of phlebitis formation involves an increase in capillary permeability, which allows proteins and fluids to leak into the interstitial space. The traumatized tissue continues to be irritated mechanically or chemically (Table 8–2).

The immune system causes leukocytes to gather at the inflamed site. When leukocytes are released, pyrogens stimulate the hypothalamus to raise body temperature. Pyrogens also stimulate bone marrow to release more leukocytes. Redness and tenderness increase with each step of the phlebitis (Maki & Ringer, 1991). When local inflammation is viewed under a microscope, histologic changes are marked, with loss of endothelial cells, edema, and presence of neutrophils in the vein wall. Inspection of the affected site reveals a similar appearance regardless of the underlying cause (Fig. 8–2).

TABLE 8–2

TYPES OF PHLEBITIS

Mechanical Phlebitis

Mechanical irritation, causing a phlebitis or inflammation of the vein can be attributed to use of too large a cannula in a small vein. A large cannula placed in a vein with a smaller lumen than the cannula irritates the intima of the vein, causing inflammation and phlebitis. Large veins with thick walls hold up better during an infusion. In addition, veins higher on the forearm are less likely to develop phlebitis. The other cause of mechanical phlebitis is improper taping, in which the catheter tip rubs the vein wall, damaging the endothelial cell. Manipulation of the catheter during infusion causes irritation of vein wall. Securely affix catheter hub and tubing using the Chevron method to prevent wiggling of the catheter.

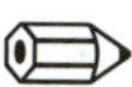

NOTE: The technical expertise of the person inserting the cannula influences the risk for mechanical phlebitis. In comparative trials (Maki & Ringer, 1991), a twofold lower rate of infusion-related phlebitis and reduction of catheter-related sepsis occurred when experienced nurses on an I.V. therapy team inserted I.V. catheters and provided close surveillance of infusion sites.

Chemical Phlebitis

Chemical phlebitis occurs when a vein becomes inflamed by irritating or vesicant solutions or medication. This is the result of contact with infusates with high or low osmolarities or pH or if very small veins are used for venous access (Josephson, 1999).

Several factors contribute to chemical phlebitis. Generally, these include administration of:

- Irritating medications or solutions
- Improperly mixed or diluted medications
- Too-rapid infusion
- Presence of particulate matter in solution

The more acidic the I.V. solution, the greater is the risk of the patient's developing chemical phlebitis. I.V. solutions have a pH of 3 to 6, which helps to prevent them from caramelizing during sterilization and helps to maintain stability. Dextrose solutions have a pH of 3.5 to 6.5 or lower, whereas saline solutions have a pH of 5.5 (USP, 1995). The pH falls further with storage; pH values of 3.4 have been found in date-expired 5% dextrose solutions (Hecker, 1988). Additives such as vitamin C, doxorubicin (Adriamycin), and cimetidine can further decrease the pH. Some drugs such as heparin, which has a pH of 5 to 7.5, can raise the pH. Hypertonic fluids such as 10% dextrose, which have a tonicity of greater than 375, increase the hazards of phlebitis. An increase in electrolytes also adds to the increased tonicity of the solution.

Additives such as potassium chloride (KCl) and various I.V. medications can produce severe venous inflammation (Perdue, 1995) found that phlebitis developed in 27.2 percent of patients who received continuous infusion of KCl in addition to intermittent medications. It was reported that patients who received more than 30 mEq of KCl/L of solution have a greater risk of developing phlebitis.

(Continued)

TABLE 8–2

TYPES OF PHLEBITIS ***(Continued)***

Chemical Phlebitis

Another factor contributing to chemical phlebitis is particulate matter in a solution, such as drug particles that do not fully dissolve during mixing and are not visible to the eye. The use of a 1.0- to 0.5-micron particulate matter filter eliminates this problem.

The use of catheters for peripheral I.V. therapy can predispose patients to phlebitis. Several different materials are used in the manufacturer of catheters. Catheters made of silicone elastomer and polyurethane have a smoother microsurface, are thermoplastic, are more hydrophilic, become more flexible than polytetrafluoroethylene (Teflon) at body temperature, and induce less venous irritation. Maki and Ringer (1991) showed that the incidence of phlebitis increased progressively with the increasing period of cannulation. Their study revealed the risk to be 30 percent by day 2 and 39 to 40 percent by day 3.

Intermittent infusions with heparin locks cause less irritation to the vein wall over time than continuous infusions. The slower the rate of infusion, the less irritating the solution is to the vein wall because cells of the vein are exposed for a shorter period of time to solutions with less than normal pH. The fact that heparin is used to maintain the lock might have further significance in the reduction of phlebitis rates.

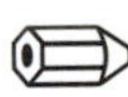

NOTE: Examples of three common I.V. solutions and their pH and osmolarity:

Solution	pH	Osmolarity, mOsm/L
5% dextrose in water	3 to 5	252
5% dextrose in water with 0.45% sodium chloride	4	406
5% dextrose in water with Ringer's lactate	5	524

Bacterial Phlebitis

Bacterial phlebitis, also referred to as septic phlebitis, is the least common type of phlebitis. It is an inflammation of the intima of a vein that is associated with a bacterial infection. Factors contributing to the development of bacterial phlebitis include poor aseptic technique, failure to detect breaks in the integrity of the equipment, poor cannula insertion technique, inadequately taped cannula, and failure to perform site assessments.

Bacterial phlebitis can be prevented by preparing solutions aseptically under a laminar flow hood. All solution containers should be inspected carefully before hanging; in addition, handwashing and preparing skin carefully are necessary to prevent bacterial phlebitis.

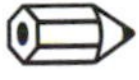

NOTE: Handwashing is the most important procedure for preventing nosocomial infections and thus bacterial phlebitis (Wenzel, 1993). All equipment should be inspected for integrity, particulate matter, cloudiness, and any signs indicating a break in sterility.

Shaving is not recommended because of the potential for microabrasion, which allows microorganisms to enter the vascular system.

(Continued)

TABLE 8–2

TYPES OF PHLEBITIS *(Continued)*

Postinfusion Phlebitis
Postinfusion phlebitis is associated with inflammation of the vein that usually becomes evident within 48 to 96 hours after the cannula has been removed. Factors that contribute to its development are cannula insertion technique; condition of vein used; type, compatibility, and pH of solution or medication being infused; gauge, size, length, and material of cannula; and cannula indwelling time.
Postinfusion phlebitis can occur without the usual signs or symptoms. There is no way to anticipate this type of phlebitis; however, after it appears, the treatment is the same as for any other phlebitis (Bohony, 1993).

Factors that influence the development of phlebitis, include but are not limited to:

- The insertion technique
- The condition of patient; vein condition compatibility (type and pH) of the medication or solution ineffective filtration
- The gauge, size, length, and material of cannula (Table 8–3)

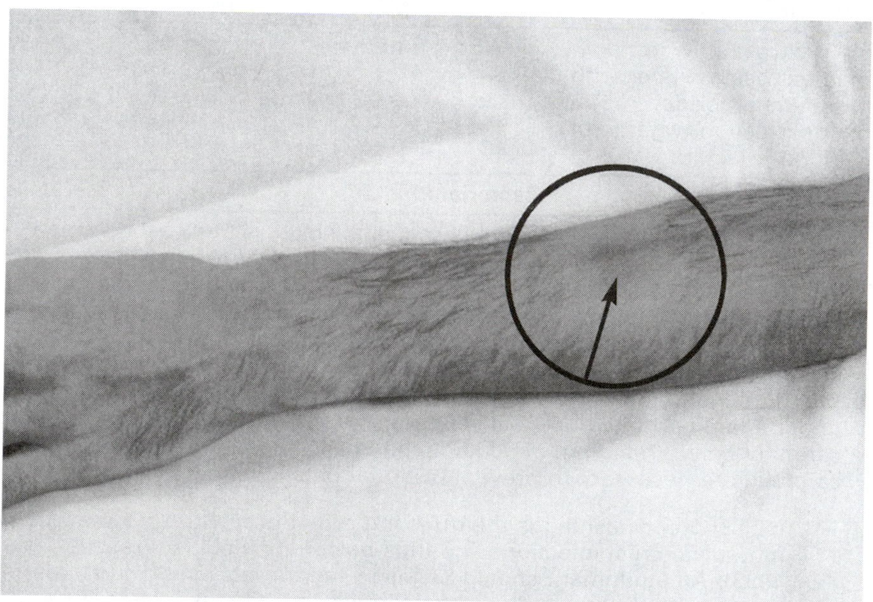

FIG. 8–2. Phlebitis. (Courtesy of Johnson & Johnson Medical Inc., Arlington, Texas.)

TABLE 8–3

FACTORS AFFECTING PHLEBITIS FORMATION

1. Catheter material
   - Polypropylene > Teflon
   - Silicone elastomer > polyurethane
   - **Teflon > polyurethane**
   - Teflon > steel needles
2. Catheter size
   - Large bore > small bore
3. **Insertion in emergency room > inpatient unit**
4. **Increasing duration of catheter placement**
5. **Infusate**
   - Low pH
   - Potassium chloride
   - Hypertonic glucose, amino acids, lipids
   - **Antibiotics** (especially β-lactams, vancomycin, metronidazole)
   - High flow rate of I.V. fluid (>90 mL/h)
6. Daily I.V. dressing changes > dressing changes every 48 hours
7. Host factors
   - Poor-quality peripheral veins
   - **Insertion in the upper arm or wrist > hand**
8. Age
   - Children: older > younger
   - Adults: younger > older
   - **Women > men**
   - White > Black
9. **Individual biologic vulnerability**

> denotes a significantly greater risk for phlebitis.

Terms in bold print are significant predictors of risk in this study.

Source: Adapted from Maki, D.G., & Ringer, M. (1991). Risk factors for infusion-related phlebitis with small peripheral venous catheters: A randomized controlled trial. *Annals of Internal Medicine,* 114, 845–854. By permission.

Signs and Symptoms

Signs and symptoms associated with phlebitis include:

- Redness at site
- Site warm to touch
- Local swelling
- Palpable cord along the vein
- Sluggish infusion rate
- Increase in basal temperature of 1°C or more

The phlebitis scale is recommended to establish a uniform standard for assessing and measuring degrees of phlebitis (Table 8–4).

TABLE 8-4

PHLEBITIS SCALE

Grade	Clinical Criteria
0	No clinical symptoms
1	Erythema at access site with or without pain
2	Pain at access site, with erythema and/or edema
3	Pain at access site with erythema and/or edema, streak formation, and palpable venous cord
4	Pain at access site with erythema and/or edema, streak formation, palpable venous cord >1 inch in length, purulent drainage

Source: *Revised Standards of Practice.* (2000). Cambridge, MA: Intravenous Nurses Society; with permission.

INS STANDARDS The Intravenous Nurses Society (INS) recommends a phlebitis scale to provide a uniform standard for measuring degrees of phlebitis.

Phlebitis always requires corrective action and documentation

The phlebitis rate is calculated according to a standards formula:

$$\frac{\text{Number of phlebitis incidents} \times 100}{\text{Total number of I.V. peripheral lines}} = \text{Percent of peripheral phlebitis}$$

(INS, 2000, 59)

Prevention

Techniques for the prevention of phlebitis include:

1. Use larger veins for hypertonic solutions.
2. Use central lines or long-arm catheters for long-term hypertonic solutions.
3. Choose the smallest I.V. cannula appropriate for the infusate.
4. Rotate the I.V. site every 72 hours, a practice that has been shown to significantly decrease the risk of phlebitis.
5. Stabilize the catheter to prevent mechanical irritation.
6. Use a 0.22-micron inline final filter, which removes air, bacteria, and harmful particulate matter.
7. Venipuncture should be performed by skilled professionals.
8. Observe good handwashing practices.
9. Add a buffer to known irritating medications and to hypertonic solutions.
10. Change solution containers every 24 hours.

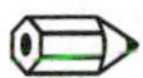 **NOTE:** Be aware that:

- *Phlebitis risk factors in I.V. therapy increase after 24 hours.*
- *All peripheral I.V.s should be changed every 48 to 72 hours.*
- *A 3+ phlebitis (see Table 8–4) takes from 10 days to 3 weeks to heal.*
- *Dextrose solutions, potassium chloride (KCl), antibiotics, and vitamin C have a lower pH and are associated with a higher risk of phlebitis.*

Treatment

1. Discontinue the infusion at the first sign of phlebitis (1+).
2. Apply warm or cold compresses to the affected site. Cold significantly decreases intradermal skin toxicity for 45 minutes.
3. Consult the physician if the patient has a phlebitis rating of 3+.
4. Depending on agency policy, notify infection control.

Documentation

Documentation is critical when phlebitis has been detected. Document the site assessment, the phlebitis rating (1, 2, 3, or 4), whether the physician was notified, and the treatment provided.

THROMBOPHLEBITIS

Thrombophlebitis denotes a twofold injury: thrombosis and inflammation. A painful inflamed vein promptly develops from the point of thrombosis. Thrombophlebitis causes the patient unnecessary discomfort (Weinstein, 1997). Chemical or mechanical phlebitis can also precipitate a thrombophlebitis.

Thrombophlebitis is related to:

- Use of veins in the legs for infusion therapy
- Use of hypertonic or highly acidic infusion solutions
- Causes similar to those of phlebitis (i.e., insertion technique; condition of patient; vein condition; compatibility [type and pH of medication or solution]; ineffective filtration; and the gauge, size, length, and material of the cannula).

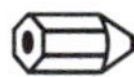 **NOTE:** Thrombophlebitis is often the sequela of phlebitis.

Signs and Symptoms

Signs and symptoms of thrombophlebitis include:

- Sluggish flow rate
- Edema in the limbs
- Tender and cordlike vein
- Site warm to touch
- Visible red line above venipuncture site

- Diminished arterial pulses
- Mottling and cyanosis of the extremities

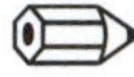 **NOTE:** If the inflammation is the result of bacterial phlebitis, a much more serious condition leading to septicemia may develop if the patient is not treated.

Prevention

Techniques used to prevent thrombophlebitis include:

1. Use the veins in forearm rather than in the hands when infusing any medication.
2. Do not use veins in joint flexion areas.
3. Check the infusion site for signs and symptoms of redness, swelling, or pain at the site at least every 4 hours in adults and every 2 hours in children.
4. Anchor the cannula securely to prevent mobility of the catheter tip.
5. Infuse solutions at prescribed rate. Do not attempt to catch up on delayed infusion time.
6. Use the smallest sized catheter that meets the needs of the patient.
7. Dilute irritating medications.

Septic thrombophlebitis can be prevented with:

- Appropriate skin preparation
- Aseptic technique in the maintenance of infusion
- Good handwashing procedures

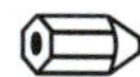 **NOTE:** Thrombophlebitis can lead to a potential embolism owing to the thrombus formation in the vein wall.

Treatment

1. Remove the entire I.V. catheter and restart the infusion in the opposite extremity using all new equipment.
2. Consult the physician.
3. Provide comfort by applying warm, moist compresses to the area for 20 minutes.

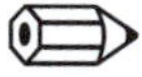 **NOTE:** You must discontinue the infusion and restart the infusion to prevent progression of thrombophlebitis.

Documentation

Document all observable symptoms and the patient's subjective complaints such as "feels tender to touch" and "it hurts." State your actions to resolve the problem and the time at which you notified the physician. Document the site in which you restarted the infusion.

INFILTRATION

Infiltration is the seepage of nonvesicant solution or medication into surrounding tissue. Infiltration occurs from the dislodgement of the cannula from the intima of a vein. It can also occur from phlebitis, causing the vein to become threadlike when the lumen along the cannula shaft narrows, so fluid leaks from the site where the cannula enters the vein wall. Infiltration is second to phlebitis as a cause of I.V. therapy morbidity.

Infiltration is related to:

- Puncture of the distal vein wall during venipuncture
- Puncture of any portion of the vein wall by mechanical friction from the catheter or needle
- Dislodgement of the catheter or needle from the intima of the vein
- Poorly secured infusion device
- High delivery rate or pressure (psi) from an electronic infusion device
- Overmanipulation of an I.V. device

Signs and Symptoms

Signs and symptoms of infiltration include:

- Coolness of skin around site
- Taut skin
- Dependent edema
- Absence of blood backflow
- A “pinkish” blood return
- Infusion rate slowing but continuing to infuse

Prevention

Prevention of infiltration includes performing adequate and continuous assessment of the site. Checking for a blood return, or backflow of blood, is not a reliable method of determining the patency of a cannula. A blood return may be present when small veins are used because they may not permit blood flow around the cannula. Use of veins that have had previous punctures or veins that are very fragile may cause a seeping of fluid at the site above or below the vein cannula entry point; a blood return may be present, yet an infiltration is occurring (Fig. 8–3).

Infiltration and swelling below the I.V. site may be caused by hands underneath the patient during turning. Occlusion or restriction of blood flow caused fluid to back up in the vessels, resulting in infiltration and dependent edema below the I.V. site rather than above.

The most accurate method of checking for infiltration is assessment of the site: With infusion running, apply pressure 3 inches above the catheter site in front of the catheter tip. If infusion continues to run, suspect infiltration. When the vein is compressed and the catheter is in proper

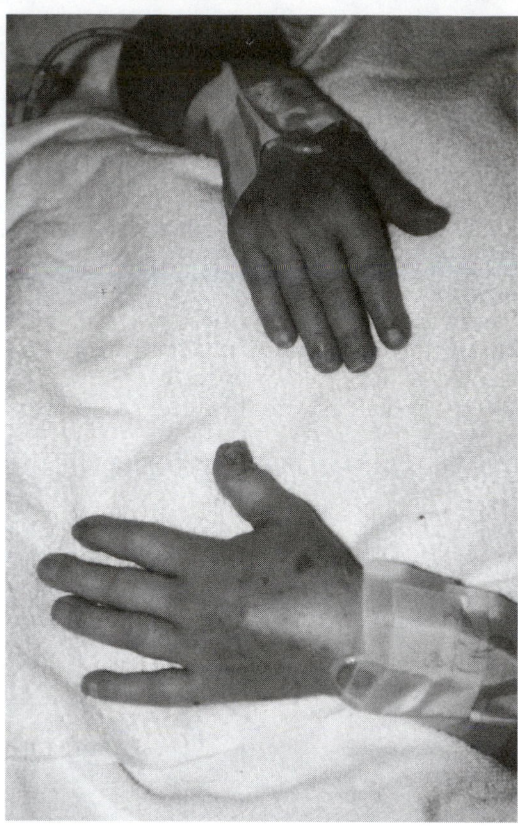

FIG. 8–3. Infiltration and swelling below the I.V. site because of hands underneath the patient during turning. Occlusion or restriction of blood flow caused fluid to back up in the vessels, resulting in infiltration and dependent edema below the I.V. site rather than above. (Courtesy of Beth Fabian, CRNI.)

alignment in the vein, the I.V. solution will stop because of occlusion. In addition, compare both of the patient's arms when assessing for infiltration (Fig. 8–4).

INS STANDARDS The INS has a classification for infiltration using a 0 to 4 scale. (INS, 2000, 60) (Refer to Table 8–5.)

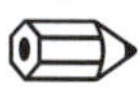

NOTE: Immobilized patients and patients with muscular weakness or paralysis of an extremity may have edema of an extremity that is not related to infiltration of an I.V. site. Accurate assessment of the cannula and infusion site is the key to differentiation.

Treatment

Use of warm compresses to treat infiltration has become controversial. It has been found that cold compresses may be better for some infiltrated infusates and warm compresses may be more effective for others. Elevation of the infiltrated extremity may be painful for the patient. Consult with the physician for orders regarding treatment (Masoorli, 1997).

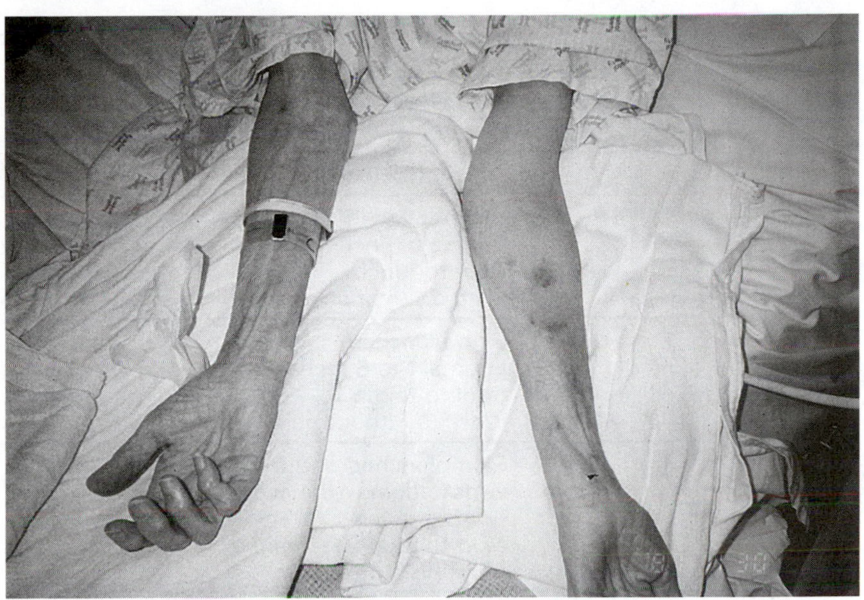

FIG. 8–4. Infiltration. Compare both arms when assessing for infiltration (note that left arm is swollen compared with the right arm).

Documentation

Document the assessment findings, any written and verbal communications, nursing and medical interventions, and patient response patterns.

EXTRAVASATION

Extravasation is infiltration of a vesicant medication. A **vesicant** solution is a fluid or medication that causes the formation of blisters, with subsequent sloughing of tissues occurring from the tissue necrosis (Tabor, 1993) (Figs. 8–5 and 8–6).

Patients who have a high risk for extravasation injury are presented in Table 8–6.

Extravasation injury is related to:

- Puncture of the distal vein wall during venipuncture and administration of irritating or vesicant medications or solutions
- Puncture of any portion of the vein wall by mechanical friction from the catheter or needle while infusing irritating or vesicant solutions
- Dislodgement of the catheter or needle from the intima of the vein
- Poorly secured infusion device
- High delivery rate or pressure from an electronic infusion device

TABLE 8–5

INFILTRATION SCALE

Grade	Criteria
0	No symptoms
1	Skin blanched Edema <1 inch Cool to touch With or without pain
2	Skin blanched Edema 1 to 6 inches Cool to touch With or without pain
3	Skin blanched and translucent Gross edema >6 inches Cool to touch Mild to moderate pain Possible numbness
4	Skin blanched and translucent Skin tight, leaking Gross edema >6 inches Deep, pitting tissue edema Circulatory impairment Moderate to severe pain

Source: *Revised Standards of Practice.* (1998). Cambridge, MA: Intravenous Nurses Society; with permission.

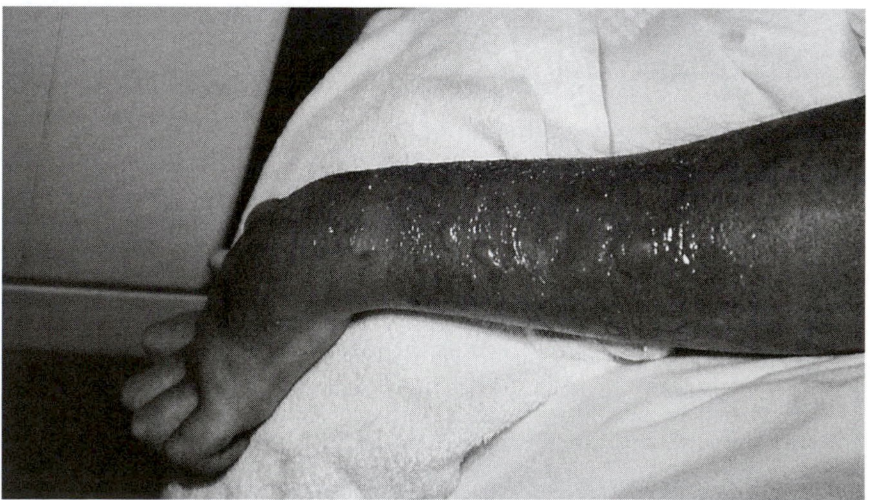

FIG. 8–5. Infiltration of vancomycin into subcutaneous tissue, causing blistering of skin. (Courtesy of Beth Fabian, CRNI.)

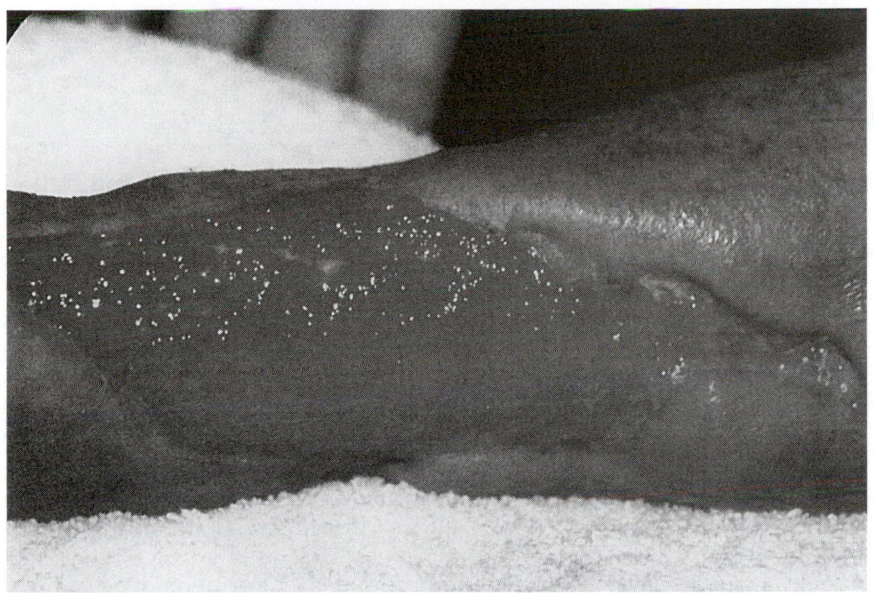

FIG. 8–6. Extravasation with tissue necrosis. (Courtesy of Johnson & Johnson Medical Inc., Arlington, Texas.)

- Overmanipulation of the I.V. device
- Thrombus or fibrin sheath formation at the vascular access device (VAD) catheter tip

Signs and Symptoms

Sign and symptoms of extravasation include:

- Complaints of pain or burning
- Swelling proximal to or distal to the I.V. site

TABLE 8–6

FACTORS AFFECTING RISK FOR EXTRAVASATION INJURY

Age
Neonate
Geriatric patient
Condition
Oncology patient
Comatose patient
Anesthetized patient
Patients with peripheral or cardiovascular disease
Diabetic patient
Equipment
High-pressure infusion pumps

- Puffiness of the dependent part of the limb
- Skin tightness at the venipuncture site
- Blanching and coolness of the skin
- Slow or stopped infusion
- Damp or wet dressing

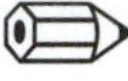 **NOTE:** Never increase the flow rate to determine the infiltration of a vesicant. Checking for blood return is not a reliable method of determining an infiltration (Perdue, 1995).

The severity of damage is directly related to the type, concentration, and volume of fluid infiltrated into the interstitial tissues. The endothelium is particularly sensitive to pH and osmolarity differences found in physiologic and nonphysiologic solutions. These fluids may induce cellular injury through irritation, stimulating the inflammatory process. The damaged tissue release precipitating proteins with an increase in capillary permeability, which allows fluid and protein shifts to interstitial space. Edema, ischemia, vasoconstriction, pain, and erythema are responses to these cellular changes and may lead to tissue necrosis (Hastings-Tolsma et al., 1993).

The most harmful vesicant medications are antineoplastic agents, doxorubicin (Adriamycin, which causes the most severe tissue necrosis), dopamine hydrochloride (Dopastat, Intropin), norephinephrine (levarterenol bitartrate, Levophed), potassium chloride in high doses, amphotericin B (Fungizone), calcium, and sodium bicarbonate in high concentrations.

Prevention

To prevent vesicant extravasations, the following should be considered:

1. The use of skilled practitioners. Registered nurses specifically trained and supervised in chemotherapy administration should administer irritating and vesicant medications. Practitioners should also be skillful in venipuncture and skillful and competent in using VADs.
2. The practitioner's knowledge of vesicants. The practitioner should have an understanding of the signs and symptoms of extravasation and be able to perform appropriate management.
3. The condition of patient's vein. Patients with small, fragile veins; limited access; long-term therapy; and multiple vein sticks are prone to infiltration.
4. The drug administration technique.
   - Give continuous vesicant administration into a long-term VAD.
   - Avoid giving vesicant through a VAD without a good blood return.
   - Always use a free-flowing I.V. to give push medications.
   - Avoid using a controlled infusion device for vesicants given peripherally.

- Assess for blood return frequently (such as every 2 to 5 mL or hourly).

5. The site of venous access. Avoid the large veins of the forearm, especially the posterior basilic vein, and the metacarpal veins of the dorsum of the hand. Avoid the use of the antecubital fossa and avoid using the lower extremity veins. Remove dressings to fully visualize the vein during administration.
6. The condition of the patient. Vomiting, coughing, or retching can cause excessive movement, resulting in a loss of access. Sedation from antiemetics or pain medications limit a patient's ability to report pain during infusion. Patients who are unable to communicate, such as infants and obtunded patients, also need to be observed closely (Camp-Sorrell, 1998).

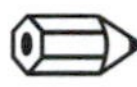

NOTE: Restraints must be applied with extreme caution and within the guidelines established by the Joint Commission on Accreditation of Healthcare Organizations (JCAHO) and by the Food and Drug Administration (FDA). Immobilization devices should be well padded and applied so that they do not cause nerve damage, constrict circulation, or cause pressure areas; they should be removed at frequent intervals, and nurse-assisted range-of-motion exercises should be performed. Inadequate or improper use of immobilization devices can cause very serious complications; policies and procedures should be established to guide their use (JCAHO, 1995).

INS STANDARDS Treatment of infiltration should be established in organizational policy and procedure. (INS, 2000, 60)

Treatment

Treatment depends on the severity of the infiltration. Refer to Table 8–5 for the infiltration scale. Consideration should be given to the completion of an unusual occurrence report on type of infusate and severity of the infiltration. (INS, 1998, 35)

INS STANDARDS The infiltration of any amount of blood product, irritant, or vesicant is classified as a grade 4. (INS, 2000, 60)

The most effective treatment for extravasation is prevention. However, if extravasation is suspected:

1. Stop the I.V. flow and leave the cannula in place until after any residual medication and blood are aspirated and an antidote particular to the vesicant is instilled into the tissues.
2. Administer the prescribed antidote (this cannot be delayed).
3. Remove the cannula.
4. Apply thermal manipulation to alter the temperature in the superficial skin for 24 to 72 hours. Cold topical applications are used for all extravasations except those of the Vinca alkaloids.

5. Photograph the suspected area of extravasation according to institutional policy.
6. Elevate the arm 4 inches. (Note: Elevation of the extremity with infiltration or extravasation is controversial. Research is showing that using small quantities of infiltrated I.V. solutions followed by magnetic resonance imaging decreases hypotonic solutions in volume; hypertonic solutions increase in volume with elevation. A 4-inch (10-cm) elevation of the extremity made no difference in the rate of fluid reabsorption for either solution. Elevating the arm may be uncomfortable for some patients (Yucha, 1994; Hadaway, 1999).
7. Consult the physician. Request a plastic surgery consultation if a vesicant drug has infiltrated.
8. Document all details of the incidence (Camp-Sorrell, 1998; Hadaway, 1999).

Antidotes

Antidotes for extravasation injury fall into four categories: (1) those that alter local pH, (2) those that alter DNA binding, (3) those that chemically neutralize, and (4) those that dilute extravasated drug (Table 8–7.)

If you are going to instill an antidote, do so through the existing I.V. catheter or use a 1-mL tuberculin syringe, injecting small amounts subcutaneously in a circle around the infiltrated area (Camp-Sorrell, 1998).

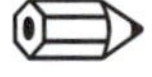

NOTE: If you work with high-risk patients, a copy of Table 8–7 could be posted in the medication area for quick reference.

Documentation

It is important to document the following when extravasation occurs:

- Patient demographics
- Insertion site; any difficulty in previous venipuncture attempts; number and location of previous venipuncture attempts
- Drug dose and dilution (mg/mL)
- Method of drug administration (i.e., peripheral, central, push, continuous)
- Clinical signs of suspected extravasation
- Amount infiltrated
- Amount aspirated
- Patient symptoms
- Assessment of extravasated area
- Physician notification
- All interventions (Camp-Sorrell, 1998)

TABLE 8–7

ANTIDOTES FOR EXTRAVASATED DRUGS

Extravasated Drug Class	Medications	Antidote, Dose*	Nursing Tip
	Adrenergic Agents		
Usually sloughing and tissue necrosis with extravasation	Amrinone (Inocor) Dobutamine (Dobutrex) Dopamine (Intropin) Epinephrine (Adrenaline) Isoproterenol (Isuprel) Metaraminol (Aramine) Methoxamine (Vasoxyl) Norepineprine (Levophed) Phenylephrine (NeoSynephrine)	5 to 10 mg phentolamine mesylate	Discontinue infusion Apply cold compresses Slightly elevate† extremity only if the elevation does not cause pain Use small intradermal needle (27 to 25 g)
	Alkalinizing Agents		
Usually cause ulceration, sloughing, cellulitis, and tissue necrosis	Sodium bicarbonate	Inject 1% procaine to reduce venospasm	Discontinue infusion
	Tromethamine (Tham-E)	Hyaluronidase 150 U/mL 0.2 mL × 5 SQ	Use small intradermal needle (27 to 25 g) Apply cold compresses Elevate slightly†
	Alkylating Agents		
Usually causes sloughing and tissue necrosis	Carmustine (BCNU) irritant	Inject long-acting dexamethasone or other corticosteroid	Discontinue infusion Apply cold compress Elevate slightly†

(Continued)

TABLE 8–7

ANTIDOTES FOR EXTRAVASATED DRUGS *(Continued)*

Extravasated Drug Class	Medications	Antidote, Dose*	Nursing Tip
	Alkylating Agents ***(Continued)***		
	Stretptozocin (Zancosar)	Dimethylsulfoxide (DSM) applied topically	Apply every 3, 4, 6 ,or 8 hours for 7 to 14 days
	Mechlorethamine (nitrogen mustard) vesicant	Sodium thiosulfate Dilute 4 mL with 6 mL of sterile water inject 1 to 4 mL through existing cannula; give 1 mL for each milliliter extravasated	Use ice compresses for 20 min/h until inflammation dissipates
	Antihypertensive Agents		
	Nitroprusside sodium (Nipride)	Sodium thiosulfate Dilute 4 mL with 6 mL of sterile water inject 1 to 4 mL through existing cannula; give 1 mL for each milliliter extravasated	Discontinue infusion Use cool compress Elevate slightly†
	Dobutamine (Dobutrex) Dopamine (Dopastat) Epinephrine Metaraminol (Aramine) Norepinephrine	Phentolamine (Regitine), 5 to 10 mg SQ diluted in 10 to 15 mL of sodium chloride	Treatment must start immediately Use cool compresses

(Continued)

TABLE 8–7

ANTIDOTES FOR EXTRAVASATED DRUGS *(Continued)*

Extravasated Drug Class	Medications	Antidote, Dose*	Nursing Tip
	Antineoplastic Agents		
(DNA/RNA inhibitors or mitotic inhibitors) Usually causes severe tissue sloughing and necrosis	Dacarbazine (DTIC) vesicant Etoposide (VePeside) irritant Vinblastine (Velban) vesicant Vincristine (Oncovin) vesicant Vindesine (Eldisine) vesicant	Inject long-acting dexamethasone or other corticosteroid	Discontinue infusion Apply warm compress Elevate slightly†
	Antibiotic Antineoplastic Agents		
Generally cause stinging, burning, severe cellulitis, and tissue necrosis	Dactinomycin (Actinomycin D) vesicant Daunorubicin (Daunomycin) vesicant Doxorubicin (Adriamycin) vesicant	Flush the extravasated area with 0.9% sodium chloride Inject long-acting OR Inject hyaluronidase (15 U/mL 0.2 mL × 5 SQ throughout the area)	Discontinue infusion Use small gauge (27 to 25) needle Apply cold compresses Elevate slightly†
	Idarubicin (Idamycin) vesicant	Aspirate as much of drug as possible from tissue Flush with 0.9%sodium chloride Inject long-acting OR Inject hyaluronidase 15 U/mL 0.2 mL × 5 SQ	Discontinue infusion Apply ice compresses Elevate slightly†

(Continued)

TABLE 8–7

ANTIDOTES FOR EXTRAVASATED DRUGS *(Continued)*

Extravasated Drug Class	Medications	Antidote, Dose*	Nursing Tip
	Antibiotic Antineoplastic Agents ***(Continued)***		
	Mitomycin C (Mutamycin) vesicant Plicamycin (Mithramycin) vesicant	Inject long-acting dexamethasone	Discontinue infusion after sodium bicarbonate (neutralizing agent is instilled into cannula) Apply cool compresses
Vein irritants that generally cause necrosis, sloughing, cellulitis, and tissue necrosis	Calcium salts Calcium carbonate Calcium chloride Calcium gluconate Calcium lactate Calcium gluceptate Potassium solutions	Inject hyaluronidase through 150 U/mL 0.2 mL × 5 SQ	Discontinue infusion Apply cool compresses Elevate slightly†
Hypertonic (>10%) solutions	Dextrose solutions	Inject hyaluronidase through 150 U/mL 0.2 mL × 5 SQ	Discontinue infusion Apply cool compresses Elevate slightly†

*Side effects of antidotes:
Dimethyl sulfoxide (DMSO): Mild side effects, mild burning, skin scaling and unpleasant garlic odor. Use with local cooling measures
Hyaluronidase (Wydase): Rash, urticaria
Phentolamine (Regitine): Hypotension, tachycardia, flushing, nausea and vomiting
Sodium thiosulfate: Rash, hypersensitivity
Hydrocortisone sodium or dexamethasone: Delayed wound healing, various skin eruptions

†Research on small quantities of infiltrated I.V. solutions followed by magnetic resonance imaging found that hypotonic solutions decreased in volume and hypertonic solutions increased in volume with elevation. A 4-inch (10-cm) elevation of the extremity made no difference in the rate of fluid reabsorption for either solution. Elevating the arm may be uncomfortable for some patients.

NOTE: Soft tissue damage from extravasation can lead to prolonged healing, potential infections, necrosis, multiple debridement surgeries, cosmetic disfiguration, loss of limb function, and amputation.

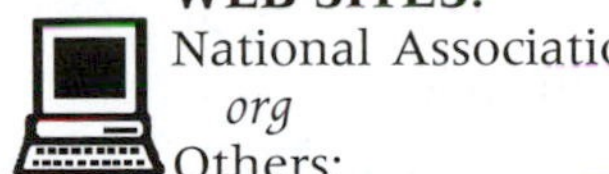
WEB SITES:
National Association of Vascular Access Networks: *www.navannet.org*
Others:______

LOCAL INFECTIONS

Infections related to the use of I.V. therapy consist of those related to microbial contamination of the cannula or infusate. One of the most serious forms of intravascular device-related infection occurs when intravascular thrombus surrounding the cannula becomes infected. This causes septic thrombophlebitis, or **suppurative** phlebitis (Maki & Mermel, 1998).

Local infections are preventable by maintaining aseptic technique and following guidelines established by the INS or Centers for Disease Control and Prevention for the duration of infusion, length of time of catheter placement, and tubing change criteria.

Local infections are related to:

- Catheters left in place for more than 72 hours
- Field sticks that are not changed after 24 hours
- Poor technique in placing the catheter
- Poor technique in maintaining and monitoring the peripheral site

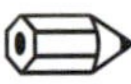
NOTES: In any patient with an intravascular catheter who develops high-grade bloodstream infection that persists after an infected cannula has been removed, it is likely the patient has infected thrombus in recently cannulated vein (Maki & Mermel, 1998).

Suppurative phlebitis of peripheral I.V. catheters is now rare, and the syndrome of I.V. suppuration is predominately a complication of central venous catheters.

Signs and Symptoms

Signs and symptoms of local infection include:

- Redness and swelling at the site
- Possible exudate of purulent material
- Increased quantity of white blood cells
- Elevated temperature (chills are not associated with local infection)

The ways a catheter tip may acquire bacteria are:

- During introduction of venipuncture
- During removal of stylet
- From colonization from skin
- From contaminated I.V. solutions
- From air inlet filter malfunction
- From microorganisms entering system at catheter or administration set junction.

Prevention

Techniques used to prevent local infections include:

1. Inspect all solution containers for cracks and leaks before hanging.
2. Change solution containers every 24 hours.
3. Maintain aseptic technique during cannula insertion, I.V. therapy, and catheter removal (Perdue, 1995).

The risk of local infection is affected by the choice and preparation of site. The venipuncture site should be scrubbed with 70 percent alcohol to remove blood or dirt, which can interfere with disinfectant prepping solution. Then for excellent bactericidal activity, perform a 20-second circular preparation with 1 to 2 percent tincture of iodine, iodophor or 70 percent isopropyl alcohol or chlorhexidine, and allow the site to dry. If the patient is allergic to iodine, use 70 percent alcohol for a 1-minute vigorous scrub. I.V. cannulae contaminated during the time of insertion by microorganism on the hands of hospital personnel contribute significantly to local infections. Washing hands with soap and water with mechanical friction for at least 15 seconds removes most transient acquired bacteria (Wenzel, 1993). See Chapter 2 for further information on infections at cannula sites.

Treatment

1. Consult with the physician.
2. Remove the cannula.
3. Culture the cannula tip and insertion site.
4. Apply a sterile dressing over the site.
5. Use systemic antibiotic therapy, which may be necessary.
6. Monitor the site.

Documentation

Document the assessment of the site, culture technique, sources of culture, notification of the physician, and any treatment initiated. Culture techniques are discussed in Chapter 2.

VENOUS SPASM

Venospasm can occur suddenly and for a variety of reasons. The spasm usually results from the administration of a cold infusate, an irritating solution, or a too-rapid administration of I.V. solution or viscous solution such as a blood product.

Venous spasm is related to:

- Administration of cold infusates
- Mechanical or chemical irritation of intima of vein

Signs and Symptoms

Signs and symptoms of venous spasms include:

- Sharp pain at I.V. site that travels up the arm, which is caused by a piercing stream of fluid that irritates or shocks the vein wall
- Slowing of the infusion

Prevention

Techniques used to prevent vasospasm include:

1. Dilute the medication additive adequately.
2. Keep the I.V. solution at room temperature.
3. Wrap the extremity with warm compresses during the infusion.
4. Give the solution at the prescribed rate.

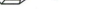

NOTE: If a rapid infusion rate is desired, use a larger cannula.

Treatment

1. Apply warm compresses to warm the extremity and decrease flow rate until the spasm subsides.
2. Restart the I.V. if venospasm continues.

Documentation

Document the patient complaints, duration of complaints, treatment, and length of time to resolve the problem. Also document whether the I.V. site needed to be rotated to resolve the problem.

HYPERSENSITIVITY REACTIONS

A hypersensitivity reaction is the response of the body to an antigen. An antigen is an agent that is capable of stimulating antibodies. It is a protein that coats the surface of specific tissue cells and then identifies them as part of the body rather than as foreign.

With I.V. infusion, hypersensitivity to the infusate, its preservatives, or I.V. medications can occur. The patient may be allergic to the cannula material, tape, or the antiseptic used to prepare the venipuncture site. Depending on the specific allergic reaction, the signs and symptoms range from rashes, itching, and hives to bronchial spasm and anaphylaxis (Josephson, 1999).

Prevention

1. A thorough history is needed in eliciting information about allergy status.
2. Proper patient identification in acute and home care settings.

3. Verify allergies to over-the counter medications, foods, and topical preparations, especially iodine and tape.

Treatment

1. Discontinue the infusion and keep the vein open with sodium chloride.
2. DO NOT REMOVE THE CANNULA until the new line is started.
3. Monitor vital signs.
4. Have emergency equipment ready.
5. Administer drugs according to agency policy and physician orders.

Documentation

Document assessments, type of catheter in place, the medication or solutions that were infusing, and nursing interventions.

SYSTEMIC COMPLICATIONS

Systemic complications can be life threatening. Such complications include septicemia, circulatory overload, pulmonary edema, air embolus, speed shock, and catheter embolus.

SEPTICEMIA

Septicemia is the leading cause of death in intensive care units (ICUs), where an estimated 600,000 patients are aggressively treated and only 50 to 60 percent of them survive (White, 1997). Septicemia is a febrile disease process that results from the presence of microorganisms or their toxic products in the circulatory system (Guyton & Hall, 1997). Neither the intravascular device nor the infusate are cultured in most of these infections; consequently, the source remains unknown.

The microorganism most frequently implicated in catheter-related bloodstream infections is coagulase-negative staphylococcus (Maki & Mermel, 1998). I.V. infusion–related sepsis is most often attributed to *Staphylococcus aureus* and *S. epidermidis* bacteria, the *Candida albicans* yeast, and the coliform species *Escherichia, Enterobacter,* and *Klebsiella*. Vascular system septicemia introduced with I.V. catheters is generally caused by the *Enterobacter, Serratia, S. epidermidis, Pseudomonas,* enterococci *and Candida* pathogens (Stanford, Gilbert, & Sande, 1996).

Nurses must be aware of risk factors, prevention techniques, and the presence of an infected catheter tip because bacteremia, fungemia, or septicemia could occur. Risk factors include:

- Patient factors: age, alteration in host defense, underlying illness, presence of other infectious processes

- Infusion factors: solution container, stopcocks, catheter material and structure, insertion site, hematogenous seeding, manipulation of the infusion system, certain transparent dressings, and duration of cannulation (Maki & Ringer, 1991)

Septicemia is related to:

- Irrigation of clogged I.V. catheters can propel a clot, which is a high source of bacterial contamination, into the systemic circulation.
- Break in aseptic technique during venipuncture and maintenance of cannula.
- Contaminated infusate.
- Use of stopcocks can be a source or entry site for contaminants.

Signs and Symptoms

Signs and symptoms of septicemia include:

- Fluctuating fever, tremors, chattering teeth
- Profuse, cold sweat
- Nausea and vomiting
- Diarrhea (sudden and explosive)
- Abdominal pain
- Tachycardia
- Altered mental status
- Hypotension
- Tachypnea and tachycardia

Table 2–5 lists the microbial pathogens associated with intravascular line-related infections.

Prevention

Techniques used to prevent septicemia include:

1. Good handwashing. Handwashing and sterile technique are imperative to minimize the risk of technique-induced septicemia.
2. Careful inspection of solutions for abnormal cloudiness, cracks, and pinholes.
3. Use of only freshly opened solutions.
4. Protein solutions, such as albumin and protein hydrolysates, should be used as soon as the seal is broken.
5. Use iodine-containing antiseptics rather than alcohol-containing antiseptics, which have a superior spectrum of antimicrobial activity. They are inexpensive, well tolerated, and highly reliable.
6. Use Luer-lock connections when possible.
7. Cover infusion sites with a sterile dressing.
8. Limit use of add-on devices.

9. Inspect the site and assess the patient routinely to ensure early recognition of symptoms.
10. Change peripheral cannulae according to the INS standards of practice.

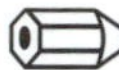 **NOTE:** The key to prevention of septicemia is staff education.

Treatment

It is sometimes difficult to differentiate between infusion-associated sepsis and septicemia of other causes, unless associated with phlebitis (Maki & Mermel, 1998).

The steps in treating suspected septicemia based on patient signs and symptoms are:

1. Consult the physician.
2. Restart a new I.V. system in the opposite extremity.
3. Obtain cultures from the administration set, container, and catheter tip site, as well as the patient's blood.
4. Initiate antimicrobial therapy as ordered.
5. Monitor the patient closely.
6. Determine whether the patient's condition requires transfer to the ICU.

Documentation

Document the signs and symptoms assessed, the time the physician was notified, and all treatments instituted. Document the time of transfer to ICU, the time the new I.V. infusion and system was started, and how the patient is tolerating interventions.

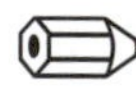 **NOTE:** Fluids temporarily discontinued to administer blood components should be discarded and fresh solutions restarted after transfusion is terminated.

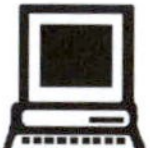

WEB SITES:
Association of Professionals in Infection Control: *www.apic.org*
Others:____

FLUID OVERLOAD

Overloading the circulatory system with excessive I.V. fluids causes increased blood pressure and central venous pressure. Circulatory overload is caused by infusing excessive amounts of isotonic crystalloid solutions too rapidly, failure to monitor the I.V. infusion, or too-rapid infusion of any fluid in a patient compromised by cardiopulmonary or renal disease.

Fluid overload is related to:

- Rapid infusion of an I.V. solution
- Hepatic, cardiac, or renal disease

AGE-RELATED COMPLICATIONS: FLUID OVERLOAD

Risk for fluid overload and subsequent pulmonary edema is especially increased in elderly patients with cardiac disease.

Signs and Symptoms

Signs and symptoms of circulatory overload include:

- Weight gain
- Edema
- Puffy eyelids
- Hypertension
- Wide variance between intake and output
- Rise in central venous pressure (CVP)
- Shortness of breath and crackles in lungs
- Distended neck veins

Prevention

Techniques used to prevent circulatory overload include:

1. Monitor the infusion, especially sodium chloride, and know the solution's physiologic effects on the circulatory system.
2. Maintain flow at prescribed rate.
3. Do not "catch up" on I.V. solutions that are behind schedule; instead, recalculate all infusions that are not on time.
4. Monitor the intake and output on all patients receiving I.V. fluids.
5. Know the patient's cardiovascular history.

Treatment

Consult the physician if you suspect circulatory overload.

1. Decrease the I.V. flow rate.
2. Place the patient in the high Fowlers position.
3. Keep the patient warm to promote peripheral circulation.
4. Monitor vital signs.
5. Administer oxygen as ordered.
6. Consider changing the administration set to a microdrip set.

Documentation

Document patient assessment, notification of physician, and treatments instituted by physician order. Monitor the patient and record vital signs on an interval flow sheet.

PULMONARY EDEMA

Fluid overload can lead to pulmonary edema. Fluids too rapidly infused increase venous pressure and lead to pulmonary edema. Pulmonary edema is an abnormal accumulation of fluid in the lungs. In pulmonary edema, fluid leaks through the capillary wall and fills the interstitium and alveoli. "The pulmonary vascular bed has received more blood from the right ventricle than the left ventricle can accommodate and remove. The slightest imbalance between inflow on the right side and outflow on the left side may have drastic consequences" (Smeltzer & Bare, 2000).

Patients at risk for pulmonary edema are those with cardiovascular disease, those with renal disease, and elderly patients. It is important to identify patients at risk for pulmonary edema and provide nursing care that decreases the heart's workload. Sodium chloride given to correct profound sodium deficits can lead to pulmonary overload and must be monitored closely (Metheny, 1996). Pulmonary edema is related to:

- Overzealous infusion of parenteral fluids, especially those that contain sodium
- Patients with compromised cardiovascular or renal systems

Signs and Symptoms

Initial signs and symptoms of pulmonary edema include:

- Restlessness
- Slow increase in pulse rate
- Headache
- Shortness of breath
- Cough
- Flushing

As fluid builds in the pulmonary bed, later signs and symptoms include hypertension, severe dyspnea, gurgling respirations, coughing up frothy fluid, and moist crackles.

Prevention

Techniques used to prevent pulmonary edema include:

1. Obtain a baseline assessment before starting I.V. therapy.
2. Review the patient's history of cardiac or respiratory problems before starting I.V. therapy.

3. Maintain a consistent infusion rate.
4. Monitor lung sounds for crackles.

Treatment

Consult the physician if you suspect pulmonary edema. Treatment is the same as for circulatory overload.

Documentation

Document patient assessment, notification of physician, and treatments instituted by physician order. Monitor the patient and record vital signs on an interval flow sheet.

AIR EMBOLISM

Air embolism is a rare but lethal complication, especially involving VADs. The problem is treatable with prompt recognition, but prevention is the key. The pathophysiologic consequences of air emboli are a result of air's entering the central veins, which is quickly trapped in the blood as it flows forward. Trapped air is carried to the right ventricle, where it lodges against the pulmonary valve and blocks the flow of blood from the ventricle into the pulmonary arteries (Richardson & Bruso, 1993). Less blood is ejected from the right ventricle, and the right heart overfills. The force of right ventricular contractions increases in an attempt to eject blood past the occluding air pocket. These forceful contractions break small air bubbles loose from the air pocket. Minute air bubbles are subsequently pumped into the pulmonary circulation, causing even greater obstruction to the forward flow of blood as well as local pulmonary tissue hypoxia. Pulmonary hypoxia results in vasoconstriction in the lung tissue, which further increases the workload of the right ventricle and reduces blood flow out of the right heart. This leads to diminished cardiac output, shock, and death.

The same intrathoracic pressure changes that allow for pulmonary ventilation are responsible for air emboli associated with subclavian line removal. Pressure in the central veins decreases during inspiration and increases during expiration. If an opening into a central vein exposes the vessel to the atmosphere during the negative inspiratory cycle, air can be sucked into the central venous system in much the same manner that air is pulled into the lungs.

The causes of air embolism include:

- Allowing the solution container to run dry
- Superimposing a new I.V. bag to a line that has run dry without clearing the line of air
- Loose connections that allow air to enter the system
- Poor technique in dressing and tubing changes for central lines
- Air in administration tubing cassettes of electronic infusion devices

Signs and Symptoms

Initial signs and symptoms of air embolism include:

- Patient complaints of palpitations
- Lightheadedness and weakness
- Pulmonary findings: dyspnea, cyanosis, tachypnea, expiratory wheezes, cough, and pulmonary edema
- Cardiovascular findings: "mill wheel" murmur; weak, thready pulse; tachycardia; substernal chest pain; hypotension; and jugular venous distention
- Neurologic findings: change in mental status, confusion, coma, anxiousness, and seizures

If untreated, these signs and symptoms lead to hemiplegia, aphasia, generalized seizures, coma, and cardiac arrest.

Prevention

Techniques used to prevent air embolism include:

1. Remove air from administration sets. To do so, wrap tubing around a pencil to force air bubbles upward into drip chamber infusing.
2. Vent air from port using a syringe attached to needleless system.
3. Use a 0.22-micron air-eliminating filter.
4. Follow the protocol for dressing and tubing changes of central lines.
5. Superimpose I.V. solutions before the previous solution runs completely dry.
6. Attach piggyback medications to high injection port so the check valve will prevent air from being drawn into the line after the infusion of medication.
7. Use Luer-lock connectors whenever possible.
8. Do not bypass the "pump housing" of electric volumetric pumps.

Treatment

If you suspect an air embolus, do the following:

1. Call for help.
2. Place the patient in Trendelenburg's position on left side (left lateral decubitus position) with the head down. This causes the air to rise in the right atrium, preventing it from entering the pulmonary artery.
3. Administer oxygen.
4. Monitor vital signs.
5. Have emergency equipment available.
6. Notify the physician immediately.

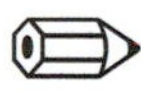

NOTE: A pathognomonic indicator of an air embolism is a loud, churning, drumlike sound audible over the precordium, called a "mill wheel murmur." This symptom may be absent or transient.

Documentation

Document patient assessment, nursing interventions to correct the cause of embolism if apparent, notification of physician, and treatment. If emergency treatment was necessary, use an interval flow sheet to document the management of the air embolism, record interval vital signs, and indicate patient response.

SPEED SHOCK

Speed shock occurs when a foreign substance, usually a medication, is rapidly introduced into the circulation. Rapid injection permits the concentration of medication in the plasma to reach toxic proportions, flooding the organs rich in blood—the heart and the brain. Syncope, shock, and cardiac arrest may result.

Speed shock is related to administration of I.V. medications or solution at a rapid rate.

Signs and Symptoms

Signs and symptoms of speed shock include:

- Dizziness
- Facial flushing
- Headache
- Tightness in the chest
- Hypotension
- Irregular pulse
- Progression of shock

Prevention

Techniques used to prevent speed shock include:

1. Reduce the size of drops by using microdrop sets for medication delivery.
2. Use an electronic flow control with high-risk drugs.
3. Monitor the infusion rate for accuracy before piggybacking in the medication.
4. Be careful not to manipulate the catheter; cannula movement may speed up the flow rate.

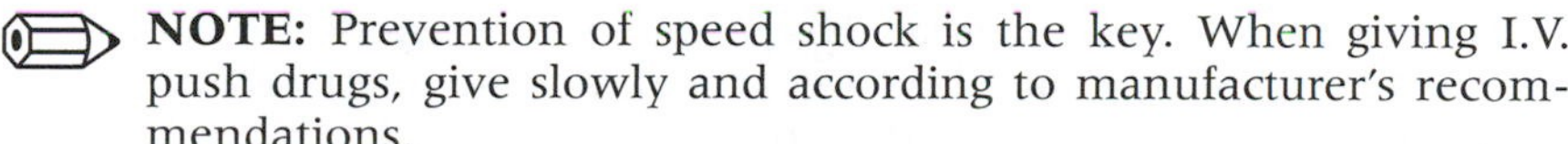

NOTE: Prevention of speed shock is the key. When giving I.V. push drugs, give slowly and according to manufacturer's recommendations.

Treatment

If you suspect speed shock, do the following:

1. Get help.
2. Give antidote or resuscitation medications as needed.
3. Have naloxone (Narcan) available on the unit if giving I.V. narcotics.

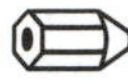 **NOTE:** See Chapter 10 for appropriate steps in delivery of I.V. push medications.

Documentation

Document the medication or fluid administered and the signs and symptoms the patient reported and those assessed. Also document the physician notification, the treatment initiated, and the patient response.

CATHETER EMBOLISM

Catheter embolism is an infrequent systemic complication of over-the-needle catheters. In this situation, a piece of the catheter breaks off and travels through the vascular system. It may migrate to the chest and lodge in the pulmonary artery or the right ventricle.

Catheter embolism is related to:

- Reinsertion of same catheter used in an unsuccessful venipuncture
- Removing a stylet and reinserting it, sheering off the catheter tip
- Pressure directly over the catheter during discontinuation of therapy
- Placement of the catheter in a joint flexion

Signs and Symptoms

Signs and symptoms include:

- Sharp, sudden pain at the I.V. site
- Minimal blood return, short
- Rough and uneven catheter noted on removal
- Cyanosis
- Chest pain
- Tachycardia
- Hypotension

Pulmonary embolism, cardiac dysrythmia, sepsis, endocarditis, thrombosis, and death may result if the catheter embolism migrates to the chest and lodges in the pulmonary artery or the right ventricle.

Prevention

Techniques used to prevent catheter embolism include:

1. Never reinsert a needle in a catheter (over-the-needle) after removal.
2. Avoid inserting the catheter over joint flexion when movement causes catheter to bend back and forth.
3. Splint the arm if the patient is restless.
4. Do not apply pressure over the site while removing a catheter.

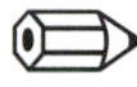 **NOTE:** Always use radiopaque catheters, so the catheter will be detectable on radiograph.

Treatment

If the patient is cooperative, have him or her apply digital pressure on the vein above the insertion site. This may prevent the catheter from migrating. Other techniques include:

1. Applying a tourniquet above the elbow.
2. Contacting the physician and radiologist.
3. Starting a new I.V. line.
4. Preparing the patient for radiographic examination.
5. Measuring the remainder of the catheter tip to determine the length of the embolized tip.

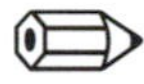 **NOTE:** Be sure to assess circulation of extremity while the tourniquet is on the arm.

Documentation

Document the patient's subjective complaints in quotes. Document the discontinuation of the catheter, the technique used, and the length of catheter removed. State the nursing interventions and the time the physician was notified.

ERRATIC FLOW RATES

According to a survey (Cohen, 1993), free-flow incidents are common occurrences in delivery of infusion therapy. In this survey of more than 400 nurses, 42 percent knew of free-flow incidents at their institutions.

There are many factors to consider in determining flow rate (Table 8–8). These include body size, fluid type, patient's age and condition, physiologic responses as reflected by urinary output, pulmonary status, and specific drugs being infused. The very young and the very old often need a slower rate of infusion and small volumes of solution. Patients with cardiac or renal diseases may also have problems tolerating large fluid volumes or fast rates. Situations in which flow rates have been poorly

TABLE 8–8

FACTORS IN FLOW-RATE CONTROL

Patient-Related	Vein-Related
Patient or family intervention	Infiltration
Patient blood pressure	Phlebitis
	Venous spasm
Tubing-Related	**Clot formation**
"Cold flow" of plastic tubing	**needle or catheter position**
Drop formation rate	
Final in-filters kinked or pinched tubing	**Other**
Rate of fluid flow	Height of I.V. standard
Slipping of roller clamp	Bed position
Electronic infusion device malfunction	

Source: Adapted from Steele, J. (1983). Too fast or too slow: The erratic I.V. *American Journal of Nursing, 6,* 898–900, with permission.

regulated can have serious consequences, especially with I.V. solutions containing medications such as epinephrine, theophylline, meperidine, lidocaine, sodium bicarbonate, amphotericin B, potassium chloride magnesium, and heparin (Cohen, 1993).

Accurate flow rate is imperative when a drug level must be kept constant. If the rate is too slow:

- The patient is not receiving the desired amount of drug or solution.
- It can lead to a clogged I.V. needle or catheter and perhaps the loss of a premium vein.

If the rate is too fast:

- Hypotonic solutions can lead to the development of pulmonary edema or congestive heart failure.
- Rapid infusion of hypertonic glucose can result in osmotic diuresis, leading to dehydration.
- Hypertonic solutions are also irritating and phlebitis can result.
- Free-flow administration of drugs can cause serious cardiovascular and respiratory complications.

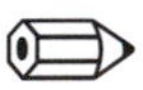

NOTE: A fast rate is considered more dangerous than a rate that is too slow.

Prevention

Prevention of erratic flow rates and the complications they cause include:

1. Allowing only experienced nurses to set up, adjust, or remove I.V. administration sets.

2. Using pumps that provide free-flow protection; checking with each manufacturer.
3. Properly closing clamps if removing administration set from pump.
4. Checking or recalculating infusion rates.
5. Providing or attending staff development education on electronic infusion devices.
6. Reporting all free-flow incidents.

Treatment

Treatment techniques for erratic flow rates include the following:

1. Stopping the flow and recalculating the drip rate.
2. Treating the patient symptomatically.
3. Consulting the physician.
4. Recalculating the infusion rate.

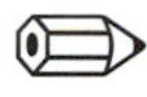

NOTE: In addition, notify the product evaluation committee or central services if cause of erratic flow is an electronic infusion device.

Table 8–9 presents a summary of the complications of peripheral I.V. therapy.

TABLE 8–9

COMPLICATIONS OF PERIPHERAL I.V. THERAPY

Complication	Signs and Symptoms	Treatment	Prevention
		Local	
Hematoma	Ecchymoses Swelling Inability to advance catheter Resistance during flushing	Remove catheter if indicated Apply pressure with 2 × 2s Elevate extremity	Use indirect method of venipuncture Apply tourniquet just before venipuncture
Thrombosis	Slowed or stopped infusion Fever and malaise Inability to flush device	Discontinue catheter Apply cold compresses to site Assess for circulatory impairment	Use pumps Choose microdrip sets with gravity flow if rate is below 50 mL/h Avoid flexion areas

(Continued)

TABLE 8–9

COMPLICATIONS OF PERIPHERAL I.V. THERAPY *(Continued)*

Complication	Signs and Symptoms	Treatment	Prevention
		Local *(Continued)*	
Phlebitis	Redness at site Site warm to touch Local swelling Palpable cord along vein Sluggish infusion rate	Discontinue catheter Apply cold compresses initially, then warm Consult physician if 3+	Use larger veins for hypertonic solutions Choose smallest I.V. cannula that is appropriate for infusion Good handwashing practices Add buffer to irritating solutions Change solution containers every 24 hours Rotate infusion sites every 48 to 72 hours
Infiltration (extravasation)	Coolness of skin around site Taut skin Dependent edema Backflow of blood absent Infusion rate slowing	Discontinue catheter Apply cool compresses Elevate extremity slightly Follow guidelines if extravasation occurs Have antidote chart available	Stabilize the catheter Place catheter in appropriate site Avoid antecubital fossa
Local infection	Redness and swelling at site Possible exudate of purulent material Increased WBC count Elevated temperature	Discontinue catheter and culture site and cannula Apply sterile dressing over site Administer antibiotics as ordered	Inspect all solutions Good technique during venipuncture and site maintenance

(Continued)

TABLE 8–9

COMPLICATIONS OF PERIPHERAL I.V. THERAPY ***(Continued)***

Complication	Signs and Symptoms	Treatment	Prevention
		Local	
Venous spasm	Sharp pain at I.V. site Slowing of infusion	Apply warm compress to site with infusion still running Restart infusion if spasm continues	Dilute medications Keep I.V. solution at room temperature
Hypersensitivity reactions	Vary depending on reaction Rashes, itching, bronchial spasm, anaphylaxis	Stop infusion and keep I.V open with sodium chloride DO NOT use DC cannula Have emergency equipment available Administer drugs according to agency policy	Thorough history Verify allergies Proper patient identification
		Systemic	
Septicemia	Fluctuating fever Profuse sweating Nausea and vomiting Diarrhea Abdominal pain Tachycardia Hypotension Altered mental status	Restart new I.V. system Obtain cultures Notify physician Initiate antimicrobial therapy ordered Monitor patient closely	Good handwashing technique Careful inspection of solutions Use Luer locks Cover infusion sites with sterile dressings Follow standards of practice related to rotation of sites and hang time of infusions Use iodine-based prepping solutions

(Continued)

TABLE 8-9

COMPLICATIONS OF PERIPHERAL I.V. THERAPY *(Continued)*

Complication	Signs and Symptoms	Treatment	Prevention
		Systemic *(Continued)*	
Fluid overload	Weight gain Puffy eyelids Edema Hypertension Changes in I & O Rise in CVP Shortness of breath Crackles in lungs Distended neck veins	Decrease I.V. flow rate Place patient in high Fowler position Keep patient warm Monitor vital signs Administer oxygen as ordered Consider changing to microdrip set	Monitor infusion Maintain flow at prescribed rate Monitor I & O Know patient's cardiovascular history Do not "catch up" infusions; instead, recalibrate
Air embolism	Lightheadedness Dyspnea, cyanosis, tachypnea, expiratory wheezes, cough Mill wheel murmur, chest pain, hypotension Change in mental status, confusion, coma, seizures	Call for help Place patient in Trendelenburg position Administer oxygen Monitor vital signs Notify physician	Remove all air from administration sets Use locks Attach piggyback
Speed shock	Dizziness Facial flushing Headache Tightness in chest Hypotension Irregular pulse Progession of shock	Get help Give antidote or resuscitation medications	Reduce the size of drops by using a microdrip set Use electronic infusion device Monitor infusion rate Dilute I.V. push medications if possible

(Continued)

TABLE 8–9

COMPLICATIONS OF PERIPHERAL I.V. THERAPY *(Continued)*

Complication	Signs and Symptoms	Treatment	Prevention
		Systemic	
Catheter embolism (Note: Use only radiopaque catheters)	Sharp sudden pain at I.V. site Rough, uneven catheter noted on removal Chest pain Tachycardia	Apply tourniquet above elbow Contact physician Start a new I.V. line Measure remainder of catheter	Do not apply pressure over site Never reinsert a stylet that has been removed from sheath Avoid joint flexions

NURSING PLAN OF CARE

PREVENTION OF COMPLICATIONS

Focus Assessment

Subjective

- Patient reports signs and symptoms of discomfort at the I.V. site

Objective

- Evaluate for anxiety or fear
- Assess intake and output ratios
- Assess cardiac and renal functions
- Assess for age-related risks
- Determine baseline weight
- Assess vital signs
- Inspect skin for integrity

Patient Outcome Criteria

The patient will:

- Express fears related to infusion therapy.
- Remain free of complications related to the administration of I.V. therapy.
- Report any changes in comfort of I.V. site.
- Demonstrate care in maintaining the I.V. system.

Nursing Diagnoses

- Anxiety (mild, moderate, severe) related to threat to or change in health status; misconceptions regarding therapy
- Altered tissue perfusion (peripheral) related to infiltration of fluid or medication

(continued)

(continued)

- Decreased cardiac output related to sepsis contamination; infusion of isotonic or hypertonic fluids
- Fear related to insertion of catheter; fear of needles
- Hyperthermia related to increased metabolic rate, illness, dehydration
- Impaired gas exchange related to ventilation–perfusion imbalance; embolism
- Impaired skin integrity related to I.V. catheter, irritating I.V. fluids, inflammation, infection, infiltration
- Impaired tissue integrity related to altered circulation; fluid deficit or excess; irritating I.V. fluids; inflammation; infection; infiltration
- Impaired physical mobility related to pain or discomfort resulting from placement and maintenance of I.V. infusion
- Alteration in comfort, pain, related to physical trauma (e.g., catheter insertion)
- Risk of infection related to broken skin or traumatized tissue

Nursing Management

1. Maintain strict aseptic technique.
2. Examine the solution for type, amount, expiration date, character of the fluid, and lack of damage to container.
3. Select and prepare an electronic infusion device as indicated.
4. Administer fluids at room temperature.
5. Administer I.V. medications at prescribed rate and monitor for results.
6. Monitor I.V. flow rate and site during infusion.
7. Replace I.V. cannula, administration set, and dressing every 48 to 72 hours.
8. Maintain occlusive dressing.
9. Perform I.V. site checks and document at regular intervals.
10. Limit I.V. potassium to 20 mEq per hour or 120 mEq per 24 hours as appropriate.
11. Record intake and output.
12. Use serial weight to assess for fluid overload.

PATIENT EDUCATION

- Instruct the patient to perform routine activities: bathing, movement in bed, and ambulation to maintain I.V. system.
- Instruct the patient to report any signs or symptoms of common local complications (e.g., redness, swelling, pain at site).
- Instruct the patient to report any interruption in flow rate.
- Instruct the patient on the purpose of the electronic infusion device.

The new JCAHO standards address the broad range of home health care services: Standard P.L. 100-203 establishes mandates affecting the home health industry:

- Establish home health hotlines in each state.
- Place more emphasis on client outcomes.
- Document questions about complaints.
- Develop, maintain, and update a database containing the results of each agency's certification and survey.

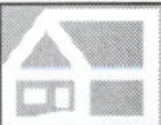

HOME CARE ISSUES

Home care practitioners must be aware of the potential danger that exists in I.V. drug administration and must be able to handle emergency situations. Adverse reactions, such as drowsiness, dizziness, nausea, diarrhea, and local and systemic complications, can occur with delivery of medications in the home setting.

Allergic reactions from hypersensitivity to a specific antigen can also occur. An emergency kit, including epinephrine, diphenhydramine (Benadryl), and dexamethasone (Decadron) or hydrocortisone (Solu-Cortef), should be available to clinicians delivering medication in the home setting. The emergency kit should also include an airway, unused tubing, and additional catheters in the event that a new I.V. access must be established.

Potential problems and complications encountered in home infusion therapy include:

- Mechanical problems
- Nonrunning I.V. lines
- Inability to flush lines
- Electronic infusion device alarms

KEY POINTS

After reading this chapter, you have increased your awareness about the risks to patients receiving I.V. therapy. Remember, you have observation skills to assess for local complications, as well as cognitive skills to assess for systemic complications.

- There are two divisions of complications, local and systemic.
- Local complications can become dangerous systemic adverse processes.
- Prevention is the best intervention for avoiding complications of infusion therapy.

KEY TIPS FOR PREVENTING LOCAL COMPLICATIONS

- Maintain INS guidelines regarding tubing change, cannula change, and length of time I.V. solutions remain hanging.
- Follow aseptic technique in skin preparation and venipuncture techniques.
- Wash hands. Choose appropriate dressings.
- Secure tubing and cannula with good taping technique.
- Use a 0.22-micron inline filter as an extra safeguard.
- Keep solutions at prescribed rate.
- Document observed I.V. site every 4 hours for adults and every 2 hours for infants and children.
- Phlebitis (bacterial, chemical, or mechanical) is a frequently encountered problem associated with infusion therapy and can lead to cellulitis, thromboembolic complications, or sepsis.

KEY TIPS FOR PREVENTING SYSTEMIC COMPLICATIONS

- Use good handwashing procedures.
- Inspect solutions and equipment for breaks in integrity.
- Use Luer-lock connectors.
- Limit the use of add-on devices.
- Maintain flow rates at the prescribed rate.
- Use a 0.22-micron filter when appropriate.
- Use electronic infusion devices.

CHAPTER ACTIVITIES

COMPETENCY CRITERIA: Assessment of Patients for Local Complications Related to Peripheral Infusion Therapy
COMPETENCY STATEMENT: Competent I.V. nurses will be able to assess for complications associated with I.V. therapy.
Note: The cognitive (knowledge) information that is embedded within this performance-based competency includes aseptic technique, fluid and electrolyte balance, risk factors of extravasation injury, phlebitis scale, infiltration scale, and prevention techniques.
This competency *links* to the competency of infection control, management of intravenous equipment, parenteral solutions, and initiation of peripheral I.V. therapy

Performance	Skilled	Needs Education
Critical Action Statements		
1. Performs assessment skills related to local complications A. Site inspection B. Comparison of extremities C. Dependent edema		
2. Demonstrates treatment for local complications A. Application of warm compress B. Application of ice compress C. Elevation of extremity		
3. Demonstrates use of antidote for extravasation injury A. Subcutaneous wheals using TB syringe B. Through the I.V. line		
4. Performs steps to correct erratic flow rate A. Check for kinks B. Retaping C. Milking tubing D. Recalculation		
5. Demonstrates removal of air from administration set		
6. Demonstrates culturing technique A. Site B. Cannula		

(continued)

(continued)

Performance	Skilled	Needs Education
Critical Action Statements		
7. Demonstrates the use of phlebitis scale		
8. Demonstrates use of infiltration scale		

EVALUATION CRITERIA

1. Observation of treatment of local complication
2. Return demonstration of culturing technique
3. Return demonstration of use of antidote of extravasation injury
4. Return demonstration of I.V. infusion problems
5. Recalculation problems
6. Implementation of nursing interventions (i.e., discontinuation of IV cannula, application of heat or cold where appropriate, elevation of extremity, notification of physician)

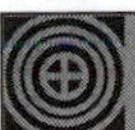

CRITICAL THINKING ACTIVITY

1. Check the policy and procedure manual in the facility in which you are working. Is there a policy that addresses the:
   A. Length of time the I.V. catheter is to be left in the patient?
   B. Frequency of tubing changes?
   C. Type of solution used for preparing site before venipuncture?

2. Do you feel that more attention should be paid to the quality management of the I.V.s in your hospital, extended care facility, or home care setting? Why?
   If yes, how can you contribute to safer I.V. therapy?

3. Have you ever detected a case of phlebitis? Describe the changes that you found.

4. The infusion slows on your patient. What are the steps in checking or managing this situation?

POST-TEST

1. Which of the following are local complications associated with I.V. therapy?
   a. Speed shock, septicemia, and venous spasm
   b. Phlebitis, venous spasm, and hematoma
   c. Septicemia, thrombophlebitis, and hematoma
   d. Phlebitis, pulmonary edema, and speed shock
2. Nurses can avoid a thrombosis formation by:
   a. Avoiding injury to the vein wall
   b. Avoiding multiple punctures
   c. Avoiding through-and-through punctures
   d. All of the above
3. A patient states that his I.V. site is sore. You assess the site and note redness and swelling but no signs of palpable cord or streak. Using the criteria for infusion phlebitis, what is the severity of this phlebitis?
   a. 3+
   b. 2+
   c. 1+
   d. 0
4. The highest risk factor for phlebitis is among patients who are:
   a. Immunosuppressed
   b. Neonates
   c. Receiving total parenteral nutrition
   d. Receiving medications through multiple lines
   e. All of the above
5. While a solution is infusing, which of the following is a treatment for venous spasm?
   a. Apply a cold pack to site
   b. Increase the flow rate of solution
   c. Apply a warm compress to site
   d. Administer pain medication
6. An air embolism can be caused by:
   a. A severed I.V. line
   b. I.V. administration set that is improperly primed
   c. Bypassing the pump housing
   d. All of the above
7. You check an infusion site on a patient and find swelling and cool skin temperature. Also, the patient's skin feels rigid with blanching, and the infusion rate has slowed. These are signs of:
   a. Phlebitis
   b. Catheter embolus
   c. Hematoma
   d. Infiltration
8. You are performing a venipuncture and an ecchymosis forms over and around the insertion area with a raised and hardening of area. You are unable to advance the cannula into the vein. These are signs of:
   a. Phlebitis

b. Infiltration
c. Hematoma
d. Occlusion

9. What is the one MOST important nursing intervention that is key to the prevention of many I.V.-related complications?
   a. Reading the policy and procedure manuals
   b. Handwashing procedures
   c. Using microdrip sets
   d. Competency testing
10. To prevent damage to the intima of the vein wall, which of the following syringe barrels should be used on a peripheral I.V. line?
   a. 1 mL or smaller
   b. 3 mL or smaller
   c. 3 mL or larger
   d. 10 mL or larger

REFERENCES

Bohony, J. (1993). 9 common I.V. complications and what to do about them. *American Journal of Nursing,* 93(10), 45–49.

Camp-Sorrell, D. (1998). Developing extravasation protocols and monitoring outcomes. *Journal of Intravenous Nursing,* 21(4), 232–241.

Centers for Disease Control and Prevention. (1996). *Guideline for Prevention of Intravascular Infections.* Atlanta: US Department of Health and Human Services.

Cohen, M.R. (1993). Recognizing the dangers of free flow. *Nursing 93,* 6, 56–59.

ECRI. (1992). Emergency Care Research Institute. *IV Free Flow Still a Cause For Alarm,* 21(9), 323–328.

Goetz, A.M., Miller, J., Wagener, M., & Muder, R. (1998). Complications related to intravenous midline catheter usage. *Journal of Intravenous Nursing,* 21(2), 76–80.

Guyton, A.C., & Hall, J.C. (1996). *Textbook of Medical Physiology* (9th ed). Philadelphia: W.B. Saunders.

Hadaway, L. (1998). Infiltration vs extravasation: Identification and interventions. Annual Conference Intravenous Nurses Society, May, 1998.

Hadaway, L. (1999). I.V. infiltration: Not just a peripheral problem. *Nursing 99,* 99(9), 41–47.

Hastings-Tolsma, M.T., Yucha, C.B., Tompkins, J., et al. (1993). Effect of warm and cold applications on the resolution of I.V. infiltrations. *Research in Nursing & Health,* 16, 171–178.

Intravenous Nursing Society. (2000). *Revised Standards of Practice.* Philadelphia: Lippincott, Williams & Wilkins.

Joint Commission on Accreditation of Health Care Perspective. (1995). *Joint commission perspectives: Interpretations: Limitations on hospital patient movement that constitute restraint.* Joint Commission on Accreditation of Health Care Organizations, 11–12, 15–16.

Josephson, D.L. (1999). *Intravenous Infusion Therapy for Nurses: Principles & Practice.* Albany: Delmar Publishers, 81–107.

Kuwahara, T., Asanami, S., Tamura , T., & Kaneda, S. (1998). Effects of pH and osmolality on phlebitic potential of infusion solutions for peripheral parenteral nutrition. *Journal of Toxicol Science,* 23(1), 77–85.

Maki D.G. & Mermel (1998). Infections due to infusion therapy. In Bennett, J.V., & Brachman, P.S. (eds.). *Hospital Infections* (3rd ed.) Philadelphia: Lippincott-Raven.

Maki, D.G., & Ringer, M. (1991). Risk factors for infusion-related phlebitis with small peripheral venous catheters. *Annals of Internal Medicine,* 114, 845–854.

Masoorli, S. (1997). Consult stat: Never assume anything when a patient IV infiltrates. *Nursing 97,* 60(7), 65.

Messner, R.L., & Pinkerman, M.L. (1993). Preventing a peripheral I.V. infection. *Nursing 93,* 6, 34–41.

Metheny, N.M. (1996). *Fluid and Electrolyte Balance: Nursing Considerations* (3rd ed.). Philadelphia: J.B. Lippincott.

Nightingale, F. (1859). *Notes on Nursing: What It Is, And What It Is Not.* London: Harrison, 59, Pall Mall, 59.

Perdue, M. (1995). Intravenous complications. In Terry, J., Baranowski, L., Hedrick, C., & Recker, D. (1992). Catheter-related sepsis: An analysis of the research. *Research Analysis,* 11 (5), 249–261.

Powers, F.A. (1999). Your elderly patient needs I.V, therapy: can you keep her safe? *Nursing 99,* 99(7), 54–55.

Richardson, D., & Bruso, P. (1993). Vascular access devices: Management of common complications. *Journal of Intravenous Nursing,* 16(1), 44–48.

Sanford, J.P., Gilbert, D.N., & Sande, M.A. (1996). *Guide to Antimicrobial Therapy* (26th ed). Dallas, TX: Antimicrobial Therapy, Inc.

Tipton, J.M., & Skeel, R.T. (1995). *Management of Acute Side Effects of Cancer Chemotherapy.*

Skeel, R.T., & Lachant, N.A. (eds.). *Handbook of Cancer Chemotherapy* (4th ed.). Boston: Little, Brown, 573–574.

Smeltzer, S.C., & Bare, B.G. (2000). *Brunner and Suddarth's Textbook of Medical-Surgical Nursing* (9th ed). Philadelphia: J.B. Lippincott.

United States Pharmacopeia (USP) (1995). *Drug Information for the Health Care Professional,* 15(1). Rockville, MD: United States Pharmacopedial Convention.

Weinstein, S. (1997). *Plumer's Principles and Practices of Intravenous Therapy* (6th ed.). Philadelphia: Lippincott.

Wenzel, R.P. (1993). *Prevention and Control of Nosocomial Infection* (2nd ed.). Baltimore: Williams & Wilkins, pp. 450–451.

White, K.M. (1997). Understanding the hemodynamics of sepsis. *Critical Care Choices,* 1997. Springhouse, PA: Springhouse Corp.

Wood, L.S. & Gullo, M. (1993). IV vesicants: How to avoid extravasation. *American Journal of Nursing,* 93(4), 42–45.

Yucha,C. (1993). Differences among intravenous extravasations using four common solutions. *Journal of Intravenous Nursing,* 16(5). 277–281.

Yucha, C. (1994). Effect of elevation on intravenous extravasations. *Journal of Intravenous Nursing,* 17(5), 231–234.

ANSWERS TO CHAPTER 8

Pre-Test

1. a, **2.** b, **3.** b, **4.** a, **5.** a, **6.** a, **7.** a, **8.** c, **9.** e, **10.** b, **11.** d

Post-Test

1. b, **2.** d, **3.** c, **4.** e, **5.** c, **6.** d, **7.** d, **8.** c, **9.** b, **10.** c

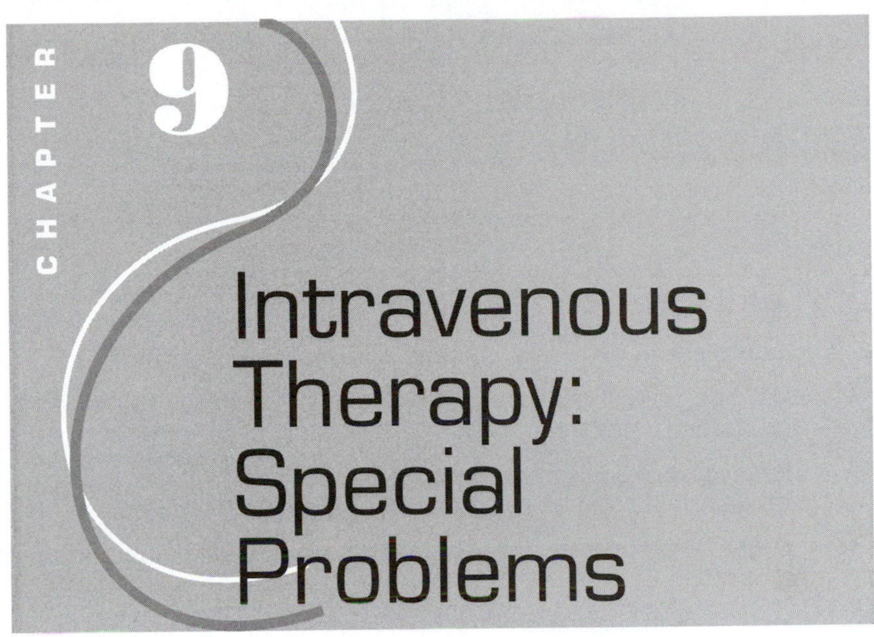

CHAPTER 9 Intravenous Therapy: Special Problems

Children are not little adults.

Virginia Turner, 1995

CHAPTER CONTENTS

LEARNING OBJECTIVES

Upon completion of this chapter, the reader will be able to:

1. Describe terms related to delivery of I.V. therapy to pediatric and geriatric patients.
2. Identify physiologic characteristics of neonates, infants, children, and geriatric patients related to their venous structure.
3. Locate common sites for venipuncture in pediatric and geriatric patients.
4. Identify common reasons for neonate and infant infusions.
5. List the formulas available for calculating the fluid needs of an infant.
6. Contrast the stages of development and fears through the life span as related to the performance of invasive procedures.
7. Identify the types of needles and catheters available for pediatric patients.
8. Describe special considerations for successful venipuncture of neonates, infants, and geriatric patients.
9. Describe the use of intraosseous infusions in pediatric patients.
10. Identify the complications related to intraosseous infusions.
11. List the risk factors associated with infusions in pediatric and geriatric patients.
12. Describe techniques for venipuncture in patients with sclerotic veins, alterations in skin integrity, obesity, and edema.

GLOSSARY

Body surface area Surface area of the body determined through use of a nomogram
Caloric method Calculation of metabolic expenditure of energy
Infant Child younger than age 2 years

Intraosseous infusion Infusion within the bone marrow cavity
Meter square method Use of a nomogram to determine surface areas of a patient
Neonate Infant in the period of extrauterine life up to the first 28 days after birth
Oncotic Tissue pressure within the tissue
Purpura Condition in which spontaneous bleeding occurs in the subcutaneous tissue, causing purple patches to appear on the skin
Tangential lighting Light touching a curve; indirect lighting
Weight method Formula based on weight in kilograms to estimate the fluid needs

PRE-TEST

1. Risk factors affecting the need for infusion therapy in neonates include:
   a. Prematurity
   b. Catabolic disease
   c. Hypothermia
   d. Acid–base imbalance
   e. All of the above
2. The three methods for assessment of 24-hour fluid needs in an infant are:
   a. Meter square, diaper weight, and urinary output
   b. Meter square, weight, and caloric methods
   c. Meter square, specific gravity, and head circumference
3. Common sites for venipuncture in infants younger than age 9 months include:
   a. Dorsum of the hand, dorsum of the foot, and scalp veins
   b. Dorsum of the foot, external jugular vein, and saphenous vein
   c. Dorsum of the hand, dorsum of the foot, and the external jugular vein
   d. Scalp veins, antecubital space, and external jugular vein
4. Intraosseous infusions are useful for:
   a. Emergency delivery of medication and fluids
   b. Long-term nutritional support
   c. Home antibiotic therapy
5. Complications of intraosseous infusions include all of the following **EXCEPT:**
   a. Osteomyelitis
   b. Cellulitis
   c. Damage to the epiphyseal plate
   d. Fractured humerus
6. Physiologic changes in geriatric patients that affect I.V. placement include:
   a. Arteriosclerosis
   b. Increased density and amount of collagen in the vessel walls
   c. Loss of subcutaneous fat
   d. Thinning of the skin
   e. All of the above
7. How many superficial veins in the infant's head are accessible for venipuncture?
   a. 1
   b. 2
   c. 4
   d. 6
8. To perform an I.V. infusion on a preschool child, the nurse should:
   a. Explain the procedure in simple terms
   b. Explain the procedure completely
   c. Restrain the child
   d. Provide reading materials to the child before performing the venipuncture

9. To perform a venipuncture on a toddler, it is helpful if the nurse:
    a. Provides pictures for the child to color during the procedure
    b. Provides a doll or stuffed animal in which to start the I.V. infusion before venipuncture
    c. Has assistance for the venipuncture
    d. Has the parents assist with the procedure
10. Tangential lighting should be used with patients who have:
    a. Alterations in skin surfaces
    b. Burned skin surfaces
    c. Edematous tissue
    d. Easily palpable and visible veins
11. The use of multiple tourniquets can be helpful with:
    a. Pediatric patients
    b. Frail geriatric patients
    c. Patients with sclerosed veins
    d. Patients with dark skin
12. Techniques to dilate a vein for venipuncture in an elderly person with fragile veins include all of the following **EXCEPT:**
    a. Apply the tourniquet loosely over the patient's sleeve
    b. Apply multiple tourniquets
    c. Use digital pressure to enhance vein filling
    d. Use warm compresses before venipuncture

Children, older adults, and persons with certain disorders can create challenges to the safe administration of I.V. therapy. Understanding these problems and ways to overcome them can help I.V. nurses ensure safe delivery with minimal risk to patients.

PEDIATRIC I.V. THERAPY

Intravenous therapy for pediatric patients requires special considerations to safeguard children. When assessing a child before administration, the practitioner must be aware of the body composition of an infant and the homeostatic differences between children and adults. In addition, the calculation of small doses, low infusion rates, and choice of appropriate venipuncture site and equipment need to be taken into consideration.

PHYSIOLOGIC CHARACTERISTICS

A **neonate** is a child in the period of extrauterine life up to the first 28 days after birth. Low-birth-weight and premature infants have decreased energy stores and increased metabolic needs compared with those of full-term, average-weight newborns.

A premature infant's body is made up of approximately 90 percent water; the newborn infant's is 70 to 80 percent, and the adult's is about 60 percent. **Infants** have proportionately more water in the extracellular compartment than do adults. Therefore, any depletion in these water stores may lead to dehydration. As an infant becomes older, the ratio of extracellular to intracellular fluid volume decreases.

Although infants have a relatively greater total body water content, this does not protect them from excessive fluid loss. Infants are more vulnerable to fluid volume deficit because they ingest and excrete a relatively greater daily volume of water than adults (Metheny, 1996). Any condition that interferes with normal water and electrolyte intake or that produces excessive water and electrolyte losses will produce a more rapid depletion of water and electrolyte stores in an infant than it will in an adult.

CULTURAL AND ETHNIC CONSIDERATIONS: NEWBORN INFANTS

Newborn body proportions differ among racial groups. It has been thought that newborn body proportions appear to be genetically programmed to conform to the pelvic shape of the mother (Giger & Davidhizar, 1999).

Illness, increased muscular activity, thermal stress, congenital abnormalities, and respiratory distress syndrome influence metabolic demands as well. The metabolic demand of an infant is two times higher per unit of weight than that of adults (Wong, 1998).

In most cases, 100 to 120 cal/kg/d maintains a normal infant and provides sufficient calories for growth. For high-risk infants who require increased handling for procedures, the calorie requirement is up to 100 percent higher than that of a normal newborn. Heat production increases calorie expenditure by 7 percent per degree of temperature elevation. Infants and young children cannot store protein as well as adults; therefore, preventive nutritional support is needed.

Young children have immature homeostatic regulating mechanisms that need to be considered when water and electrolyte replacement is needed. Renal functioning, acid–base balance, body surface area differences, and electrolyte concentrations all must be taken into consideration when planning fluid needs.

Newborns' renal functions are not yet completely developed. Infants' kidneys appear to become mature by the end of the neonatal period. An infant's kidneys have a limited concentrating ability and require more water to excrete a given amount of solutes. Infants are less likely to be able to regulate fluid intake and output.

The buffering capacity to regulate acid–base balance is lower in the newborn than in older children. Neonates, with an average pH of 7.0 to 7.38, are slightly more acidotic than adults. This base bicarbonate deficit is thought to be related to high metabolic acid production and to renal immaturity.

The integumentary system in neonates is an important route of fluid loss, especially in illness. This must be considered when determining fluid balance in infants and young children because their body surface area is greater than those of older children and adults. Any condition that produces a decrease in intake or output of water and electrolytes affects the body fluid stores of the infant. Because the gastrointestinal (GI) membranes are an extension of the body surface area, relatively greater losses occur from the GI tract in sick infants (Wong, 1998).

Plasma electrolyte concentrations do not vary strikingly among infants, small children, and adults. The plasma sodium concentration changes little from birth to adulthood. The potassium and chloride concentrations are higher in the first few months of life than at any other time.

Magnesium and calcium are both low in the first 24 hours after birth. The serum phosphate level is elevated in the early months of infancy, which contributes to a low calcium level. Newborn infants are vulnerable to disrupted calcium homeostasis when stressed by illness or by an excess phosphate load and are at risk for hypocalcemia (Metheny, 1996). Table 9–1 provides normal laboratory values in newborns.

CULTURAL AND ETHNIC CONSIDERATIONS: DECISION MAKING

In many cultures, women can express an option regarding the care of a child; however, many consider woman to be subservient to men; and the men (e.g., the husband or the eldest son) make all decisions. Be sure to be sensitive to lines of communication.

TABLE 9–1

NORMAL LABORATORY VALUES FOR CHILDREN

Laboratory Value	Neonate	Infant	2–5 years	6–12 years	Adolescent
Blood Count					
Red blood cells (million/μL)		2.7–5.4	4.27	4.31	4.60
Whole blood cells (per μL)		6000–17,000	5000–15,500	4500–13,500	4500–11,000
Platelet count (per μL)	84,000–479,000	150,000-400,000/mm all remaining ages			
Partial thromboplastin time and prothrombin time		<17 s		18–22 s	
Hemoglobin (g/dL)	14.5	9.0–14.0		11.5–15.5	Male 13–16 Female 12-16
Serum Electrolytes					
Sodium (mEq/L)		139–146	138–145		136–146
Potassium (mEq/L)		4.1–5.3		3.4–4.7	3.5–5.1
Magnesium (mEq/L)		1.4–1.9 . . . same for all ages			
Calcium (mg/dL)	7.5–11	8.8–10.8		8.4–10.8	
Chloride (mEq/L)			98–106 . . . same for all ages		
Phorphorus (mg/dL)	4.0–10.5		5.0–7.8		

PHYSICAL ASSESSMENT

A physical assessment should be performed on pediatric patients before I.V. therapy is begun. Table 9–2 presents the components of a pediatric assessment.

Risk factors that must be considered during the assessment phase include prematurity, catabolic disease state, hypothermia, hyperthermia, metabolic or respiratory alkalosis or acidosis, and other metabolic derangements.

Candidates for neonatal I.V. therapy include those with:

- Congenital cardiac disorders
- GI defects
- Neurologic defects

TABLE 9–2

COMPONENTS OF THE PEDIATRIC PHYSICAL ASSESSMENT

Measurement of head circumference (up to 1 year)
Height or length
Weight
Vital signs
Skin turgor
Presence of tears
Moistness and color of mucous membranes
Urinary output
Characteristics of fontanelles
Level of child's activity related to growth and development

Candidates for infant I.V. therapy include those with:

- Fluid volume deficit (dehydration)
- Electrolyte imbalance (diarrhea)
- Antibiotic therapy for treatment of serious infections
- Need for nutritional support for maintenance of growth and development
- Antineoplastic therapy for treatment of cancer

ASSESSMENT OF FLUID NEEDS

There are three methods for assessment of 24-hour maintenance of fluids: meter square, caloric, and weight.

Meter Square Method

A nomogram is used to determine the **body surface area (BSA)** of the patient in the **meter square method.** To use a nomogram in this method, draw a straight line between the point representing the patient's height on the left vertical scale to the point representing the patient's weight on the right vertical scale. The point at which the line intersects indicates the body surface area in square meters.

Advantages

- Provides calculation of body surface area to help determine the amount of fluid and electrolytes to be infused and assists with computing rate of infusion
- Helps to calculate adult and pediatric dosages of I.V. medications
- Is simple to calculate

Disadvantage

- Difficulty in accessibility to visual nomogram

To calculate the maintenance of fluid requirements, use the following:

Formula: 1500 mL/m^2 per 24 hours

Example
If child's surface area is $0.5m^2$, then 1500 mL × 0. 5 m^2 = 750 mL/24 hours.

Weight Method

The **weight method** uses the child's weight in kilograms to estimate fluid needs. This method uses 100 to 150 mL/kg for estimating maintenance fluid requirements and is most useful in children weighing less than 10 kg. (Use of the square meter method is recommended in children weighing more than 10 kg.)

Advantage

- Simple to use

Disadvantage

- Inaccurate in children who weigh more than 10 kg

Example
For a child weighing 10 kg, 100 × 10 kg = 1000 mL in 24 hours.

Caloric Method

The **caloric method** calculates the usual metabolic expenditure of fluid. It is based on the following metabolic expenditure:

- Child weighing 0 to 10 kg expends approximately 100 cal/kg/d.
- Child weighting 10 to 20 kg expends approximately 1000 calories plus 50 cal/kg for each kg over 10 kg.
- Child weighing 20 kg or more expends approximately 1500 calories, plus 20 cal/kg for each kg over 20 kg.

Advantage

- Simple to calculate

Disadvantage

- Not totally accurate unless actual calorie requirements and energy intake are continuously assessed

Formula:
The formula for calculating fluid requirement is
100 to 150 mL/100 calories metabolized.

Example

If the weight of the child is 30 kg and the child expends 1700 cal/d, fluid requirement is 1700 to 2550 mL/24 hours.

FACTORS AFFECTING FLUID NEEDS IN PEDIATRIC PATIENTS

The most common cause of increased fluid and calorie needs in children is temperature elevation. An increase in temperature of 1 degree increases a child's calorie needs by 12 percent. Fluid requirements of a child who is hypothermic decrease by 12 percent (Wong, 1998). In children, loss of GI fluids, ongoing diarrhea, and small intestinal drainage can seriously affect fluid balance.

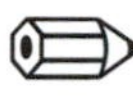

NOTES: To ensure the accuracy of fluid needs, most pediatric patients should be on strict intake and output monitoring, including diaper weighing.

When weighing an infant's diaper, consider the weight of the diaper before it was wet. The weight difference in a dry and a wet piece of linen represents the amount of liquid that it has absorbed. The weight of the fluid measured in grams is the same as the volume measured in milliliters (Wong, 1998).

SITE SELECTION

When selecting the venipuncture site, keep in mind that the main goal of I.V. therapy is to provide the treatment with safety and efficiency while meeting the child's emotional and developmental needs (Wheeler & Frey, 1995). Consider the following factors before selecting a site for venipuncture:

- Age of child
- Size of child
- Condition of veins
- Reason for therapy
- General patient condition
- Mobility and level of activity of child
- Gross and fine motor skills (e.g., sucks fingers, plays with hands, holds bottle, draws)
- Sense of body image
- Fear of mutilation
- Cognitive ability of the child (i.e., understands and follows directions) (Wheeler & Frey, 1995).

PERIPHERAL ROUTES

Peripheral routes for pediatric I.V. therapy include scalp veins and the veins in the dorsum of the hand, forearm, and foot (Fig. 9–1).

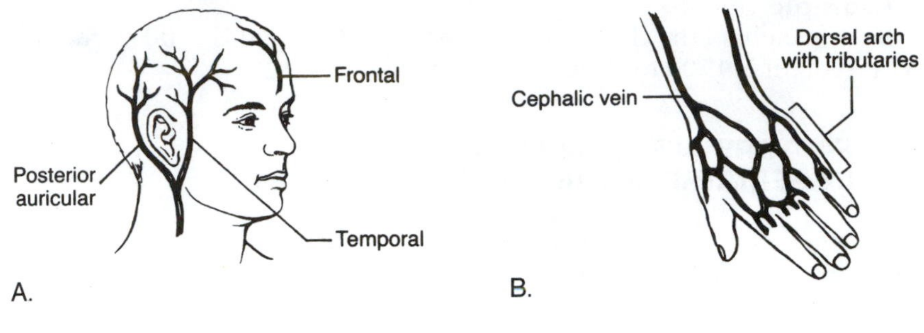

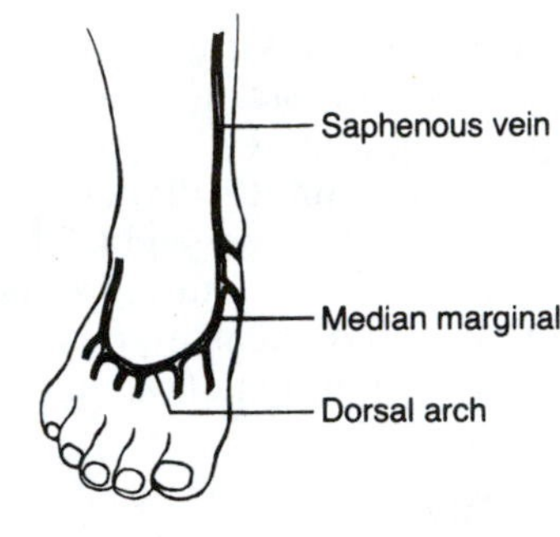

FIG. 9–1. Superficial veins of the scalp (*A*) and dorsum of hand (*B*) and foot (*C*). (From Kuhn, M.: *Pharmacotherapeutics: A Nursing Process Approach,* 4th ed. Philadelphia: F. A. Davis, with permission.)

Scalp Veins

The major superficial veins of the scalp can be used. Scalp veins can be used in children up to age 18 months; after that age, the hair follicles mature and the epidermis toughens. There are four scalp veins used most commonly for I.V. access: frontal (best access), preauricular, supraorbital, and occipital.

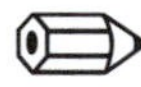 **NOTE:** The choice of scalp vein for placement of I.V. therapy is often traumatic for the parents because removal of hair may have cultural as well as religious significance. In addition, maintaining patency of this site can be difficult at times.

Advantages

- Easily visualized
- Readily dilates because it has no valves
- Hands kept free
- Head easily stabilizes

Disadvantages

- Shaving of hair
- Infiltrates easily
- Disfigurement with infiltration
- Difficult to secure device
- Increased family anxiety

The I.V. needle must be placed in the direction of blood flow to ensure that the I.V. fluid will flow in the same direction as that of the blood returning to the heart. In the scalp, venous blood generally flows from the top of the head down.

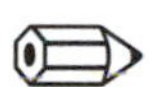

NOTES: A rubber band with a piece of tape attached can be used as a tourniquet (or pressure can be applied with the finger to distend the vein). Place the rubber band low on the forehead like a headband. It is also recommended that the rubber band be cut to decrease the chances of dislodging the I.V. after cannulation (Wheeler & Frey, 1995).

Shaving is not recommended; if necessary, clip the hair on infants.

CULTURAL AND ETHNIC CONSIDERATIONS: USING SCALP VEINS

People in the Hmong culture believe the spirit (soul) of the child can be released from the head. Be sure to check with an elder family member before choosing a site for venipuncture.

Dorsum of the Hand and Forearm

Because the veins over the metacarpal area are mobile and not well supported by surrounding tissue, the limb must be immobilized with a splint and tape before cannulation. This site can be used in all ages.

The antecubital fossa should not be routinely used because of the use of the antecubital area for blood drawing and the mobility problems resulting from use of this site. However, the antecubital area can be used for placement of peripherally inserted central catheters (PICCs).

Advantages

- Easily accessible
- Readily visible
- Large enough for a larger-gauge cannula
- Bones act as natural splints

Disadvantages

- Increased nerve endings
- Difficult to anchor cannula on infant
- Interferes with child's activity

Dorsum of the Foot

The foot is used as a venipuncture site for infants and toddlers but should be avoided in children who are walking. The curve of the foot, especially around the ankle, makes entry and cannula advancement difficult. The veins used are the saphenous, median, and marginal dorsal arch. Because neonates have very little subcutaneous adipose tissue, the veins are easily identified and cannulated just beneath the skin.

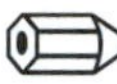

NOTE: The foot should be secured on a padded board with a normal joint position.

Advantages

- Readily dilates
- Hands kept free
- Less rolling of vein
- Increased visibility in chubby infants
- Easy to splint

Disadvantages

- Decreased mobility in walking
- Limited to smaller-gauge cannulas
- Located near arteries
- Difficult to advance cannula

SELECTING THE EQUIPMENT

A nurse must be aware of the special needs of pediatric patients when selecting appropriate equipment for administering fluids and medication. When choosing administration equipment, the safety of the child requires that the activity level, age, and size of the patient be considered. For safe delivery of I.V. therapy in pediatric patients, the following equipment is recommended:

- An electronic infusion device for administration of therapy.
- The volume of solution container used should be based on the age, height, and weight of the patient and should contain no more than 500 mL of fluid (preferably 250 mL).
- Special pediatric equipment, such as volume control chamber for the delivery of therapy.
- Plastic fluid containers (preferable to glass because of possible breakage).
- Microdrip tubing (60 drops/min).
- Monitoring at least every 2 hours and more frequently, depending on patient's age and size or type of therapy.

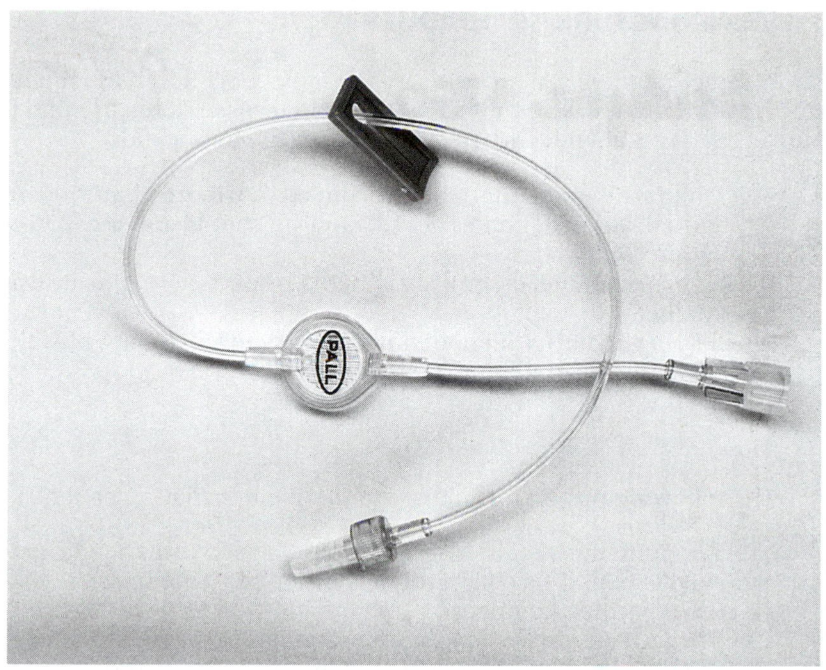

FIG. 9–2. Neonatal and infant 0.2-micron air-eliminating filter set. (Courtesy of Pall Corporation, Port Washington, New York.)

- Visible cannula site.
- A 0.2-micron air-eliminating filter set (Fig. 9–2) is available for neonates and infants to provide 96-hour bacterial and associated endotoxin retention for patient protection.

NEEDLE SELECTION

The choice of needle depends on the site selected. Peripheral cannulas, gauges 26 to 21, can be used in children. A 27- to 19-gauge scalp vein (butterfly) needle is easy to insert but has the risk of infiltrating easily. The scalp vein needle has been replaced by more contemporary types of peripheral venous access devices.

Over-the-needle catheters, 26- to 14-gauge, are now used more frequently than metal needles. For neonates, 26- to 24-gauge needles are used; for children, 24- to 22-gauge are most common. Over-the-needle cannulas usually last longer than scalp vein needles These catheters are also easier to stabilize.

VENIPUNCTURE TECHNIQUES

The methods for venipuncture are the same for children as for adults (see Chapter 7); a direct or indirect method can be used. Keep in mind the following safety guidelines when setting up an I.V. for a child.

- A child's I.V. container should contain no more than 500 mL. Children younger than age 12 months should have a 250-mL solution container.
- Obtain a volume control chamber. Connect it to the infusion container.
- Fill the cylinder with enough fluid to prime the tubing plus fluid for a *maximum* of 2 hours (Josephson, 1999).

Tips

The following tips on technique are unique to pediatric patients:

1. Venipuncture should be performed in a room separate from the child's room. The child's room is his or her "safe space."
2. Use a pacifier for neonates and infants.
3. Use mummy and clove-hitch immobilizers as needed. Infants should be covered with a blanket to minimize cold stress. If the dorsum of the hand is used, place the extremity on an armboard before venipuncture.
4. A flashlight or transilluminator device placed beneath the extremity helps to illuminate tissue surrounding the vein; the veins are then outlined for better visualization (Wheeler & Frey, 1995).
5. Warm hands by washing them in hot water before gloving.
6. Omit tourniquet use if possible. Use a rubber band to dilate scalp veins.
7. Use a saline-filled syringe with a scalp vein infusion device.
8. Minimizing pain during venipuncture is a goal of nursing care. Two commonly used methods are the use of a topical cream (EMLA or Numby Stuff) or the use of ethyl chloride spray (an assistant is needed to spray) (Harvey, 1998).
9. Flush the needle immediately with saline when a backflow of blood occurs.
10. Use surgical lubricating jelly to help secure the tape around a scalp I.V. by applying a small amount under the tape.
11. Use only hypoallergenic or paper tape. When you are ready to remove the tape, apply warm water; the tape will then lift off easily (Wheeler & Frey, 1995).
12. Stabilize the cannula with a padded tongue blade. Collect laboratory specimens at the time of I.V. insertion.
13. Use colored stickers or drawings on the I.V. site as a reward.
14. Always have extra help.

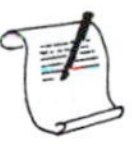

INS STANDARDS The site selected should be readily visible and roller bandages should never be used around the cannula site. (INS, 2000, 49)

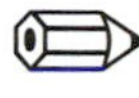

NOTES: When securing a child's extremity to an armboard, use clear tape for visualization of the I.V. site and digits or skin immediately adjacent to the site.

Use of a paper cup to cover the infusion site on the scalp is not recommended. A clear medicine cup can offer the needed protection.

Stabilizing and maintaining the patency of I.V. cannula sites can be a challenge. Poorly secured I.V. access sites may result in dislodgements or infiltrations requiring I.V. restarts. Some commercial products are available to help protect I.V. sites. For example, the Bubbles and Boards System (Acme United Corporation) is a three-piece system designed to meet the needs for I.V. cannula protection, site visibility, limb stabilization, and maintenance of skin integrity (Stifter & Shanahan, 1994). The I.V. House (Progressive IVs, Inc.) is a one-piece unit that protects any I.V. site (Fig. 9–3).

For children, illness and hospitalization constitute major life crises. Children are vulnerable to the crises of illness and hospitalization because stress represents a change from the usual state of health and environmental routine and because children have a limited number of coping mechanisms to resolve the stressful events.

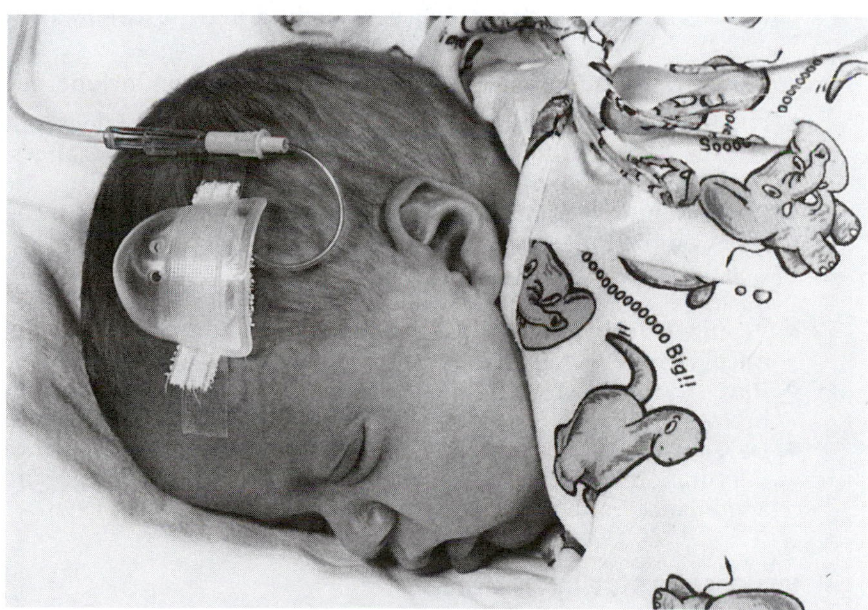

FIG. 9–3. Protection of the I.V. site by one-piece IV House. Courtesy of Progressive IVs, Inc., Hazelwood, Missouri.

Children's understanding of, reaction to, and methods of coping with illness or hospitalization are influenced by the significance of individual stressors during each developmental phase. The major stressors are separation, loss of control, and bodily injury. Table 9–3 summarizes the principal behavioral responses to each stressor as related to the function of I.V. therapy.

MEDICATION ADMINISTRATION

Delivering medication to children requires that the nurse have expert knowledge of the techniques for the delivery of medication and for the calculation of formulas. The most common methods of calculation are covered in the beginning of this chapter: body weight and body surface area are most frequently used. Dosages of pediatric medications are usually recommended in terms of body weight. The dose and volume can be different in children, and drugs are frequently calculated to the tenth of a milligram or milliliter (Wheeler & Frey, 1995).

INS STANDARDS Most infusion complications in pediatric patients are attributed to dosing, fluid administration, or both. A nurse administering infusion therapy to pediatric patients must posses the knowledge necessary to verify, calculate, administer, and accurately control the rate of the prescribed therapy.

Consideration should be given to the use of smaller volume containers in infants and premature infants because of complications of fluid volume overload and special pediatric equipment for the delivery of therapy. (INS, 2000, 2)

Prevention strategies for delivering medication to children include:

- Purchase and use scales that only measure weight in kilograms.
- Have a method (flow sheets) of documenting weight changes. Include weight changes in shift reports.
- Perform annual competency checks on weighing children using scales on the unit.
- Collaborate with biomedical engineers regarding the frequency of quality assurance and calibration checks of scales.
- Require nurses to verify accuracy in dose recommendations and calculations on original drug and I.V. fluid prescription forms.
- Have available a current medication manual that provides necessary information for safe administration of I.V. medications.
- Develop charts of frequently used drugs that provide practical information of medication concentrations, drug dosing, and administration requirements. Post the charts (Kennedy, 1996).

INTERMITTENT INFUSIONS

The in-line calibrated chamber is commonly used in the general pediatric setting. The medication is injected into the in-line chamber and infused at a prescribed rate.

TABLE 9–3

NURSING INTERVENTIONS FOR THE CHILD REQUIRING I.V. THERAPY AS RELATED TO PHYSICAL AND PSYCHOLOGICAL DEVELOPMENT

Age	Development/ Stressor	Behavior	Intervention
Infant	Trust versus mistrust *Stressor:* Pain	Cries, screams, clings in protest Neonate: easily distracted—total body reaction Infant: localized reaction; often uncooperative	Consistency in assigning caregivers Encourage parents to assist with care Explain I.V. to parents Have assistance starting I.V.
Toddler	Autonomy versus shame and doubt *Stressor:* Loss of control Physical restriction Loss of routine and rituals Bodily injury and pain	Protests verbally Cries for parents Kicks, bites, tries to escape to find parents Resists Verbally unco-operative	Allow to express feelings Encourage parental help Allow as much mobility as possible in securing I.V. Encourage pres-ence of favorite toy or blanket during procedure Use comfort after procedure
Preschool	Initiative versus guilt *Stressor:* Loss of control Sense of own power Bodily injury—intrusive proce-dure, mutilations	Protests less directly Anxiety, guilt, shame, physio-logic responses Immature behavior	Allow child to express protest Provide play and diversional activity Encourage to play out feelings and fears Allow as much mobility as possible; limit invasive procedures Explain procedure in simple terms; start pretend I.V. on doll

(Continued)

TABLE 9–3

NURSING INTERVENTIONS FOR THE CHILD REQUIRING I.V. THERAPY AS RELATED TO PHYSICAL AND PSYCHOLOGICAL DEVELOPMENT *(Continued)*

Age	Development/ Stressor	Behavior	Intervention
School-age	Industry versus inferiority *Stressor:* Loss of control Enforced dependency Altered family roles Bodily injury and pain Illness and death—intrusive procedures in genital area	Loneliness, boredom, isolation, hostility, and frustration Depression and displaced anger Seeks information Passively accepts Communicates about pain	Allow to express feelings both verbally and nonverbally Involve in starting I.V. by tearing tape or holding tubing Encourage peer contacts Use diversional activities
Adolescent	Identity versus role diffusion *Stressor:* Loss of control Loss of identity Enforced dependency Bodily injury and mutiliation	Rejection Uncooperativeness Self-assertion Overconfidence Boredom	Explore feelings regarding hospitalization Help to adjust to authority Explain all procedures Allow choices in sites Provide privacy

Source: From Wong, D.L. (1997). *Whaley and Wong's Essentials of Pediatric Nursing,* 5th ed. St. Louis: Mosby, Inc. Reprinted with permission.

Advantage

- Simplicity

Disadvantages

- Not practical for small infants
- Necessity of drug compatibility with primary solution or requirement of a second tubing setup
- Flushing of the chamber with a certain volume is insufficient to clear the chamber of medication

RETROGRADE INFUSION

Retrograde infusion is used in the general pediatric area and neonatal intensive care units and often in infants or children who cannot tolerate rapid infusion rates or additional fluid volume. A specific retrograde administration set is required for this purpose. The tubing volume varies but generally holds less than 1 mL. A three-way stopcock or access port is at each end of the tubing. To use retrograde infusion, follow these steps:

1. Attach the retrograde tubing and prime along with the primary administration set. The tubing functions as an extension set when it is not used to administer medication.
2. To administer the medication, attach a medication-filled syringe to the port proximal to the patient and connect an empty syringe to the port most distal from the patient.
3. Make sure the clamp between the port and the child is closed and then inject the medication distally up the tubing. The fluid in the retrograde tubing is displaced upward into the tubing and the empty syringe.
4. Remove both syringes and open the lower clamp. The medication is then infused into the patient at the prescribed rate.

SYRINGE PUMP

Using syringe pumps is an increasingly popular and accurate method of delivery of I.V. medications in children. They can be connected by an extension set into a primary line. (See Chapter 6 for information on syringe pumps.)

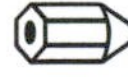

NOTE: Parenteral nutrition and transfusion therapy are also frequently administered to the pediatric client; special considerations for the delivery of blood products and parenteral nutrition are discussed in Chapters 12 and 14.

FORMULAS FOR DELIVERY OF PEDIATRIC THERAPIES

The following are formulas used in calculating the delivery of pediatric therapies.

Body Weight

Doses of drugs based on kilograms of body weight require that nurses use the weight (in kg) of the child in dosage administration (1 kg = 2.2 lb). Many drugs are ordered as milligram per kilogram of body weight. Multiply the milligrams of the drug by the kilograms of body weight.

$$\text{mg of drug} \times \text{kg of child's body weight} = \text{Child's dose}$$

Body Surface Area (BSA)

Doses of drugs based on BSA are determined by multiplying the child's BSA (m^2) times the recommended adult dose, divided by the adult's BSA (1. 73 m^2).

$$\frac{\text{BSA of child } (m^2) \times \text{Recommended adult dose}}{\text{BSA of adult } (1.73\ m^2)} = \text{Child's dose}$$

Bastedo's Rule

This rule determines the child's dose based on the child's age plus 3, times the average adult dose, divided by 30.

$$\frac{\text{Age (years)} + 3 \times \text{Average adult dose}}{30} = \text{Child's dose}$$

Clark's Rule

This rule determines the child's dose based on the child's weight in relation to the average adult body weight and dose.

$$\frac{\text{Weight (lb)} \times \text{Average adult dose}}{(\text{Average adult weight} = 150\text{ lb})} = \text{Child's dose}$$

Cowling's rule

This rule determines the child's dose based on the child's age and the average adult dose, divided by 24.

$$\frac{\text{Age (years on next birthday)} \times \text{Average adult dose}}{24} = \text{Child's dose}$$

Fried's Rule

This rule determines the infant's dose based on the infant's age in relation to the average adult body weight and dose.

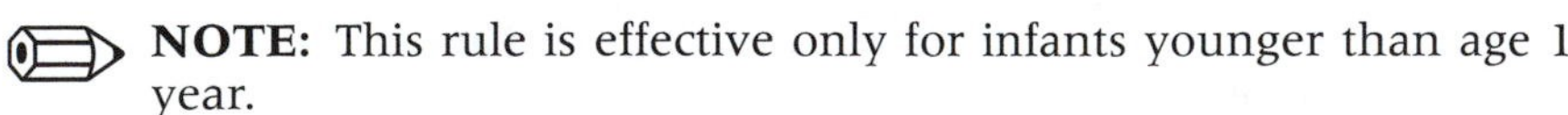

NOTE: This rule is effective only for infants younger than age 1 year.

Young's Rule

This rule determines the child's dose based on the child's age and average adult dose, divided by the child's age plus 12.

$$\frac{\text{Age in years} \times \text{Average adult dose}}{\text{Age (in years)} + 12} = \text{Child's dose}$$

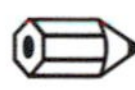 **NOTE:** Using a calculator is advisable for all pediatric doses; **always** double-check calculations with another licensed nurse (Henke, 1999).

ALTERNATIVE ADMINISTRATION ROUTES

Alternative routes for administration of I.V. therapy in pediatric patients are intraosseous and umbilical veins and arteries.

Intraosseous Route

The intraosseous route is a safe alternative for fluid and drug administration in infants and children. From 1940 to 1950, the **intraosseous infusion** for both adults and children was widely used. By the late 1950s, it was replaced by plastic catheters and newer infusion techniques.

The revised standards and guidelines outlined in the *Textbook of Pediatric Advanced Life Support* by the American Heart Association (1998) recognized intraosseous infusion as an effective route for the administration of emergency medications or fluids to children younger than age 6 years. These guidelines further emphasize the importance of establishing and maintaining an infusion route during the resuscitation of critically ill children.

Intraosseous infusion uses the rich vascular network of the long bones to transport fluids and medications from the medullary cavity to the circulation. The medullary cavity is composed of a spongy network of venous sinusoids that drain into a central venous canal. Blood exits the venous canal by the nutrient and emissary veins into the circulation. Fluids infused into the medullary space diffuse a short space and then are absorbed into the venous circulation; the distribution is similar to that in I.V. injection (Fig. 9–4).

Advantages

- Provides quick access in emergency cases when life-sustaining medication must be administered
- In patients with difficult venous access, provides alternative access for delivery of volume resuscitation
- Useful in patients with cardiac arrest, shock, trauma, or any situation in which the potential benefits of rapid venous access outweigh the low incidence of complications

Disadvantages

- Potential for osteomyelitis (low incidence reported).
- Potential for cellulitis; however, studies have reported only a 0.6 percent incidence of cellulitis.
- Potential damage to the epiphyseal plate.

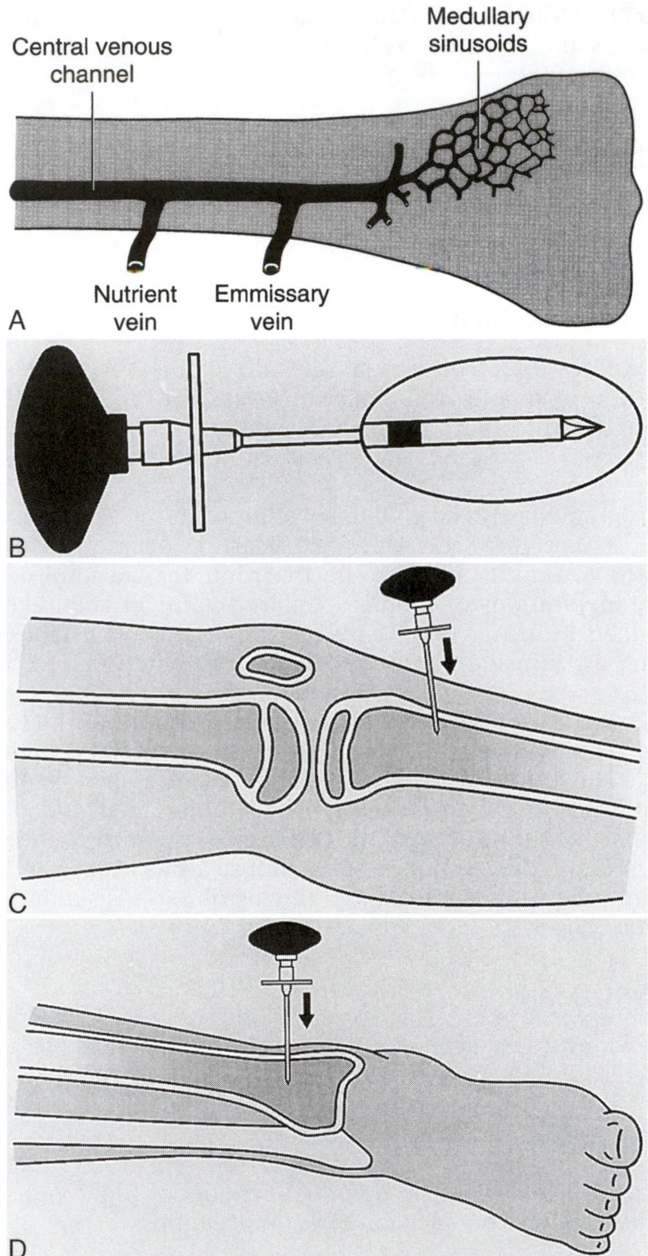

FIG. 9–4. Intraosseous infusion. (*A*) Intramedullary venous system. (From Spivey, W.H., [1987]. Intraosseous Infusions, *Journal of Pediatrics 111,* 639. Used with permission.) (*B*) Intraosseous needle, (*C*) placement of intraosseous needle in proximal tibia, (*D*) placement of intraosseous needle in distal tibia. (Courtesy of Cook Critical Care. Ellettsville, Indiana.)

- Potential embolus caused by fat dislodged from the marrow cavity is (Josephson, 1999).

Intraosseous Insertion Technique

The appropriate sites for intraosseous infusion are the distal tibia, the proximal tibia, and the distal femur. The distal tibia is used most frequently because of the flat area proximal to the malleolus and the thin covering of bony cortex (Wheeler & Frey, 1995).

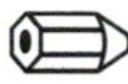 **NOTE:** This method of infusion should be used only in children younger than age 6 years.

PROCEDURE 9–1: INTRAOSSEOUS INSERTION

Equipment Needed

- Povidone-iodine solution (Betadine)
- Jamshidi Bone Marrow Biopsy Needle or 16- or 19-gauge straight-gauge needle with stylet, short shaft, and sturdy handle
- Commercially prepared disposable intraosseous infusion needle
- One 10-mL syringe filled with saline
- Fluid and medications to be administered with administration set
- Tape or Elastoplast

Instructions to Patient

- Explain procedure and location of intraosseous needle to child's parents. Explain that procedure is limited in time until venous access can be established by another route. Verify parents' understanding of explanations.

Procedure

- Prepare the child's skin using the povidone-iodine solution.
- Wear gloves, mask, gown, and goggles.
- Select the site.
- Use local anesthesia, 1 percent lidocaine hydrochloride, if the patient is awake and alert.
- Access the anteromedial tibia, 1 to 2 cm below the tibial tuberosity. (Using the sternum in children is discouraged because it is too thin and poorly developed to guarantee safe placement.)
- Insert the needle at a 90-degree angle to the bone. A twisting or boring motion is used until penetration through the cortex is achieved. Placement is confirmed by feeling the needle "pop" as it advances into the marrow, aspirating marrow into the needle, or visualizing free flow of fluid through the needle.
- Remove the stylet.
- Infuse saline by the syringe to clear the needle of marrow, as well as to check for placement.

(continued)

(continued)

- Start infusion of fluid or medications under gravity pressure.
- Apply a sterile dressing.
- Regulate infusion.

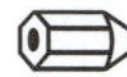

NOTE: The following guidelines should be used to ensure that the needle is in the bone marrow cavity:

1. The needle remains erect without support.
2. Bone marrow is aspirated (although its absence does not mean incorrect placement).
3. I.V. fluid flows easily without signs of infiltration.

Documentation

- Chart the site, needle type and size, type of fluid and medication, and patient response to the treatment. (Smith, 1998).

INS STANDARDS This access route shall only be performed as an emergency, short-term procedure when vascular access by the I.V. route cannot be achieved.

Intraosseous needles shall be removed within 24 hours. Intraosseous ports are removed within 30 days or immediately if complications develop. (INS, 2000, 68)

Contraindications

Patients who have areas of cellulitis or infected burns or those with recently fractured bones should not undergo intraosseous infusion. Patients with osteogenesis imperfecta or osteoporosis are not good candidates for this route (Smith, 1998).

Nursing Management

The nursing staff is responsible for managing the site and assessment, administration of the fluid or medication, proper use of I.V. equipment, and documentation.

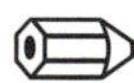

NOTE: After the needle is removed, a sterile gauze pad should be placed over the puncture site and direct pressure applied. The site should be inspected daily and redressed. If no drainage is seen after 48 hours, the dressing may be removed (Wheeler, 1989).

UMBILICAL VEIN AND ARTERIES

There are three vessels in the umbilical cord: one vein and two arteries. These vessels provide alternative routes for vascular access in neonates. These routes are reserved for emergency access in the delivery room and for hemodynamic monitoring in the neonatal intensive care unit.

The goals of arterial catheterization are different from those of venous catheterization. The main goals of arterial umbilical catheterization are:

- Monitoring arterial pressure
- Obtaining blood samples for arterial pH and blood gases
- Performing aortography
- Performing exchange transfusions

The vein of the umbilicus can be catheterized up to 4 days of life. However, it is usually inserted in the delivery room in a compromised infant. The goals of venous catheterization include:

- Administering emergency medications and fluids
- Obtaining venous blood sampling
- Performing exchange transfusion (Wheeler & Frey, 1995)

There is a risk of vascular compromise, hemorrhage, air embolism, infection, thrombosis, and vascular perforation with umbilical catheterization. The risk of infection is greater with the venous catheter and becomes a significant risk after 24 hours. The umbilical venous catheter is removed as soon as an alternative access route has been established (usually within 48 to 72 hours).

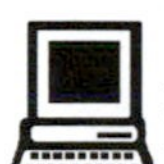

WEB SITES:
Society of Pediatric Nurses: *www.pednurse.org*
American Academy of Pediatrics: *www.aap.org*
Intravenous Nurses Society: *www.ins1.org*
Transcultural Nursing Society: *www.tcns.org*
Other sites:____

GERIATRIC I.V. THERAPY

The older population, 33.9 million in 1996, represents about one in every eight Americans. The older population itself is getting older. In 1996, the 65- to 74-year-old age group was eight times larger than in 1900, the 75- to 84-year-old age group was 16 times larger, and the 85 years of age and older group was 31 times larger (Smeltzer & Bare, 2000). Healthcare practitioners need a heightened awareness and understanding of the special needs of elderly patients.

PHYSIOLOGIC CHANGES

Aging occurs on all levels of bodily function: cellular, organic, and systemic. "Loss of cells and loss of physiologic reserve make up the dominant processes of aging" (Smeltzer & Bare, 2000). The major system changes the nurse must be aware of related to infusion therapy are homeostatic changes, immune system and cardiovascular changes, and skin and connective tissue changes.

Homeostasis is the body's ability to maintain a stable internal environment. As a person ages, his or her homeostatic mechanism become less efficient, and reserve power is lost. For example, when external stressors such as trauma or infection occur, there is minimal reserve capacity. This creates a situation in which the person is more vulnerable to disease.

Two immune processes change with aging:

1. The immune system becomes hyporesponsive to foreign antigens (e.g., decreased numbers of circulating lymphocytes and cells have fewer receptors to decrease ability to generate energy).
2. The immune system becomes hyperresponsive to itself.

Cardiovascular changes related to arteriosclerosis become clinically recognizable. With aging, three functions of the heart are affected: (1) the ability to oxygenate the cardiac muscle decreases, (2) diastolic filling decreases, and (3) left ventricular wall thickness increases. Arteries show progressive chemical and anatomic changes, with an increase in cholesterol, other lipids, and calcium. The intima increases, which increases resistance and decreases compliance of veins and arteries. The elastic fibers progressively straighten, fray, split, and fragment. There is an increase in density and amount of collagen fibers in the vessel walls, along with decreasing elasticity of these walls.

The skin is one of the first systems to show signs of the aging process. The epidermis and dermis are visible markers of aging and greatly affect the placement of peripheral catheters. As a person ages, a loss of subcutaneous supporting tissue and resultant thinning of the skin occur. The turnover rate for the production of new cells slows: at the age of 20 years, turnover of new cells takes 3 weeks; at age 30 years, 6 weeks; and after age 30 years, 2 months. Folds, lines, wrinkles, and slackness appear as the skin ages. **Purpura** and ecchymoses may appear owing to the greater fragility of the dermal and subcutaneous vessels and the loss of support for the skin capillaries. Minor trauma can easily cause bruising.

A common symptom in older people is pruritus or "itchiness." This is usually caused by dry skin and by medications and should be considered when preparing for parenteral therapy.

NOTE: Alcohol as a preparatory aid will add to the drying effect of the skin (Whitson, 1996).

The dermis becomes relatively dehydrated and loses strength and elasticity. This layer has underlying papillae that hold the epidermis and dermis together; this means that as one ages, the older skin loosens. Older skin has decreased flexibility in the collagen fibers, increased fragility of the capillaries, and fewer capillaries. Older skin feels dryer because of loss of subcutaneous fat and decreased production of sebum and sweat (Smeltzer & Bare, 2000).

FLUID BALANCE IN ELDERLY PERSONS

Fluid balance in elderly persons is affected by the physiologic changes associated with aging. Older people do not possess the fluid reserves of younger individuals or the ability to adapt readily to rapid changes. Alterations in fluid and electrolyte balance frequently accompany illness.

Renal structural changes associated with the aging process result in a decreased glomerular filtration rate. When fluid is restricted for any reason, nurses must be aware that there will be a slower conservation of fluids in response to the fluid restriction.

The total body water is reduced by 6 percent, which creates a potential for fluid volume deficit. GI changes such as decreased volumes of saliva and gastric juice as well as calcium absorption cause the mouth to be drier in the aged, in addition to the potential for sodium and potassium deficit during episodes of vomiting and gastric suction, and calcium deficit.

Cardiovascular and respiratory changes combine to contribute to a slower response to the stress of blood loss, fluid depletion, shock, and acid–base imbalances (Metheny, 1996). Elderly patients should be assessed for potential fluid volume disturbances (Table 9–4).

Careful assessment and monitoring of elderly patients for complications related to infusion therapy can help avoid systemic complications. Monitor electrolyte, blood urea nitrogen (BUN), and creatinine levels throughout therapy. Assess regularly signs and symptoms of fluid overload: distended neck veins, full bounding pulse, elevated blood pressure, and moist crackles. Weigh the patient daily (Powers, 1999).

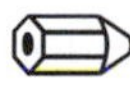

NOTES: Dextrose administered without a pump to elderly patients can lead to cerebral edema more rapidly than in younger patients.

Many elderly patients take digoxin for cardiac problems. Be

TABLE 9–4

ASSESSMENT GUIDELINES FOR FLUID VOLUME DISTURBANCES IN THE ELDERLY

Skin turgor of forehead or sternum
Temperature (normal body temperature often below 98.6°F)
Rate and filling of veins in hand or foot
Daily weight possibly a more accurate measure of patient's fluid balance
Intake and output
Tongue—center should be moist, with observable pool of saliva beneath the tongue (even though the aged have decreased saliva, this method is useful in evaluating hydration)
Orthostatic (postural) blood pressure changes
Swallowing ability
Functional assessment of patient's ability to obtain fluids

careful with administering fluids that do not contain potassium over a lengthy period of time to elderly patients. Hypokalemia can potentiate the action of digitalis glycosides, causing toxicity.

VENIPUNCTURE TECHNIQUES

Elderly patients require special venipuncture techniques to successfully place and maintain I.V. therapy. The potential complications associated with trauma, surgery, and illness in elderly people, along with the physiologic changes mentioned previously, require that nurses be knowledgeable in the special skills associated with delivery of care.

INS STANDARDS Geriatric patients may be at greater risk for potential complications related to infusion therapy and may require more frequent monitoring. (INS, 2000, 13)

VASCULAR ACCESS DEVICE SELECTION

Consider the skin and vein changes of older adults before initiating I.V. therapies. Also, consider catheter design and gauge size. Softer, more flexible materials and those that soften after insertion into the vein may allow increased indwelling time and prevent or reduce complications. The bevel-tip design of the peripheral catheter's needle may help to decrease trauma to vein.

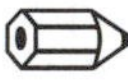

NOTE: Use of a 22- to 24-gauge catheter is appropriate for delivery of I.V. therapy in elderly patients. These sizes help reduce insertion-related trauma (Fabian, 1995).

SELECTING ADMINISTRATION EQUIPMENT

Because of the risk of overadministration or underadministration of I.V. therapy, the type of infusion equipment selected should provide safe, consistent delivery of medication and fluids. Advanced technology provides uses of stationary and ambulatory electronic monitoring devices. Monitoring devices must have safety features to protect high-risk patients from fluid volume overload.

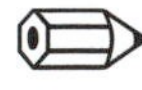

NOTES: To prevent fluid overload, use a microdrip administration set when appropriate.

Because of the fragile nature of the veins of elderly patients, be aware of the potential complications associated with pressures generated from mechanical infusion devices (see Chapter 6 for a discussion of safety features associated with programmable pumps).

SELECTING A VEIN

Selecting a vein that can support I.V. therapy for at least 72 hours can be a challenge for nurses. Initial venipuncture should be in the most distal portion of the extremity, allowing for subsequent venipunctures to move progressively upward. However, in older adults, the veins of the hands may not be the best choice for the initial site because of the loss of subcutaneous fat and thinning of the skin. Physiologic changes in the skin and veins must be considered when a site is selected. Areas for I.V. access should have adequate tissue and skeletal support. Avoid flexion areas and areas with bruising because the oncotic pressure is increased in these areas and causes vessels to collapse.

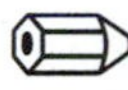

NOTE: To enhance vein location, use adequate lighting. Bright, direct overhead examination lights may have a "washout" effect on veins. Instead, use side lighting, which can add contour and "shadowing" to highlight the skin color and texture and allow visualization of the vein shadow below the skin.

Use a tourniquet to help distend and locate appropriate veins but avoid applying it too tightly because it can cause vein damage when the vein is punctured. During venous distention, palpate the vein to determine its condition. Veins that feel ribbed or rippled may distend readily when a tourniquet is applied, but these sites are often impossible to access, causing pain for the patient (Fabian, 1995).

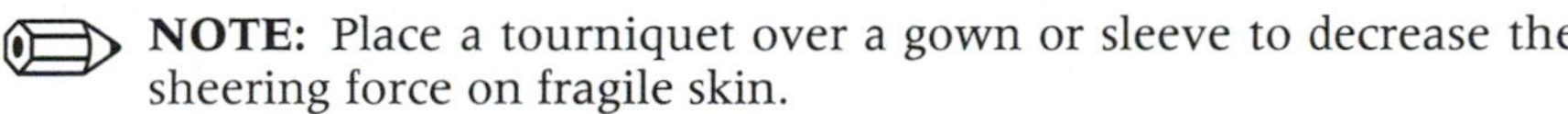

NOTE: Place a tourniquet over a gown or sleeve to decrease the sheering force on fragile skin.

Valves become stiff and less effective with age. Bumps along the vein path (i.e., valves) may cause problems during attempts at vein access. Venous circulation may be sluggish, resulting in slow venous return, distention, venous stasis, and dependent edema. A catheter may not thread into a vein with stiff valves.

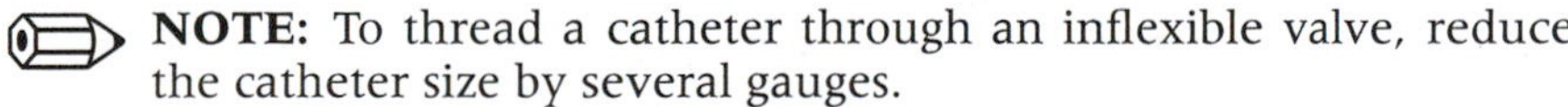

NOTE: To thread a catheter through an inflexible valve, reduce the catheter size by several gauges.

Small surface veins appear as thin tortuous veins with many bifurcations (Fig. 9–5). Appropriate catheter gauge and length selection is critical to successful I.V. access placement in these veins.

CANNULATION TECHNIQUES

In elderly patients, stabilization of the vein is critical. The vessels may lack stability as a result of the loss of tissue mass and may tend to roll. Techniques to perform a venipuncture in elderly patients include:

1. Use of traction by placing the thumb directly along the vein axis about 2 to 3 inches below the intended venipuncture site. The

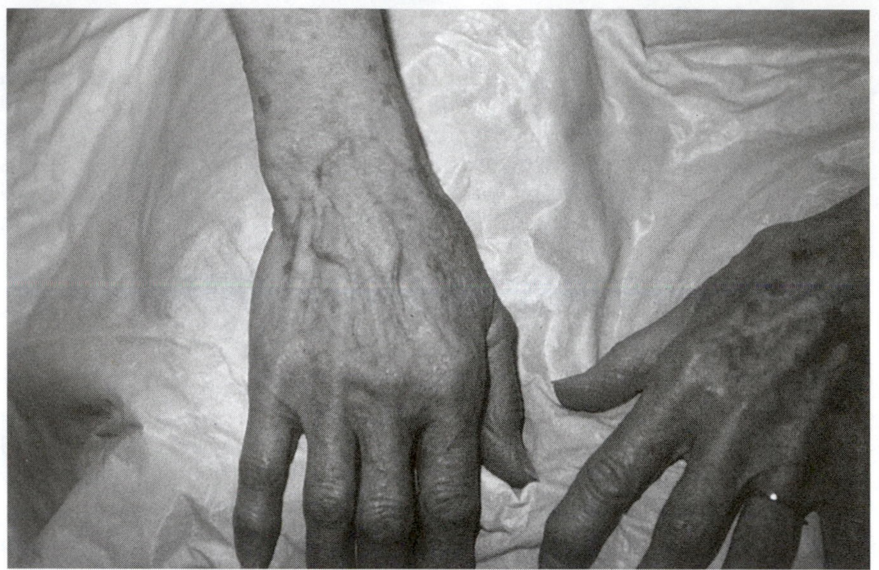

FIG. 9–5. Fragile veins of the elderly patient.

palm and fingers of the traction hand serve to hold and stabilize the extremity. Using the index finger of the hand, provide traction to further stretch the skin above the intended venipuncture site. Maintain traction throughout venipuncture.

2. Insert the catheter, using either the direct or indirect technique. When the direct technique is used, insert the catheter at a 20- to 30-degree angle in a single motion, penetrating the skin and vein simultaneously. Do not stab or thrust the catheter into the skin; this could cause the catheter to advance too deeply and accidentally damage the vein. Use the indirect method (two-step) for patients with small, delicate veins. An alternative method is to have another nurse apply digital pressure with the hand above the site of venipuncture and release it after the vein has been entered.
3. For patients with very small, spidery veins, preflush the catheter before access is attempted. Preflushing enhances the backflow.

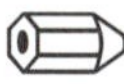 **NOTE:** If the veins are fragile or if the patient is taking anticoagulants, avoid using a tourniquet; constricted blood flow may overdistend fragile veins, causing vein damage, vessel hemorrhages, or subcutaneous bleeding.

TIPS FOR FRAGILE VEINS

The following are tips for elderly patients with fragile veins:

- Avoid overdistention to prevent hematoma.
- Avoid multiple tapping of the vein.

- Use the smallest gauge needle necessary.
- Lower the angle of approach.
- Pull the skin taut and stabilize the vein throughout venipuncture.
- Use the one-handed technique: advance the catheter off the stylet into the vein (Whitson, 1996).

OTHER SPECIAL PROBLEMS

Before initiating I.V. therapy, the nurse must know the patient's diagnosis and allergies. Conditions involving alterations in skin surface (e.g., in patients with systemic lupus erythematosus, dermatitis, skin lesions, and burns); hard sclerosed veins (e.g., in patients with renal failure or sickle cell disease, and those who are I.V. drug abusers), obesity, and edema affect the technique that the therapist will use for a successful venipuncture.

ALTERATIONS IN SKIN SURFACES

Take precautions in patients with alterations in skin surfaces caused by lesions, burns, or a disease process. Patients with altered skin integrity are often photosensitive and need additional protection of their already damaged tissue. **Tangential lighting** is recommended (Fig. 9–6). This indirect lighting does not flatten veins or cause damage to the skin. Use a

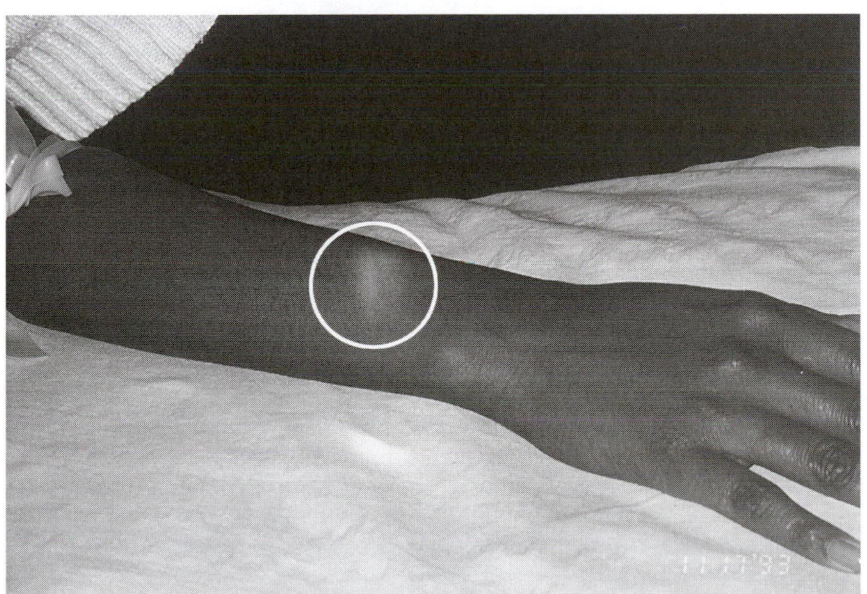

FIG. 9–6. Tangential lighting.

light directed toward the side of the patient's extremity to illuminate the blue veins and provide a guide for venipuncture. This technique can also be used on dark-skinned individuals.

> **CULTURAL AND ETHNIC CONSIDERATIONS: SKIN COLOR**
> Skin color is the most significant biological variation in terms of nursing care. When caring for clients with highly pigmented skin, establish the baseline color by daylight. Give dark-skinned individuals a window to provide access to sunlight (Giger & Davidhizar, 1999).

HARD SCLEROSED VESSELS

If the peripheral vessels are hard and sclerosed because of a disease process, personal misuse, or frequent drug therapy, venous access is difficult. The practitioner should assess for collateral circulation. To find collateral veins, a nurse can use the multiple tourniquet technique. By increasing the **oncotic** pressure inside the tissue, blood is forced into the small vessels of the periphery (Fig. 9–7).

The multiple tourniquet technique helps novices learn the differences between collateral veins and sclerosed vessels. Usually, veins appear in the hand with this approach (Fabian, 1995).

PROCEDURE 9–2: MULTIPLE TOURNIQUET TECHNIQUE

Equipment Needed

- I.V. start equipment and fluids

Instructions to Patient

- Explain reasons for use of multiple tourniquet technique and that there may be some pressure discomfort. Verify patient's understanding of explanation.

Procedure

- Place one tourniquet high on the arm for 2 minutes and leave in place. The arm should be stroked downward toward the hand.
- After 2 minutes, place a second tourniquet at midarm just below the antecubital fossa for 2 minutes.
- If soft collateral veins do not appear in the forearm, place a third tourniquet at the wrist.

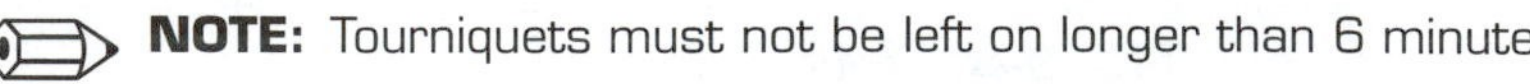

NOTE: Tourniquets must not be left on longer than 6 minutes.

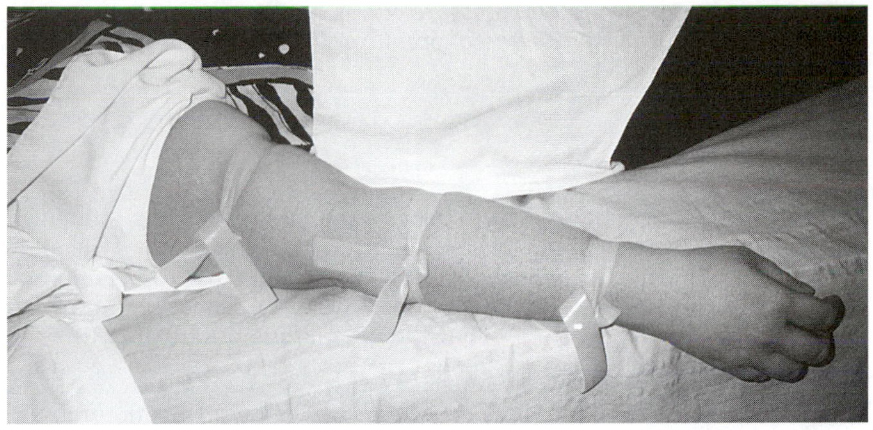

FIG. 9–7. Multiple-tourniquet technique.

Documentation

- Chart the site, needle type and size, type of fluid and medication, and patient response to the treatment.

OBESITY

In patients with excessive adipose tissue, the veins in the extremities react one of two ways to the subcutaneous fat:

- The vessels will be buried deep in the tissue, thereby requiring a 2-inch catheter to access the vein.
- The vasculature will be forced to the surface because the veins have been displaced by the adipose tissue. A vessel can usually be located below the antecubital site on the lateral dorsum of the forearm.

CULTURAL AND ETHNIC CONSIDERATIONS: OBESITY

African-Americans have heavier bones and muscle mass than European-Americans. African-American women are consistently heavier at every age group than their European-American counterparts.

Although ethnicity does appear to have an influence on body weight, a predictor of obesity is socioeconomic status. The average obesity is more pronounced in the low class, less pronounced in the middle class, and even less pronounced in the upper class (Giger & Davidhizar, 1999).

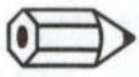 **NOTE:** Use of a blood pressure cuff is not recommended for obese patients because increased pressure from the cuff can cause a backflow of blood.

EDEMA

In locating accessible vasculature in a patient with edema, the nurse must displace tissue fluid with digital pressure. Often this will allow visualization of an accessible vein. Care must be taken not to contaminate the site after the area is prepared. Venipuncture must be done quickly after the area is prepped to prevent the edematous fluid from obscuring the site.

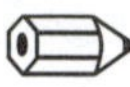 **NOTE:** Edematous fluid causes an increase in oncotic pressure. Therefore, if the fluid is not infusing after the catheter is in place, suspect that the vein may have collapsed as a result of the oncotic pressure in the tissue (Fabian, 1995).

NURSING PLAN OF CARE

PEDIATRIC PATIENTS

Focus Assessment

Subjective

- Interview the patient's parents for the patient's current health status.

Objective

- Measure height and weight for calculation of body surface area and drug dosage.
- Note developmental level.

Patient Outcome Criteria

The patient will:

- Maintain hydration status, with decreased edema.
- Demonstrate beneficial effects from I.V. therapy.
- Return to preillness weight.
- Have normal vital signs for his or her age.
- Participate in activities appropriate to his or her age.
- Demonstrate reduced fear behaviors.
- Participate in decision-making process about self-care when appropriate.

Nursing Diagnoses

1. Impaired skin integrity related to I.V. infiltration, diarrhea, edema, or dry skin
2. Alteration in comfort or pain related to the position of the I.V.

(continued)

(continued)

3. Risk for infection related to invasive procedures
4. Potential anxiety related to the procedure of I.V. therapy
5. Altered body image related to the placement of I.V. therapy equipment
6. Alteration in family process related to the hospitalization of family member
7. Parental role conflict related to illness or hospitalization of a child
8. Sensory and perceptual alterations related to fluid imbalances
9. Ineffective thermoregulation related to newborn transition to extrauterine environment
10. Fear related to loss of control, autonomy, independence, competence, and self-esteem

Nursing Management

1. Monitor intake and output.
2. Explain procedures and equipment.
3. Provide opportunities for non-nutritive sucking in infants.
4. Encourage parents to provide daily care of the child.
5. Instruct the parents in performing special care for the child.
6. Inform the parents about the child's progress.
7. Explain the rationales for treatment and procedures to parents and pediatric patient when appropriate.
8. Comfort infant after painful procedures.
9. Maintain daily routine during hospitalization.
10. Provide quiet, uninterrupted environment during nap time and night time as appropriate.
11. Immobilize when appropriate for venipuncture.
12. Use appropriate equipment for delivery of safe I.V. therapy.
13. Perform I.V. checks every 2 hours and document.
14. Monitor for fluid overload.
15. Monitor vital signs.
16. Maintain universal precautions.
17. Calculate drug dosage correctly and double check with another nurse before administration.

PATIENT EDUCATION: PEDIATRIC AND ELDERLY PATIENTS

Pediatric Patients

- Provide age-appropriate instructions.

Infants

- Encourage parents to keep in infant's line of vision and encourage parents to comfort child.

Toddlers

- Instruct to allow child to participate during instruction; give simple explanations; explain procedures in relation to what the child sees, hears, tastes, smells, and feels; emphasize the aspects of procedures that require cooperation (e.g., lying still).
- Communicate using behaviors; use play by demonstrating with dolls and small replicas of equipment.
- Limit teaching sessions to 5 to 10 minutes.
- Prepare immediately before procedure.

Preschoolers

- Explain procedures in simple terms and in relation to how they affect the child.
- Demonstrate the uses of and allow child to play with equipment.
- Encourage "playing out" on a doll.
- Avoid overestimating the child's comprehension; encourage the child to verbalize.
- Limit each teaching session to 10 to 15 minutes.
- Explain unfamiliar situations such as noises and lights.

School-age Children

- Explain procedures using correct terminology; explain reasons for procedures using anatomic drawings.
- Explain function and operation of equipment in clear terms.
- Allow manipulation of and practice with equipment.
- Allow for questions and discussion.
- Limit teaching sessions to 20 minutes.
- Instruct in advance of procedures.
- Use small groups or encourage teaching of peers.
- Instruct parents.
- Provide ways to maintain control (e.g., deep breathing, counting, relaxation).

Adolescents

- Involve patient in all decisions.
- Discuss how procedure may affect physical appearance.
- Be aware of adolescent's difficulty with accepting authority.
- Instruct in groups and encourage peer instruction.
- Teaching session can be as along as 45 minutes (Wong, 1998).

- Be sensitive to cultural issues, especially related to nursing care of children in the home care setting:
  - Communication channels
  - Spatial behaviors (tactile and visual space)
  - Social (family system) organization
  - Perception of time
  - Use of folk medicine and health-seeking behaviors of the parent (Giger & Davidhizar, 1999)
  - Remember that in most Asian cultures, nursing care must be directed to the family as a whole as well as to the individual family member.

Elderly Patients

- Speak slowly, clearly, and directly to elderly patients with sensory deficits.
- Address the patient by his or her proper name.
- Explain the steps of any procedure to increase cooperation and decrease anxiety.
- Do not use terminology that is unfamiliar.

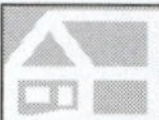

HOME CARE ISSUES

Pediatric Patients

- The home care environment must be assessed to be sure that I.V. therapy can be carried out safely. The parents must be educated about the use and care of I.V. therapy and accept involvement in and responsibility for the treatment regimen.
- Focus on the psychosocial and developmental needs of the child and family in planning home infusion therapy.
- A child is more mobile and active in the home; use a portable infusion device that is easy for the child and family to operate.
- Encourage parents to spend private time with each of their children.
- Keep in mind that parents need support from a home care agency in case the hospital unit nurses are not available; this may increase anxiety and fear.
- Identify alternate caregivers.

Elderly Patients

- Specific challenges of the elderly patient in administration of home infusion therapy:
  - The patient may be less ready to adapt to environmental changes, especially relating to independence.
  - The teaching of complex drug admixtures, tubing connections, I.V. maintenance, I.V. pump programming, and accessing and de-accessing devices requires patience and step-by-step approaches. All equipment should be user friendly. Written teaching materials, video programs, and demonstrations with return demonstrations can be helpful (Weinstein, 1993).
- Evaluation of language or cultural differences can dramatically affect understanding of necessary health care concepts.
- Sensory changes occur with aging (e.g., in vision, hearing, and manual dexterity). Observe the patient working with various devices (the needleless system may eliminate the risk of needlestick injuries) to ensure proficiency.

KEY POINTS

PEDIATRIC I.V. THERAPY

- Children are not small adults. Physiologic differences must be kept in mind with particular focus on total body weight (85–90% water) and heat production (increases caloric expenditure by 7% for each degree of temperature), and immature renal and integumentary systems important in regulation of fluid and electrolyte needs.
- Physical assessment of a pediatric patient includes measuring the head circumference (for patients up to 1 year of age) and checking height or length, vital signs, skin turgor, presence of tears, moistness and color of membranes, urinary output, characteristics of fontanels, and level of child's activity.
- Dehydration is a common cause of fluid and electrolyte imbalance; assessment of fluid needs includes the meter square weight or caloric method.
- Peripheral routes include the four scalp veins, dorsum of the hand and forearm, and dorsum of the foot.
- Selection of I.V. equipment must keep in mind safety, activity, age, and size.
- Needle selection depends on the age of child: 26 to 24 gauge for neonates; 24 to 22 gauge for children.
- Use small volume solutions (250 or 500 mL). Use a volume control chamber and, when indicated, infusion pumps.
- Always have extra help when starting an I.V. in a child.
- Perform venipuncture in a separate room, use pacifier for neonates and infants, warm hands before applying gloves, use rubber band to dilate scalp veins, use surgical lubricating jelly under adhesive tape, and use stickers or drawing as rewards.
- Delivery of medications to children can be by intermittent infusion, retrograde infusion, or syringe pump.
- Alternate routes include intraosseous and umbilical vein and arteries.
- Intraosseous route: use only for 24 hours; use for children younger than 6 years of age. Contraindicated in patients with cellulitis or infected burn, fractured bone, osteoporosis, or osteogenesis imperfecta.

GERIATRIC I.V. THERAPY

- Physiologic changes include homeostatic mechanisms becoming less efficient; immune system becoming hyporesponsive to foreign antigens; cardiovascular changes, including a change in elasticity of the vein walls; skin losses; subcutaneous support; and thinning of skin.
- Assessment guidelines include skin turgor, temperature, rate and filling of veins in hand or foot, daily weight, intake and output, center of tongue should be moist, postural blood pressure, swallowing ability, and functional assessment of patient's ability to obtain fluids if not NPO.
- Venipuncture techniques should take into consideration the skin and vein changes of elderly persons; use small-gauge catheters, use blood pressure cuff, or place loose tourniquet over clothing. Use warm compresses to visualize veins. Consider microdrip administration sets.

OTHER SPECIAL PROBLEMS

- Alterations in skin surfaces: Use tangential lighting.
- Hard sclerosed vessels: Use multiple tourniquet technique.
- Obesity: Use 2-inch catheter, lateral veins, and multiple tourniquet technique.
- Edema: Displace edema with digital pressure.
- Fragile veins: Maintain traction using one-handed technique. Be gentle.

CHAPTER ACTIVITIES

COMPETENCY CRITERIA: Delivery of Infusion Therapy to Pediatric Patients
COMPETENCY STATEMENT: Competent I.V. nurses will be able to initiate peripheral I.V. therapy to pediatric patients.
Note: The cognitive (knowledge) information that is embedded within this performance-based competency includes aseptic technique, physiologic characteristics of children, factors affecting fluid needs, physiology of fluid balance in pediatric patients, venous anatomy, and developmental age criteria.
This competency *links* to the competency of infection control, management of intravenous equipment, parenteral solutions, and initiation of peripheral I.V. therapy

Performance	Skilled	Needs Education
Critical Action Statements		
1. Chooses age-appropriate site for venous access A. Scalp vein B. Dorsum of hand C. Dorsum of foot		
2. Demonstrates choice of equipment appropriate for safe infusion to pediatric patient A. 250- to 500-mL container B. Volume control device C. Electronic infusion device		
3. Chooses age-appropriate cannula device A. Type and size		
4. Evaluates the need for pain management before the procedure:		
5. Applies topical anesthetic cream according to manufacturer's recommendations. A. EMLA cream B. Numby Stuff		
6. Performs venipuncture with assistance A. Parents B. Other healthcare personnel		
7. Demonstrates appropriate use of immobilizers to perform venipuncture A. Mummy wrap		

(continued)

Performance	Skilled	Needs Education
Critical Action Statements		
8. Performs venipuncture in separate room from child's "safe space"		
9. Demonstrates formulas for calculation of pediatric medication administration A. Body weight formula B. Body surface area C. Clark's rule D. Bastedo's rule E. Young's rule		
10. Documentation of site assessments A. Every 2 hour		

EVALUATION CRITERIA

1. Validation of initiation of pediatric intravenous therapy with preceptor
2. Calculation of pediatric infusion problems
3. Review of documentation of site assessments

CRITICAL THINKING ACTIVITY

1. You are working on a pediatric ward and assigned a 6-month-old baby with meningitis. The I.V. is placed in the baby's scalp. You assess the baby and find the site covered with a white paper cup and lots of tape; the baby's eye beneath the cup is swollen. What is the problem? How do you remedy this situation?

2. You must start an I.V. on a 70-year-old obese person with a diagnosis of systemic lupus erythematosus. What do you need to consider before venipuncture? What techniques should you use to be successful?

3. You must start an I.V. on a 10-year-old boy who has never been hospitalized. His diagnosis is osteomyelitis. How would you approach this patient?

4. You are working in an emergency room and a 2-year-old near-drowning victim is brought in and is in respiratory distress. Would you consider intraosseous infusion?

POST-TEST

In 1 through 5, fill in the missing term in the following sentences.

1. ____________ infusion is the delivery of fluids and electrolytes into the medullary cavity in the bone.
2. The ____________ method calculates the metabolic expenditure of energy in figuring fluid replacement.
3. The period of extrauterine life up to the first 28 days of life is called the ____________ period.
4. The breakdown of chemical compounds into more elementary principles by the body is referred to as ____________.
5. The ____________ is determined through use of a nomogram.
6. The preferred choice for I.V. site in the young infant younger than age 9 months is the:
   - a. Frontal vein in the scalp
   - b. Dorsum of the foot
   - c. Dorsum of the hand
   - d. Occipital vein on the head
7. The weight method of estimating fluid requirements in a child refers to:
   - a. Weighing diapers and estimating output to replace sensible losses
   - b. A formula based on weight in kilograms to estimate fluid needs
   - c. A calculation of metabolic expenditure of energy based on weight
   - d. Use of a nomogram
8. In a dark-skinned person, the best method for locating an accessible vein is:
   - a. Multiple tourniquets
   - b. Tangential lighting
   - c. Direct overhead lighting
   - d. Light application of a tourniquet
9. Which of the following is the most appropriate cannula size for use on a 2-month-old infant?
   - a. 18-gauge over-the-needle catheter
   - b. 23- to 25-gauge scalp vein needle
   - c. 16-gauge scalp vein needle
   - d. 22- to 24-gauge over-the-needle catheter
10. The most common site for intraosseous infusion is the:
    - a. Proximal humerus
    - b. Distal humerus, 6 cm below the acromion process
    - c. Anterior tibia, 1 to 3 cm below the tibial tuberosity
    - d. Proximal posterior femur
11. When performing an I.V. on a toddler, methods that can be used to assist the therapist in this invasive procedure based on developmental age include:
    - a. Letting the child express feelings and scream
    - b. Encouraging the child to hold a favorite toy or blanket
    - c. Performing the procedure quickly with assistance from other staff or parents
    - d. All of the above

12. The most appropriate equipment for an infant receiving I.V. fluids includes:
    a. Microdrip tubing connected to a 50-mL infusate container
    b. Microdrip volume control cylinder attached to a 250-mL infusate container
    c. Macrodrip tubing connected to a volume control cylinder
    d. Any tubing or container as long as it is regulated with an electronic infusion device

REFERENCES

Aehlert, B. (1996). *Pediatric Advanced Life Support Study Guide.* St. Louis: Mosby Year Book.

American Association of Retired Persons (AARP) (1985). *A Profile of Older Americans.* U.S. Department of Health & Human Services.

Centers for Disease Control and Prtevention (1995). *Intravascular device-related infections prevention: Guideline availability notice.* Fed. Reg., Part II, 60(187), Atlanta P49978-50006.

Fabian, B. (1995). Intravenous therapy in the older adult. In Terry, J., Baranowski, L., Lonsway, R., & Hedrick, C., eds. *Intravenous Therapy: Clinical Principles and Practice.* Intravenous Nurses Society. Philadelphia: W.B. Saunders.

Giger, J.N., & Davidhizar, R. (1999). *Transcultural Nursing Assessment & Intervention* (3rd ed). St. Louis: Mosby.

Harvey, P. (1998). *Local Anesthesia and the Pediatric Patient.* Intravenous Nursing Annual Convention. Houston, Texas.

Henke, G. (1999). *Med-Math* (3rd ed.). Philadelphia: Lippincott, pp. 241–257.

Hodge, D. (1985). Intraosseous infusions: A review. *Pediatric Emergency Care,* 1, 215–218.

Intravenous Nursing Society. (2000). Revised Standards of practice. *Journal of Intravenous Nursing,* 21 (1S).

Josephson, D.L. (1999). *Intravenous Infusion Therapy for Nurses.* Albany: Delmar Publishers.

Kennedy, D. (1996). Medication "Safety Checks" in pediatric acute care. *Journal of Intravenous Nursing,* 19(6), 295–302.

Metheny, N.M. (1996). *Fluid and Electrolyte Balance: Nursing Considerations* (3rd ed.). Philadelphia: J.B. Lippincott.

Powers, F.A. (1999). Your elderly patient needs I.V. therapy. . . Can you keep her safe? *Nursing 99,* 99(7), 54–55.

Smeltzer, S.C., & Bare, B.G. (2000). *Brunner and Suddarth's Textbook of Medical-Surgical Nursing* (9th ed.). Philadelphia: J.B. Lippincott, pp. 150–165.

Stifter, J., & Shanahan, N. (1994). The IV bubbles and boards system. *Journal of Pediatric Nursing,* 9(6), 417–419.

Smith, M.F. (1998). Emergency access in pediatrics. *Journal of Intravenous Nursing,* 21(3), 149–159.

Taylor, S. (1992). Lost in the system. *Journal of Intravenous Nursing* (supplement 15), S2–S6.

Wheeler, C.A., & Frey, A.M. (1995). Intravenous therapy in children. In Terry, J., Baranowski, L., Lonsway, R., & Hedrick, C. *Intravenous Therapy: Clinical Principles and Practice.* Intravenous Nurses Society. Philadelphia: W.B. Saunders, pp. 467–494.

Weiner, E.S., & Albanese, C.T. (1998). Venous access in pediatric patients. *Journal of Intravenous Nursing,* supplement 21(5S), S122–S133.

Whitson, M. (1996). Intravenous therapy in the older adult: Special needs and considerations. *Journal of Intravenous Nursing,* 19(5), 251–255.

Wong, D.L. (1998). *Whaley & Wong's Nursing Care of Infants and Children* (6th ed). St. Louis: Mosby-Year Book.

United States Department of Health and Human Services. (1990). *Healthy People 2000.* Washington: U.S. Government Printing Office.

ANSWERS TO CHAPTER 9

Pre-Test

1. e, **2.** b, **3.** a, **4.** a, **5.** d, **6.** e, **7.** c, **8.** a, **9.** c, **10.** a, **11.** c

Post-Test

1. Intraosseous, **2.** Caloric, **3.** Neonatal, **4.** Catabolism, **5.** Body surface area, **6.** c, **7.** b, **8.** b, **9.** d, **10.** c, **11.** d, **12.** b

UNIT THREE

Advanced Infusion Practice

CHAPTER 10

Administration of Intravenous Medications

In the future, which I shall not see, for I am old, may a better way be opened! May the methods by which every infant, every human being will have the best chance of health, the methods by which every sick person will have the best chance of recovery, be learned and practiced! Hospitals are only an intermediate state of civilization never intended, at all events, to take in the whole sick population.

Florence Nightingale, 1860

CHAPTER CONTENTS

LEARNING OBJECTIVES

Upon completion of this chapter, the reader will be able to:

1. Define the terminology related to administration of I.V. medications.
2. Identify the advantages of I.V. medications.
3. List the hazards associated with I.V. medications.
4. Identify the methods through which medications may be delivered by the I.V. route.
5. Identify three incompatibilities related to I.V. therapy.
6. Describe the proper technique in delivery of I.V. bolus medication.
7. Describe the treatment of adverse effects of I.V. medications.
8. State the precautions to be followed when medication is infused via the epidural route.
9. List the key steps in dressing management of an intraspinal catheter.
10. Describe the method of delivery and nursing considerations for intraperitoneal therapy.
11. Describe the special considerations when administering anti-

infective therapy, chemotherapeutic agents, and narcotics via the I.V. route.

12 List the key points in delivering medications intravenously for pain control.

13 Describe nurses' roles in the delivery of investigational drugs.

GLOSSARY

Adsorption Attachment of one substance to the surface of another

Admixture Combination of two or more medications

Bolus Concentrated medication or solution given rapidly over a short period of time; may be given by direct I.V. injection or I.V. drip

Chemical incompatibility Change in the molecular structure or pharmacologic properties of a substance, which may or may not be visually observed

Clinical trial Planned experiment that involves patients and is designed to evoke an appropriate treatment of future patients with a given medical condition

Compatibility Capable of being mixed and administered without undergoing undesirable chemical or physical changes or loss of therapeutic action

Delivery system A product that allows for the administration of medication

Distribution Process of delivering a drug to the various tissues of the body

Drug interaction An interaction between two drugs; also, a drug that causes an increase or decrease in another drug's pharmacologic effects

Epidural Situated on or over the dura mater

Incompatibility Chemical or physical reaction that occurs among two or more drugs or between a drug and the delivery device

Intermittent drug infusion: I.V. therapy administered at prescribed intervals

Intraspinal: Spaces surrounding the spinal cord, including the epidural and intrathecal spaces

Intrathecal Within a sheath, surrounded by the epidural space and separated from it by the dura mater; contains cerebrospinal fluid

Intravenous push Manual administration of medication under pressure over 1 minute or as manufacturer of medication recommends

Multiple-dose vial Medication bottle that is hermetically sealed with a rubber stopper and designed to be entered more than once

Physical incompatibility An undesirable change that is visually observed

Single-dose vial Medication bottle that is hermetically sealed with a rubber stopper and is intended for one-time use

Therapeutic incompatibility Undesirable effect occurring within a patient as a result of two or more drugs being given concurrently

PRE-TEST

1. Which of the following are advantages of I.V. medications?
   a. Provides a route for irritating substances, has instant drug action, and has better control administration.
   b. Encourages speed shock, has a rapid onset of action, and allows for absorption of drugs in gastric juices.
   c. Prevents errors in compounding of medication, has a low risk of infiltration, and has a low risk of phlebitis.
   d. Allows for uninterrupted control of rate, has a low risk of side effects, and has a low risk of adsorption.
2. Incompatibilities of drugs fall into which of the following three classes?
   a. Physical, incompatible, and chemical
   b. Physical, chemical, and therapeutic
   c. Therapeutic, absorption, and distribution

For 3, 4, and 5, match the description of the catheter in column II with the term in column I.

COLUMN I	COLUMN II
3. Epidural	a. Catheter is placed over the dura mater.
4. Intrathecal	b. Needle is inserted into the tissue spaces.
5. Subcutaneous	c. Catheter is within a sheath that contains spinal fluid.

6. The role of the registered nurse in investigational drugs include(s):
   a. Communicating with the Institutional Review Board
   b. I.V. administration of investigational drugs
   c. Assisting with final study report
   d. Participating in data collection
   e. All of the above
7. Alcohol is contraindicated for site preparation or maintenance of epidural catheters because of the potential for:
   a. Migration into the epidural space
   b. Obliterating the catheter
   c. Possible nerve damage
   d. Breakdown of the catheter material
8. Delivery of morphine by the epidural route has been associated with a high incidence of:
   a. Pruritus
   b. Nausea
   c. Diarrhea
   d. Urinary incontinence

9. Pain management may be provided by all of the following **EXCEPT:**
   a. Systemic analgesic
   b. The subcutaneous route
   c. The intraspinal route
   d. The intraperitoneal route
10. To reduce the hazards of vascular irritation with delivery of medication, nurses should:
   a. Use the largest cannula possible
   b. Use a cannula smaller than the lumen of a vessel
   c. Administer most medications via the intramuscular route
   d. Use electronic infusion devices with a PSI of 10 or above

PRINCIPLES OF INTRAVENOUS MEDICATION ADMINISTRATION

ADVANTAGES

The infusion of I.V. medication provides a direct access to the circulatory system, a route for administration of fluids and drugs to patients who cannot tolerate oral medications, a method of instant drug action, and a method of instant drug administration termination. This route offers pronounced advantages over the subcutaneous (S.Q.), intramuscular (I.M.), and oral routes (Table 10–1.)

Drugs that cannot be absorbed by other routes because of the large molecular size of the drug or destruction of the drug by gastric juices can be administered directly to the site of **distribution,** the circulatory system, with I.V. infusion. Drugs with irritating properties that cause pain and trauma when given by the intramuscular or subcutaneous route can be given intravenously. When a drug is administered intravenously, there is instant drug action, which is an advantage in emergency situations. The I.V. route also provides instant drug termination if sensitivity or adverse reactions occur. This route provides for control over the rate at which drugs are administered; prolonged action can be controlled by administering a dilute medication infusion intermittently over a prolonged time period (Weinstein, 1997).

Intravenous medications are provided for rapid therapeutic or diagnostic responses or a delivery route for solutions or medications that cannot be delivered by any other route. Nurses administering the solution or medication are accountable for achieving effective delivery of prescribed therapy and for evaluating and documenting deviations from an expected outcome, including the implementation of corrective action.

INS STANDARDS Nurses are responsible for assessing the appropriateness of prescribed therapy, including patient assessment, patient age and condition, appropriateness of solution and medication prescribed, and appropriateness of drug and its dose, route, and rate. Before administration

TABLE 10–1

ADVANTAGES AND DISADVANTAGES OF INTRAVENOUS MEDICATION ADMINISTRATION

Advantages
1. Provides a direct access to the circulatory system
2. Provides a route for drugs that irritate the gastric mucosa
3. Provides a route for instant drug action
4. Provides a route for delivering high drug concentrations
5. Provides for instant drug termination if sensitivity or adverse reaction occurs
6. Provides for better control over the rate of drug administration
7. Provides a route of administration in patients in whom use of the gastrointestinal tract is limited
Disadvantages
1. Drug interaction because of incompatibilities.
2. Adsorption of the drug is impaired, which is caused by leaching into I.V. container or administration set.
3. Errors in compounding (mixing) of medication
4. Speed shock
5. Extravasation of a vesicant drug
6. Chemical phlebitis

of the solution or medication, the nurse must be knowledge in indications, actions, use, side effects, and adverse reactions associated with the solution or medication. (INS, 2000, 73)

DISADVANTAGES

Despite the many advantages of I.V. medication, there are also disadvantages associated with this venous route; these disadvantages are not found with other drug therapies (see Table 10–1).

The number of drug combinations, along with the ever-increasing production of drugs and parenteral fluids, has compounded these disadvantages. The disadvantages specific to the administration of I.V. drugs include **drug interactions;** drug loss via **adsorption** of I.V. containers and administration sets; errors in mixing techniques; and the complications of speed shock, extravasation of vesicant drugs, and phlebitis.

Drug Interactions

Drug interactions are not always clear cut. Many factors affect drug interactions, including drug solubility and drug **compatibility.** Mixing of two drugs in a solution can cause an adverse interaction called drug

incompatibility. Factors affecting drug solubility and compatibility include:

- Drug concentration
- Brand of I.V. fluid or drug
- Type of administration set
- Preparation technique, duration of drug–drug or drug–solution contact
- pH value
- Temperature of the room and light

Drugs can be compatible when mixed in certain solutions but incompatible when mixed with others. Mixing two incompatible drugs in solution in a particular order may be enough to avoid a potentially adverse interaction (Gahart & Nazareno, 1999).

The pH of both the solution and the drug must be considered when compounding medications. Drugs that are widely dissimilar in pH values are unlikely to be compatible in solution. For example, dextrose solutions are slightly acidic, with a pH of 4.5 to 5.5. Several antibiotics on the market have an acidic pH that is stable in dextrose; however, alkaline antibiotics, such as carbenicillin, are unstable when mixed with dextrose. Dextrose, with a pH of 4.5 to 5.5, should be used as a base for acidic drugs; sodium chloride solution, with a pH value of 6.8 to 8.5, should be used for alkaline medication dilution.

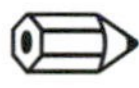

NOTE: When in doubt about I.V. drug compatibilities, a good practice is to flush the I.V. administration set with sodium chloride before and after medications are infused.

Adsorption

Adsorption is the attachment of one substance to the surface of another. Many drugs adsorb to glass or plastic. The disadvantage associated with adsorption is that the patient receives a smaller amount of the drug than was intended. The amount of adsorption is difficult to predict and is affected by the drug concentration, solution of the drug, amount of surface contacted by the drug, and temperature changes.

An example of adsorption is the binding of insulin to plastic and glass containers. The insulin rapidly adsorbs to I.V. containers and tubing until all potential adsorption sites are saturated. During the initial part of an infusion, very little insulin may reach the patient; later, after adsorption sites are saturated, more of the insulin in the solution is delivered to the patient. To prevent this from occurring, injecting the drug as close to the I.V. insertion site as possible will promote better therapeutic drug effects.

Polyvinyl chloride (PVC) in plastic flexible I.V. bags promotes drug adsorption. There are several drugs that have significant loss during infusion in PVC plastic solution containers; these include:

- Vitamin A acetate (not the palmitate form)
- Insulin

- Phenothiazine tranquilizers (e.g., chlorpromazine, prochlorperazine)
- Hydralazine (Apresoline)
- Warfarin (Coumadin)

A phthalate (DEHP) is a plasticizer that is added to PVC that allows PVC to be flexible. Some drug formulations leach this plasticizer out of the plastic matrix and into the solution. DEHP is fat-soluble, I.V. fat emulsion products that extract the plasticizer from the PVC bags and tubing. DEHP is also leached from PVC bags by organic solvents and surfactants contained in some drugs, which may result in DEHP-induced toxicity. Many drug manufacturers recommend nonphthalate **delivery systems** in the package inserts. Many companies are manufacturing nonphthalate I.V. bags and tubing to prevent this problem. (Chapter 6 provides further information on DEHP leaching and a list of nonphthalate products.)

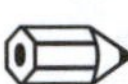 **NOTE:** When mixing medications into glass or plastic systems, refer to the manufacturer's guidelines to prevent adsorption.

ERRORS IN MIXING

Drug toxicity, subtherapeutic infusion, or erratic therapeutic effects can result from inadequate mixing of a drug into the infusion container. Inadequate mixing can contribute to a **bolus** of medication being delivered to the patient, which may cause adverse effects.

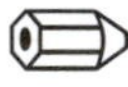 **NOTE:** Burning at the I.V. site from a presumably dilute drug is a warning that the concentration of the drug is too high and needs to be further diluted.

Factors that contribute to inadequate mixing include:

- Length of time required to adequately mix drugs in flexible bags
- Addition of a drug to a hanging flexible bag
- Additives injected at a slow rate into the primary bag (the turbulence of fast flow promotes mixing, especially in glass containers)
- Inadequate movement of the additive from the injection port (e.g., the long, narrow sleeve-type additive ports on some flexible bags, as opposed to the button type, hinder effective mixing)
- Tendency of very dense drugs to settle at the bottom of infusion container

Ten key recommendations for adequate mixing of I.V. medications are presented in Table 10–2.

NOTE: Because of the complexity of this function, many hospitals allow only registered pharmacists to prepare admixtures.

TABLE 10–2

TEN KEY RECOMMENDATIONS FOR ADEQUATE MIXING OF I.V. MEDICATIONS

1. Gently invert the I.V. container several times to adequately mix the medication with the solution, taking care to avoid foaming the solution.
2. When inversion is impossible, gently swirl or rotate to mix to prevent the drug from settling to the bottom of the container.
3. When agitating an intermittent infusion set, clamp off the air vent; if the vent becomes wet, the solution will not infuse properly after mixing.
4. Vacuum devices can facilitate mixing in plastic flexible bags by creating a vacuum and drawing any drug left in the port into the body of the bag.
5. When possible, use premixed solutions from the manufacturer; for example, using premixed heparin or potassium chloride solutions can save time and avoid dose errors as well as preclude mixing problems.
6. Add one drug at a time to the primary I.V. solution. Mix and examine thoroughly before adding the next drug.
7. Add the most concentrated or most soluble drug to the solution first because some incompatibilities, such as precipitates, require a certain concentration or amount of time to develop. Mix well, and then add the dilute drugs.
8. Add colored additives last to avoid masking possible precipitate cloudiness.
9. Always visually inspect containers after adding and mixing drugs; hold the container against a light or a white surface and check for particulate matter, obvious layering, or foaming.
10. If you do not have a clear understanding of the compatibility or stability of the admixtures you are using, check the manufacturer's recommendation or consult a pharmacist.

SPEED SHOCK

Nurses must be aware that speed shock can be caused by too-rapid administration of a drug. Rapid onset of action is a double-edged sword: on one hand, it is to the patient's advantage to have rapid action in certain clinical situations; on the other hand, after it is infused, the rapid onset cannot be recalled. (See Chapter 8 for additional information on speed shock.)

EXTRAVASATION

Nurses must be aware of the patency of the I.V. cannula before initiating an infusion to prevent extravasation of a vesicant or irritating medication or solution. (See Chapter 8 for additional information on extravasation.)

CHEMICAL PHLEBITIS

Chemical phlebitis can occur from the pH of the medication; a pH greater than 11.0 or lower than 4.3 is most irritating to vein walls. Antibiotics, chemotherapeutic agents, potassium chloride, and diazepam (Valium) are known to cause irritation to vein walls and promote chemical phlebitis. (See Chapter 8 for further information on phlebitis.)

INTRAVENOUS DRUG SAFETY

Getting the right solution or medication to a patient is often a complicated, error-prone process. The order has to be properly written on the correct medical record, read, and properly interpreted and transcribed. The drug has to be retrieved and labeled correctly. The proper patient has to be identified and the infusion rate correctly set. A study by Johnson and Bootman (1995) found that medication and solution errors cost the United States as much as $76.6 billion each year.

To reduce errors, hospitals should support programs that use premixed, commercially manufactured I.V. solutions or an I.V. preparation process that is centralized to the pharmacy where proper quality assurance controls for drug preparation have been implemented and are constantly monitored (Cohen, 1997).

PREVENTING MEDICATION ADMINISTRATION ERRORS

If an error is made or found, follow the formal reporting procedure used in your institution.

NOTE: Medication errors must be reported and documented as they are made.

Common causes of medication errors often revolve around the five "rights" of medication administration that have turned into "wrongs":

- Wrong patient
- Wrong dose
- Wrong time
- Wrong route
- Wrong mediations

To prevent medication errors, **ALWAYS:**

- Check ambiguous drug orders.
- Check ambiguous drug names.
- Beware of atypical drug names.
- When using a dropper, never use the dropper of one medication to administer another medication.
- Question the use of multiple ampules or vials to provide a single dose.

- Question unusually small or large doses.
- Be suspicious of abrupt and excessive increase and decreases of medication.
- Question the term "midnight" on an order to determine the date.
- Refuse to interpret illegible handwriting (Kuhn, 1998).

AGE-RELATED CONSIDERATIONS: OLDER ADULTS AND THE EFFECTS OF GENDER

Almost 60 percent of older adults fear adverse drug reactions or overmedication, which leads to noncompliance in taking their medications. This fear discourages compliance (Kuhn, 1999). Drug side effects in elderly persons are often mistaken for signs of aging.

Gender can have a profound effect on metabolism of drugs. For example, women have the potential for higher blood plasma levels of psychotropic drugs, especially when used with oral contraceptives. Also, women have a greater likelihood of adverse reactions to antipsychotic agents.

There are a number of ways that medication errors can occur during the administration of I.V. medications. Common errors in administering medications include:

- Lack of knowledge about drugs.
- Errors in drug identity checking (e.g., selecting the wrong drug because it is similar in packaging to another).
- Mistakes in calculations.
- Use of pumps and controllers: The use of modern electronic infusion devices can dramatically increase accuracy and safety and has significant patient benefits; it also introduces new problems of potential errors, including improper setting of pumps, which can have serious consequences in terms of drug delivery (Hunt & Rapp, 1996).

The Emergency Care Research Institute (ECRI) has performed extensive studies on the mechanical and safety features of pumps and controllers.

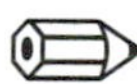

NOTE: Nurses are the last line of defense to detect and correct a potential medication error.

DRUG COMPATIBILITY

Compatibility is required for a therapeutic response to prescribed therapy. Chemical, physical, and therapeutic compatibilities must be identified before admixing and administering I.V. medications.

An incompatibility results when two or more substances react or interact and change the normal activity of one or more components. Incompatibility may be manifested by harmful or undesirable effects and is likely to result in a loss of therapeutic effects. Incompatibility may occur when:

- Several drugs are added to a large volume of fluid to produce an **admixture.**
- Drugs in separate solutions are administered concurrently or in close succession via the same I.V. line.
- A single drug is reconstituted or diluted with the wrong solutions.
- One drug reacts with another drug's preservative.

Specific incompatibilities fall into three categories: physical, chemical, and therapeutic.

PHYSICAL INCOMPATIBILITY

A **physical incompatibility** is also called a pharmaceutical incompatibility. Physical incompatibilities occur when one drug is mixed with other drugs or solutions to produce a product that is unsafe for administration.

Insolubility and absorption are the two types of physical incompatibility. Insolubility occurs when a drug is added to an inappropriate fluid solution, creating an incomplete solution or a precipitate. This risk occurs more frequently with multiple additives, which may interact to form an insoluble product. Signs of insolubility include visible precipitation, haze, gas bubbles, and cloudiness. Some precipitations may be microcrystalline (i.e., smaller than 50 microns) and not apparent to the eye. The use of micropore filters is intended to prevent such particles from entering the vein. The use of a 0.22-micron inline filter reduces the amount of microcrystalline precipitates.

The presence of calcium in a drug or solution usually indicates that a precipitate might form if mixed with another drug. Ringer's solution preparations contain calcium, so check carefully for incompatibility before adding any drug to this solution.

Other physical incompatibilities caused by insolubility include the increased degradation of drugs added to sodium bicarbonate and the formation of an insoluble precipitate when sodium bicarbonate is combined with other medications in emergency situations.

The following are important recommendations regarding physical drug incompatibilities:

- Never administer a drug that forms a precipitate.
- Do not mix drugs prepared in special diluents with other drugs.
- When administering a series of medications, prepare each drug in a separate syringe. This will lessen the possibility of precipitation. Insolubility may also result from the use of an incorrect solution to reconstitute a drug.

- Follow the manufacturer's directions for reconstituting drugs (Kuhn, 1998).

CHEMICAL INCOMPATIBILITY

A **chemical incompatibility** is a reaction of a drug with other drugs or solutions, which results in alterations of the integrity and potency of the active ingredient. The most common cause of chemical incompatibility is the reaction between acidic and alkaline drugs or solutions, resulting in a pH level that is unstable for one of the drugs. A specific pH or a narrow range of pH values is required for the solubility of a drug and for the maintenance of its stability after it has been mixed.

THERAPEUTIC INCOMPATIBILITY

A **therapeutic incompatibility** is an undesirable effect occurring in a patient as a result of two or more drugs being given concurrently. An increased therapeutic or a decreased therapeutic response is produced.

This incompatibility often occurs when therapy dictates the use of two antibiotics. For example, in the use of chloramphenicol and penicillin, chloramphenicol has been reported to antagonize the bacterial activity of penicillin. If prescribed, penicillin should be administered at least 1 hour before the chloramphenicol to prevent therapeutic incompatibility.

Therapeutic incompatibility may go unnoticed until the patient fails to show the expected clinical response to the drug or until peak and trough levels of the drug show a lack of therapeutic levels. If an incompatibility is not suspected, the patient may be given increasingly higher doses of the drug to try to obtain the therapeutic effect.

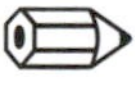

NOTE: When more than one antibiotic is prescribed for intermittent infusion, stagger the time schedule so that each can be infused individually.

CULTURAL AND ETHNIC CONSIDERATIONS: I.V. DRUG ADMINISTRATION

In ethnic and cultural groups (i.e., African-Americans and Asian-Americans) with a high incidence of glucose-6-phosphate dehydrogenase (G6PD) deficiency, some drugs may impair red blood cell metabolism, leading to anemia. Caffeine, a component of many drugs, is excreted more slowly by Asian-Americans. Asian-Americans may require smaller doses of certain drugs (Giger and Davidhizar, 1999).

INTRAVENOUS MEDICATION ADMINISTRATION

There are several methods used to administer I.V. medications, including continuous, intermittent infusions, and I.V. push. Nursing responsibilities of I.V. drug administration include:

- Identifying whether a prescribed route (i.e., continuous, intermittent, or push) is appropriate
- Using aseptic technique when preparing an admixture
- Identifying the expiration date on solutions and medications
- Following the manufacturer's guidelines for the preparation and storage of the medication
- Being knowledgeable of the pharmacologic implications relative to patient clinical status and diagnosis
- Verifying that all solution containers are free of cracks, leaks, and punctures
- Monitoring the patient for therapeutic response to the medication

CONTINUOUS INFUSION

Continuous infusion occurs when large-volume parenteral solutions of 250 to 1000 mL of infusate are administered over 2 to 24 hours. Medications added to these large-volume infusates are administered continuously. An I.V. pump or controller to ensure an accurate flow rate should regulate these infusions.

Advantages

- Admixture and bag changes can be performed every 8 to 24 hours
- Constant serum levels of the drug are maintained

Disadvantages

- Monitoring the drug rate can be erratic if not electronically controlled
- Higher risk of drug incompatibility problems
- Accidental bolus infusion can occur if medication is not adequately mixed with the solution

---

PROCEDURE 10–1: ADMINISTRATION OF CONTINUOUS INFUSIONS

Verify the physician's order, educate the patient regarding purpose of therapy, and document the procedure and any patient teaching that you performed.

Step 1. Spike the I.V. container with an I.V. administration set.

Step 2. Regulate the flow rate.

Step 3. Based on the type of drug being administered, monitor the patient

at the recommended time intervals for therapeutic and nontherapeutic effects of the drug.
Step 4. Place time tape on the bag even when a pump or controller is used to verify the administration rate at a quick glance.

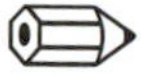

NOTE: When adding medication to an infusion container, use **single-dose vials** instead of **multiple-dose vials** to decrease the potential for infection, complications, and medication errors.

AGE-RELATED CONSIDERATIONS: PEDIATRIC PATIENTS

Continuous infusions in pediatric patients should have in-line volume-control chambers and be controlled by infusion pumps. No more than 1 to 2 hours' worth of solution should be placed in the chamber at any one time.

INS STANDARDS After adding an administration set, a solution or medication container must be infused or discarded within 24 hours. (INS, 2000, 73)

INTERMITTENT INFUSION

Intermittent infusion is any administration of a medication or an infusion that is not continuous. Technological advances have produced alternatives for the administration of intermittent doses. Types of intermittent infusions are piggybacked through the established pathway of the primary solution, simultaneous infusion, use of volume control set, and intermittent infusions through a locking device.

Piggyback through Primary Pathway

A secondary I.V. line used intermittently is commonly called a piggyback set. Piggyback infusion through an established pathway of the primary solution is the most common method for drug delivery by the intermittent route. A piggyback set includes a small I.V. container, short administration set without ports, and a macrodrip system. The drug is diluted in 50 to 250 mL of 5 percent dextrose in water or 0.9 percent sodium chloride and administered over 15 to 90 minutes (Baldwin, 1995). When infusing medications with this method, the secondary infusion is administered via the piggyback Y port with the backcheck valve (Fig. 10–1A).

This Y port is located on the upper third of the primary line. Although the primary infusion is interrupted during the piggyback infusion, the drug from the intermittent infusion container comes in contact with the primary solution below the piggyback injection port; therefore, the drug and the primary solution should be compatible.

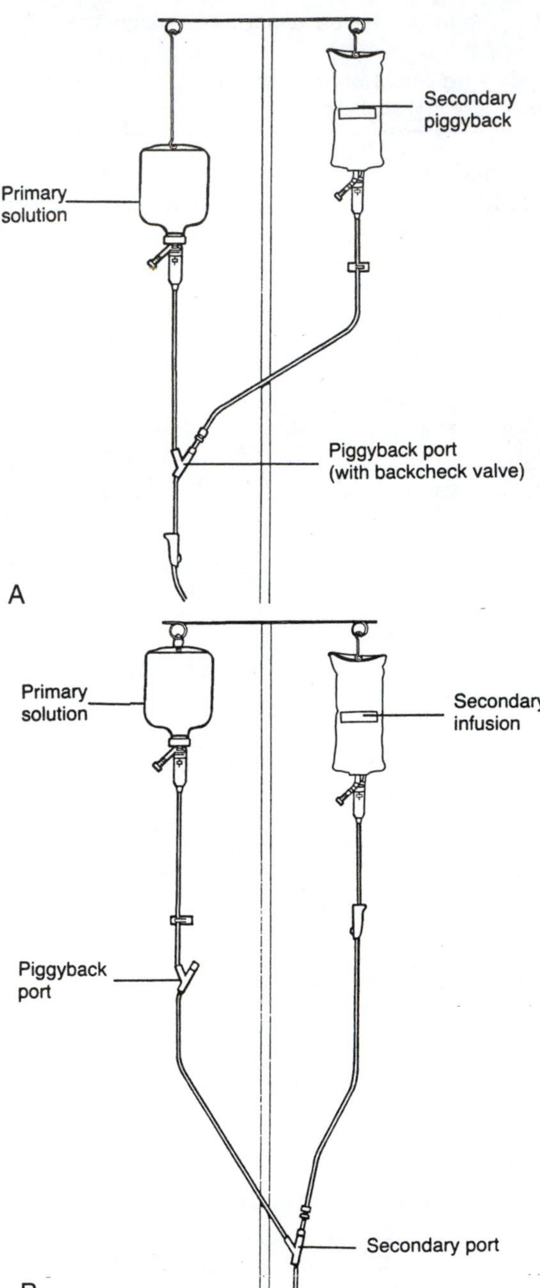

FIG. 10–1. Methods of delivery of secondary infusions. (*A*) Secondary piggyback infusion. (*B*) Simultaneous infusion.

The Occupational Safety and Health Administration (OSHA) has recently recommended the use of needleless systems to connect secondary infusions to primary administration sets. The needle-free system aims to reduce the risk of accidental needlestick injuries.

I.V. pumps may be used to maintain constant infusion rates and maintain accurate titration of drug dosages.

Advantages

- Risk of incompatibilities is reduced.
- Larger drug dose can be administered at a lower concentration per milliliter than with the I.V. push method.
- Peak flow concentrations occur at periodic intervals.
- There is a decreased risk of fluid overload.

Disadvantages

- The administration rate may not be accurate unless electronically monitored.
- The high concentration of drug in intermittent solution may cause venous irritation.
- I.V. set changes can result in wasting a portion of the drug.
- If the patient is not properly monitored, fluid overload or speed shock may result.
- Drug incompatibility can occur if the administration set is not adequately flushed between medication administrations.

INS STANDARDS When preparing solutions or medications for administration, single-use medication vials or ampules are recommended. The use of multiple-dose vials increases the potential for infection, complications, and medication errors. If multiple-dose vials are used, they should be labeled with date and time the vial is initially entered. (INS, 2000, 73)

AGE-RELATED CONSIDERATIONS: ELDERLY PATIENTS

Consider the volume used for dilution of piggyback medication when planning intake for elderly patients (Josephson, 1999).

PROCEDURE 10–2: ADMINISTRATION OF PIGGYBACK SECONDARY INFUSION

Verify the physician's order, educate the patient regarding purpose of therapy, and document the procedure and any patient teaching that you performed.

Step 1. Add drug to secondary I.V. infusion solution (making sure that the base solution is compatible with the drug).

(continued)

(continued)

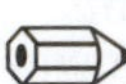 **NOTE:** Most pharmacists prepare the admixture before dispensing.

Step 2. Spike the secondary administration set into the piggyback solution container. Prime the set.
Step 3. Confirm the patient's identity.
Step 4. Confirm that the primary solution is compatible with the secondary infusion.
Step 5. Hang the secondary piggyback set container and wipe the upper injection port of the primary line (i.e., port closest to the drip chamber) with an alcohol sponge.
Step 6. Insert the needleless tip from the secondary line into the injection port.

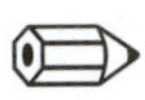 **NOTE:** Most needle-free systems have a Luer-Lok device that secures the secondary administration set to the primary set port.

Step 7. To run the secondary set container by itself, lower the primary set container with the extension hook that comes in the secondary administration box.
Step 8. Open the clamp and adjust the drip rate.

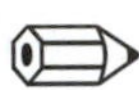 **NOTE:** As the secondary infusion begins, the backcheck valve will close from pressure, stopping the primary solution from infusing. When the secondary infusion has emptied, the backcheck valve will open, allowing the primary solution to begin infusing.

SIMULTANEOUS INFUSION (PRIMARY AND SECONDARY)

Secondary infusions can be infused concurrently with the primary solution. Rather than connecting the intermittent infusion at the piggyback port, it is attached to the lower Y site (Fig. 10–1B). Disadvantages of administration of secondary concurrent with primary solution include the tendency for blood to back up into the tubing after the secondary infusion has been completed, causing occlusion of venous access device and increased risk of drug incompatibility. Drug incompatibility is a greater risk with the simultaneous infusion method.

INTERMITTENT INFUSIONS THROUGH A LOCKING DEVICE

Medication administered by intermittent infusion is usually diluted in 1 to 50 mL of infusate and infused over a 1 to 15 minutes. An intermittent infusion is attached directly to an I.V. lock. Saline or heparinized saline is used to maintain patency of the lock.

Advantages

- Incompatibilities are avoided.
- A minimal amount of fluid is provided to the patient on restricted intake.
- Minimal drug is wasted.

Disadvantages

- If the fluid container runs dry, blood backs into the cannula and tubing and could cause a clot.
- After each infusion of medication, the lock must be flushed with heparinized saline or saline (depending on agency policy) to maintain patency.

PROCEDURE 10–3: ADMINISTRATION OF INTERMITTENT MEDICATION THROUGH LOCKING DEVICES

Verify the physician's order, educate the patient regarding the purpose of therapy, and document the procedure and any patient teaching you may have performed.
Step 1. Wash hands.
Step 2. Flush lock with 1 to 2 mL of 0.9 percent sodium chloride.
Step 3. Infuse the drug at the prescribed rate.
Step 4. After the drug delivery, flush the lock with 0.9 percent sodium chloride.

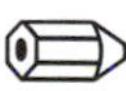 **NOTE:** In the absence of an antireflux valve, exert positive pressure on the syringe when withdrawing from the I.V. lock to prevent a backflow of blood into the I.V. catheter.

VOLUME CONTROL CHAMBER

The volume control chamber method of intermittent delivery of medication is used most frequently with pediatric patients or when the delivery of small amount of well-controlled drug needs to be administered to critical care patients. Medication is added to the volume control chamber and diluted with I.V. solution. The infusion is generally over 15 minutes to 1 hour. Volumes delivered vary from 25 to 150 mL per drug dose (Fig. 10–2).

Advantages

- Runaway infusions are avoided without the use of electronic infusion devices.
- Volume of fluid in which the drug is diluted can be adjusted.

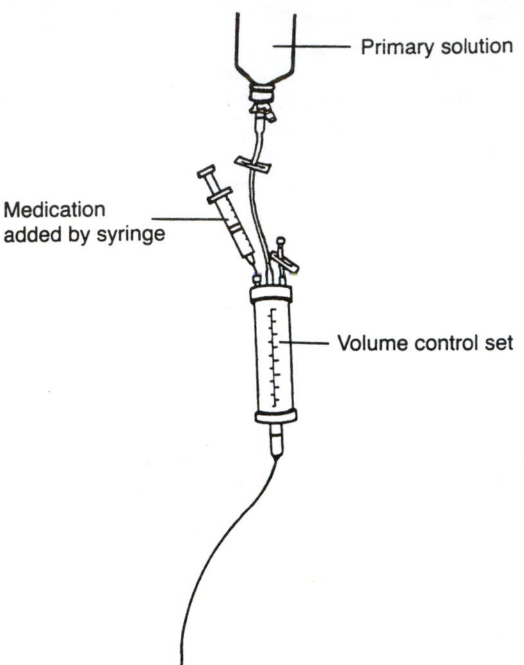

FIG. 10–2. Administration of medication via a volume control chamber.

Disadvantages

- Medication must travel the length of the tubing before it reaches the patient, causing a significant time delay.
- A portion of the medication can be left in the tubing after the chamber empties.
- Incompatibilities may develop when the chamber, which is usually within the primary line, is used for multiple drug deliveries.
- Labeling of the chamber must coincide with the drug's being delivered. If multiple drugs are delivered, this could present a problem.

DIRECT INJECTION (I.V. PUSH)

Intravenous push administration of a medication provides a method of administering high concentrations of medication. Administration through this route can be accomplished by direct penetration of a vein, by penetration of vein using a syringe, and needle scalp vein infusion set or over-the-needle infusion device, or by access of low injection port of primary administration sets. The purpose is to achieve rapid serum concentrations.

Direct injection requires that the drug be drawn into a syringe before administration or that the drug be available in a prefilled syringe. Needle protector or needle-free systems can be used connected to the venous access device or with administration sets to deliver the medication (Baldwin, 1995).

Advantages

- Barriers of drug absorption are bypassed.
- Drug response is rapid and usually predictable.
- The patient is closely monitored during the full administration of the medication.

Disadvantages

- Adverse effects occur at the same time and rate as therapeutic effects.
- The I.V. push method has the greatest risk of adverse effects and toxicity because serum drug concentrations are sharply elevated.
- Speed shock is possible from too-rapid administration of medication.

Adverse effects that can occur during administration of a medication directly into a vein include changes in the patient's level of consciousness, vital functions, and reflex activity.

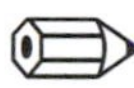

NOTE: If adverse effects occur, supportive care is the basis for treatment of most symptoms because specific antidotes are available for only certain drugs.

PROCEDURE 10–4: DIRECT ADMINISTRATION (I.V. PUSH)

Verify the physician's order, educate the patient regarding the purpose of therapy, and document the procedure and any patient teaching that you may have performed.

Step 1. Check the compatibility of the drug with the primary solution.

Step 2. Dilute opioid narcotics and follow the recommendation of the manufacturer for administration.

Step 3. Swab the lowest Y port with alcohol.

Step 4. Insert a needleless tip with a syringe attached into the medication port.

Step 5. Pinch the tubing to the primary solution.

Step 6. Inject one fourth of the medication into the patient over a 15- to 20-second period.

Step 7. Unpinch the tubing, allowing the primary solution to flush. Watch the patient for any adverse effects.

Step 8. Repeat steps 5 to 7, delivering one fourth of the drug each time for three more times.

Step 9. When all of the desired drug is delivered, remove the syringe.

(continued)

(continued)

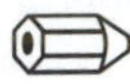

NOTE: This procedure should take at least 1 minute; however, always follow the recommendations of the manufacturer for the delivery of the drug. For example, drugs such as phenytoin and diazepam must be delivered over a lengthy period of time; the manufacturer provides specific guidelines for administration.

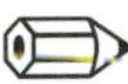

NOTE: The Centers for Disease Control and Prevention (CDC, 1995) recommended that heparin only be used when intermittent infusion devices are used for blood sampling. Heparin is no longer routinely recommended for intermittent flushing.

CONTINUOUS SUBCUTANEOUS MEDICATION ADMINISTRATION

Continuous subcutaneous infusion is a practical and simple approach to pain management. Two factors that contribute to unsatisfactory pain management are (1) inadequate dosage and titration of available pain medications and (2) limited resources to properly educate and advise physicians and nurses on pain management. Patients who require parenteral narcotics are candidates for continuous subcutaneous infusion. This type of infusion therapy can be established for the following types of patients who require intermittent injection, usually longer than 48 hours:

- Patients unable to take medications by mouth
- Patients who require subcutaneous injections for more than 48 hours
- Patients who require parenteral narcotics but have poor venous access

Advantages

- Easy care for home management of pain
- Decreased number of times tissue is traumatized by repeated injections
- Better home management of pain, which decreases hospital time
- Decrease in central nervous system (CNS) side effects associated with intermittent drug therapy, such as nausea, vomiting, and drowsiness
- Decrease in pain breakthrough

Disadvantages

- Local irritation at infusion site
- Rapidly escalating pain of dying patients requiring larger volumes of drug; this route is inappropriate for volumes larger than 1 mL/h

PROCEDURE 10–5: ADMINISTRATION OF CONTINUOUS SUBCUTANEOUS INFUSION

Verify the physician's order, educate the patient regarding the purpose of therapy, and document the procedure and any patient teaching you may have performed.

Step 1. Establish baseline vital signs.
Step 2. Have the patient rate his or her pain on a scale of 1 to 10.
Step 3. Establish subcutaneous access per hospital policy and use continuous infusion guidelines.
Step 4. Use a 24-gauge catheter with a 26-gauge insertion needle. The Soft-set (MiniMed Technologies) also has a 42-inch microbore tubing attached to the infusion device, which can then be attached to a PCA pump. This system has a Luer-Lok hub. The tubing is made of polyfin, which is compatible with most drug deliveries.
Step 5. Prime tubing if needed.

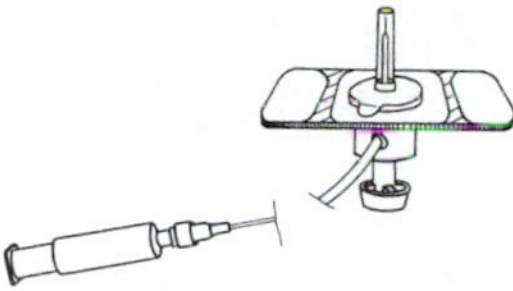

1. Fill syringe and Sof-set. ™

Step 6. Cleanse site with povidone-iodine swab stick.

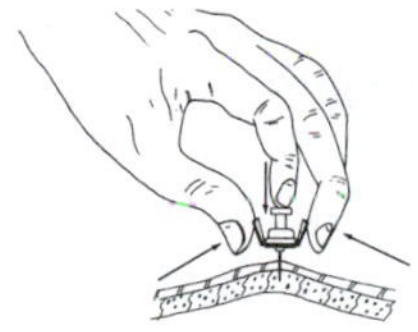

2. Cleanse and pinch skin.

Step 7. Insert the needle perpendicular to the skin.

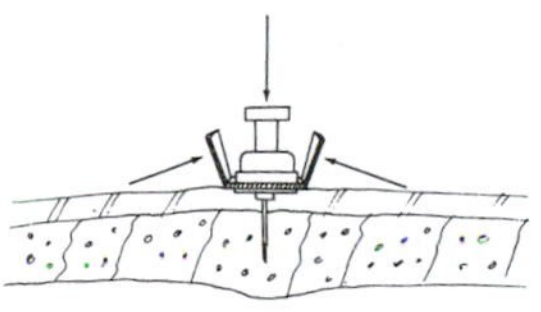

3. Insert needle.

(continued)

(continued)

Step 8. Stabilize the needle or catheter following manufacturer recommendations.

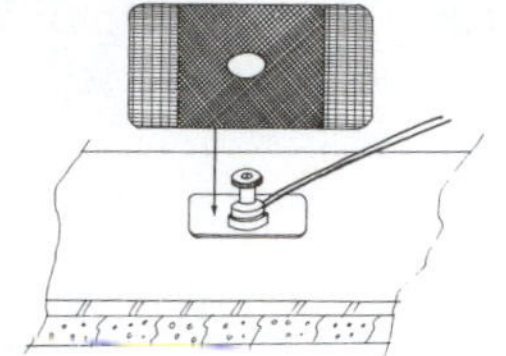
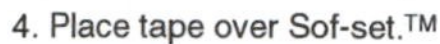

4. Place tape over Sof-set.TM

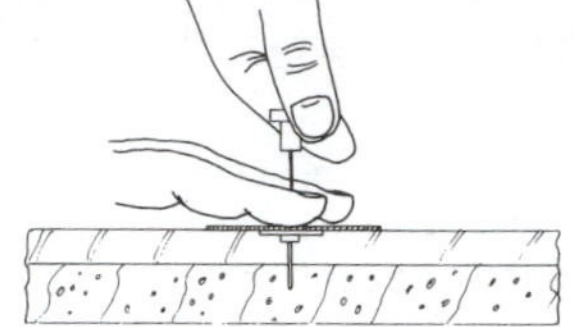

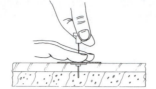

5. Remove introducer needle.

Step 9. Administer the prescribed bolus dose and immediately begin the continuous infusion.

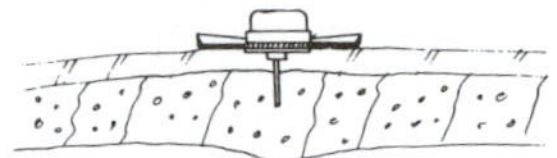

6. Begin pumping.

Step 10. Obtain vital signs and assess neurologic status and pain level every 30 minutes (four times) and as needed.

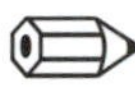

NOTE: The character of the skin is important; the skin surface must be dry, and body hair may need to be clipped, not shaved. Use an adhesive bandage to secure subcutaneous device.

(Figures Courtesy of MiniMed Technologies, Sylmar, California.)

INTRAPERITONEAL MEDICATION ADMINISTRATION

An intraperitoneal catheter has been developed for the treatment of patients with intra-abdominal malignant tumors. A Tenckhoff dialysis catheter or port is surgically placed and chemotherapeutic agents are instilled directly into the intraperitoneal cavity. Access to the peritoneal cavity can be achieved through the use of a temporary catheter. Ovarian and colorectal cancers often have a high incidence of peritoneal seeding when a patient undergoes surgical treatment for intra-abdominal adenocarcinoma or sarcoma (West, 1998). (The intraperitoneal route is discussed in Chapter 13.)

INTRAOSSEOUS MEDICATION ADMINISTRATION

Intraosseous infusion, or the administration of drugs or solutions through a needle inserted into the bone marrow of children younger than age 6 years is common practice in the emergency room setting. This route is used when conventional routes cannot be used. Indications for the use of intraosseous route include patients with extensive burns or trauma for which diffuse edema causes difficult peripheral access; profound shock resulting in poor circulatory system; and combative behavior, making any catheter insertion difficulty. (The intraosseous route is discussed in Chapter 9.)

INTRAVENTRICULAR MEDICATION ADMINISTRATION

Intraventricular access sites using an Ommaya reservoir are used for:

1. The delivery of antifungal agents to treat fungal meningitis and brain abscesses
2. The delivery of antibacterial drugs for the treatment of chronic CNS infections
3. The delivery of chemotherapy for treatment of meningeal leukemia and neoplastic infiltration of the CNS
4. Intrathecal administration of methotrexate to patients who have primary intraocular lymphoma with CNS spread
5. Intractable pain control in patients with advanced head and neck cancer
6. Administration of medications through a temporary ventriculostomy to relive rapid increases in intracranial pressure
7. In patients with unresectable tumors as a means to drain excessive fluid accumulation caused by cystic brain tumors
8. The regular intrathecal removal of cerebrospinal fluid (CSF) to monitor drug levels in patients receiving antibiotic therapy

The intraventricular route related to administration of chemotherapeutic agents is discussed in Chapter 13.

INTRA-ARTERIAL MEDICATION ADMINISTRATION

The intra-arterial route is used for the delivery of chemotherapy through the blood supply to a tumor. The arteries most commonly used are the hepatic artery (for colorectal metastasis to the liver), the celiac artery (for liver tumors), and the carotid artery (for tumors of the head, neck, and brain). The pelvic arteries have been used to infuse high concentration of antineoplastic medications to treat patients with advanced cervical cancer (West, 1998). (The intra-arterial route is discussed in Chapter 13.)

INTRASPINAL MEDICATION ADMINISTRATION

There are two types of intraspinal catheters: epidural and intrathecal. Intraspinal catheters are used:

1. For postoperative acute pain
2. For pain management when chronic pain cannot be controlled by

conventional treatment modalities or when conventional methods restrict a patient's mobility
3. When treating cancer cells that cross the blood-brain barrier
4. To treat severe spasticity in neurologically impaired patients

Intraspinal catheters can be temporary external catheters or more permanent tunneled catheters, ports, or implanted pumps. The type of catheter chosen is based on the patient's diagnosis and medical condition.

A temporary catheter is in place for several hours to no more than 14 days. This type of catheter places patients at risk for infection. For patients receiving therapy longer than 14 days, a catheter may be tunneled from the intraspinal space to an exit onto the abdominal wall (Fig. 10–3). Ports are used with epidural catheters and accessed with noncoring needles. Implanted pumps are used for administering intraspinal medications (West, 1998). Intraspinal analgesia does not cause the CNS side effects that systemic narcotic delivery may cause.

THE EPIDURAL AND INTRATHECAL SPACES

The spinal anatomy consists of two spaces, the **epidural** space and the **intrathecal** space. **Intraspina**l is the term used to encompass both the epidural and intrathecal spaces surrounding the spinal cord. The intrathecal space is surrounded by the epidural space and separated from it by the dura mater; the intrathecal space contains CSF, which bathes the spinal cord. The epidural and intrathecal spaces share a common center, the spinal cord. The epidural space surrounds the spinal cord and intrathecal space and lies between the ligamentum flavum and the dura mater. This is a potential space because the ligamentum flavum and the dura mater are not separated until medication or air is injected between them. This potential space contains a venous network of veins that are large and thin walled and has a strong leukocytic activity to reduce the risk of infection. Dividing epidural and intrathecal spaces is a tough, fatty membrane called the dura. The dura's permeability is important in determining how fast epidural drugs cross into the intrathecal space and how long they remain there to be active. The epidural space also contains fat in proportion to a person's body fat. Opiate receptor sites are cells contained in the dorsal horn of the spinal cord, at which point opioids combine with their respective receptor site to generate analgesia.

Local anesthetic agents are frequently used with intraspinal narcotics and are instrumental in controlling pain and reducing postoperative complications. When a patient experiences acute pain, the sympathetic system (part of the autonomic nervous system) is activated, increasing the workload of the heart. When intraspinal local anesthetic agents are administered, a sympathetic block results, which produces a decrease in blood pressure, pulse, and respirations. The advantages of adding local anesthetic agents to an epidural narcotic are that it produces a sympathetic block, resulting in decreased workload on the heart, and decreases the incidence of thrombophlebitis and paralytic ileus (St. Marie, 1995).

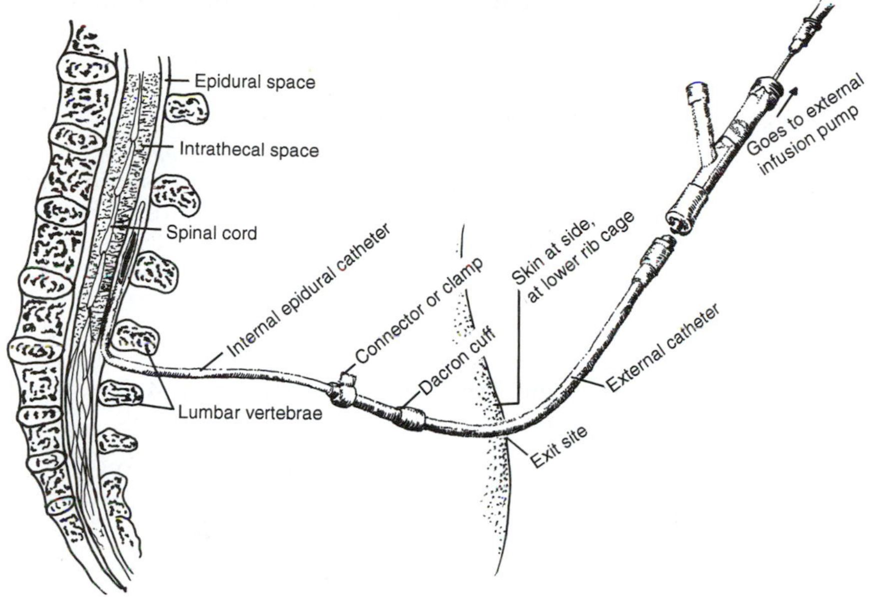

FIG. 10–3. Epidural catheter for pain relief. (From St. Marie, B. [1989]. Administration of intraspinal analgesia in the home care setting. *National Intravenous Therapy Association, 12*[3], 166. Copyright 1989 by the National Intravenous Therapy Association. Reprinted by permission.)

GENERAL SIDE EFFECTS OF INTRASPINAL MEDICATION DELIVERY

The goal of managing side effects with intraspinal narcotic infusions is early intervention. Common side effects include nausea, vomiting, urinary retention, pruritus, and respiratory depression. Nausea and vomiting can be controlled with antiemetics such as prochlorperazine (Compazine).

Excessive drowsiness or confusion can occur when too much narcotic is being administered. This is usually improved by decreasing the amount of epidural narcotic infusion. Titrating an opioid antagonist, such as naloxone (Narcan), 0.2 mg I.V., or an agonist/antagonist, such as nalbuphine (Nubain), 5 to 10 mg subcutaneously, may reverse side effects without eliminating the analgesia (St. Marie, 1995).

Urinary retention is a common side effect and may occur 10 to 20 hours after the first injection of intraspinal narcotic. This may require either administration of bethanecol (Urecholine) or intermittent catheterization.

Pruritus is caused by the opiate's interacting with the dorsal horn and not by a histamine release. This is best treated with an antagonist rather than with diphenhydramine (Benadryl). After an epidural injection, 8.5

percent of all patients experience pruritus; after an intrathecal injection *46 percent experience pruritus.*

EPIDURAL MEDICATION ADMINISTRATION

The epidural route can be used for acute and cancer pain management. There are various approaches to the administration of narcotics by the epidural route: a single-bolus injection of narcotic or local anesthetic, a continuous infusion of narcotic with or without local anesthetics, or a continuous infusion of narcotic with a patient-activated bolus. Medications commonly administered through the epidural route include preservative-free morphine (Astromorph and Duramorph), sublimaze (Fentanyl) and bupivacaine (Marcaine). See Figure 10–4 for various methods of epidural administration.

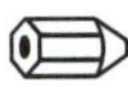

NOTE: Preservatives in narcotics or local anesthetics used in the epidural or intrathecal space need to be avoided to prevent nerve damage.

Advantages

- Permits control or alleviation of severe pain without the sedative effects
- Permits delivery of smaller doses of a narcotic to achieve desired level of analgesia
- Prolongs the analgesia (average about 14 hours)
- Allows for continuous infusion, if needed
- Allows terminal cancer patients treated with epidural narcotics to be more comfortable and mobile
- Can be used for short-term or long-term therapy
- Does not produce motor paralysis or hypotension

Disadvantages

- Nurses' lack of understanding of pharmacologic agents; nurses must be educated in the use of these agents.
- Only preservative-free narcotics can be used.
- Complications such as paresthesia, urinary retention, and respiratory depression (greatest 6 to 10 hours after injection) can occur.
- Catheter-related risks (e.g., infection, dislodgement, and leaking) can occur.
- Pruritus can occur on the face, head, and neck or may be generalized.

INS STANDARDS Placement of an epidural catheter, port, or pump is a medical act. Administration of medication by a registered nurse (RN) shall be in accordance with the state Nurse Practice Act. (INS, 2000, 67)

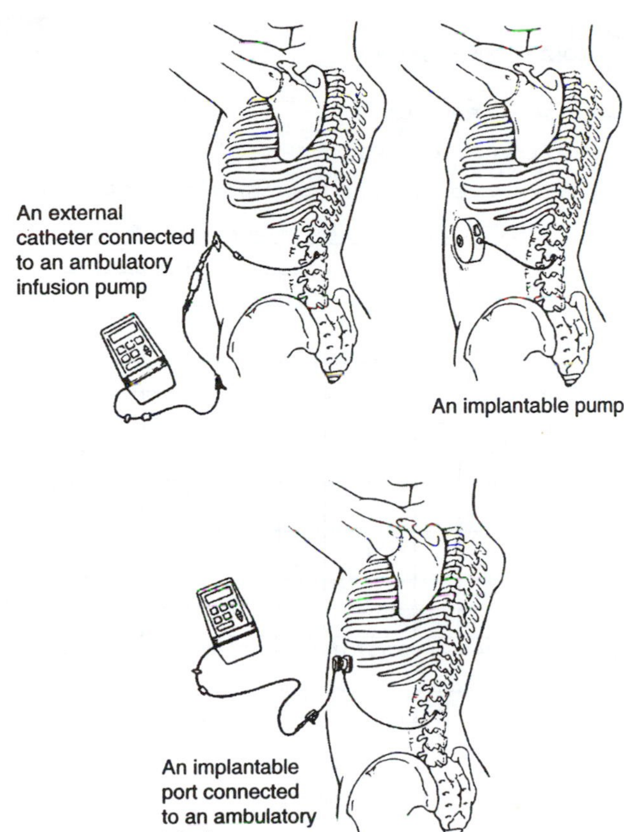

FIG. 10–4. Methods of epidural administration. (Courtesy of SIMS Deltec, Inc., St. Paul, Minnesota.)

Key Points in Epidural Catheter Management

The insertion of the epidural catheter is a sterile procedure and is a function performed by a physician or anesthesiologist. Administration of medication by a nurse through an epidural catheter must be in accordance with each state's Nurse Practice Act.

Nursing responsibilities include: (1) patient and family education, (2) site and dressing management, (3) medication administration (depending on State Practice Acts), and (4) evaluation of pain relief.

Key points in management include:

1. Avoid the use of preservatives (mainly alcohol, phenol, sodium metabisulfite) in medications because they have a destructive effect on neural tissue (West, 1998).
2. After insertion, lay the exposed catheter length cephalad along the spine and over the shoulder. Tape the entire length of the

EPIDURAL FLOWSHEET
INTERMITTENT OR CONTINUOUS INFUSION

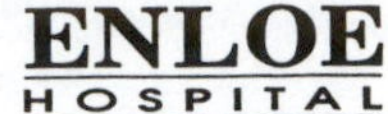

DATE ____________ MEDICATION ____________

EDUCATION: CHART ON BACK OF FLOW SHEET

1) INTERMITTENT INJECTIONS: VS Q 15" X 2 THEN Q 4 HOURS
2) CONTINUOUS INFUSION: VS Q 15" X THEN Q 4 HOURS
A) RESP., SEDATION LEVEL, MOTOR RESPONSE, DERMATOMES (ANESTHETICS) Q 1 HOUR X 4, THEN Q 2 HOURS

FOR ANY INFUSION RATE INCREASE RETURN TO INITIAL ASSESSMENT FREQUENCIES

TIME															
TERMPERATURE															
BLOOD PRESSURE															
PULSE															
RESPIRATIONS															
SEDATION LEVEL															
PAIN SCALE															
SITE ASSESS .Q8°															
MOTOR RESPONSE NO DEFICIT															
DERMATOMES LEVEL/RESPONSE															
S/SX TOXICITY															
INITIALS															

ASSESS PAIN Q 4 HOURS FOR ALL TYPES OF EPIDURAL ANALGESIA

SEDATION LEVEL

3 – Alert/Awake
2 – Occassionally drowsy, easy to awake
1 – Frequently drowsy, easy to arouse
0 – Somnolent, difficult to arouse
S – Normal sleep, easy to arouse

ANESTHETICS S&SX TOXICITY

Circumoral tingling
Muscle twitching
"Metallic" taste/tinnitus

PAIN

0 – 10 scale
0 – no pain
10 – worst pain

DERMATOMES
(Anesthetics only)

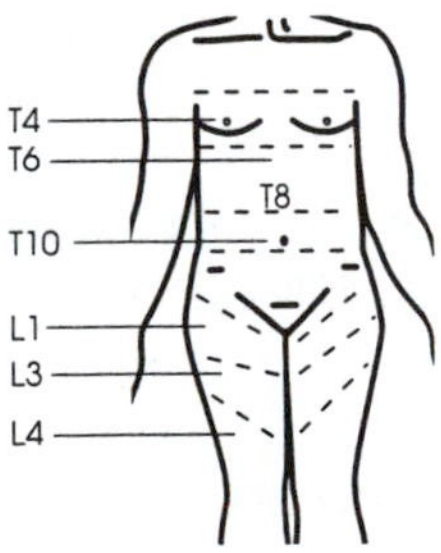

Signatures
(07–15) ____________
(15–23) ____________
(23–07) ____________

Addressograph

S6002277 5/93 PRINTED BY THE GRAPHIC FOX, INK., CHICO

FIG. 10–5. Example of continuous or intermittent epidural flowsheet. (Courtesy of Enloe Medical Center, Chico, California.)

exposed catheter in place to provide stability and protection. The end of the catheter and the filter are generally placed on the patient's chest wall and taped securely in a position that allows the patient or family member to access the catheter for use.

3. To prevent particulate matter from infusing into the spinal fluid, an inline filter should always be used when accessing any intraspinal catheter.
4. Clearly label the epidural catheter after placement to prevent accidental infusion of fluids or medications.
5. Understand the lipid and water solubility properties of the drugs being administered. (This better prepares the nurse to work with patients receiving epidural or intrathecal analgesic agents through the various methods of administration.)
6. Evaluate the effects of the drug on the patient's alertness; caregivers should also be taught to observe for levels of sedation.

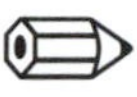

NOTES: Site care must be done carefully to avoid dislodgement of the catheter.

Ineffective pain control should be reported to the physician or anesthesiologist that is managing care of the epidural catheter.

INS STANDARDS A 0.22-micron filter without surfactant should be utilized for medication administration.

The epidural device should be aspirated to ascertain the absence of spinal fluid before administration of medication. (INS, 2000, 67)

Monitoring

A flowsheet (Fig. 10–5) should be used to monitor the patient's response to epidural medication. This allows tracking of the patient's analgesia and any side effects. Included on the flow sheet are:

- Evaluation of mental status
- Respiratory status
- Indication of numbness in the lower extremities
- Signs of infection
- Bowel function
- Bladder function
- Integrity of the epidural system
- Narcotic dose
- Patient's pain rating
- Site care

PROCEDURE 10–6: ADMINISTRATION OF MEDICATION VIA AN EPIDURAL CATHETER

Verify the physician's order, educate the patient regarding the purpose of therapy, and document the procedure, including any patient teaching you may have performed.

(continued)

(continued)

Step 1. Check the anesthesiologist's order, narcotic dosage, and route. Ensure that naloxone (Narcan) or ephedrine is readily available. Double check for correct medication (preservative-free diluent), dose, and route before administration.

Step 2. Verify that the estimated level of the catheter tip and the initial dose are documented by the anesthesiologist.

Step 3. Inform the patient of the procedure.

Step 4. Assemble the equipment; wash hands with chlorhexidine.

Step 5. Complete a patient assessment including inspection of the catheter site for signs of injection and cerebral spinal fluid drainage; pain level; baseline vitals signs; response to previous injection; and urinary bladder fullness.

Step 6. Secure the entire hub apparatus by sandwiching with transpore tape.

Step 7. Draw up the dose into a 10-mL or larger size syringe using a filter needle.

Step 8. Attach pulse oximetry monitor to the patient (if ordered).

Step 9. Don gloves, scrub the injection port with a povidone-iodine swab, and allow 2 minutes of contact time. Wipe with sterile 2 × 2 gauze to remove any excess povidone-iodine.

Step 10. Enter the injection cap using the 10-mL empty syringe. Gently aspirate to verify catheter location by observing that less than 1 mL of fluid returns.

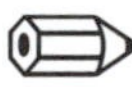

NOTE: If the aspirate is blood, blood-tinged fluid, or greater than 1 mL of fluid, notify the anesthesiologist and do not continue the procedure. Save the aspirated fluid.

Step 11. Rescrub the injection cap with a povidone-iodine solution for 20 seconds. Wipe with a sterile 2 × 2 gauze to remove any excess povidone-iodine. Enter the injection port with the 10-mL syringe that contains the prescribed preservative-free analgesia. Slowly inject the narcotic at a rate of approximately 5 mL/min.

Step 12. Check the catheter cap and hub assembly connection for fluid leakage.

Step 13. Closely monitor the patient's vital signs, and pain level every 15 minutes × 2, then every 4 hours.

Step 14. Document initial and ongoing assessments in the nurses' notes; any changes in the patient's condition; all communication with the physician; and education provided to the patient.

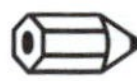

NOTES: Have naloxone (Narcan) available, 0.4 mg, to treat respiratory depression or increased sedation.

Never use alcohol for site preparation or for accessing the catheter because of the potential for alcohol migration into the epidural space.

Dressing Management of Epidural Catheter

Epidural catheter dressings should only be changed if they loosen and are no longer occlusive. Temporary epidural catheters are not sutured into place and can become dislodged very easily. During the dressing change, the nurse must carefully stabilize the epidural catheter. This is a sterile procedure.

1. Wash hands with antimicrobial soap and water for at least 1 minute.
2. Remove old dressing. Use a cotton ball soaked in sterile water to assist in lifting the edge of dressing.
3. Wet a cotton-tipped applicator in povidone-iodine solution; clean the area starting at the catheter, working outward in a circular motion. Repeat two more times and allow the area to dry. (Note whether any crusted areas are around the catheter; if so, remove them by using a swab dipped in hydrogen peroxide before using the povidone-iodine or Hibiclens.)
4. Apply a new transparent dressing.
5. Remove the tape holding the catheter end, clean skin under the tape, allow to dry, and retape for comfort and safety (St. Marie, 1995).
6. The catheter should be coiled near the insertion site to prevent accidental dislodgement.

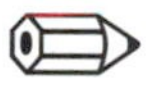

NOTE: Do not use alcohol on skin or at dressing site because of the risk of migration of alcohol into the epidural space and the possibility of neural damage.

Complications Associated with Epidural Pain Management

Complications associated with epidural analgesia are not common. Complications may arise form several sources. Patients may have a reaction or side effect to the medication being administered or a problem resulting from the placement or displacement of the catheter. Conditions requiring **immediate** physician notification include:

- Respiratory depression
- Extreme dizziness as a result of inadequate orthostatic hypotension or excessive narcotic effect
- New onset of paresthesia or paresis
- Difficulty or inability to infuse epidural medication
- Pain at the insertion site
- Disruption or displacement of the epidural catheter
- Signs and symptoms of local or systemic infection
- Inadequate pain relief
- Signs and symptoms of coagulopathies
- Inability to remove the catheter
- Circumoral tingling
- Tremulousness

- Tinnitus
- Metallic taste
- Ascending loss of sensation in patients receiving an anesthetic medication

Other complications that may not warrant immediate physician notification but need to be reported at the earliest convenience include the inability to urinate and pruritus, which may be treated with parenterally administered medication while the epidural infusion continues.

Nurses must assess adequate pain control carefully. Inadequate pain relief can occur for three reasons: epidural catheter migration, insufficient dosages of narcotics and local anesthetics, and undetermined surgical complication.

Respiratory depression from epidural or intrathecal narcotic administration is a risk. Vital signs should be assessed and naloxone should be available to reverse the depressant effects of a narcotic.

Infections are rare from epidural catheters, but precautions should be instituted to keep the catheter insertion process and exit site sterile. If an infection develops elsewhere in the body, the patient should be evaluated for removal of the epidural catheter (St. Marie, 1995).

Catheter migration may occur in two ways: (1) the catheter may migrate through the dura mater into the intrathecal space, creating an overdose of narcotic, or (2) the catheter may migrate into an epidural vein or subcutaneous space, creating inadequate pain relief.

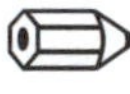
NOTE: If catheter migration is suspected, the physician should be notified and the placement check should be verified by an anesthesiologist.

INTRATHECAL MEDICATION ADMINISTRATION

The intrathecal injection of a narcotic requires approximately 10 times less medication than is needed in the epidural space. The intrathecal space, however, is associated with a greater risk for infection. Intrathecal narcotic infusions may be considered for cancer patients who have a life expectancy of more than a few months who do not receive adequate pain relief with systemic narcotics, tricyclic antidepressants, or nonsteroidal anti-inflammatory drugs (NSAIDs) and who have pain located below the midcervical dermatomes. Intrathecal narcotics given as a single injection is commonly administered for cesarean surgeries, vaginal hysterectomies and some orthopedic surgeries. Intrathecal infusions of narcotics require an implanted infusion pump, not an external pump, because of the risk of infection (St. Marie, 1995).

Advantages

- Useful for delivery of certain antineoplastic agents, antibiotics, analgesics, and anesthetic agents.
- Effective alternative to oral or parenteral therapy for abatement of

pain associated with cancer because of direct delivery of narcotic to opiate receptors in the brain and spinal column.
- Allows for low doses of drug to produce the same degree of analgesia as high doses required systemically.

Disadvantages

- Possible life-threatening side effects.
- Potential for spinal fluid leak.
- Potential infection.

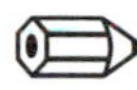

NOTE: When an intrathecal catheter is attached to an implanted pump, the manufacturer's guidelines regarding aspiration must be followed.

INS STANDARDS Mask and sterile gloves are worn for access and maintenance procedures (INS, 2000, 67). A 0.2 micron filter without surfactant should be utilized for medication administration (INS, 2000, 67).

Complications Associated with Intrathecal Medication Delivery

Parameters for monitoring site care and managing complications and side effects are the same as for epidural infusions. There is a greater risk of infection with intrathecal medication administration because the CSF is a good medium for bacteria. Spinal headache may occur, especially in young women.

The most effective remedy for spinal headache is a blood patch. This is performed by drawing approximately 10 mL of blood from the patient's arm and injecting the blood epidurally near the level of the original insertion of the intrathecal needle. This blood gels over the dural puncture and prevents CSF from leaking out of the dural hole, stopping the headache (St. Marie, 1995).

Implanted Pumps

Design features of an implanted pump include a pump reservoir designed to continuously infuse a specific volume of medication over a specific period of time. A sterile occlusive dressing should be placed over the noncoring needle.

INS STANDARDS The smallest gauge noncoring needle that can deliver the prescribed therapy should be used. (INS, 2000, 51)

ARTERIOVENOUS FISTULA

An arteriovenous (AV) fistula facilitates accessing of the vascular system. AV fistulas are used for administration of parenteral therapies.

INS STANDARDS The nurse should determine the integrity of the fistula by palpation and/or auscultation before cannulation. (INS, 2000, 52)

KEY POINTS IN THE DELIVERY OF ARTERIOVENOUS PARENTERAL THERAPY

- The nurse must be knowledgeable regarding the type of fistula that is in place: synthetic, bovine graft, or anastomosis.
- The integrity of the graft site must be determined before venipuncture by palpation and auscultation.
- Sterile technique must be used; wear sterile gloves.
- Potential complications include, but are not limited to, infection, occlusion, and thrombosis.

INS STANDARDS Arterial pressure within the AV fistula increases the potential for bleeding. Therefore when removing the stylet from the catheter, or removing the cannula from the fistula, techniques should be employed to reduce the potential for bleeding. (INS, 2000, 52)

SPECIAL DRUG ADMINISTRATION CONSIDERATIONS

ANTI-INFECTIVES

Before administering antibiotic, antifungal, and antiviral agents intravenously, it is essential to understand the pharmacotherapeutics related to these drugs. Manufacturer recommendations for administration should be followed carefully. Anti-infectives are administered to achieve therapeutic coverage based on culture and sensitivity reports.

Key Questions

1. Has the infecting organism been identified (suspected or confirmed by culture)?
2. Is the organism resistant to any antimicrobials?
3. Is the site of infection identified?
4. What is the status of the host (patient) defenses?
5. Is the nurse familiar with the antimicrobial pharmacokinetics?
6. What is the status of the patient's renal and hepatic function?
7. Is monitoring the patient's blood levels necessary to avoid toxicity of dosage?
8. Does the patient have an allergy to the anti-infective agent? (Kuhn, 1998)

Table 10–3 provides anti-infective I.V. medication guidelines.

Antibiotics

Antibiotic's action is bacteriostatic, inhibiting bacterial cell wall synthesis and producing a defective cell wall, or bactericidal, altering intracellular function of the bacteria. Knowledge of each antibiotic administered is essential for safe delivery of the medication.

TABLE 10–3

ANTI-INFECTIVE I.V. MEDICATION GUIDELINES

Category	Drug	Key Points
Antibiotics	Aminoglycosides	● Assess for muscle weakness. ● Assess blood urea nitrogen (BUN) and serum creatinine levels. ● Assess balance and hearing functions for any damage to the eighth cranial nerve.
	Cephalosporin	● Be aware of nephrotoxic effects. ● Do not administer if patient is sensitive to penicillin. ● Rotate sites often; high risk for phlebitis. ● Monitor renal function with BUN and creatinine. ● Use cautiously in pregnant and lactating women.
	Chloramphenicol	● Only administer I.V. ● Assess for bone marrow suppression.
	Erythromycin	● High risk of phlebitis. ● One of the safest antibiotics.
	Fluoroquinolones	● Maintain fluid intake to prevent crystalluria. ● Can cause venous irritation; administer over 60 minutes.
	Macrolides	● Can cause phlebitis (erythromycin); dilute in at least 100 mL of sodium chloride or 5% dextrose ● Beware of transient hearing loss. ● Interaction: Aminophyllin and tetracycline can cause toxic theophylline levels.
	Penicillins	● Can cause phlebitis. ● Never administer procaine penicillin I.V. ● Interaction: Aspirin increases blood levels. ● Concomitant use of bacteriostatic agents decreases the activity of penicillin.

(Continued)

ANTI-INFECTIVE I.V. MEDICATION GUIDELINES *(Continued)*

Category	Drug	Key Points
Antibiotics *(Continued)*	Tetracycline	● Do not administer to patients with liver dysfunction or renal failure. ● Assess patient for superinfections. ● I.V. site must be rotated frequently because of potential venous irritation and thrombophlebitis.
Antifungals	Amphotericin B	● Light sensitive, but protection is not necessary. ● Use in hospitalized patients only. ● Monitor vital signs, intake, and output. ● During therapy, frequently test renal and liver function. ● To reduce nephrotoxic effects: Administer mannitol, 12.5 g, before and after each dose. ● Incompatibility*:* Not compatible with any solution with a pH below 4.2. ● Do not mix with any drug unless absolutely necessary; there are many incompatibilities.
	Fluconazole	● Administer in a glass system. ● Inadequate treatment may lead to recurrent infection. ● Hepatotoxicity may occur; if any signs and symptoms of liver disease exist, laboratory analysis should be done and the drug discontinued. ● Incompatibility*:* Manufacturer states: "Do not add supplemental medication."
	Miconazole	● Monitor blood counts, electrolytes, and lipids. ● Can be administered intrathecally and as bladder irrigant. ● Pruritus is a common side effect. ● Incompatibility: Incompatible in syringe or solutions with any other drug.

(Continued)

TABLE 10–3

ANTI-INFECTIVE I.V. MEDICATION GUIDELINES ***(Continued)***

Category	Drug	Key Points
Antivirals	Acyclovir	● Can cause renal tubular damage if too rapidly infused; make sure patient is adequately hydrated. ● Incompatibility: Blood products, dobutamine, protein solutions, or dopamine.
	Cidofovir	● Dilute in 100 mL of 0.9% sodium chloride; solution is stable for 24 hours. ● Prehydrate patient before administration to minimize renal toxicity.
	Ganciclovir	● Follow guidelines for handling cytotoxic drugs. ● Maintain hydration. ● Assess renal function; frequent blood counts. ● Do not use during pregnancy unless justified. ● Incompatibility: Any other drug or solution because of alkaline pH, blood products, and protein solutions. ● Has numerous side effects, such as anemia, which may be life threatening. ● Use caution in cerebral edema or potential fluid overload. ● Toxicity may be increased by nephrotoxic or cytotoxic drugs. ● Protect from light.
	Foscarnet	● Monitor patient for renal impairment. ● Prehydration required before infusion.
Antiretrovirals	Zidovudine	● I.V. infusion only until oral therapy can be administered. ● Dilute dose with D5W or 0.9% NaCl for concentration of <4 mg/mL. ● Infuse at a constant rate over 1 hour. ● Monitor CBC every 2 weeks during the first 8 weeks because of the potential for developing anemia.

General Nursing Considerations

1. Be knowledgeable of the antibiotic ordered, it's normal dosage, side effects, and compatibilities, and the purpose of the antibiotic in treatment of the patient's infection.
2. Be sure the drug has not expired.
3. Be familiar with reconstitution, dilution, and storage information.
4. Correctly label the admixture with drug name, concentration, diluent, date, time, and initials.
5. Be familiar with potential adverse effects of the drug.
6. Use strict aseptic technique throughout administration.
7. Be aware that the drug must be delivered at specified times to ensure maintenance of the proper drug levels and to identify therapeutic, subtherapeutic, and toxic drug levels.
8. Use assessment skills to monitor functions of the organ or organs that metabolize the antibiotic.
9. Evaluate the patient every shift for sensitivity to the drug.
10. Be prepared to respond to anaphylaxis.

Antifungals

The method of action of antifungal agents is injury to the cell wall of the fungi. The drugs in this classification are specifically targeted for fungi. Two antifungals, amphotericin B and fluconazole, can be given by the I.V. route. The most frequently administered antifungal agent by I.V. route is amphotericin B.

Key points in delivery of antifungal agents include: (1) most are infused as a suspension; (2) these drugs should not be filtered, and (3) they should be administered slowly over 2 to 6 hours.

Antivirals

Antiviral agents are selectively toxic to viruses. A safe, broad-spectrum antiviral drug has yet to be discovered. Most chemicals administered by the I.V. route to combat virus growth are antimetabolites or are related to the antimetabolites used in treating malignant tumors. These drugs tend to be toxic and usefulness is limited. They are administered in selected situations. For all antivirals, avoid use in patients with a previous hypersensitivity reaction. Use cautiously in patients with renal impairment, in pregnant patients, and in children. Presently there are five antiviral agents that are infused by the I.V. route: acyclovir, cidofovir injection, foscarnet, ganciclovir, and zidovudine (Gahart & Nazareno, 1999).

NARCOTICS

Pain management begins with complete assessment of the patient's pain, including location, intensity, quality, frequency, onset, duration, aggravating and alleviating factors, associated symptoms, and coping mechanisms. Pain perception and tolerance are highly individual responses. According to McCafferty and Beebe (1989), the definition of pain is "whatever the experiencing person says it is, existing whenever he says it does."

Many therapeutic approaches are available for pain including behavioral approaches, application of heat and cold, massage, physical therapy, management with narcotics and non-narcotics by oral, subcutaneous, or I.V. routes, neurosurgery, and anesthetics.

The World Health Organization and the American Pain Society (1989) have grouped analgesia into three types: options, non-narcotic analgesics and nonsteroidal anti-inflammatory drugs (NSAIDs), and adjuvants.

Opioids include narcotic analgesics and narcotic agonists. Non-narcotic analgesics, nonopioids, and NSAIDs provide relief of mild to moderate pain. Adjuvants include drugs to treat other signs and symptoms of pain, such as depression, anxiety, and nausea; often these are referred to as coanalgesics.

Parenteral narcotics can be delivered by continuous infusion or by intermittent dosing. The routes for continuous infusion include the I.V., subcutaneous, and intraspinal (epidural or intrathecal) routes (Table 10–4).

Continuous Infusion

Morphine is the narcotic most commonly used for continuous infusion for pain management. Continuous infusions lead to a continuous level of pain control without the peaks of side effect development and the troughs of breakthrough pain. A smaller amount of the drug is generally needed to prevent the recurrence of the pain. Continuous infusions of narcotics are appropriately used in trauma, postsurgical, and terminal care settings.

Intermittent Dosing (Patient-Controlled Analgesia)

The concept of patient-controlled analgesia (PCA) began in 1970. PCA is a pain management strategy that allows a patient to self-administer I.V. narcotic pain medication by pressing a button that is attached to a computerized pump. Patients may receive intermittent doses of narcotics when they state that the pain is episodic. It is desirable to treat pain only when experienced, with fast-acting narcotics that are effective for short periods. The goal of PCA is to provide the patient with a serum analgesia level for comfort with minimal sedation. Putting patients in charge of their own pain management makes sense because only the patient knows how much he or she is suffering.

NOTE: It is more desirable to use small doses of narcotics frequently than large doses of narcotics infrequently.

New Joint Commission on Accreditation of Healthcare Organizations (JCAHO) standards that integrate pain assessment and management into

TABLE 10–4

I.V. NARCOTIC ADMINISTRATION GUIDELINES

Category	Drug	Key Points
Narcotic agonists	Meperidine	• Avoid in patients with impaired renal function. • Must be diluted. • Shorter acting than morphine. • Not recommended I.V. in children. • Use with caution in patients with glaucoma, head injuries, chronic obstructive pulmonary disease. • Cough reflex is suppressed.
	Morphine	• Use with caution in patient with impaired ventilation, bronchial asthma, increased intracranial pressure, liver failure. • Should be diluted.
	Hydromorphone	• Use with caution in patients with head injuries, respiratory depression, and increased intracranial pressure. • Slightly shorter duration than morphine. • Should be diluted.
	Levorphanol	• Accumulates on days 2 to 3, long half-life. • I.V. is not usual route of choice; subcutaneous is the usual route.
Narcotic agonist/ antagonists	Pentazocine	• May cause psychotomimetic effect. • Contraindicated in patients with previous myocardial infarction. • Low addictive element. • Contraindicated in children under age 12 years. • May be given undiluted.
	Nalbuphine	• Use with caution in patients with head injuries, pregnancy, lactation. • May be given undiluted.
	Butorphanol	• Use with caution in patients with respiratory depression, head injuries, and impaired liver or kidney function. • May be given undiluted.

(Continued)

TABLE 10–4

I.V. NARCOTIC ADMINISTRATION GUIDELINES *(Continued)*

Category	Drug	Key Points
Narcotic partial agonists	Buprenorphine	● May produce withdrawal in narcotic-dependent patients. ● Use with caution in patients with asthma, respiratory depression, or impaired renal or hepatic function. ● Contraindicated in children younger than age 12 years. ● May be given undiluted.

the JCAHO accreditation standards have been approved. These new standards will appear in all of the year 2000 to 2001 accreditation manuals. The standards call on accredited hospitals, home care agencies, long-term care facilities, behavioral health facilities, outpatient clinics, and health plans to:

- Recognize the right of patients to appropriate assessment and management of their pain.
- Assess pain in all patients.
- Record the results of the assessment in a way that facilitates regular reassessment and follow up.
- Educate relevant providers in pain assessment and management.
- Determine competency in pain assessment and management during the orientation of all new clinical staff.
- Establish policies and procedures that support appropriate prescription or ordering pain medications.
- Ensure that pain does not interfere with participation in rehabilitation.
- Educate patients and their families about the importance of effective pain management.
- Include the patient's needs for symptom management in the discharge planning process.
- Collect data to monitor the appropriateness and effectiveness of management (JCAHO, 1999).

Key points in providing safe, adequate pain relief include:

1. Define the types of patients to use the PCA device.
2. Develop teaching tools.
3. Select the appropriate equipment.
4. Select the medications used and establish consistency of use and dosage.
5. Define who will handle the side effects and provide an appropriate method of communication (St. Marie, 1991).

Candidates for whom PCA should be considered include:

1. Patients who are anticipating pain that is severe yet intermittent (e.g., patients suffering from kidney stones)
2. Patients who have constant pain that worsens with activity
3. Pediatric patients who are older than age 7 years who are capable of being taught to manage the PCA machine
4. Patients who are capable of manipulating the dose button
5. Patients who are motivated to use PCA

Key concepts of PCA include:

1. In the first 24 hours after surgery, the patient has the greatest need for pain control.
2. Studies have shown that the best results for PCA occur when the patient can administer a bolus every 5 to 10 minutes.
3. When patients have control of their narcotic doses, they will keep the narcotic within therapeutic levels.
4. When patients are in control and know they can get more immediate pain relief by pushing a button, they are more relaxed.
5. Analgesia is most effective when a therapeutic serum level is consistently maintained.
6. Postoperative patients can easily titrate doses according to need and avoid peaks and troughs associated with conventional I.V. and intramuscular administration of narcotics.
7. Studies have found that orthopedic patients seemed more tolerant of repositioning when on PCA.
8. Patients with abdominal surgery ambulate sooner after surgery.
9. Patients whose pain is controlled are better able to cough and deep breathe.

WEB SITES: American Academy of Pain management: *www.aapainmanage.org*
American Pain Society: *www.ampainsoc.org*
Other:____

INVESTIGATIONAL DRUGS

Administration of investigational medications shall be in accordance with state and federal regulations. Signed informed patient consent is required before patient participation in the investigation.

Investigational drugs are defined as medications that are not approved for general use by the Food and Drug Administration (FDA). Many **clinical trials** are conducted as a form of planned experiment that evoke appropriate treatment of future patients with a given medical condition. Clinical trials are designed to discover a drug's efficacy in selected patient populations.

Following are the phases of FDA drug studies:

Phase I: Clinical pharmacology and therapeutics

- Evaluate drug safety.
- Determine an acceptable single drug dosage for levels of patient tolerance for acute multiple dosing.

Phase II: Initial clinical investigation for therapeutic effect

- Evaluate drug efficacy.
- Conduct a pilot study.

Phase III: Full-scale evaluation of treatment

- Evaluate the patient population for which the drug is intended.

Phase IV: Postmarketing surveillance

- Provide additional information about the efficacy or safety profile.

The role of the registered nurse in investigational drugs is to assist the investigator (physician) in conducting the study.

Key points in the role of the nurse in investigational drugs include:

1. Communicating with Institutional Review Board (IRB); being familiar with their policies and federal regulations (copies of communication between the investigator and the IRB should be given to the sponsor)
2. Writing informed consent, explaining to patient, and obtaining signature
3. Communicating with the hospital's legal counsel and ethics committee to complete protocols
4. Administering the investigational drug by the I.V. route (or as indicated)
5. Participating in collection of data
6. Assisting with blood sampling when required
7. Assisting with final study report, which is a requirement of the U.S. federal regulations for the sponsor

General ethical requirements of clinical research worldwide are outlined in the Declaration of Helsinki, issued by the World Medical Association in 1960 and revised in 1975. This document has been accepted internationally as the basis for ethica l research.

NURSING PLAN OF CARE

ADMINISTRATION OF I.V. MEDICATIONS

Focus Assessment

Subjective

- Review present illness.
- Review current drug therapy.
- Review previous drug therapy and side effects.
- Review lifestyle for home care.
- Note any allergies before starting medication.

Objective

- Observe the patient's ability to ingest and retain fluids.
- Monitor vital signs.
- Weigh the patient.
- Assess patient-related factors that may alter the patient's response to drug, such as age or renal, liver, and cardiovascular function.
- Assess current medications for clues to drug interaction and incompatibility.

Patient Outcome Criteria

The patient will:

- Respond therapeutically to the drug.
- Demonstrate improved fluid balance.
- Verbalize understanding of the purpose of the medication.
- Demonstrate absence of complications associated with I.V. therapy.

Nursing Diagnoses

1. Altered health maintenance related to limited skills of family members with I.V. medications
2. Anxiety (mild, moderate, severe) related to threat to or change in health status; misconceptions regarding therapy
3. Diarrhea related to side effects of medication
4. Impaired physical mobility related to pain and discomfort resulting from placement and maintenance of I.V. catheters
5. Risk for injury related to altered electrolyte balance resulting from drug administration
6. Fluid volume deficit related to inadequate oral intake secondary to nausea and vomiting
7. Impaired tissue integrity related to adverse reaction to medication

Nursing Management

1. Develop and use an environment that maximizes safe and efficient administration of medications.
2. Follow the five rights of medication administration.
3. Verify the prescription or medication order before administering the drug.

(continued)

(continued)

4. Select the appropriate sizes of syringes and needles.
5. Determine the correct dilution, amount, and length of administration time as appropriate.
6. Monitor drug infusion at regular intervals.
7. Monitor for irritation, infiltration, and inflammation at the infusion site.
8. Maintain I.V. access.
9. Administer drugs at selected times.
10. Monitor the therapeutic range of drug levels.
11. Note the expiration date on the medication container.
12. Administer medication using the appropriate technique.
13. Monitor for therapeutic response.
14. Monitor renal function for adequate excretion of drug through the kidneys.
15. Monitor for allergies, drug interactions, and drug incompatibilities.
16. Dispose of unused or expired drugs according to agency policy.
17. Monitor intake and output.
18. Maintain strict aseptic technique.
19. Monitor for need of pain relief medications, as needed.
20. Sign narcotics and other restricted drugs according to agency protocol.
21. Document medication administration and patient responsiveness.

PATIENT EDUCATION

- Patient education on I.V. medication administration is vital for the acute care and alternative settings. When possible, patient education should begin before a patient's discharge from the hospital to facilitate a smooth transition to home care.
- The education should begin with instructions outlining the insertion of the I.V. catheter and step-by-step details of the procedure for all peripheral, midline, and peripherally inserted central catheter (PICC) line insertions. All potential complications after insertion and the patient or responsible party should sign an informed consent.
- Routine maintenance care involved in central line management for medication infusions should be provided.
- Fully instruct the patient about the infusion pump; written step-by-step instruction with diagrams or pictures and manufacturer manuals are excellent tools. Include troubleshooting instructions and telephone numbers to call for 24-hour assistance.
- Instructions on proper handwashing, setting up the infusion pump with medication, flushing the catheter, and self-administration of the medication must be included in patient training sessions.
- Instruct the patient on the expected actions and adverse effects of medication.
- The patient or caregiver must be taught the procedure of drug administration clearly and in simple terminology.
- Provide a checklist to help evaluate the steps in the learning process; this also provides a method of documenting the completion of self-drug administration.
- Instruct the patient on administration of anti-infectives around the clock to maintain blood levels (Hammond, 1998).

HOME CARE ISSUES

The rapidly growing home care infusion industry now provides many I.V. drugs. Medications that are now being delivered in the home include cardiovascular drugs, antihypertensives, antibiotics, heparin, interferon, colony-stimulating factors, chelation therapy (deferoxamine), growth hormones, gammaglobulin, and medications for pain management.

Individuals can receive medical therapies outside the hospital to maximize their independence. A number of methods exist for delivery of medication intravenously in the home environment: gravity, I.V. push, or ambulatory pump.

Safety. Patients who are able to care for themselves are the best candidates for using ambulatory pumps and usually make the adjustment quickly.

Effectiveness. To ensure effective treatment, coordination of care among the patient, nurse, physician, and pharmacist is essential.

Acceptance. Unless the patient understands the treatment, procedure, and administration regimen and accepts them into his or her lifestyle, home drug therapy will not be successful.

Cost. Delivering drug therapy at home is cost-effective as long as it effectively treats the problem. Medicare and third-party payers have recognized financial savings using this method (Brown, 1988).

ANTI-INFECTIVES

Computerized ambulatory infusion devices (drug pumps) have enabled antimicrobial therapy to be safely and effectively administered in the home with minimal disruption in the patient's life. When administering antimicrobials in the home, safety, effectiveness, acceptance, and cost need to be considered.

Cost savings assist the growth of outpatient intravenous antibiotic therapy each year. The basic models for delivery of outpatient intravenous antibiotic therapy (OPIVAT) can be divided into three types: (1) the visiting nurse model, (2) the infusion center model, and (3) the self-administration model (Tice, 1996).

HOME NURSING

Advantages: Opportunity for home inspection, supervised drug administration

Disadvantage: The costs of nurse time and travel

OUTPATIENT INFUSION CENTERS

Advantages: Medial resources readily available and can be combined with visits to the physician

Disadvantage: The patient has to travel to the clinic and the cost of clinic overhead

(continued)

HOME CARE ISSUES *(continued)*

SELF-ADMINISTRATION

Advantage: Reduced staff costs and overhead, patient autonomy

Disadvantage: Unsupervised administration and patient education and training

The I.V. push method in the home for anti-infective drug delivery has become a safe and effective route with properly trained staff using standardized policies and procedures. Low incidences of complication exist with all types of access device using the I.V. push method. It was found that there was no significant difference in phlebitis rates among delivery methods. The I.V. push method was found to be cost-efficient for delivery of anti-infectives in the alternative setting (Markel-Poole, Nowobilski-Vasilios & Free, 1999).

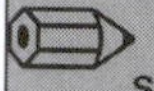

NOTES: As with any I.V. medication delivery, emergency drugs should be readily available and protocols established for their use.

Clinical assessment of the patient on antibiotics is based on the same standards regardless of the treatment environment, including monitoring for adverse reactions, disease processes, and laboratory tests.

PAIN MANAGEMENT

For home use, the epidural catheter may be attached to a preprogrammed infusion pump containing a medication cassette that requires replacing on a weekly basis.

Teach the patient and caregiver on how the intraspinal catheter works and the importance of keeping appointments for pump refills.

WHEN THE PATIENT SHOULD CALL THE HOME CARE NURSE

- Side effects from the drug
- Particles floating in the medication
- Discoloration of the medication
- Leaking medication bags
- Instructions when medication schedule has been altered for any reason
- Pump malfunction
- Problems with intravenous line (e.g., inability to flush, bleeding at site, pain, redness, swelling)
- I.V. dressing becomes loose
- I.V. line out of the vein
- Medication label does not match the orders from the physician

KEY POINTS

- Advantages of I.V. medications include provides a direct access to the circulatory system; provides a route for drugs that irritate the gastric mucosa; provides a route for instant drug action; provides a route for delivering high drug concentrations; provides for instant drug termination if sensitivity or adverse reaction occurs; provides a route of administration in patients in whom use of the GI tract is limited.
- Disadvantages of I.V. medications include drug interaction because of incompatibilities; adsorption of the drug being impaired because of leaching into the I.V. container or administration set; errors in compounding of medication; speed shock; extravasation of a vesicant drug; chemical phlebitis.
- Common errors in administering medications include: lack of knowledge about drugs, errors in drug identity checking, mistakes in calculations, and improper use of pumps and controllers.
- Drug incompatibility fall into three broad categories: physical, chemical and therapeutic.
- I.V. medication can be delivered by continuous infusion, intermittent infusion, and I.V. push through a locking device.
- The subcutaneous infusion route is used for 48 hours for patients unable to take medications by mouth and who have poor venous access.
- The intraventricular route via an Ommaya reservoir can be used for delivery of medications directly to the brain.
- There are two types of intraspinal catheters: epidural and intrathecal.
- Epidural and intrathecal administrations provide superior pain control, require small doses, and produce longer periods of relief between doses while preventing many systemic side effects.
- Alcohol must **NEVER** be used for site preparation or for accessing an intraspinal catheter. Only preservative-free medications can be delivered by the intraspinal routes.
- The intraperitoneal route is used when high concentrations of medication need to be delivered directly into the peritoneal cavity.
- Administration of investigational medications must be in accordance with state and federal regulations
- Phases of FDA drug studies:
  Phase I: Clinical pharmacology and therapeutics
  Phase II: Initial clinical investigation
  Phase III: Full-scale evaluation and treatment
  Phase IV: Postmarketing surveillance

CHAPTER ACTIVITIES

COMPETENCY CRITERIA: Epidural Management
COMPETENCY STATEMENT: Competent I.V. nurses will demonstrate management of epidural catheters.
Note: The cognitive (knowledge) information embedded within this performance-based competency includes spinal anatomy and physiology; actions and side effects of morphine, sublimaze, dilaudid, and demerol; and complications associated with epidural medication administration. This competency *links* to the competency of infection control.

Performance	Skilled	Needs Education
Critical Action Statements		
1. Confirms catheter tip placement and affirms test dose administered by physician		
2. Confirms emergency equipment available at bedside or on unit		
3. Demonstrates use of preservative-free medications		
4. Labels epidural catheter as designated line		
5. Demonstrates use of electronic infusion device to administer continuous medication		
6. Demonstrates use of 0.22-micron filter on epidural catheter		
7. Performs patient assessment of: A. Site and catheter integrity B. Level of pain, baseline vital signs C. Patient response to injection		
8. Demonstrates use of povidone-iodine to scrub injection port		
9. Completes epidural flow sheet to monitor patient's response to epidural medication		

EVALUATION CRITERIA
1. Validation of management of epidural catheter with preceptor.

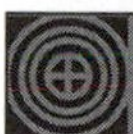

CRITICAL THINKING ACTIVITY

1. The patient requires pain medication and the order is for 2 mg of morphine I.V. every 2 hours as needed for pain. Discuss the key points to remember when delivering this medication by the I.V. push route.

2. You are working in a small rural outpatient clinic. A patient comes in in respiratory distress with electrolyte imbalance. The physician orders a primary solution of 5 percent dextrose and 0.45 percent normal saline with vitamins B and C and aminophyllin. Also ordered is 20 mEq of potassium chloride to be administered over 2 hours. No pharmacist is available to assist you with this admixture. How do you infuse these medications and how do you check for compatibility?

3. You are mixing two medications in one syringe for an I.V. push administration. The solution has turned a pale yellow. Can you safely administer this drug? If not, what type of incompatibility is this?

4. A patient complains of burning from the antibiotic that was just started. The antibiotic is diluted in 100 mL of 5 percent dextrose in water piggybacked to run 45 minutes. What alternatives do you have for dealing with this complaint?

POST-TEST

1. Which of the following are incompatibilities of I.V. therapy?
   a. Intermittent, physical, and biotransformation
   b. Drug interaction, drug synergism, and drug tolerance
   c. Physical, chemical, and therapeutic
2. Methods by which a registered nurse can deliver medication via the I.V. route include all of the following **EXCEPT:**
   a. I.V. push (bolus)
   b. Continuous subcutaneous infusion
   c. Continuous infusion
   d. Piggyback
   e. Epidural
3. The key point(s) in infusion of I.V. antifungal drugs is(are):
   a. Most are infused as a suspension
   b. They should not be filtered
   c. They should be administered slowly
   d. All of the above
4. WHO and the American Pain Society have grouped analgesics into which three categories?
   a. Opioids, non-narcotic nonsteroid, and adjuvants
   b. Anesthetics, non-narcotic, and cholinergics
   c. Adrenergics, opioids, and opiates
5. I.V. push medications should be administered according to manufacturer's recommendations but not faster than:
   a. 10 minutes
   b. 5 minutes
   c. 1 minute
   d. 30 seconds
6. The goal of patient-controlled analgesia is to provide the patient with:
   a. A serum analgesia level for comfort without sedation
   b. A serum analgesia level to achieve sedation
   c. A method of euthanasia
   d. Limited control over pain management
7. Which of the following agencies is involved in investigational drug protocols?
   a. FDA
   b. CDC
   c. IRB
   d. EPA
8. Which of the following are side effects of epidural pain medication?
   a. Urinary retention, pruritus, and respiratory depression
   b. Respiratory depression, peptic ulcer, and hemiparesis
   c. Pruritus, nausea, and urinary incontinence

9. Clear fluid in the syringe after aspiration of an epidural catheter is an indication of catheter:
   a. Patency
   b. Kinking
   c. Migration
   d. Damage
10. All of the following are key points in the delivery of epidural infusions **EXCEPT:**
   a. Use only alcohol swabs to prepare site
   b. Use only povidone-iodine swabs to prepare site
   c. Use a 0.2-micron filter without surfactant for medication administration
   d. Aspirate the catheter to ascertain the presence of spinal fluid

REFERENCES

American Pain Society (1989). *Principles of Analgesic Use in the Treatment of Acute Pain and Chronic Cancer Pain. A Concise Guide to Medical Practice* (2nd ed.). Skokie, IL: American Pain Society.

Baldwin, D.R. (1995). Pharmacology. In Terry, J., Baranowski, L., Lonsway, R., & Hedrick, C., eds. *Intravenous Therapy: Clinical Principles and Practice.* Philadelphia: W.B. Saunders, pp. 192–195.

Boger, J.E., DeLuca, S.T., Watkins, D.F., et al. (1997). Infusion therapy with milrinone in the home care setting for patients who have advanced heart failure. *Journal of Intravenous Nursing,* 20(3), 148–154.

Cohen, M.R. (1997). IV drug safety. *INS Newsline,* September/October, 3.

Deglin, J.H., & Vallerand, A.H. (1999). *Davis's Drug Guide for Nurses* (6th ed.). Philadelphia: F.A. Davis.

Gahart, B.L., & Nazareno, A.R. (1999). *Intravenous Medications* (15th ed.). St. Louis: Mosby.

Giger, J.N., & Davidhizar, R.E. (1999). *Transcultural Nursing: Assessment & Intervention.* St. Louis: Mosby, pp. 138–139.

Hammond, D. (1998). Home intravenous antibiotics: The safety factor. *Journal of Intravenous Nursing,* 21(2), 81–95.

Holland, M.S., Gammill, B.G., & Mackey, D.C. (1990). New technologies in anesthesia: Update for nurse anesthetists: Alternatives for postoperative pain management. American Association Nurse Anesthetists AANA journal course, 58, 210–211.

Hunt, M.L., & Rapp, R.P. (1996). Intravenous medication errors. *Journal of Intravenous Nursing*, supplement 19(3S), S9–S15.

Johnson, J.A., & Bootman, J.L. (1995). Drug-related morbidity and mortality. *Archives Internal Medicine,* 155, 1949–1956.

Joint Commission on Accreditation of Health Care Organizations (1999). *New JCAHO Pain Standards.* Available: *www.jcaho.org/standard/pm-frm.html*

Josephson, D.L. (1999). *Intravenous Infusion Therapy for Nurses: Principles and Practice.* Albany: Delmar Publishers.

Kennedy, D. (1996). Medication "safety checks" in pediatric acute care. *Journal of Intravenous Nursing,* 19(6), 295–306.

Kuhn, M. (1998). *Pharmacotherapeutics: A Nursing Process Approach* (4th ed.). Philadelphia: F.A. Davis.

Markel-Poole, S., Nowobilski-Vasilios A., & Free, F. (1999). Intravenous push medications in the home. *Journal of Intravenous Nursing,* 22(4), 209–215.

Nightingale, F. (1860). *Notes on Nursing.* New York: Appleton & Co.

Noah, V.A., & Godin, M. (1994). A perspective on di-20ethyl-hexyphthalate in intravenous therapy. *Journal of Intravenous Therapy,* (4), 210–211.

Pearson, S.D., & Trissel, L.A. (1993). Leeching of diethylhexylphalate for polyvinylchloride containers by selected drugs and formulation components. *American Journal of Hospital Pharmacy,* 50, 1405–1409.

Ryder, E. (1991). All about patient-controlled analgesia. *Journal of Intravenous Nursing,* 14(6), 372–379.

Snyder, E.L., Hedber, S.L., & Napychank, P.A. (1993). Stability of red cell antigens and plasma coagulation factors stored in a nondiethylhexyl phthalate-plasticized container. *Transfusion,* 33, 515–519.

St. Marie, B. (1995). Pain management. In Terry, J., Baranowski, L., Lonsway, R., & Hedrick, C, eds. *Intravenous Therapy Clinical Principles and Practices.* Philadelphia: W.B. Saunders, pp. 277–297.

Tice, A.D. (1996). Alternate site infusion: The physician-directed, office based model. *Journal of Intravenous Therapy,* 19(4), 188–193.

Weinstein, S.M. (1997). Plumer's principles and practices of intravenous therapy (6th ed.). Philadelphia: J.B. Lippincott.

West, V.L. (1998). Alternate routes of administration. *Journal of Intravenous Nursing,* 21(4), 221–231.

ANSWERS TO CHAPTER 10

Pre-Test

1. a, **2.** b, **3.** a, **4.** c, **5.** b, **6.** e, **7.** c, **8.** a, **9.** d, **10.** b

Post-Test

1. c, **2.** b, **3.** d, **4.** a, **5.** c, **6.** a, **7.** c, **8.** a, **9.** a, **10.** a

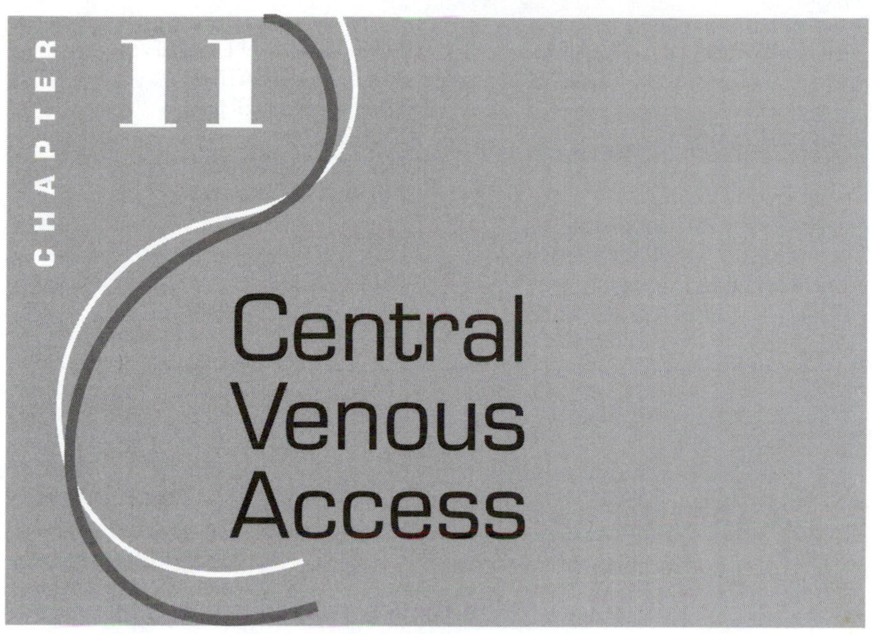

CHAPTER 11 Central Venous Access

As long as the beginner pilot, language learner, chess player, or driver is following rules, his performance is halting, rigid, and mediocre. But with the mastery of the activity comes the transformation of the skill, which is like the transformation that occurs when a blind person learns to use a cane. The beginner feels pressure in the palm of the hand, which can be used to detect the presence of distinct objects such as curbs. But, with mastery the blind person no longer feels pressure in the palm of the hand, but simply feels the curb. The cane has become an extension of the body.

Expert Performance, Dreyfus and Dreyfus, 1997

A similar transformation occurs with the expert nurse clinician's tools.

CHAPTER CONTENTS

LEARNING OBJECTIVES

Upon completion of this chapter, the reader will be able to:

1. Define the glossary of terms as related to central venous devices.
2. Discuss the hazard associated with percutaneous insertion of central lines: intravascular malpositioning and extravascular malpositioning.
3. Differentiate between short- and long-term access devices.
4. Identify the advantages of peripherally inserted central catheters (PICCs), tunneled catheters, and implanted ports.
5. Identify candidates for central line insertion.
6. Discuss the procedure for insertion of PICCs.
7. List the steps in dressing management of PICCs, tunneled catheters, and implanted ports.
8. Identify the complications associated with placement of PICCs, tunneled catheters, and implanted ports.
9. Identify the signs and symptoms of post-insertion complications associated with central lines.
10. Compare the advantages and disadvantages of tunneled catheters with the advantages and disadvantages of implanted ports.
11. Explain the differences in pressure gradients associated with the use of small- and large-barrel syringes in irrigating central lines.
12. Discuss the nursing management of tunneled catheters and implanted ports.

13 State the catheter tip location of PICCs and midclavicular line placements.

14 Discuss process for declotting of thrombotic and nonthrombotic occlusions of central lines.

15 Use the nursing process in providing nursing care to the patient with a central venous access device.

GLOSSARY

Anthropometric measurement Measurement of the size, weight, and proportions of the human body

Biocompatibility The quality of not having toxic or injurious effect on biological systems

Broviac catheter Tunneled venous catheter with one Dacron cuff with an outer diameter of 1.0; useful for infusion of nutrient solutions

CVC Central venous catheter

CVTC Central venous tunneled catheter

Distal Farthest from the heart; farthest from the point of attachment; below previous site of cannulation

Extravascular malpositioning Introducer of the central venous percutaneous catheter is passed out of the vessel and into the pleural space or the mediastinum

Groshong catheter Surgically implanted, long-term tunneled Silastic catheter; unique in that it has a two-way valve adjacent to the closed tip, which prevents backflow of blood

Hickman catheter Long-term tunneled Silastic catheter inserted surgically

Implanted port Catheter surgically placed into a vessel, body cavity, or organ and attached to a reservoir, which is placed under the skin

Infraclavicular Situated below a clavicle

Intravascular malpositioning Catheter tip of a percutaneous, tunneled, or implanted port coils in the vessel, which advances into a venous tributary other than the superior vena cava or does not reach the superior vena cava

Iontopheresis Method of delivering anesthesia without injection through the skin via an electronic device

Lymphedema Swelling of an extremity caused by obstruction of lymphatic vessels

Midclavicular Peripherally inserted catheter with the tip location in the proximal axillary or subclavian veins

Peripherally inserted central venous catheter (PICC) Long (20 to 24 in) I.V. access device made of a soft flexible material (silicone or a polymer); PICCs are usually inserted into one of the superficial veins of the peripheral vascular system with the tip location in the superior vena cava

Silicone Material containing silicone carbon bond, used as lubricants, insulating resins, and waterproofing materials

Thrombogenicity Generating or production of thrombosis

Trendelenburg position Position in which the head is lower than the feet; used to increase venous distention

Tunneled catheter Catheter designed to have a portion lie within a subcutaneous passage before exiting the body

VAD Vascular access device

Valsalva maneuver The process of making a forceful attempt at expiration with the mouth nostrils and glottis closed

PRE-TEST

Match the term in column I with the definition in column II.

COLUMN I	COLUMN II
1. CVC	a. Peripherally inserted central catheter
2. CVTC	b. Vascular access device
3. VAD	c. Central venous tunneled catheter
4. PICC	d. Central venous catheter

5. The advantage(s) of the peripherally inserted catheters include:
   - a. Decreases risk of pneumothorax and air embolism on insertion
   - b. Preserves peripheral vascular system in the upper extremity
   - c. Eliminates the pain of frequent venipunctures
   - d. Decreases cost and is time-efficient
   - e. All of the above
6. Which of the following is the best site selection for a PICC?
   - a. Basilic vein
   - b. Innominate vein
   - c. Jugular vein
   - d. Subclavian vein
7. The key point(s) in dressing management of PICCs include:
   - a. Change dressing after the first 24 hours
   - b. Inspect the catheter insertion site for redness, swelling, and drainage
   - c. Use care not to dislodge the catheter during the dressing change
   - d. Transparent dressing is recommended after the first 24 hours
   - e. All of the above
8. Complications related to the insertion of PICCs include:
   - a. Bleeding, malposition of the catheter, and nerve damage
   - b. Phlebitis, infection, and air embolism
   - c. Bleeding, cardiac arrhythmias, and infection
9. The advantage(s) of CVTCs include:
   - a. Can be repaired if catheter breaks or leaks
   - b. Is useful for all I.V. therapies
   - c. Eliminates multiple venipunctures
   - d. All of the above
10. When irrigating a CVC, the barrel capacity of the syringe should be:
    - a. 1 cc
    - b. 3 cc
    - c. 5 cc
    - d. 10 cc

ANATOMY OF THE VASCULAR SYSTEM

To understand the placement of central venous catheters (CVCs), it is important to understand the anatomy of the upper extremity venous system, arm, and axilla. The important veins include the basilic, cephalic, axillary, subclavian, internal and external jugular, right and left innominate (brachiocephalic) veins, and superior vena cava (SVC). It is also imperative that registered nurses are fully aware of the anatomic position and structures of the arm and axilla venous system when insertion of PICCs is desired.

VENOUS STRUCTURES OF THE ARM

The superficial veins of the upper extremities lie in the superficial fascia and are visible and palpable. Superficial veins include the cephalic and the basilic veins. The cephalic vein ascends along the outer border of the biceps muscle to the upper third of the arm. It passes in the space between the pectoralis major and deltoid muscles. The vein decreases in size just a few inches above the antecubital fossa and may terminate in the axillary vein or pass above or through the clavicle in a descending curve. Normally, the cephalic vein turns sharply (90 degrees) as it pierces the clavipectoral fascia and passes beneath the clavicle. Near its termination, the cephalic vein may bifurcate into two small veins, one joining the external jugular vein and one joining the axillary vein. Valves are located along the cephalic vein's course.

The basilic vein is larger than the cephalic vein. It passes upward in a smooth path along the inner side of the biceps muscle and terminates in the axillary vein. The origins of these veins in the lower arm are most often used for short-term peripheral devices. At and above the antecubital fossa, these veins are appropriate for the placement of **PICCs** and arm ports (Sansivero, 1998).

Valves are present in the venous system until approximately 1 inch before the formation of the brachiocephalic vein. The presence of valves within veins helps to prevent the reflux of blood and is especially important in the lower extremities, where venous return is working against gravity (Fig. 11–1).

VENOUS STRUCTURES OF THE CHEST

The venous structures of the chest include the subclavian, the internal and external jugular, and brachiocephalic veins (formerly called the innominate veins), and the SVC. Large veins in the head, neck and chest do not have valves. Gravity helps blood to flow properly from the head and neck, and negative intrathoracic pressure promotes flow from the head and neck and the inferior vena cava (Sansivero, 1998).

The subclavian vein extends from the outer border of the first rib to the sternal end of the clavicle and measures about 4 to 5 cm in length; the

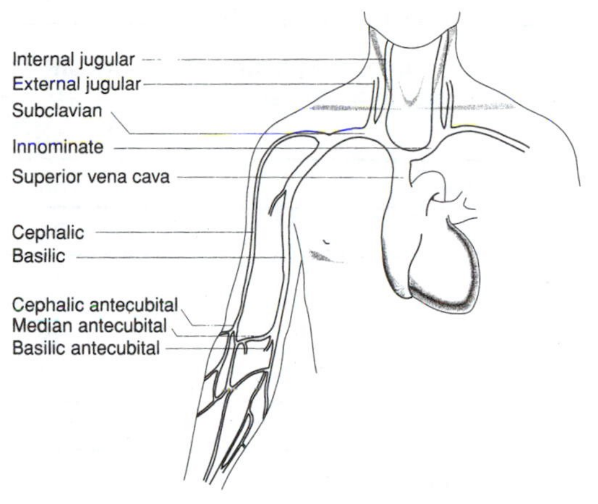

FIG. 11–1. Anatomic venous structures of the arm and chest. (Source: Markel, S., & Reynan, K. [1990]). Impact on patient care: 2652 PIC catheter days. *Journal of Intravenous Nursing, 13(6),* 349. Copyright 1990 by the *Journal of Intravenous Nursing.*)

right brachiocephalic vein measures about 2.5 cm, and the left brachiocephalic vein measures about 6 to 6.5 cm. The external jugular lies on the side of the neck and follows a descending inward path to join the subclavian vein along the middle of the clavicle. The internal jugular vein descends first behind and then to the outer side of the internal and common carotid arteries; it joins the subclavian vein at the root of the neck.

The right brachiocephalic vein is about 1 inch long and passes almost vertically downward to join the left innominate vein just below the cartilage of the first rib. The left brachiocephalic vein is about 2.5 inches long and is larger than the right innominate vein. It passes from left to right in a downward slant across the upper front of the chest. It joins the right brachiocephalic vein to form the SVC. The SVC receives all blood from the upper half of the body. It is composed of a short trunk 2.5 to 3.0 inches long. It begins below the first rib close to the sternum on the right side, descends vertically slightly to the right, and empties into the right atrium of the heart. The right atrium receives blood from the upper body via the SVC and from the lower body via the inferior vena cava. The venae cavae are referred to as the great veins. Table 11–1 summarizes the **anthropometric measurements** of the upper extremity veins.

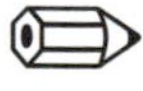 **NOTE:** Poiseuilleu's law (fourth power law) states that flow through a single vessel is most affected by the vessel diameter, and as vessel diameter increases, the flow rate increases by a factor of 4. For example, when the diameter doubles, flow rate increases 16 times (24); with a fourfold increase, the flow rate increases 256 times (44).

Central catheters should never be placed in the right atrium. When CVCs are placed in the right atrium, the risk of dysrhythmias, pericardial puncture, and fluid entry into the pericardial space can cause cardiac tamponade, a complication with a mortality rate of 78 to 98 percent.

TABLE 11–1

ANTHROPOMETRIC MEASUREMENTS OF VENOUS ANATOMY

Vein	Length, cm	Diameter, mm
Cephalic	38	6
Basilic	24	8
Axillary	13	16
Subclavian	6	19
Right brachiocephalic	2.5	19
SVC	7	20

SVC = superior vena cava.

CHOOSING THE VENOUS ACCESS DEVICE

Choosing the most appropriate **venous access device (VAD)** for a patient is a collaborative process involving the patient, the practitioner placing the device, and the patient's referring physician. Knowledge of venous anatomy and physiology, VAD technology, and the patient's current health status and infusion plan are important aspects in this process. The goal of VAD selection and placement should be to deliver safe, efficient therapy that maximizes the patient's quality of life.

ASSESSMENT PARAMETERS

Assessment parameters that must be considered before device selection and placement include patient characteristics, therapy characteristics, and device characteristics.

Patient characteristics include the suitability of target vessels that should be evaluated for size and patency. The vein must be large enough to accommodate the selected VAD to minimize the risk of phlebitis and thrombosis. The vein should fill when a tourniquet is applied, feeling firm but pliable to palpation. Patients who are very thin may benefit from the newer "low profile" devices.

Patient preference of the nondominant arm for ease of self-care should be considered if appropriate. The patient's lifestyle is an important consideration in choosing an implanted versus an external device. Take into consideration activity restrictions, maintenance requirements, body image distortion, and ease of use. The patient's usual occupational and recreational activities need to be included in the assessment process.

The ability of the patient or designated caregiver to manage day-to-day VAD care and infusions should be assessed before device selection and placement. The ability to see, hear, perform fine motor tasks, read and

TABLE 11–2

CONDITIONS AFFECTING VASCULAR ACCESS DEVICE SITE PLACEMENT

Previous surgical interventions	Lymph node dissections Subclavian vein stenting or resection Vena cava filters Myocutaneous flap reconstruction Skin grafts Previous vein harvesting Presence of A-V grafts and hemodialysis fistulas Presence of intravascular stents
Cutaneous lesions in proximity to VAD exit or puncture site	Herpes zoster Malignant cutaneous lesions Bacterial or fungal lesions Burns Extensive scarring or keloids
Disease process or conditions	Severe thrombocytopenia (<50,000 platelets) Other coagulopathy (i.e., hemophilia, idiopathic thrombocytopenia purpura, thrombotic thrombocytopenia purpura) Concurrent anticoagulation therapy Lymphedema Allergies Extremity paraplegia Preexisting vessel thrombosis or stenosis
Other considerations	Site within current radiation port Infection near exit site (e.g., tracheostomy) Morbid obesity Patient inability to position desired site for placement Patient inability to tolerate insertion procedure

understand written instructions, and emotionally cope with the demands of site care and therapy are important considerations.

Conditions That Limit VAD Placement

Conditions that may limit VAD site placement are listed in Table 11–2. These challenges can be overcome with careful device selection and placement.

Knowledge of the type of therapy can help identify the desired VAD and the number of lumens that will be necessary to deliver safe infusions. The number of concurrent and intermittent infusions along with drug compatibility and stability need to be considered (Sansivero, 1998). Nutritional solutions with final concentrations of 10 or 5 percent protein (or both) should be infused through a central line with the tip in the distal one third of the SVC (INS, 2000, 43).

Selection of Device

Selection of a device is influenced by the cost, risk factors, and benefits of various VADs in relation to any conditions that could limit VAD access, as well as patient and therapy characteristics.

The least expensive and invasive device is not necessarily the most appropriate selection, depending on the risks associated with peripheral infusions of irritant or vesicant agents. Using a venous access device selection algorithm along with a thorough patient assessment can help with device selection (Fig. 11–2).

CENTRAL VENOUS CATHETER MATERIALS

Most VADs are made of silicone elastomers, thermoplastic urethane (TPU), or polyvinyl chloride (PVC). Over the past 10 years, many technical advances in polymer research have provided medical manufacturers with a wide variety of new materials for catheter manufacturer. All catheters, whether they are used for short- or long-term access, should have a radiopaque lateral strip or a radiopaque distal end for visualization on radiography.

Polyvinyl Chloride

Polyvinyl chloride was the first catheter material. The material is stiff, can cause damage to the tunica intima, and carries with it a risk of platelet aggregation and subsequent thrombus formation. Current technology has provided other materials for CVCs that are less thrombogenic materials (Weinstein, 2000).

Silicone Elastomers

Silicone elastomers (Silastic) are soft and pliable and cannot be inserted by the conventional over-the-needle technique. Catheters made of Silastic require special insertion procedures with or without guidewires. Because of its soft, flexible nature, silicone is less likely to damage the intima of the vein wall and is reported to be less thrombogenic. Many PICCs are made of this biocompatible material.

Although **silicone** rubber posses a wide range of desirable properties, it is not well suited to blood-contacting applications because of its high degree of thrombogenicity. The surface "tackiness" and high coefficient of friction typical of silicone often result in difficulty with device insertion and a possibility of catheter fragmentation (Brown, 1995). There can be fibrin sheath formation when particulate matter is present.

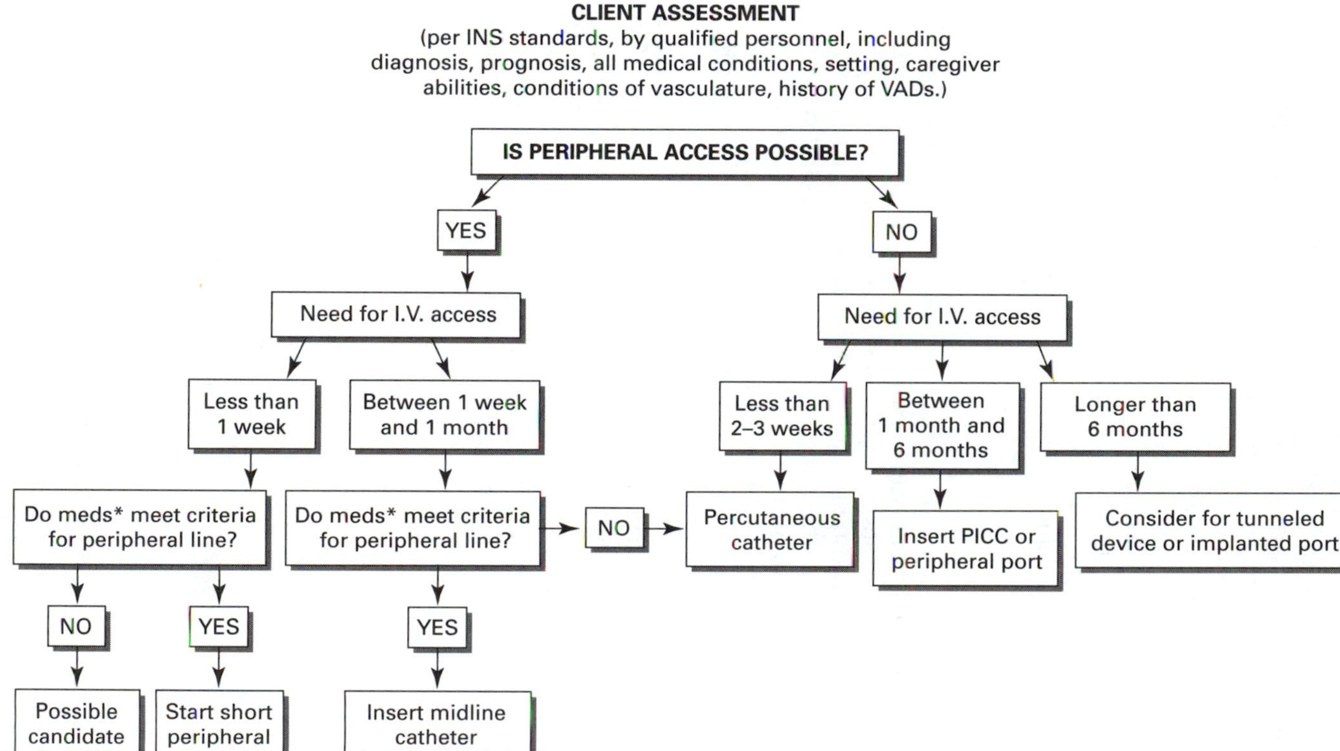

Medication criteria: Final osmolarity < 500 mOsm/L, pH between 5 and 9, not an irritant or vesicant.

FIG. 11–2. Venous access device selection algorithm.

Thermoplastic Polyurethane

TPU catheters may be emerging as the most commonly used catheters because of the material's versatility, malleability (i.e., tensile strength and elongation characteristics), and **biocompatibility.** TPU catheters do not have any plasticizers or other harmful additives that can be readily extracted (Brown, 1995). Polyurethane is a commonly used material for short-term percutaneously placed CVCs and is more frequently being used in long-term CVCs and PICCs. Polyurethane is stiffer than silicone and softens after insertion, making threading of the catheter easier. Polyurethane catheters have thinner walls than silicone catheters owing to greater tensile strength. Polyurethane is similar to silicone in biocompatibility and is thrombus resistant.

Coatings

To further decrease the risk of complications inherent with even the most biocompatible materials, catheters coated or bonded with hydrophilic materials, antiseptic substances, antibiotics, or heparin are available. The quest for bacteria-resistant materials has led to studies in which antibiotics were bonded to the catheter insertion site. Central catheters, such as the ARROWgard, were developed that have a colonization-resistant chlorhexidine and silver sulfadiazine antiseptic surface molecularly bonded into the polyurethane catheter along its entire indwelling length.

The VitaCuff is a stand-alone add-on device made of silver ions in a biodegradable collagen matrix that is placed around the catheter (Fig. 11–3.) The cuff works in conjunction with the Dacron cuff, an inherent component of some catheters, and is positioned beneath the skin surface during catheter placement.

The device's collagen band is impregnated with silver ions that are released over several weeks, creating a physical barrier to bacteria. Silver

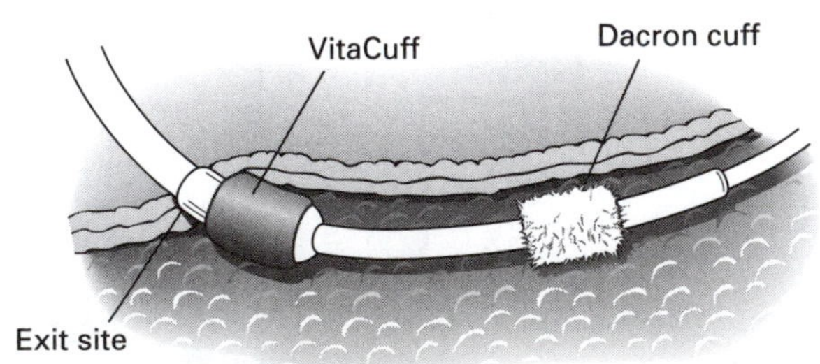

FIG. 11–3. Positioning of VitaCuff antimicrobial cuff. (Courtesy of BARD Access Systems, Salt Lake City, Utah.)

ions have broad-spectrum activity against many of the bacteria and fungi that are related to catheter infections.

The CDC states that "of the studies reported to date, antimicrobial-coated catheters do not appear to pose any greater risk of adverse effects than do noncoated catheters, but additional controlled trials need to be done to evaluate their efficacy fully, to determine the appropriate situations or their use, and to assess the risk of toxicity and emergence of resistant blood stream pathogens" (CDC, 1995).

LUMENS

Catheters are available in single, double, triple, and the recently created quadruple lumens. The diameter of each lumen varies because of the need for larger diameters for administering hypertonic or viscous solutions. Refer to each particular manufacturer's information to ascertain which lumen is the largest if you are administering vesicant or hypertonic solution through one lumen (Fig. 11–4).

For most solutions and medications, any lumen may be selected for infusion. It is recommended that the distal lumen be used for administering vesicant solutions. The proximal lumen should be used for blood

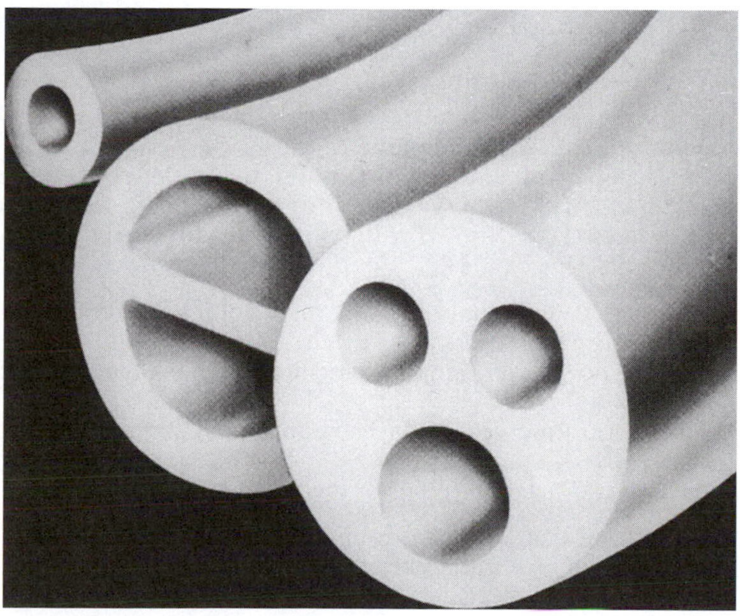

FIG. 11–4. Single, double, and triple lumens. (Courtesy of Bard Access Systems, Salt Lake City, Utah.)

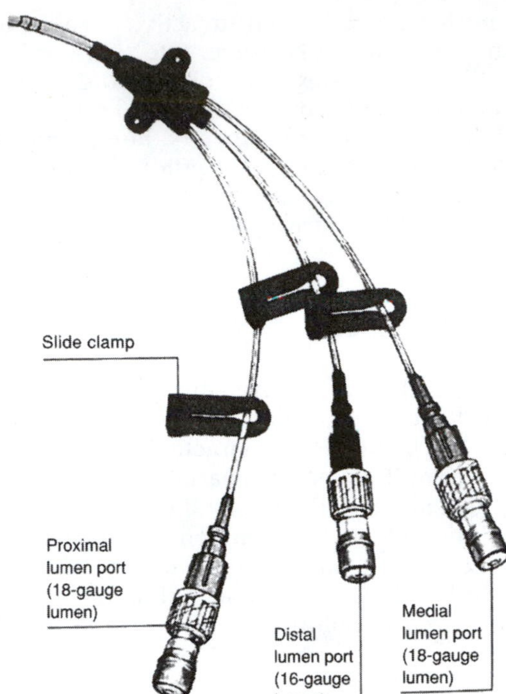

FIG. 11–5. Injection ports of the triple-lumen catheter include the proximal lumen port, distal lumen port, and medial lumen port. The distal port (middle line) is usually the largest of the three lines.

withdrawal, when possible, to avoid contamination of the specimen from solutions infusing into the other lumens.

The lumens open at different points on the catheter to allow for adequate dilution within the vessel during simultaneous administering different infusates (Fig. 11–5). Port (lumen) protocols currently used are based on the following:

Distal port: CVP monitoring and high volume or viscous fluids, colloids, or medications

Proximal port: Blood sampling, medications, or blood component administration

Medial port: Reserved exclusively for total parenteral nutrition (TPN)

Fourth port: Infusion of fluids or medications.

NOTE: The CDC (1995) recommends using a single-lumen CVC unless multiple ports are essential for the management of the patient.

Table 11–3 compares the features, advantages, and disadvantages of CVCs, and Table 11–4 discusses the care and maintenance of CVCs.

TABLE 11–3

COMPARING CENTRAL VENOUS CATHETERS

Type and Use	Features	Advantages	Disadvantages
		Short Term	
Percutaneous Up to several weeks Intended for days to several weeks	Material: Polyurethane (most common), Silastic Length: 6–30 cm Gauge: 14–27 Available features: Heparin, hydromere, antibiotic and antiseptic coatings and antimicrobial cuff available Preattached extensions with clamps Multiple lumens	Inserted at bedside; cost effective, easy to remove, easy to exchange over guidewire	Placement time limited (usually 7 days) Requires sterile dressing changes; requires daily heparin flushes; catheter may break; requires activity restrictions
PICC Up to several months	Material: Polyurethane, Silastic (most common) Length: 33.5–60.0 cm Gauge: 14–25 Lumen: Double Groshong valve	Insertion trays, spare needles, spare catheters, and repair kits available Preattached extension with clamps Inserted at bedside by specially trained RN; cost effective; easy to remove; reliable for long-term use; eliminates risks associated with chest or neck insertion; preserves integrity of peripheral vascular system	Requires sterile dressing changes; requires routine heparin flushes except with Groshong valve in place; catheter may break; requires activity restrictions; may not be possible to withdraw blood for sampling

(Continued)

TABLE 11–3

COMPARING CENTRAL VENOUS CATHETERS *(Continued)*

Type and Use	Features	Advantages	Disadvantages
	Long Term		
Tunneled Long-term intermittent continuous or daily I.V. access	Material: Silastic Length: 55–90 cm Gauge: 2.7–19.2 Fr Lumen: Multiple Groshong valve Detachable hub Antimicrobial collagen cuff	Can remain in place indefinitely; requires aseptic dressing changes; clean when site is healed; can be repaired externally; self-care possible	May require routine heparin flushes, except with Groshong valve; catheter may break; daily to weekly site care; may be difficult to remove
Implanted ports Long-term intermittent, continuous or daily I.V. access	Material: Catheter: Silastic, polyurethane Port: Titanium, stainless steel, plastic Height: 9.8–17.0 mm Width of base: 24–50 mm Lumen: Dual Groshong valve	Can access dome port from any angle Preattached catheter or port or two-piece system Several catheter/port locking devices available No dressing changes required, monthly heparin flushes, no activity restrictions, reduced risk of infection	Requires noncoring needle to access; expensive; requires minor surgery to remove

TABLE 11–4

CARE OF CENTRAL VENOUS CATHETERS

Type of Catheter	Flushing	Tubing Change	Dressing Change
		Short-Term	
Percutaneous	1:10 to 1:100 U heparin equal to twice the volume capacity of tubing plus any extensions	Primary and secondary sets every 48 hours; every 24 hours with TPN	Change every 48 hours for gauze dressing. Every 3–7 days or PRN for TSM dressing Use three swabs of 70% isopropyl alcohol and three swabs of povidone-iodine, wiping from site outward to cleanse site Antimicrobial ointments are recommended
PICC	1:10 to 1:100 U heparin in volume equal to twice the volume capacity of tubing (1 mL) plus any extensions daily	Same as above	Same as above Remove dressing by pulling upward to avoid dislodging the catheter

(Continued)

TABLE 11–4

CARE OF CENTRAL VENOUS CATHETERS *(Continued)*

Type of Catheter	Flushing	Tubing Change	Dressing Change
		Long Term	
Tunneled	1:10 to 1:100 U heparin in volume equal to twice the volume capacity of tubing (4 mL) plus any extensions; daily to weekly With Groshong tip, use 5 mL of 0.9% sodium chloride flush weekly	Same as above	Same as above
Implanted port	1:10 to 1:100 U heparin in volume equal to twice the volume capacity of tubing (3 mL) plus any extensions	Same as above	Same as above No dressing is needed after the incision is healed Stabilize device with Steri-Strips Change noncoring needle at least weekly

PRN = as needed; TPN = total parenteral nutrition; TSM = transparent semipermeable membrane.

SHORT-TERM ACCESS DEVICES

Short-term access devices are intended to be used for days to weeks. These devices can be single- or multiple-lumen catheters made of several materials. They are inserted by a percutaneous venipuncture and are not tunneled under the skin. The infraclavicular, jugular, or femoral veins are the sites used if performed by a physician, and the veins of the antecubital area are used if performed by a registered nurse specially trained for peripheral central venous access.

PERCUTANEOUS CATHETERS

In 1961, the first I.V. catheter for accessing the central circulation was introduced. Subclavian catheterization was initially inserted using surgical cutdown technique such as that advocated by Heimback and Ivey (1976). However, percutaneous introduction into the subclavian vein using the Seldinger through-the-needle guidewire technique is now generally preferred. The percutaneous short-term catheter is secured by suturing, and the catheter is not tunneled. This catheter may remain in place for 7 days.

The most common site for insertion of percutaneous catheters is the infraclavicular approach to the subclavian vein (Fig. 11–6). The patient is placed in the Trendelenburg position with a rolled bath blanket or towel

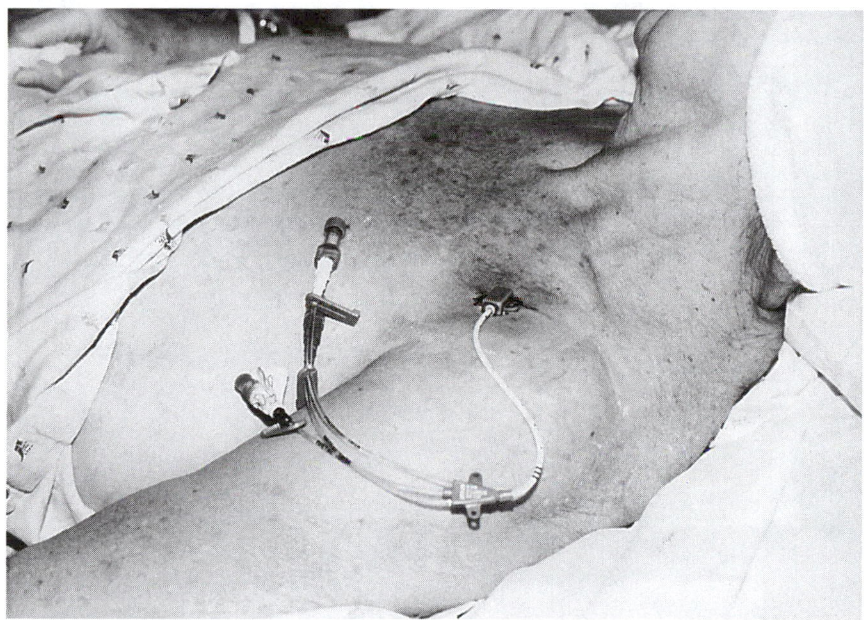

FIG. 11–6. Placement of infraclavicular percutaneous catheter.

between his or her shoulders. The patient should be instructed to perform a **Valsalva maneuver** during the venipuncture procedure to increase the size of the veins.

This exit site on the upper chest is well suited for many types of dressings, and care of the site is not complex (Fig. 11–7).

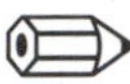

NOTE: The infraclavicular approach site requires a well-hydrated patient.

The internal jugular vein is an accessible site for the physician; however, care of this site is more difficult. The motion of the neck, a beard on men, long hair, and close proximity of respiratory secretions prevent the adequate use of transparent occlusive dressings. The femoral veins are not recommended for this type of therapy because of the difficulty of placement of the catheter tip. It is also impossible to maintain an occlusive dressing on the femoral exit site.

NOTE: After insertion of the catheter, verification by chest radiography must be obtained before any infusion. After placement of the catheter, the devices can be closed with an injection cap and heparinized while the catheter tip location is verified by radiologic examination. Do not infuse any solution but isotonic fluids without additives if the physician desires a radiograph with free-flowing solution.

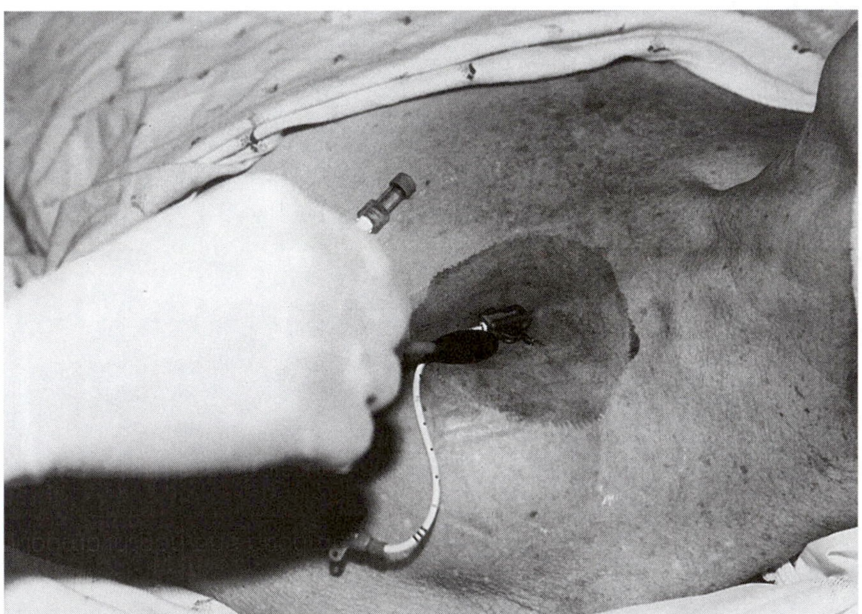

FIG. 11–7. Cleansing the central line site with povidone-iodine solution.

Dressing Management

Percutaneous catheters can be dressed in one of two ways, depending on agency policy. An occlusive gauze or tape or a transparent semipermeable membrane (TSM) dressing may be used. In today's practice, the TSM dressing has gained popularity because of its occlusive nature and ability to visualize the site.

Most protocols for frequency of dressing changes are based on empirical success and range from every other day to weekly changes, depending on the type of dressing and the patient population.

The gauze dressing should be changed every 48 hours or according to agency policy. The entire surface and all edges must be secured with tape to ensure that the dressing is closed and intact (Perrucca, 1995).

PERIPHERALLY INSERTED CENTRAL CATHETERS

Peripherally inserted central catheters were introduced in the late 1970s as a means to administer infusates when traditional routes of venous access were unachievable. The PICC is a percutaneous I.V. line composed of silicone elastomers or polyurethane. It may have a single or multiple lumens with ranges in lengths from 33 to 60 cm and diameters of 14 to 25 gauge (4 Fr/18 gauge). Insertion may be through the needle, through a peel-away introducer, through an intact cannula, or with a guidewire.

The placement of PICCs by registered professional nurses requires specialized education and demonstrated competency. PICCs are designed for delivery of therapies extending beyond 7 days to several months. The PICC was developed for use in neonates because of the catheter's small diameter and the material's flexibility.

Indications for PICC Use

The following indications for PICC use include medical-based and specific prescribed therapies.

Medical Diagnoses

Medical-based indications for PICC use include infectious diseases (e.g., osteomyelitis, endocarditis, delayed wound healing secondary to infection, meningitis, multiple abdominal fistulae), oncologic diseases, gastrointestinal (GI) diseases (e.g., pancreatitis, hyperemesis gravidarum, malabsorption syndromes), and low birth weight neonates.

Therapies

Specific prescribed therapies for PICC use include drugs or infusates with extreme variations in osmolarity; parenteral nutrition formulations with dextrose contents greater than 10 percent or osmolarity more than

500; irritating anti-infective agents such as vancomycin, nafcillin, and amphotericin B; vesicant or irritant therapies; and prolonged duration of therapy (more than 7 days), such as with pain management or chronic vasopressor infusions (INS, 1999).

Advantages

1. Peripheral insertion eliminates the potential complication of pneumothorax or hemothorax
2. Decreases risk of air embolism owing to the ease of maintaining the insertion site below the heart
3. Decreases pain and discomfort associated with frequent venipunctures for peripheral sites
4. Preserves peripheral vascular system of upper extremities
5. Cost effective and time efficient
6. Appropriate for home placement and home I.V. therapy
7. Reduced risk of infiltration and phlebitis
8. Preservation of peripheral veins
9. No age barrier

Disadvantages

1. Special training required to perform procedure
2. Forty-five minutes to 1 hour needed to complete procedure
3. Daily care required
4. Strict catheter maintenance guidelines necessary to prevent clotting of catheter
5. Small-lumen PICCs not recommended for obtaining blood samples because of possible collapse of catheter on aspiration
6. Contraindicated in patients whose lifestyles or occupations involve being in water; those with preexisting skin infections; those with anatomic distortions related to injury, surgical dissection, or trauma; and those with coagulopathies
7. Requires chest radiography for placement verification before initiation of therapy

Vein Selection

The peripheral veins in the antecubital fossa in both adults and pediatrics are the usual sites for PICC access (Fig. 11–8). Other veins that may be used include the basilic, cephalic, median-cephalic, and median-basilic veins.

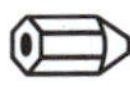

NOTE: All these sites are acceptable; however, the basilic vein and the median antecubital veins are the preferred insertion sites. Each should be assessed immediately below the antecubital space.

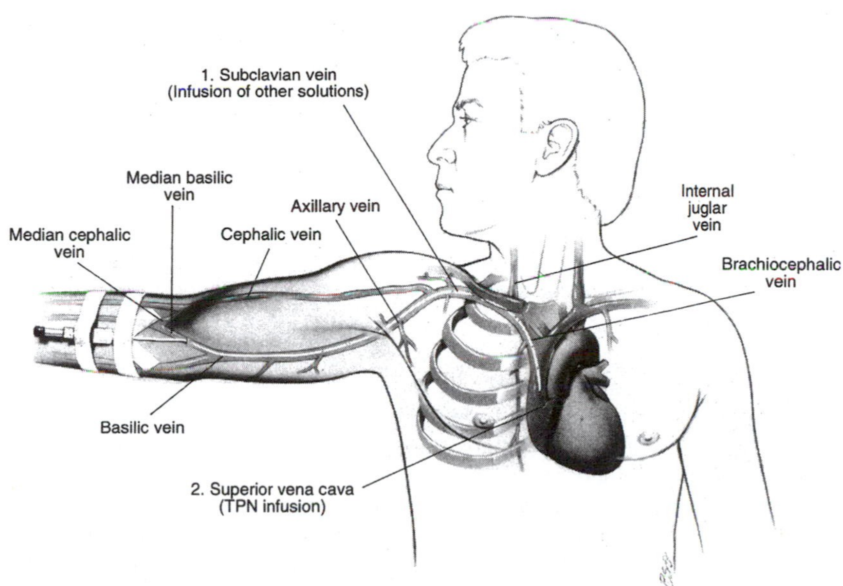

FIG. 11-8. Anatomic placement of peripherally placed central catheter. (Courtesy of Medivisuals, Dallas, Texas.)

AGE-RELATED CONSIDERATIONS: PICC VEIN SELECTION

In the neonatal and pediatric population, the external jugular, axillary, long and short saphenous, temporal, and posterior auricular veins may be appropriate site considerations (INS, 1997).

Placement

According to the recommendations of the Food and Drug Administration (FDA) Central Venous Catheter Working Group (1994) and the INS Standards of Practice 2000, PICCs should be placed in patients under sterile conditions by a specially trained registered nurse in settings such as a patient's room, outpatient area, or the patient's home. Various PICC designs are available for insertion, including the breakaway needle introducer, the peel-away sheath, the guidewire, or a slotted needle on a drum cartridge.

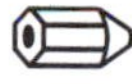

NOTE: Catheter tip placement for PICCs is the SVC (INS, 2000, 44).

INS STANDARDS The responsibilities of the registered nurse should include ascertainment of product integrity, vein selection and assessment, and use of aseptic technique (INS, 2000, 48).

Procedure

Although the actual procedure varies with different manufacturer's products, Procedure 11–1 provides a guideline for inserting a PICC.

PROCEDURE 11–1: INSERTION OF A PICC

Verify physician order, obtain history of allergies, obtain an informed consent, and conduct patient education before beginning procedure.

Gather Equipment:

- One nonsterile measuring tape
- One nonsterile tourniquet
- Two pairs of sterile gloves (powderless)
- Gown, goggles or face shield
- Tamperproof, nonpermeable sharps container
- One catheter insertion kit (write down the lot number and expiration date); select the correct PICC size according to the access needs of the patient
- One local anesthetic (bacteriostatic normal saline and 1% lidocaine)
- One sterile injection cap

Insertion Procedure:
Preinsertion Steps

1. Perform preinsertion assessment: Determine the site to be used for PICC insertion.
2. Wash the patient's arm with soap and water or chlorhexidine gluconate, rinse well, and dry thoroughly.
3. Wash hands with an antibacterial agent
4. Set up supplies and sterile field.
5. Position patient with arm to be accessed extended at 90 degrees from the trunk of the body.

Cannulation

1. Scrub hands using antiseptic soap for 60 seconds.
2. Don mask and prepare work area.
3. Position protective covering under patient's arm.
4. Place tourniquet on mid upper arm for final vein assessment.
5. Measure arm with sterile tape. For PICC placement in the SVC, measure from the antecubital insertion site up the arm to the shoulder and across the shoulder. Continue to the sternal notch and down to the third intercostal space.
6. Select vein and release tourniquet.
7. Apply nonpowdered sterile gloves.
8. Prepare site with 70 percent isopropyl alcohol, starting at insertion site and cleaning outward in a circular motion in an 8- to 10-inch diameter. Repeat three times. Allow to completely dry.

9. Anesthetize the anticipated venipuncture site. Assess for allergies before using any of the three methods.
   A. Intradermal injection: 0.1 to 0.3 mL of 1 percent lidocaine without epinephrine, using a small-gauge needle. Perform after skin preparation and immediately before venipuncture.
   B. Topical application of anesthetic after venous site selection and before skin preparation; flow manufacturer recommendations for contact time
   C. **Iontopheresis:** Method of delivering anesthesia without injection through the skin via an electronic device. Perform before skin preparation. Allow sufficient time to achieve anesthetic effect (approximately 10 to 30 minutes).
10. Cleanse with 10 percent povidone-iodine, repeating the same procedure as with isopropyl alcohol. Repeat three times.
11. Remove and discard gloves.
12. Apply tourniquet snugly.
13. Don goggles, sterile gown, and new pair of sterile powder-free gloves.
14. Drape arm with sterile towels, creating a sterile field.
15. Flush entire cannula according to manufacturer's recommendations.
16. Make venipuncture while applying reverse traction with the nondominant hand to stabilize the vein.
17. Upon confirmation of blood return, advance the introducer unit about 1/4 to 1/2 inch further into the lumen of the vein.
18. While gently pressing proximally on the tip of the introducer cannula to decrease blood spillage, remove the introducer stylet and eliminate it from the procedure field to prevent inadvertent injury.
19. Insert the cannula through the introducer device, slowly and in small increments.
20. Release the tourniquet.
21. Continue to advance the catheter. When inserted approximately halfway, instruct the patient to turn his head toward the affected arm with his chin tucked and pointed downward toward the clavicle or chest.
22. Remove the introducer.
23. Slowly advance the remaining catheter to the measured length.
24. Gently remove the guidewire from the catheter.
25. Prime and attach the extension tubing and injection cap.
26. Flush with 0.5 mL of 0.9 percent sodium chloride solution.
27. Aspirate with 0.9 percent sodium chloride to check for blood return.
28. Assess blood for type of flow, color, consistency, and pulsation.
29. Flush vigorously with remaining sodium chloride, followed by heparinized saline.
30. Secure the catheter with:
    A. Tape with sterile wound closure strips
    B. Tape supplied in manufacturer's insertion tray
    C. Catheter securement device
    D. Suture
31. Dress with sterile 2 × 2 gauze and transparent dressing, according to organizational policy and procedure.

(continued)

(continued)

32. Obtain chest radiograph for catheter tip placement.
33. Document procedure and patient response.
34. After 24 hours, assess the insertion site and upper arm by changing the initial dressing according to organizational policy and procedure. (Brown, 1989; Perucca, 1995, INS, 1999).

Key Points

Threading is often the most difficult aspect of PICC insertion. Key points in overcoming difficulties in threading of a PICC line include:

- If you meet resistance or advancement stops, try flushing while threading.
- During threading, if the flexible catheter tip kinks over onto itself, pull back on the catheter and flush. If flushing is ineffective, another vein may need to be used. Never force a kinked guidewire because it could puncture the catheter.
- If the catheter threads easily to the subclavian vein and then threading becomes difficult, have the patient turn his or her head to the side before threading the catheter with the chin on the shoulder of the PICC insertion arm to prevent malposition into the internal jugular vein. Also, flush the thread until reaching the insertion length.
- If threading progresses to a point at which the catheter abruptly stops (this may be caused by a valve, vessel narrowing, or thrombus), attempt to flush and thread past the valve or narrowing.
- If a venous spasm occurs during threading, flush to attempt to open the vein or wait up to 10 minutes while flushing intermittently before beginning rethreading attempt.

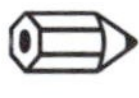

NOTE: Some PICCs are designed for suture placement to stabilize the catheter (or Steri-Strip skin closure may be used to close the exit site).

INS STANDARDS The length of time a PICC may indwell is dependent on factors related to the patient, clinical environment, skill of the inserters, skill of all caregivers, the composition of the infusate, and the VAD. With ongoing analysis of these factors, consideration may be given to leaving a PICC in place for up to 1 year (INS, 1997a).

Dressing Management

A small amount of bleeding from the insertion site occurs for the first 24 hours after insertion. After 24 hours, the original dressing must be replaced with one that can remain in place up to 7 days. Dressings have two functions: as a protective environment for the VAD and to prevent catheter migration via stabilization. Dressing change is a sterile procedure.

1. Wear nonpowdered gloves for the dressing removal.
2. Remove the transparent dressing gently by pulling in an upward direction to prevent dislodging or pulling the catheter out.
3. Assess the insertion site; the arm; and the track of the vein for redness, tenderness, edema, and drainage.
4. Remove gloves and put on a new pair of sterile nonpowdered gloves to clean the skin around the insertion site.
5. Use three alcohol swab sticks followed by three povidone-iodine swab sticks. Allow to dry.
6. Slide a 2 × 2 gauze pad under the catheter just below the insertion site if drainage is present.
7. If the catheter is not sutured, place Steri-Strips over the insertion site to prevent migration of the catheter.
8. Apply a new transparent dressing over the exposed catheter, including the hub.
9. Initial and date the dressing (Fig. 11–9).

INS STANDARDS The dressing should be changed and the site should be assessed every 24 hours until the site is epithelialized (INS, 2000, 55).

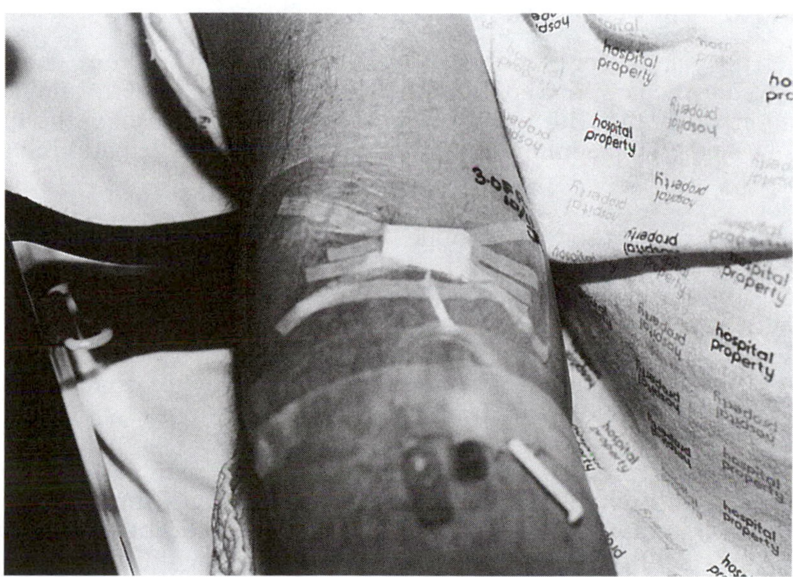

FIG. 11–9. Initial PICC dressing. The newly placed PICC has Steri-Strips to secure the line and a gauze pad under the transparent dressing for the first 24 hours.

NOTE: Avoid stretching the catheter during dressing changes and catheter removal. Stretching or excessive pressure can cause the catheter to rupture.

PICC dressing should be changed at intervals similar to those for other central line dressings. Transparent dressings are safe and efficacious up to 7 days (Maki & Mermel, 1998). Patients who are very active or perspire profusely will need more frequent dressing changes.

I.V. tubing junctions must be secured with Luer locking connections.

Monitoring

Document and communicate the following:

1. Fluid container and administration set
2. Flow rate
3. Use of electronic infusion device
4. Insertion site
5. Catheter tract and surrounding tissue
6. I.V. site dressing
7. VAD
8. Patient response

Flushing Procedure

Flushing is done routinely using 0.9 percent sodium chloride followed by heparin (except for catheters with closed distal tip and three position valve). As with many venous access devices, flushing the PICC involves the saline administering the medication-saline-heparin method (SASH):

S: 0.9 percent sodium chloride
A: Administer medication
S: 0.9 percent sodium chloride
H: Heparin

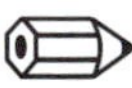

NOTE: For best results and to prevent catheter complications, flush the I.V. catheter using the "push–stop" method.

This flushing procedure is recommended to eliminate problems with incompatible drugs. The flushing volume is two times the internal fill volume of the catheter. The recommended heparin concentration is 10 to 100 U/mL (approximately 2 to 3 mL depending on the fill volume).

INS STANDARDS Flushing with a heparin flush solution to ensure and maintain patency of an intermittent central venous cannula shall be performed at established intervals. The concentration of heparin used to flush cannulas shall not alter the patient's clotting factors (INS, 2000, 56).

The frequency of the flushing procedure depends on organizational policy and patient condition. The recommendations are:

Every 4 to 6 hours for 2 Fr or smaller or after each use
Every 8 to 12 hours for larger sizes or after each use (INS, 1999)

Flushing is to be done:

1. Whenever the line needs to be locked
2. After every blood draw
3. After intermittent medication administration
4. After blood or blood component administration
5. After TPN

The technique for flushing should be the pulsatile push–pause technique to remove residues and fibrin buildup.

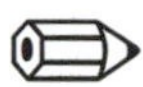

NOTE: A 10-mL or larger syringe must be used to maintain a psi (pounds per square inch) of approximately 7. A psi pressure exerted by a 1-mL syringe is greater than 300 psi, and that exerted by a 3-mL syringe is more than 25 psi (catheter burst pressure is 25 to 40 psi; Josephson, 1999).

Never force a flush.

Use of Infusion Pumps

The PICC line has been used successfully with all types of infusion pumps. With 3.0-Fr and smaller PICCs, an infusion pump may be necessary to maintain the infusion and patency of the line.

Blood Sampling

If blood sampling is needed from the PICC, a 4-Fr or larger catheter may be required. The walls of the PICC line are soft, so they collapse easily when a strong vacuum is applied; therefore, a gentle touch with a syringe is recommended. Vacutainers are not recommended.

Blood Administration

Blood products may be administered through a 4-Fr or larger PICC. Care should be taken to flush the line thoroughly after administering a blood product.

Repair

A PICC that is damaged externally can be repaired with a manufacturer-specific hub repair kit. PICCs can be temporarily repaired with a coated blunt needle inserted into the trimmed end of the broken catheter. If the catheter is damaged internally, another catheter can be placed over the existing cannula to preserve the access site. In many cases, the I.V. nurse must advocate for the patient's vascular access needs and create new techniques to preserve what may be the only access site available (Fabian, 1995).

The PICC can be replaced in one of three ways:

- Using the exchange-over-wire procedure using the Seldinger method
- Totally removing and replacing with another PICC
- Using the breakaway sheath technique

If the peripherally inserted central line is damaged, another catheter can be placed. An exchange-over-wire procedure can be used as a last resort for salvaging the line. The guidewires used for this procedure can be extremely long; therefore, strict sterile technique with gowning is recommended. The guidewire is inserted into the catheter to be removed, and the catheter is pulled out over the wire. A new catheter is then threaded back over the wire. After the new catheter is in place, the guidewire can be removed.

Dual lumen PICCs cannot be repaired. A sheath exchange allows for a damaged PICC to be removed and a new dual lumen to be placed. The application of the breakaway needle exchange procedure can be extended to replacement of midclavicular catheters. A sheath exchange can be used to preserve the access site and exchange a shorter catheter for a PICC line (Fabian, 1995).

A chest radiograph should be taken to verify the placement of the new catheter tip. This procedure should be performed only by experienced I.V. nurses certified to insert a PICC (INS, 1998). Specific manufacturer recommendations are provided for this procedure.

Discontinuation of PICC

The discontinuation of a PICC catheter must be performed by a qualified registered nurse. Minimize the risk of air embolism by positioning the patient in a dorsal-recumbent position, and instruct the patient to perform the Valsalva maneuver while the catheter is being withdrawn. The recommended procedure is as follows:

1. Abduct the patient's arm
2. Remove the dressing while wearing gloves
3. Remove the sutures if necessary
4. Remove any other securement devices
5. Withdraw the cannula with smooth, gentle pressure in small increments
6. *DO NOT STRETCH THE CATHETER* during removal

The procedure for after PICC removal is as follows:

1. Cover the site with a sterile pressure dressing
2. Leave the dressing in place for 24 hours
3. Measure the length of the catheter and compare it with the length recorder before inserting the device (INS, 1999)

Difficulty with PICC withdrawal is an uncommon but not infrequent problem, with resistance being encountered in 7 to 24 percent of removals (Macklin, 2000). Catheter removal may take several hours or more to achieve venous relaxation and total removal of cannula. The most common cause of "stuck" catheters is venospasm (Marx, 1995). Other causes include phlebitis, valve inflammation, and thrombophlebitis.

Techniques to aid in removal of catheter include:

- Apply warm moist compresses.
- Release traction on the catheter and reattempt removal in 20 to 30 minutes.
- Use mental relaxation exercises and distraction.
- Have the patient drink warm beverage to increase vasomotor tone.
- Gently massage the area of the upper arm over the PICC to relax the vein.
- Apply nitroglycerin paste to the arm over the vein where the PICC lies. (This intervention requires a physician's order.)
- Start a peripheral I.V. distal to the PICC line and infuse warm normal saline to relax the vein and increase the flow/volume within the vein.
- Sublingual administering smooth muscle relaxants, such as nitroglycerin or nifedipine, may be helpful. (This intervention requires a physician's order.)
- Wait an additional 12 to 24 hours before attempting removal again. Spasm is not sustained indefinitely and the vessel eventually relaxes, even with the continued presence of the irritating stimulus (Marx, 1995, Macklin, 2000).

PICC-associated Risks and Complications

The risks and complications associated with PICCs include arm edema, bleeding, tendon or nerve damage, cardiac dysrhythmias, malposition of catheter, catheter embolism, phlebitis, catheter sepsis, thrombosis, air embolism and Twiddler's syndrome.

Nerve damage is related to the median nerve, which lies parallel and medial to the brachial artery in the antecubital space. On the lateral side, the lateral cutaneous nerve is proximal to the cephalic vein. Because of the close proximity to these nerves, damage is a risk.

Cardiac dysrhythmias are related to irritation of the myocardial wall by an overinserted guidewire or catheter. Some institutions require the patient to be placed on a cardiac monitor during placement of a PICC in the SVC. Catheters positioned in the heart are at risk of causing myocardial erosion, perforation, cardiac tamponade, and endocardial abscess.

Intravascular and **extravascular** malpositioning of all types of short-term devices has been reported. Extravascular malpositioning can occur when the introducer slips out of the vein and the catheter is passed into the pleural space or the mediastinum (primarily during a subclavian catheterization). Intravascular malpositions are more common and can be seen with all approaches to the central vascular system. The catheter may coil in the vessel, advance into the right atrium or one of the smaller venous tributaries, or not be advanced far enough to reach the SVC from the antecubital site. The catheter must be repositioned if malpositioning occurs.

NOTE: A way to avoid intravascular malpositioning of the catheter in the jugular vein is by having the patient turn his head toward the side of the venipuncture with his chin on his shoulder. This changes the angle of the catheter to move downward toward the SVC.

Care should be taken to remove the break-away needle (introducer) before threading the catheter. Catheter shearing is the most common cause of catheter embolism, but it can also result from retraction of the catheter into the arm after external breakage, rupture of the catheter with forceful irrigation, or from the "pinch-off" syndrome. Managing catheter embolism involves retaining the fragment in the arm and preventing migration into the central veins, heart, pulmonary artery, or lung periphery. If the potential of catheter embolization occurs, immediately apply local pressure or a tourniquet proximal to the site. Obtain a radiograph to determine the location of the embolus. Radiographic visualization may be difficult if the catheter segment is short.

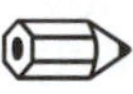

NOTE: If the patient complains of pain in the shoulder, neck, or arm at insertion site, catheter placement should be checked by radiographic examination at any time during the course of therapy.

Table 11–5 presents a summary of central venous access device complications.

MIDCLAVICULAR CATHETERS

Midclavicular catheters have been called "midline," "halfway," "PIC," and "extended peripheral" catheters. There needs to be uniform and consistent terminology to clearly reflect the peripheral device and its tip location so that appropriate care and maintenance strategies can be implemented (INS, 1997b).

Midclavicular catheters are peripherally inserted catheters with the tip location in the proximal axillary or subclavian veins. If a line intended for the SVC location falls short and ends up in the brachiocephalic (innominate) vein, it should be considered midclavicular (Fig. 11–10).

Midclavicular catheter tip placement are indicated for patients who:

1. Have limited peripheral access
2. Need I.V. fluids, electrolytes, or other medications that are isotonic when admixed

TABLE 11–5

COMPLICATIONS ASSOCIATED WITH CENTRAL VENOUS ACCESS DEVICES

Complication and Cause	Central Line Device	Signs and Symptoms	Interventions
		Insertion Complications	
Bleeding: Common with any nontunneled catheter	Percutaneous PICC Midclavicular	Oozing from site, hematoma (watch patients with thrombocytopenia), usually first 24 h after insertion Cool, mottled skin; numbness; tingling	Apply pressure dressing
Pneumothorax: Collection of air in the pleural space between the lung and chest wall; caused by puncture of the pleural covering of the lung	Percutaneous	Shortness of breath during procedure, crunching sound on auscultation, dyspnea, cyanosis, subcutaneous emphysema	Administer oxygen A chest tube may be inserted May resolve slowly without evacuation of air Monitor vital signs
Hemothorax: Blood enters the pleural cavity as a result of trauma or transection of a vein	Percutaneous PICC Midclavicular Tunneled catheter Implanted port	Sudden onset of chest pain, tachycardia, hypotension, dusky color, diaphoresis, hemoptysis	Usually noted during insertion of catheter Remove the catheter and apply pressure to site Monitor vital signs Administer oxygen
Chylothorax: Lymph (chyle) fluid enters the pleural cavity as a result of transection of the thoracic duct on the left side where it enters the subclavian vein; chyle is a milk-like substance	Percutaneous PICC Midclavicular Tunneled catheter Implanted port	Sudden onset of chest pain, dyspnea, withdrawal of a milk-like substance into the needle	Remove the catheter Monitor vital signs Administer oxygen Chest tube may be necessary

(Continued)

TABLE 11–5

COMPLICATIONS ASSOCIATED WITH CENTRAL VENOUS ACCESS DEVICES *(Continued)*

Complication and Cause	Central Line Device	Signs and Symptoms	Interventions
		Insertion Complications	
Brachial plexus injury: Network of nerves located in the lower cervical and upper dorsal spinal nerves that supply the arm, forearm, and hand	Percutaneous PICC Midclavicular	Tingling sensation in fingers, pain shooting down arm, paralysis	Pain medication Physical therapy Preventive measures
Extravascular malposition: Catheter penetrates the vessel and the tip lies outside the vascular system; occurs during threading a catheter or needle introducer	Percutaneous PICC Midclavicular	Symptoms of pneumothorax or hemothorax	Radiographic verification of catheter tip Remove catheter Monitor vital signs Oxygen, chest tube may be necessary
		Post-insertion Complications	
Air embolism: The entry of air into the circulatory system during CVC insertion, tubing changes, or caused by catheter damage or breakage; death occurs from rapid injection of air; lethal dose 70 to 150 cc	Percutaneous PICC Midclavicular Tunneled catheter Implanted port	Chest pain, dyspnea, hypotension, lightheadedness, pallor, precordial churning murmur (mill wheel), tachycardia, thready pulse, unresponsiveness	Place patient in left lateral Trendelenburg position Clamp catheter Notify physician Monitor vital signs Prepare for resuscitation Note: It only takes 1 second for 100 cc of air to be inspired by a patient sitting upright with an open 14-g CVC

Catheter migration: CVC moves from its insertion placement site to another location; may result from improper suturing, disease process, changes in intrathoracic pressure, forceful catheter flushing, tumor progression, venous thrombosis; also spontaneous (no reason when patient physically active)	Percutaneous PICC Midclavicular Tunneled catheter Implanted port	Aspiration difficulties; burning sensation, discomfort, or pain during infusion; edema of chest or neck; increased external catheter length; leaking around the insertion site; cardiac dysrhythmias; palpation of catheter in external jugular vein; patient complaints of gurgling sound in ear	Radiographic verification of tip placement Assist with CVC removal and replacement Place new PICC
Local infection: Infection at insertion site as result of break in aseptic technique; a local infection may precede or occur concomitantly with sepsis; local infection includes exit site, pocket, or tunnel infections	Percutaneous PICC Midclavicular Tunneled catheter Implanted port	Cording of vein; site drainage, redness, tenderness, warmth; increased basal temperature	Notify physician Draw blood cultures from CVC Obtain peripheral blood cultures Administer antibiotics, anticoagulants Evaluate central line for removal
Septicemia (sepsis): Systemic infection caused by contaminated infusate or break in aseptic technique; the formation of a fibrin sheath increases the potential for microbial growth or other infectious processes; occurs more frequently in patients who are immunocompromised, malnourished, or undergoing steroid and TPN therapy	Percutaneous PICC Midclavicular Tunneled catheter Implanted port	Chills, cyanosis, fever, facial flushing, explosive diarrhea, headache, nausea and vomiting, positive blood culture results, tachycardia, septic shock (altered mental function), hypotension, inadequate organ perfusion, petechiae, purpuric pustules	Assess for all sources of infection Assess vital signs Draw central and peripheral blood cultures Administer antibiotics, anticoagulants, antipyretics Prepare for respiratory support and emergency resuscitation

(Continued)

TABLE 11–5

COMPLICATIONS ASSOCIATED WITH CENTRAL VENOUS ACCESS DEVICES *(Continued)*

Complication and Cause	Central Line Device	Signs and Symptoms	Interventions
		Post-insertion Complications	
Thrombosis: The formation of blood clots within the blood vessel; causes include catheter placement outside of SVC, fibrin sheath formation, platelet aggregation on the catheter, preexisting conditions (e.g., cardiovascular disease, hematopoietic pathology, limb edema), stasis and sluggish flow rate, use of thrombogenic catheter materials (PVC), vessel wall injury at the catheter insertion site, or from mechanical irritation, or infusion of irritating products	Percutaneous PICC Midclavicular Tunneled catheter Implanted port	Earache or jaw pain, insertion site edema or redness, malaise, tachycardia, tachypnea, unilateral arm or neck pain, edema, absence of pulse distal to the obstruction, coldness, cyanosis, necrosis of digits	Administer analgesics, anticoagulants Administer oxygen if needed Apply moist, warm compresses locally Apply surgical stocking Assess vital signs Avoid use of limb affected Position patient in semi- to high Fowler's position Prepare to institute emergency resuscitative measures Prepare patient for operative thromboectomy, insertion of vena cava filter if indicated Assist with catheter removal if necessary
Nonthrombolytic: Occlusion; crystallization of TPN admixtures and drug-to-drug or drug-to-solution incompatibilities	Percutaneous PICC Midclavicular Tunneled catheter Implanted port	Sluggish flow rates, total occlusion, inability to flush or obtain blood withdrawal	Attempt to restore patency using appropriate solution (HCl or sodium bicarbonate, or ethanol)

Thrombolytic occlusions: Deposits of fibrin and blood components within and around the CVC; intraluminal blood clot, fibrin sheath totally or partially; fibrin or precipitate accumulation can occur in portal reservoir in implanted devices	Percutaneous PICC Midclavicular Tunneled catheter Implanted port	Sluggish flow rates, total occlusion, inability to flush or obtain blood withdrawal (clinically silent), fibrin (may be able to infuse solutions), but unable to aspirate blood, "ball-valve-effect"	Attempt to aspirate clot Initiate appropriate fibrinolytic treatment with t-PA
Pinch-off syndrome: CVC inserted via the percutaneous subclavian site is compressed by the clavicle and the first rib; results in mechanical occlusion; can result in complete or partial catheter transection and embolization	Percutaneous	Frequently unrecognized, catheter is positional, weak points on the catheter balloon out, difficulty in aspiration of blood, resistance to flushing or infusion (often relieved by rolling the shoulder or raising the arm), infraclavicular pain or swelling	Remove catheter Retrieve the embolized segment if necessary
SVC syndrome: Condition caused by blood clot, fibrin formation, or both that occludes the SVC	PICC Tunneled catheter Implanted port	Progressive shortness of breath; cough; sensation of skin tightness; unilateral edema; cyanosis of face, neck, shoulder, and arms; "short-cap edema" (edema of the upper extremities without edema of lower); jugular, temporal, and arm veins are engorged and distended; prominent venous pattern is present over chest	Notify physician immediately Radiographic confirmation of SVC syndrome Catheter may or may not be removed Anticoagulant therapy Place patient in semi-Fowler's position Administer oxygen Monitor fluid volume status

(Continued)

TABLE 11–5

COMPLICATIONS ASSOCIATED WITH CENTRAL VENOUS ACCESS DEVICES *(Continued)*

Complication and Cause	Central Line Device	Signs and Symptoms	Interventions
		Post-insertion Complications	
Damaged catheter: External: broken catheter caused by scissors, penetration with needle; internal: rupture caused by use of a smaller than 10-mL syringe, pinch-off syndrome	Percutaneous PICC Midclavicular Tunneled catheter Implanted port	External: Leakage from catheter, wet dressing, leakage at insertion site Internal: Swelling in chest area, infusion of solution into chest wall; swelling at point of catheter rupture (Note: Damaged external catheter can be an entry point of bacteria into the vascular system)	Monitor for pin holes, leaks, wet dressing External: Apply nonserrated clamp to proximal to damaged part of catheter Internal: Stop infusion, place patient on bedrest, prepare to repair or remove catheter

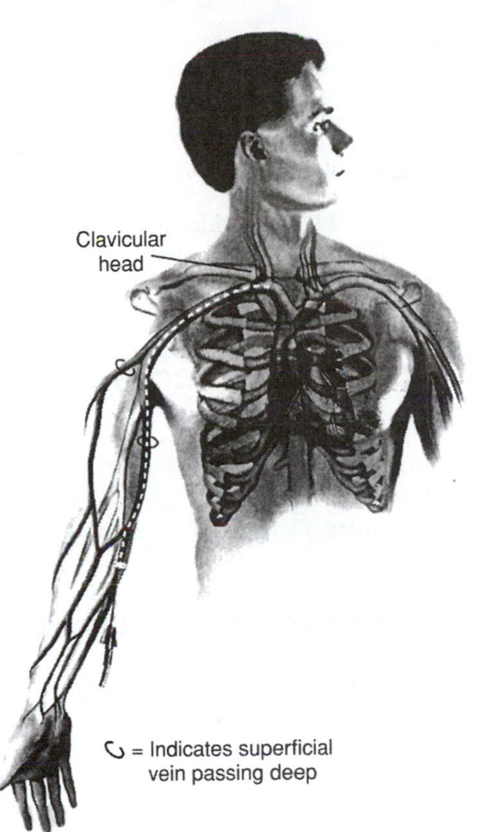

FIG. 11–10. Placement of peripherally inserted catheter in midclavicular site. (Courtesy of Bard Access Systems, Salt Lake City, Utah.)

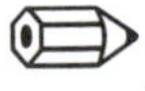

NOTE: The radiologic confirmation of midclavicular tip placement is optional.

Clinical situations in which radiologic confirmation is recommended include:

1. Difficulty with catheter advancement
2. Pain or discomfort after catheter advancement
3. Inability to flush the catheter easily
4. When the guidewire is difficult to remove or is bent after removal
5. Pain, discomfort, feelings of fullness or coldness, or the patient's hearing gurgling sounds during flushing

Care and Maintenance

Swell time for midclavicular tip placement is up to 2 to 3 months. As with all invasive lines, the patient should be monitored for objective or subjective signs of complications. The catheter should be removed by a registered nurse competent in using peripherally inserted catheters (INS, 1997b). Dressings and monitoring of the access site is the same as for PICC tip placement.

Complications

Table 11–5 provides a guide to complications associated with central lines. Midclavicular tip placement has many of the same complications as PICC placement.

LONG-TERM ACCESS DEVICES

Devices designed for long-term use can be divided into two categories: tunneled catheters and implanted ports. These catheters are made of Silastic or TPU and are available in single or multiple lumens. They require a surgical procedure for insertion.

CENTRAL VENOUS TUNNELED CATHETERS

Central venous tunneled catheters (**CVTCs**) have been available since 1975, when **Broviac** catheters were introduced for long-term TPN. The Broviac catheter was followed by a modified version, the **Hickman** catheter, which could accommodate the delivery of therapies to bone marrow transplant patients. CVTCs became the prototype for a variety of tunneled catheters currently on the market for various therapies. Inserted through a subcutaneous tunnel, these catheters are often referred to as indwelling catheters, tunneled CVCs, or right atrial catheters.

CVTCs are intended to be used for months to years to provide long-term venous access for obtaining blood samples and for administering drugs, blood products, and TPN.

CVTCs are composed of polymeric silicone with a Dacron polyester cuff that anchors the catheter in place subcutaneously. This cuff is about 2 inches from the catheter's exit site, which becomes embedded with fibroblasts within 1 week to 10 days after insertion, reducing the chances for accidental removal and minimizing the risk of ascending bacterial infection. CVTCs are available with single, double, or triple lumens. They vary in size from pediatric to adult, with most internal lumens ranging from 0.5 to 1.6 mm.

One of the advantages of CVTCs is that a break or tear in the catheter is easy to repair without adhesive. Depending on the type of catheter and the type of repair needed, adhesive may be required.

An attachable cuff, VitaCuff, is available for CVTCs. This cuff is made of biodegradable collagen impregnated with silver ion. Subcutaneous tissue grows to the cuff, providing a mechanical barrier, and the silver ion provides a chemical barrier against organisms. This cuff has proved to be cost effective in decreasing catheter-related septicemia (Maki & Mermel, 1998).

A development in CVTCs is the application of the Groshong valve feature, which has been marketed since 1984 (Fig. 11–11). This catheter has a few unique features that set it apart from other CVTCs. The Groshong catheter is made of soft, flexible Silastic material. The outer diameter dimensions are small. The catheter is available in single, double, or triple lumens. The Silastic material has a recoil memory that returns it to its original configuration if accidentally pulled. Another unique feature of the Groshong catheter is the two-way valve placed near the distal end, which restricts backflow of blood, but can be purposefully overridden to obtain venous blood samples. This valve eliminates the need for flushing with heparin. Thc valve is open inward, minimizing the risks of blood backing up the catheter lumen. The Groshong valve feature is now available on a variety of CVCs, including PICCs and ports (Fig. 11–12).

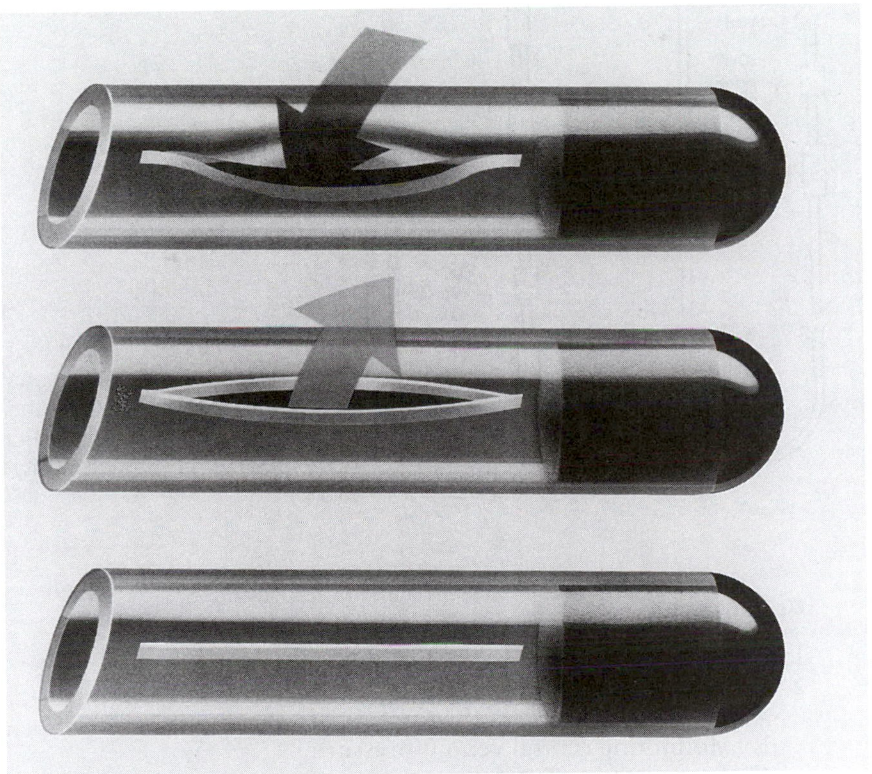

FIG. 11–11. Groshong valve. (Courtesy of BARD Access Systems, Salt Lake City, Utah.)

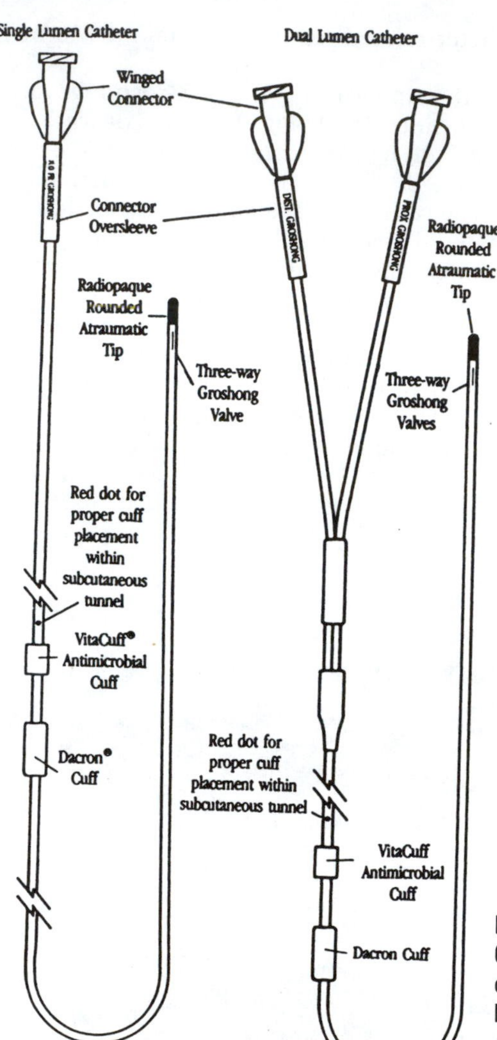

FIG. 11–12. Schematic of Groshong catheters—single and double lumen with VitaCuff and Dacron cuff. (Courtesy of BARD Access Systems, Salt Lake City, Utah.)

Advantages

1. Can be repaired if it breaks or tears
2. Can be used for many purposes including:
   A. Blood samples
   B. Monitoring central venous pressure
   C. Administering TPN
   D. Drug administration
3. Can be used for the patient with a chronic need for I.V. therapy

Disadvantages

1. Daily to weekly site care
2. Cost of maintenance supplies (dressings, materials, and changes; frequency of flushing and cap changing)
3. Surgical catheter insertion procedure that requires maintenance
4. Can affect the patient's body image

Insertion of Tunneled Catheters

Central venous tunneled catheters are inserted with the patient under local or general anesthesia by surgical **cutdown** or percutaneous puncture, and the catheter is placed by locating the subclavian vein. A separate proximal incision is made on the chest or abdominal wall, and the catheter is directed through a subcutaneous tunnel between the two incisions. The catheter is open at the distal and proximal ends and trimmed to the approximate estimated length and threaded through the subclavian vein into the SVC. The position is confirmed by fluoroscopy, adjusted if needed, and then sutured to the skin or the incision is closed with Steri-Strips. These remain in place for 10 to 14 days (Fig. 11–13).

Nursing Management of Tunneled Catheters

- Be sure the catheter is capped at all times. If it becomes uncapped, follow the steps for flushing the catheter.

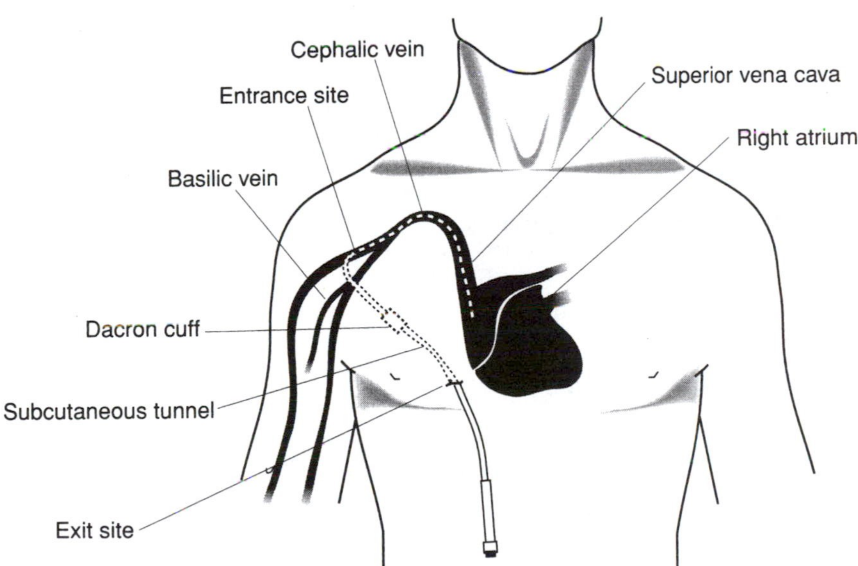

FIG. 11–13. Anatomic placement of tunneled catheter. (Courtesy of BARD Access Systems, Salt Lake City, Utah.)

NOTE: The catheter should be clamped if malfunction is suspected or when catheter breakage occurs.

- Keep all sharp objects away from the catheter.
- Never use scissors or pins on or near the catheter.
- If the catheter leaks or breaks, take a nonserrated clamp and clamp the catheter between the broken area and the exit site. Cover the broken part with a sterile gauze bandage and tape it securely. Do not use the catheter. Notify the physician.
- Protect the catheter when showering or bathing by covering the entire catheter with transparent dressing or clear plastic wrap.
- Flush after a blood drawing with 10 mL of 0.9 percent sodium chloride.
- Heparin is used to maintain the patency of the catheter, except for the Groshong catheter.

Dressing Management of Tunneled Catheters

This is a sterile procedure. To change the dressings, follow these steps:

1. Wash hands.
2. Put on mask if patient is neutropenic and then put on sterile gloves.
3. Remove the dressing from the site.
4. Inspect the site for redness, swelling, and drainage.
5. Remove gloves and put on a second pair of sterile gloves.
6. Using three alcohol swab sticks, cleanse the exit site, rotating in a circular method from inside outward. Allow to air dry.
7. Using three povidone-iodine swab sticks, cleanse the site, rotating in a circular method from inside outward; let dry 1 to 2 minutes. (Check for patient allergy to iodine before using povidone-iodine.)
8. Use TSM dressing over site.
9. Tape the catheter to the dressing and coil the remaining tubing using the Chevron technique.
10. Place the date, time, and your initials on all dressing.

Flushing Procedure

Flushing procedures vary according to the agency. Generally it is accepted practice to flush the CVTCs (except the Groshong) with twice the catheter volume of heparinized saline (volumes range from 0.8 to 1.6 mL). After medication administration or daily maintenance, flush the catheter with saline; then follow with heparinized saline.

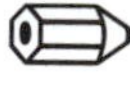

NOTE: Various care settings recommend using anywhere from 1 to 10 mL with concentrations ranging from 10 to 1000 U/mL. The frequency of flushing also varies from daily to once per week.

Changing the Injection (PRN) Cap

The injection cap must be changed at routine intervals. If the catheter is flushed every other day, cap changing may be coordinated with each third flushing (every 6 days). Using an intermittent injection cap that has a very small amount of dead space is recommended (Procedure 11–2).

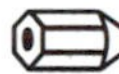
NOTE: If you have a multi-lumen catheter, remember to change all caps, even on unused lumens.

PROCEDURE 11–2: TUNNELED CATHETERS: FLUSH AND CAP CHANGE

1. Wash hands thoroughly and dry
2. Aseptically prepare sterile supplies.
3. Put on gloves.
4. Prepare air-purged heparin flush.
5. Remove tape holding catheter to chest wall and remove tape securing the cap to the catheter.
6. Cleanse the cap–catheter connection point with povidone-iodine for 30 seconds.
7. Place on sterile sponge and allow to dry.
8. Close the clamp.
9. Pick-up the catheter hub protected by sterile sponge; do not touch the cleansed connection.
10. Carefully unlock and remove.
11. Holding the new cap by the rubber injection end, connect and lock to catheter.
12. Secure connection with a strip of tape.
13. Remove clamp. Cleanse rubber end of injection cap with povidone-iodine for 30 seconds and allow to dry.
14. Carefully insert needleless syringe of heparin flush into center of rubber end. Do not force insertion.
15. Gently inject heparin. Before the syringe is completely empty, close clamp
16. Apply pressure on the plunger while withdrawing the syringe.
17. Remove the clamp.
18. Tape the catheter hub on the chest wall above heart level.

Repair of the Catheter

The CVTC can tear during reinsertion of the introducer needle, during intermittent therapy when I.V. push therapy is performed, or when using scissors near the catheter site. When this happens, blood usually backs up and fluid leaks from the site (except Groshong valve catheters). Air can enter the catheter through the tear, causing an air embolism.

Keeping up to date on repair methods can be difficult. Several types of repair kits are available. CVTCs can be repaired without a kit, but this requires a certain amount of creativity and knowledge. Types of repair include blunt-end needle repair, splicing sleeve with adhesive, manufacturer-specific hub or body repair kit, and the plastic catheter method.

To repair the catheter, you need sterile gloves, mask, sterile drapes, sterile scissors, povidone-iodine solution, extension set, and the appropriate repair kit. Follow manufacturer recommendations for external catheter repair. An example of a repair kit and instructions is shown in Figure 11–14.

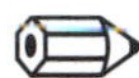

NOTE: Avoid serrated clamps on the catheter.

External clamps should not be routinely used; they are unnecessary and could damage the catheter.

Flushing a Tunneled Catheter with a Groshong Valve

Policies and procedures vary from institution to institution. The Groshong catheter should be flushed every 7 days with 0.9 percent sodium chloride when not in use. Maintain aseptic technique. After administering medications, the catheter should be flushed with 5 mL of sodium chloride. After administering viscous solutions such as lipids, flush

Connector Instructions

1. Transfer white sleeve (A) onto catheter from connector.

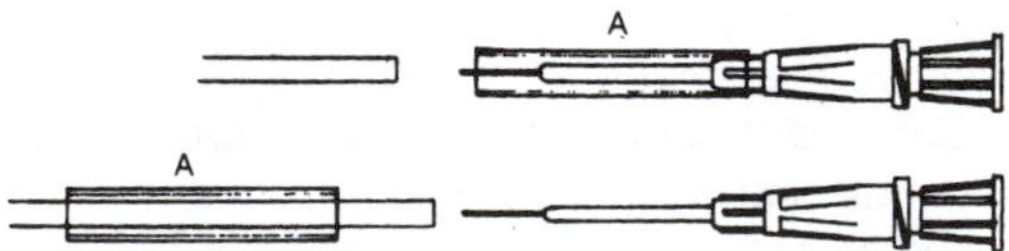

2. Firmly push catheter onto adapter to Position B.

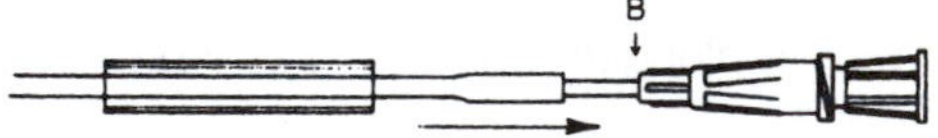

3. Slide white sleeve onto colored hub to Position C.

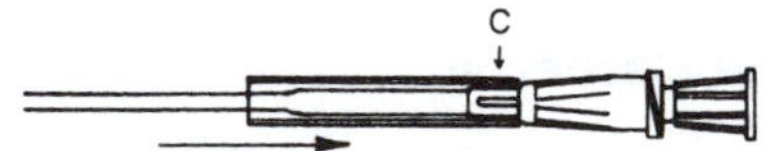

4. Remove and discard stylet.

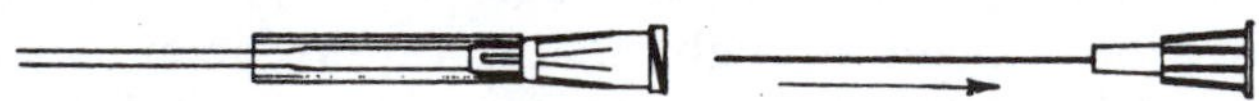

FIG. 11–14. Example of repair kit for tunneled catheter. (Courtesy of BARD Access Systems, Salt Lake City, Utah.)

briskly with 20 mL of sodium chloride to prevent crystallization of the catheter tip. Manufacturers recommend that the catheter be irrigated with a syringe attached directly to the connection hub of the catheter.

Blood Sampling from a Tunneled Catheter

To draw a blood sample from a tunneled catheter, follow these steps:

1. Flush the catheter with 0.9 percent sodium chloride.
2. Withdraw and discard 6 mL of blood.
3. Draw the blood sample.
4. Flush the catheter with 20 mL of 0.9 percent sodium chloride using the push–stop method of flushing.

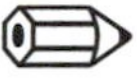

NOTE: The "push–pause" method of flushing causes a turbulent effect, cleansing the sides of the catheter as well as the end of the catheter.

An alternate method of blood sample is the push–pull method, which eliminates the need to discard any blood. Patients requiring 10 venous blood samples per day lose an additional 60 mL of blood with the discard method (Homes, 1998). With this method, the syringe is attached to the catheter and 6 mL of blood is withdrawn and pushed back into the catheter without removing the syringe. This is repeated a total of three times. This removes any residual solution within the catheter before blood collection. The push–pull method provides advantages over the discard method by reducing:

- Blood loss, particularly for patients in the pediatric, oncology, and critical care units who require frequent sample collection
- Blood loss exposure to healthcare personnel
- The risk of potential contamination of the catheter from multiple manipulations
- The risk of reporting erroneous results by eliminating the potential of confusing the laboratory sample with the discard specimen (Holmes, 1998)

Complications Associated with Tunneled Catheters

Table 11–5 is a guide to CVTC catheter complications. Common risks associated with CVTCs include exit site infections, sepsis, thrombosis, nonthrombosis occlusions, catheter migration, torn or leading catheter, and air embolism.

IMPLANTED PORTS

Implanted ports, another type of CVC, have been available for venous access since 1983. Originally, implanted ports were targeted to oncology patients who required frequent intermittent venous access.

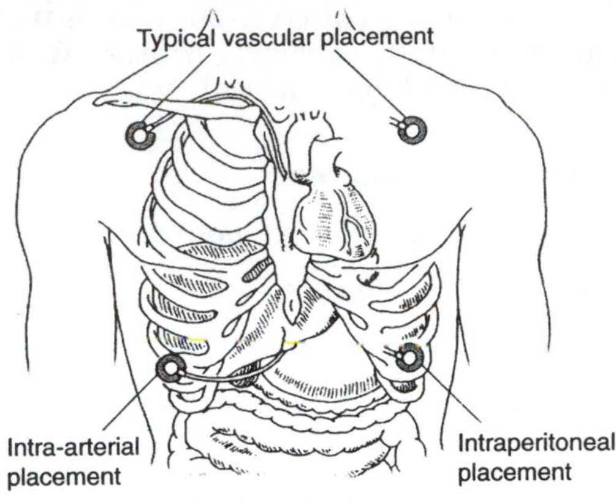

FIG. 11–15. Examples of placement sites for vascular access ports. (Courtesy of BARD Access Systems, Salt Lake City, Utah.)

Ports consist of a reservoir, silicone catheter, and central septum (Fig. 11–15).

The implanted port vascular access system provides safe and reliable vascular access; the design provides patients with an improved body image, reduced maintenance, and improved quality of life.

The self-sealing septum can usually withstand 1000 to 2000 needle punctures. Ports have raised edges to facilitate puncture with a noncoring needle. The port is made of stainless steel or titanium. The septum is connected to a silicone catheter (Riser, 1988). Many types of implanted VADs are available today, but all are inserted in the same location and have the same use. Figure 11–16 shows various types of implanted ports.

A new line of implanted ports is the CathLink 20 (Bard Access Systems), which is available in three sizes: standard profile, low profile, and ultra-low profile, allowing for placement approaches ranging from chest wall to lower arm. The CathLink 20 is designed for use with standard 20-gauge over-the-needle I.V. catheters, rather than noncoring Huber needles. The CathLink 20 port eliminates angles and large reservoirs with a layered silicone septum, which increases the septum's longevity. The port is flushed with 5 mL of heparinized sodium chloride once every 4 weeks when not in use (Fig. 11–17).

Advantages

1. Less risk of infection when used intermittently
2. Less interference with daily activities
3. Little site care
4. Needs minimal flushing
5. Easy access for fluids, blood products, or medication administration
6. Less body image disturbance owing to the lack of an external catheter device
7. Few limitations on patient activity

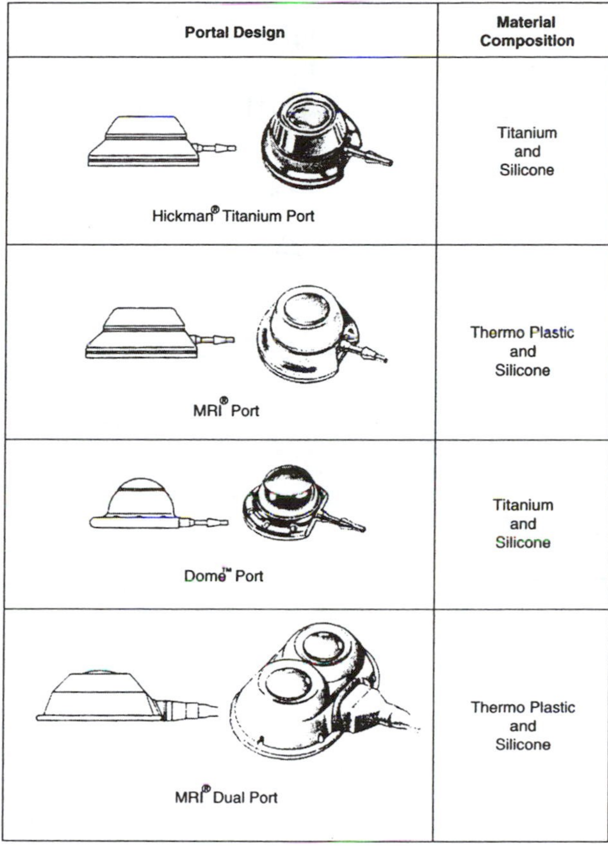

Portal Design	Material Composition
Hickman® Titanium Port	Titanium and Silicone
MRI® Port	Thermo Plastic and Silicone
Dome™ Port	Titanium and Silicone
MRI® Dual Port	Thermo Plastic and Silicone

FIG. 11–16. Examples of types of port designs. (Courtesy of BARD Access Systems, Salt Lake City, Utah.)

Disadvantages

1. Cost of insertion (considerably higher than with other VADs)
2. Postoperative care is 7 to 10 days
3. Discomfort of repeated needlesticks
4. Minor surgical procedure necessary to remove device

Insertion

The port is inserted after a local anesthetic is administered; the entire procedure takes from 30 minutes to 1 hour. An incision is made in the upper to middle chest, usually near the collarbone, to form a pocket to house the port. The Silastic catheter is inserted via cutdown into the SVC; the port is then placed in the subcutaneous fascia pocket. The port contains a reservoir leading to the catheter. The incision for the port pocket is sutured closed, and a sterile dressing is applied. The dressing may

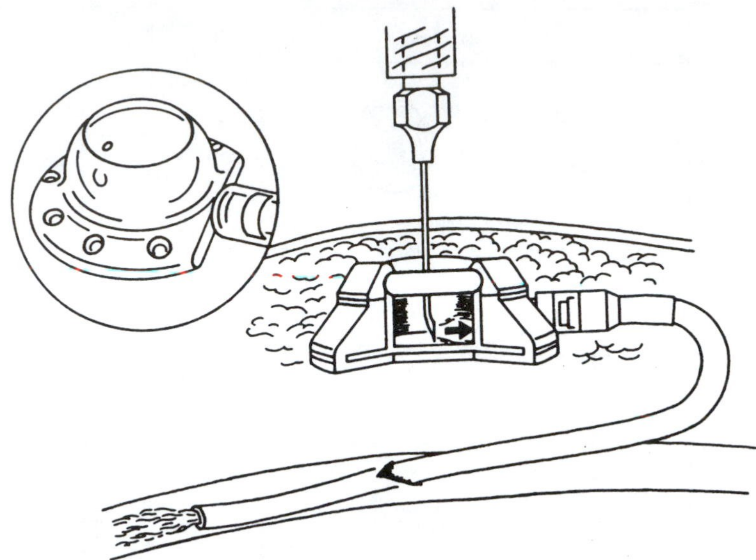

FIG. 11–17. CathLink 20 implanted port uses 20-gauge 1 3/4-in over-the-needle catheter to access the port. (Courtesy of BARD Access Systems, Salt Lake City, Utah.)

be removed after the first 24 hours. This area should be monitored until the incision has healed, about 10 days to 2 weeks after insertion.

The subcutaneous port system catheter can be placed in any of the following: SVC, hepatic artery, peritoneal space for intraperitoneal therapy, and epidural space.

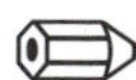 **NOTE:** Implanted ports are available in one or two septum chambers. Ports designed for peripheral access are also available.

Accessing the Port

To access an implanted port, including how to inject a bolus and inject a continuous infusion, follow the guidelines listed in Procedure 11–3.

PROCEDURE 11–3: ACCESSING AN IMPLANTED PORT

 **INS STANDARDS** Sterile gloves and masks should be used when accessing an implanted port. The smallest gauge noncoring needle that can deliver the prescribed therapy should be used. When ports are accessed, the noncoring needle should be changed at least every 7 days (INS, 2000, 51).

1. Wearing nonsterile gloves, palpate the port to find the entry septum.

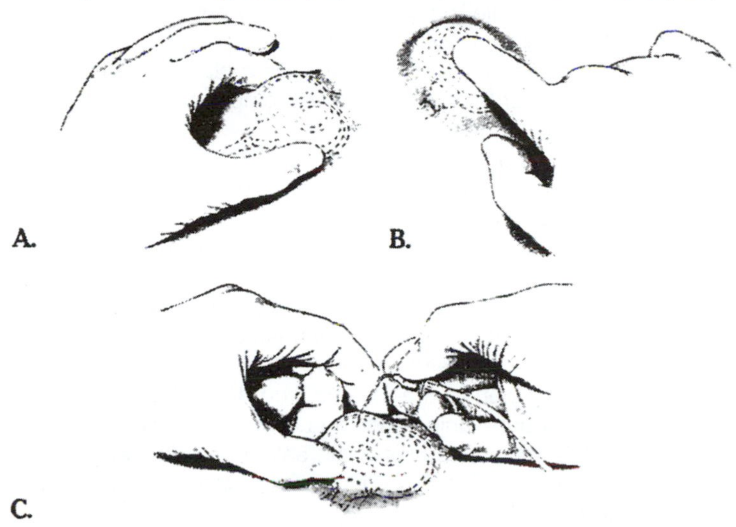

2. Put on sterile gloves.
3. Using an alcohol swabstick, cleanse exit site, rotating in a circular method from inside outward, repeat three times. Allow to air dry.
4. Using povidone-iodine swabstick, cleanse site, rotating in a circular method from inside outward, repeat three times, then let dry 1 to 2 minutes. (Check for patient allergy to iodine before use of povidone-iodine.)
5. Connect the appropriate gauge noncoring right angle needle to the Luer lock at the other end and prime the tubing.
6. Palpate the port to find the center of the septum.
7. Insert the noncoring right-angle needle into the center, pushing until the needle stops.
8. Aspirate a small amount of blood to check for patency and position.
9. Using firm, steady pressure, flush the port with approximately 10 mL of sodium chloride at the rate of less than 5 mL/min. If swelling occurs or the patient complains of pain or burning sensation, the needle is improperly positioned.
10. Attach a 10-mL syringe of heparin solution to the stopcock at the end of the extension tubing.
11. Disconnect the syringe and discard (Larouere, 1999a).
12. Inject bolus:
    - A. Attach the syringe containing the prescribed drug.
    - B. Carefully disconnect the syringe to prevent any of the drug from dripping on the patient's skin.
    - C. Attach the second 10-mL syringe of saline solution and flush the injection port and catheter.
    - D. Disconnect the syringe and discard.
    - E. Attach the 10-mL syringe of heparin solution and inject all 5 mL to prevent occlusion at the catheter tip.

(continued)

(continued)

F. Withdraw the needle, being careful not to twist or tilt.
G. Observe the injection site for signs of extravasation.
H. Use alcohol swabs, moving in a circular motion from the center of the port out to remove the povidone-iodine from the skin.

13. Inject a continuous infusion:
    A. Prepare site and access as for bolus.
    B. Roll a sterile 2 × 2 gauze pad and place under the needle hub and Luer lock to support the needle.
    C. Apply tincture of benzoin to the gauze to help the Steri-Strips adhere.
    D. Secure the needle hub and tubing by applying Steri-Strips across the hub, using a Chevron taping technique.
    E. Apply transparent dressing over the entire system.
    F. Attach the extension to the I.V. line from the infusion pump.
    G. Tape all connections unless using Luer lock connections.
14. When infusion is concluded, inject the saline and disconnect the syringe. Then attach a 10-mL syringe of heparin solution to the stopcock and flush the port.
15. Withdraw the noncoring needle without twisting or tilting.
16. Remove the tincture of benzoin with alcohol and apply a small bandage if necessary.

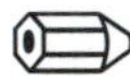 **NOTE:** I.V. tubing must be changed every 24 hours.

The dressing and extension tubing must be changed every 3 to 7 days.

Deaccessing an Implanted Port

To deaccess an implanted port, loosen the dressing covering the Huber access needle, with injection cap with alcohol and attach the syringe containing 0.9 percent sodium chloride solution. Flush the catheter.

Withdrawal of the Huber needle requires a two-handed technique. With the nondominant hand, use your thumb and index finger to stabilize the port. Steadily with an upward pull, remove the needle.

 **NOTE:** The nondominant hand securing the implanted port is particularly vulnerable to a rebound needlestick. Check the tip integrity and examine the needle for signs of occlusion or clotting. Discard in the sharps container. Cover the site with an adhesive bandage for 30 to 60 minutes (Larouere, 1999b).

Two products on the market are designed for preventing Huber needle-stick injuries. The Huber-Loc (MedCare Medical Group) is a single-use disposable device that extracts the needle and locks it inside a protective plastic housing. The Doyle Extractor (Safetech International, Inc.) uses contoured plastic blades to stabilize the port while removing the needle (Jagger, 1999).

Flushing Procedure

Flushing procedures vary from institution to institution. Flush the system with 5 mL of heparinized saline in a 10-mL syringe. If the port is not being used, flush with heparinized saline every 4 weeks. If the port is used for medication administration or blood component therapy, flush after every infusion with 10 mL of 0.9 percent sodium chloride, followed by 5 mL of sterile heparinized saline. Flush with 20 mL of 0.9 percent sodium chloride, followed by 5 mL of heparinized saline after blood withdrawal (Fig. 11–18).

Blood Sampling

To obtain a blood sample, first explain procedure to patient, then gather the equipment.

1. Aseptically prepare the injection site.
2. Insert noncoring needle attached to extension tubing and secure needle with tape.
3. Release the clamp and flush with 5 mL 0.9 percent sodium chloride in a 10-mL syringe to confirm that fluid flows through the system.
4. Withdraw at least 5 mL of blood, clamp tubing, and discard the syringe and blood.
5. Attach the syringe and release the clamp. Withdraw the desired amount of blood for sampling into a 20-mL syringe and transfer it to appropriate blood sample tube.
6. Clamp the tube and attach syringe with 20 mL of 0.9 percent sodium chloride. Release the clamp and flush the system, using the push–pause method.

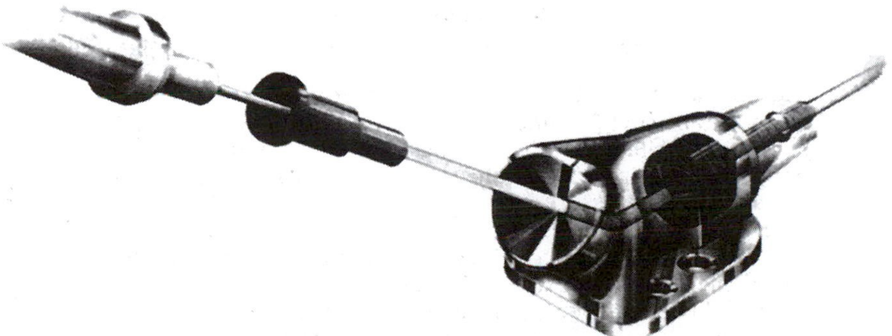

FIG. 11–18. Flushing implanted port with percutaneous needle entry. (Courtesy of BARD Access Systems, Salt Lake City, Utah.)

7. Clamp the tube and attach a syringe with 5 mL of heparinized saline in a 10-mL syringe. Release the clamp and flush the system, leaving the heparin in lock.

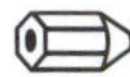 **NOTE:** Flushing with positive pressure decreases catheter complications.

Complications

The same complications associated with CVTCs can occur with implanted ports. Table 11–5 provides guidelines for dealing with central line complications. Implanted ports can also develop site infection or skin breakdown and port migration. Extravasation of vesicant medications that are infusing into the port can occur if the needle is not in place through the septum of the port and the position is not confirmed. Fluid can extravasate and collect subcutaneously, resulting in burning or swelling around the port during infusion. Patients and nurses must always verify placement, secure the needle before initiating the infusion, and observe for signs of swelling or burning.

Key Points

- Use a noncoring needle with appropriate port.
- Change the needle and extension tubing every 7 days.
- Flush the port with 0.9 percent sodium chloride and heparin every 4 weeks if the port is not in use or after every infusion, following the procedure outlined.
- For continuous infusion, change the dressing every 72 hours.
- For continuous infusion, change the tubing every 48 hours.

MANAGEMENT OF OCCLUDED CENTRAL VENOUS ACCESS DEVICES

LOSS OF PATENCY

Vascular access devices can become occluded as a result of mechanical obstruction, thrombotic occlusion, or drug precipitation (nonthrombotic). Loss of patency results from causes as simple as the patient's position to causes as involved as combinations of complex clotting processes juxtaposed on the disease process (Bagnall-Reeb, 1998).

Two criteria define CVC patency: the ability to infuse through the catheter and the ability to aspirate blood from the catheter. Withdrawal occlusion is a subset of catheter occlusions and describes the inability to freely aspirate blood from the catheter (Krzywda, 1999). The treatment must begin promptly; therefore, systematic evaluation of the catheter patency needs to be ongoing. If a VAD occlusion is left untreated, secondary complications can occur, such as loss of venous access, morbidity of recannulation, and risk of catheter infection because of a fibrin sheath for bacterial or fungal colonization.

Preventive care of clot formation and subsequent occlusion include careful catheter insertion; routine assessment of dressings, exit sites, tubing, pumps, infusion bags, and clamps; meticulous technique in blood sampling; and avoiding potential drug or solution incompatibilities. Table 11–6 presents a guide to troubleshooting occlusions.

MECHANICAL OCCLUSION

The mechanical obstruction of a catheter can be either external or internal. External causes of occlusion are a kinked or closed clamp or a tight suture at the catheter exit site. External occlusion of flow may be caused by clogged injection cap, a clogged I.V. filter, an infusion pump that has been turned off, or an empty I.V. bag. Occlusion can also occur at the catheter exit site or vein entry site if the suture used to secure the line constricts the catheter.

TABLE 11–6

TROUBLESHOOTING GUIDE FOR OCCLUDED CENTRAL VENOUS CATHETERS

Purpose of Catheter (Agent Infused)	Cause of Occlusion	Treatment
Prolonged use of catheter	Fibrin sheath or thrombosis	Thrombolytic: t-PA
Blood draw	Fibrin sheath or thrombosis	Thrombolytic: t-PA
Transfusions	Fibrin sheath or thrombosis	Thrombolytic: t-PA
Medication administration	Precipitate	$NaHCO_3$ or HCl
Cold medications or solutions	Precipitate	$NaHCO_3$ or HCl
Stability (pH of medication)	Precipitate	$NaHCO_3$ or HCl
Medication with poor solubility (e.g., Dilantin)	Precipitate	$NaHCO_3$ or HCl
Time elapse since medication mixed	Precipitate	$NaHCO_3$ or HCl
Fat emulsions (or three-in-one TPN)	Lipid aggregation	Ethanol

HCl = hydrochloric acid; $NaHCO_3$ = sodium bicarbonate.

Internal obstruction is caused by improper catheter tip placement, as well as catheter kinking or compression. The catheter can be pinched closed as a result of the patient's position by pressure of the clavicle against the first rib (pinch-off syndrome) or it can be obstructed by lodging the catheter tip against the vein wall. Catheter fracture is a partial or complete breaking of the catheter. Pinch-off syndrome is the most common cause when subclavian venipuncture is used.

Management

When I.V. flow is occluded, first determine whether the cause is internal or external. Examine the I.V. setup for kinked tubing, closed clamps, an empty infusion bag, and readjustment of the I.V. delivery system. Having the patient change position may correct the problem. Finally, chest radiography may help to confirm catheter tip placement and rule out migration.

The following interventions can be used to manage a suspected occlusion caused by mechanical forces:

1. Reposition the patient.
2. Have the patient cough.
3. Reposition the catheter, if possible.
4. Roll the patient's shoulder or raise the patient's arm on the ipsilateral side.
5. Use fluoroscopy if indicated to locate a mechanical occlusion.

THROMBOTIC OCCLUSION

Deposits of fibrin and blood components within and around the CVC can impede or disrupt flow. Thrombotic occlusions are caused by intraluminal blood clots, a fibrin sheath totally or partially around the catheter tip, or catheter abutment against the vessel wall. Implanted devices can accumulate fibrin or precipitate within the portal reservoir (Bagnall-Reeb, 1998). Thrombus formation can occur within the first 24 hours after insertion or over a period of time. A variety of thrombotic events can result in catheter occlusion.

Intraluminal Occlusion

Intraluminal occlusion occurs when the lumen of the catheter is obstructed by either clotted blood or an accumulation of fibrin. Frequently, the cause is blood remaining in the catheter after inadequate irrigation or retrograde flow (Fig. 11–19). Also, poor flushing technique after blood sampling may allow layers of fibrin to accumulate over time, narrowing or obstructing the lumen.

Fibrin Sleeve and Fibrin Tail

Platelet aggregation and fibrin deposition may completely encase the surface of the catheter and form a sac around the distal end of the catheter

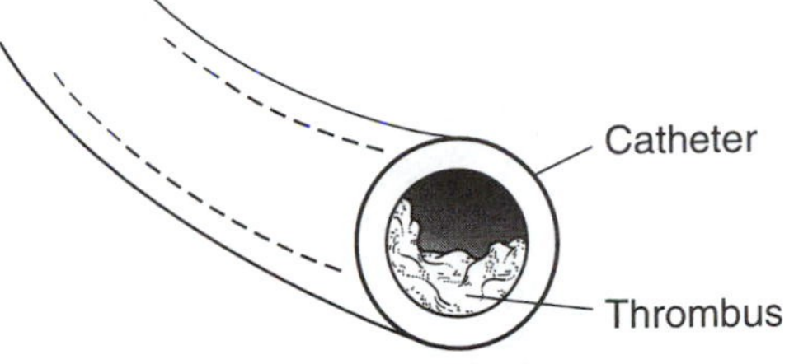

FIG. 11–19. Intraluminal occlusion. (Source: Bagnall-Reeb, Ryder, & Anglim [1994]. Venous Access Device Occlusions Independent Study Module. Illinois: Abbott Laboratories.)

(Fig. 11–20.) The sac causes retrograde flow of infusate up the catheter. The infusate may be observed on the skin (in nontunneled catheters), in the skin tunnel (in tunneled catheters), or in the subcutaneous pocket of implanted ports (Bagnall-Reeb, 1998). A "tail" of fibrin extending off the catheter tip can occur owing to platelet aggregation and fibrin accumulation. The tail usually does not interfere with infusion but may occlude the catheter on aspiration. This is commonly known as the "ball valve effect."

Venous Thrombosis

Endothelial damage to a blood vessel can result in fibrin deposition at the point of cellular damage. If the thrombus occurs along the wall of the vein, it is a mural thrombus. If the thrombus completely occludes the vein, it is a venous thrombosis.

PORTAL RESERVOIR OCCLUSION

Fluid viscosity or an improper flushing technique can produce fibrin or precipitate deposits within the reservoir of the port (Fig. 11–21.) Accumulation of deposits leads to obstruction of the tube.

Management

Gentle aspiration may dislodge the occlusive material from within the catheter lumen. Thrombolytic agents are the only available drugs to lyse existing clots. They convert plasminogen to plasmin, which acts directly on the clot to dissolve the fibrin matrix.

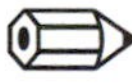 **NOTE:** Forceful flushing of the catheter to push the clot into the circulation is not recommended. The use of a guidewire or snare to manipulate the clot out of the catheter is also not recommended.

THROMBOLYTIC ADMINISTRATION

Alteplase is a recombinant form of the naturally occurring tissue plasminogen activator (tPA) that enhances the conversion of plasminogen to plasmin in the presence of fibrin. When introduced into the systemic

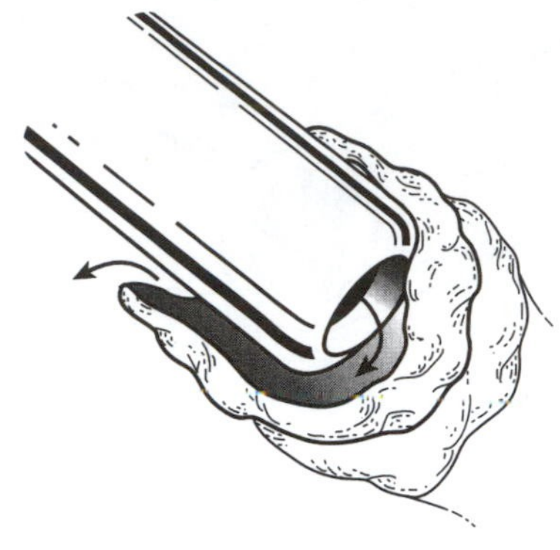

FIG. 11-20. Fibrin sleeve. (Source: Bagnall-Reeb, Ryder, & Anglim [1994]. Venous Access Device Occlusions Independent Study Module. Illinois: Abbott Laboratories.)

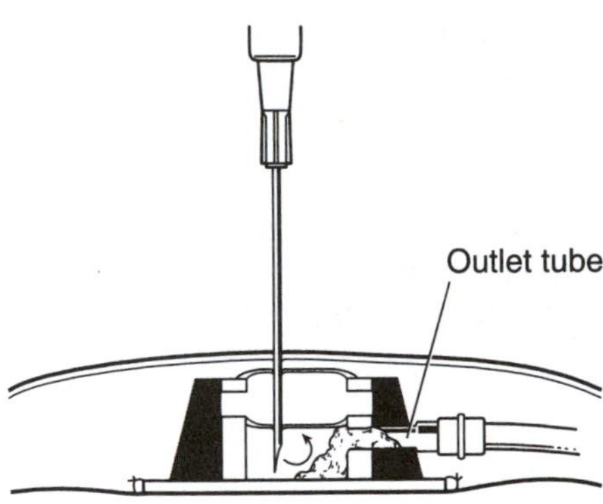

FIG. 11-21. Portal reservoir occlusion. (Source: Bagnall-Reeb, Ryder, & Anglim [1994]. Venous Access Device Occlusions Independent Study Module. Illinois: Abbott Laboratories.)

circulation, alteplase binds to the fibrin in a thrombus and converts the entrapped plasminogen to plasmin. This action initiates local fibrinolysis. Currently alteplase is FDA approved for the management of acute myocardial infarction, acute ischemic stroke, and acute massive pulmonary embolism (Postgraduate Institute for Medicine, 1999).

The optimal alteplase dose, solution volume, and indwelling time for the clearance of thrombosed CVCs have not yet been determined. Data from Haire, Atkinson, & Stephens (1994) suggest that a 2-mg dose (1 mg/mL) and a 2-hour indwelling time may be appropriate.

Contraindications to Thrombolytic Therapy

Patients who have active internal bleeding, intracranial neoplasm, hypersensitivity to thrombolytic agents, liver disease, subacute bacterial endocarditis, or visceral malignancy or who have had a cerebrovascular accident within the past 2 months, or intracranial or intraspinal surgery should not receive a thrombolytic agent.

Drug Incompatibilities

Do not mix with any other medication in any manner.

Complications of Thrombolytic Therapy

Bleeding

Bleeding may occur in two general forms: surface bleeding from invaded or disturbed sites (punctures, incision) or internal bleeding from the GI tract, genitourinary tract, vagina, or intramuscular, retroperitoneal, or intracerebral sites. Fatalities caused by cerebral or retroperitoneal hemorrhage have occurred. The antidote is administering plasma volume expanders such as fresh plasma fluids, along with whole blood if hemorrhage is unresponsive to blood replacement. Aminocaproic acid can be used.

Allergic Reactions

These reactions are rare and are usually in the form of rash, bronchospasm, or anaphylaxis.

Fever

Fever can occur and should be symptomatically controlled with acetaminophen rather than aspirin (Gahart & Nazareno, 1999).

Nursing Considerations of Thrombolytic Therapy

1. Observe the patient continuously.
2. Do not use force when instilling a thrombolytic agent into a catheter.
3. Work with declotting the catheter every 15 minutes after dwell time.
4. If necessary, obtain thrombin time, prothrombin time, or activated partial thromboplastin time to monitor.
5. Keep the physician informed.

NONTHROMBOTIC OCCLUSION

Nonthrombotic occlusions are caused by mineral precipitates. Precipitates result from poorly soluble I.V. fluid components or the interaction of the infusate with other solutions. Crystallization of TPN admixtures and drug-to-drug or drug-to solution incompatibilities are also causes of catheter occlusions.

Precipitates may occur gradually, causing sluggish flow, or they may be immediate, totally occluding the line. Determining the pH of the medication that has precipitated is the key in attempting to restore patency.

For medications at a low pH (less than 6.0), the instillation of a 0.1-M solution of hydrochloric acid (HCl) has been reported to restore catheter function. Sodium bicarbonate ($NaHCO_3$) 1 mEq/mL has been used to restore patency in catheter occluded by precipitation of medications soluble in a basic state (pH more than 7) (Bagnall-Reeb, 1998).

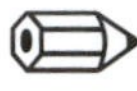

NOTE: Use of hydrochloric acid or sodium bicarbonate to clear drug precipitates is not FDA approved. Caution should be taken in using either therapy.

Catheter obstruction in patients receiving TPN may be caused by crystallization of calcium phosphate or lipid residue. This precipitation is caused by pH concentrations of dextrose, amino acid, and calcium as well as by increased temperature. To restore patency in catheters occluded with crystallized calcium phosphate, use 0.1 M of hydrochloric acid in a volume equal to the internal filling capacity and allow it to dwell for 20 minutes before being withdrawn.

Lipid occlusions may occur with three-in-one admixtures of parenteral nutrition. The buildup of lipid residue within the catheter lumen or port reservoir may cause sluggish flow or total obstruction. This residue can be dissolved with a 70 percent solution of ethanol (Hadaway, 1998).

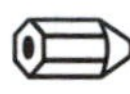

NOTE: As a preventive measure, brisk flushing of the catheter with an appropriate volume of sodium chloride after the infusion of three-in-one solutions may reduce the intraluminal lipid residue.

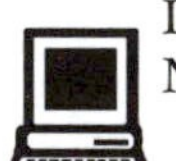

WEB SITES:

Intravenous Nurses Society: *www.ins1.org*

National Association of Vascular Access Networks (NAVAN): *www.navannet.org*

Canadian Intravenous Nurses Association (CINA): *web.idirect.com*

Others: ______________________

PEDIATRIC CENTRAL VENOUS ACCESS

The work of Dudrick et al. (1969) showed that long-term central venous access is possible in children requiring I.V. nutritional support.

Long-term central venous access is an integral part of managing children with cancer, certain congenital malformations, and GI malfunction as well as for those who need long-term access to medication or blood products.

After a decision is made to use a VAD, the device type must also be patient and disease specific. For children age 3 years and younger, totally implanted devices are used with the least frequency and most frequently in children older than age 15 years (Wiener & Albanese, 1998).

Multi-lumen devices are especially useful in the care of critically ill children or in children who experience continuous multi-use of the device. Catheter size mirrors the size of the patient. Small-lumen external catheters are commonly placed in children age 3 years or younger.

NURSING PLAN OF CARE

MANAGEMENT OF CENTRAL VENOUS ACCESS DEVICES

Focus Assessment

Objective

- Interview regarding present knowledge of illness and VADs.
- Identify learning need and ability.

Subjective

- Assess competency and dexterity of patient in managing VADs.
- Inspect site for signs of infection. Inspect dressing for integrity.
- Examine PICC and tunneled catheters for integrity.
- Obtain baseline vital signs.

Patient Outcome Criteria

The patient will:

1. Be free of complications associated with insertion and postinsertion of CVCs.
2. Describe anxiety and coping patterns.
3. Demonstrate progressive healing of tissue.
4. Demonstrate a willingness and ability to resume self-care and role responsibilities.
5. Verbalize and demonstrate acceptance of appearance.
6. Verbalize deficiency in knowledge or skill related to central VAD.

Nursing Diagnoses

- Anxiety (mild, moderate, severe) related to threat to change in health status or misconceptions regarding therapy
- Altered tissue perfusion (cardiopulmonary) related to infiltration of vesicant medication
- Body image disturbance related to perceptions of VADs
- Decreased cardiac output related to sepsis or contamination
- Fear related to insertion of catheter; fear of "needles"
- Impaired gas exchange related to ventilation-perfusion imbalance; dislodged VAD
- Impaired skin integrity related to VAD; irritation from I.V. solution; inflammation; infection
- Impaired physical mobility related to pain or discomfort resulting from placement and maintenance of VAD (knowledge deficit [VAD and maintenance of I.V. solution] relating to lack of exposure)
- Risk of infection related to broken skin or traumatized tissue from the VAD

(continued)

(continued)

Nursing Management

1. Assist with insertion of central line.
2. Insert PICC according to agency protocol.
3. Maintain central line patency and dressing according to agency protocol.
4. Monitor for fluid overload.
5. Maintain occlusive dressing.
6. Monitor for Infiltration and infection.
7. Maintain sterile technique.
8. Use an infusion pump for delivery of solutions when appropriate.
9. Monitor vital signs.
10. Monitor daily weight.
11. Monitor intake and output ratios.
12. Use 10-mL syringe to flush catheters and obtain blood samples

PATIENT EDUCATION

Patient instructions for central line devices should include:

- Type of central venous access device, purpose and length of catheter or port that will be inserted; signs and symptoms to report, such as increased temperature, discomfort, pain, and difficult breathing; site care of PICC, CVTC, or implanted port.
- Emergency measures for clamping the catheter if it breaks.
- Flushing protocol.
- Access line for administering medication, TPN, or fluids.

Nurses are instrumental in educating patients and family members that the skin area over a subcutaneously implanted VAD should not be rubbed or manipulated in any way. Twiddler's syndrome, a condition in which a patient manipulates his or her ports by habit, can cause the internal catheter attached to the port to dislodge.

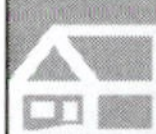

HOME CARE ISSUES

Central venous access devices are frequently used in the home for administering TPN, chemotherapy or biologic therapy, blood component therapy, and pain control, and for frequent blood sampling. Home infusion is comprehensive, beginning with principles of asepsis, handwashing, and universal precautions.

It is essential to assess whether or not the patient being considered for using a central venous line at home is interested in and motivated to learn self-care. This procedure requires a certain level of intellectual, emotional, and physical capacity and commitment to comply. If the patient is not physically or emotionally able to self-administer or monitor care, a reliable caregiver must be available.

Pretreatment assessment includes:

1. Taking a health history, including issues relevant to planned therapy
2. Verifying the medication and dosage that the patient is to receive
3. Reviewing complications and side effects of drug therapy and central line management
4. Reviewing the patient's history and past experience, if appropriate, with central lines
5. Assessing the patient's current knowledge of managing central lines
6. Providing written instruction and diagrams of accessing line, site care, and flushing protocol
7. Verifying insurance coverage for home care

The patient and family should have full instructions on how central line devices function and the safety precautions associated with their use. The home infusion patient should have step-by-step written information regarding care and maintenance.

KEY POINTS

- The tip of central venous access devices should be in the SVC, the tip should reside within 3 to 4 cm of the right atrial SVC junction. It must be free floating and lie parallel to the vessel wall without any looping or kinking.
- Central venous access devices and the length of time they may remain include:
  - Percutaneous catheters: 7 days
  - PICCs: 6 weeks to 1 year
  - Midclavicular catheters: 6 weeks
  - CVTCs: 3 years
  - Implanted ports: 3 years
- The patient should be well hydrated if using the infraclavicular approach to percutaneous catheterization.
- The optimum frequency for changing TSM dressing is unknown, but dressing should be changed at established intervals (generally every 3 to 7 days) or immediately if the integrity of the dressing is compromised.
- The basilic vein is the preferred insertion site for PICCs.
- After insertion of the central line, verification by chest radiograph must be obtained before any infusion is administered.
- To avoid intravascular malposition of the catheter in the jugular vein, have the patient turn her head toward the side of the venipuncture. This changes the angle of the catheter to move downward toward the SVC.
- Syringes with capacities of 10 mL or more must be used to access or irrigate central lines as excessive pressure from smaller-barreled syringes can cause damage or rupture of the line.
- Nurses managing central lines must be trained in their use, follow manufacturer guidelines, comply with agency protocols and policies, and be fully competent in the assessment, planning, intervention, and evaluation of the patient.
- Use Luer-locking connections on all central lines.
- Immediate complications of central lines include:
  - Bleeding
  - Pneumothorax
  - Hemothorax
  - Chylothorax
  - Brachial plexus injury
  - Extravascular malposition
- Delayed complications of central lines include
  - Air embolism
  - Catheter migration
  - Local infection
  - Septicemia
  - Thrombosis
  - Thrombolytic occlusions
  - Precipitate occlusions
  - SVC syndrome
  - Pinch-off syndrome
- Implanted ports are available in one or two septum chambers.
- Use the "push–pause" method of flushing central lines.
- Use thrombolytic agent to declot a central line of a thrombus or fibrin sheath. Use hydrochloride acid (HCl) for precipitates of drugs that have a low pH. Use $NaHCO_3$ for restoring patency of agents with high pH.
- The first step troubleshooting an occluded central line is to check for mechanical obstruction.

CHAPTER ACTIVITIES

COMPETENCY CRITERIA: Nursing Management of Central Venous Access Devices

COMPETENCY STATEMENT: Competent I.V. nurses will be able to demonstrate skill in nursing management of central venous access devices.

Note: The cognitive (knowledge) information that is embedded within this performance-based competency includes aseptic technique, knowledge of CVC design and catheter tip location, and recognition of signs and symptoms of complications of CVC devices.

This competency *links* to the competency of infection control, delivery of parenteral fluids, and management of I.V. therapy equipment.

Performance	Skilled	Needs Education
Critical Action Statements		
1. Performs baseline assessment of catheter patency A. Examines external lines for breaks or leaks B. Checks that injection caps are secure C. Verbalizes understanding of rationale for push–pause technique to irrigate CVC		
2. Maintains integrity of catheter following standards of practice A. Changes dressing (TSM) every 7 days B. Changes all injection caps every 3 to 7 days C. Changes noncoring needle every 7 days		
3. Uses 10-mL syringe to irrigate CVC device		
4. Demonstrates injection cap change A. Has patient perform Valsalva maneuver, if appropriate		
5. Demonstrates blood withdrawals for CVC A. Cleans port with alcohol B. Discards 6 mL C. Flushes catheter with 20 mL of sodium chloride after blood sample obtained		

(continued)

(continued)

Performance	Skilled	Needs Education
Critical Action Statements		
6. Demonstrates agency protocol in using thrombolytic agent to declot line A. Reviews drug allergy history B. Administers thrombolytic agent with appropriate fill volume C. Waits 15 minutes before attempting irrigation D. Verbalizes understanding of step for declotting by negative pressure technique		

EVALUATION CRITERIA

1. Preceptor observation of technique
2. Return demonstration of flushing and cap change on chest model

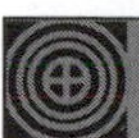

CRITICAL THINKING ACTIVITY

1. As a new graduate, you have been asked to change a complicated abdominal dressing on a patient postoperatively. This patient is receiving chemotherapy via a Hickman tunneled catheter. As you are cutting the dressing off, you accidentally puncture the catheter. What do you do? How could this have been avoided?

2. Check the flushing of central lines policy and procedure at the agency in which you are working. Does the procedure clearly give steps in the flushing of Hickman, Groshong, and implanted ports?

3. You attempt to flush a recently inserted PICC line to administer the next dose of antibiotics. The line does not flush, and resistance is felt. What do you do?

4. You are the charge nurse and a newly employed nurse assertively states that she will insert the new PICC on her patient because she has put in many PICCs in her former job as a home care I.V. nurse. How do you handle this situation?

POST-TEST

1. Implanted ports, when not in use, can be flushed every:
   a. Week
   b. 2 weeks
   c. 3 weeks
   d. 4 weeks
2. The major complication(s) of short-term central venous access devices include(s):
   a. Phlebitis or cellulitis
   b. Intravascular and extravascular malpositioning
   c. Air embolism
   d. All of the above
3. When tunneled catheters are used, the advantage(s) to the patient include(s) that they:
   a. Remain patent without flushing procedures
   b. Can be replaced easily
   c. Can be used for multiple purposes
   d. Have minimal associated body image change
4. The drug of choice for declotting a clotted short- or long-term device is:
   a. Wydase
   b. A thrombolytic agent
   c. Monoamine oxidase
   d. Acetylcholinesterase
5. The majority of central venous access devices are made of:
   a. Polystyrene
   b. Silicone
   c. PVC
   d. Titanium
6. The blunt catheter tip with a three-way valve is called a:
   a. PICC
   b. Dual lumen catheter
   c. Groshong tip
   d. Hickman catheter
7. Major complications with the implanted reservoir include all of the following **EXCEPT:**
   a. Displacement of septum
   b. Air embolus
   c. Occlusion
   d. External catheter breakage
8. Which of the following agents is used to declot a thrombus occlusion?
   a. 10 U heparin
   b. Hydrochloride acid
   c. t-PA
   d. Sodium bicarbonate

9. The nursing intervention most effective for removing a "stuck" PICC is to:
   a. Stretch the catheter and tape it to the arm for 2 to 4 hours, then remove
   b. Leave it alone, apply gently massage or moist heat to the area of the upper arm, and reattempt removal in 20 to 30 minutes after the vein relaxes
   c. Pull gently on the catheter, stretching it, then tape the stretched portion to the arm for 4 to 6 hours, and then remove it
   d. Call the physician to remove the catheter under fluoroscopy
10. When flushing a central line, all of the following flushing techniques can be used **EXCEPT:**
   a. Push–pause
   b. Use of positive pressure
   c. Gentle instillation of solution with no pressure or agitation
11. A midclavicular placement of a central line is a:
   a. PICC with the tip location in the proximal axillary or subclavian veins
   b. PICC with the tip location in the SVC
   c. Catheter surgically placed into a vessel, body cavity, or organ and attached to a reservoir, which is placed under the skin
   d. Percutaneous inserted line that is placed between the antecubital fossa and the head of the clavicle

REFERENCES

Andris, D.A., & Krzywda, E.A. (1997). Catheter pinch off syndrome: Recognition and management. *Journal of Intravenous Nursing,* 20 (5), 233–236.

Bagnall-Reeb, H. (1998). Diagnosis of central venous access device occlusion. *Journal of Intravenous Nursing,* 21 (5S), S115–S121.

Baranowski, L. (1993). Central venous access devices: Current technologies, uses, and management strategies. *Journal of Intravenous Therapy,* 16 (3), 167–194.

Brown, J.M. (1995). Polyurethane and silicone: Myths and misconceptions. *Journal of Intravenous Nursing,* 18 (3); 120–122.

Camp, D.L. (1988). Care of the Groshong catheter. *Oncology Nursing Forum,* 15 (6), 745–748.

Camp-Sorrell, D.L. (1995). Advances in tunneled and nontunneled catheters: Nursing management strategies. In Conners R., & Winters R.W. (eds.) *Home Infusion: Current Status and Future Trends* (pp. 55–70). American Hospital Publishing Company.

Centers for Disease Control and Prevention (1995). *Guideline for Prevention of Intravascular Device-Related Infections.* Notice. Atlanta, Georgia: U.S Department of Health and Human Services.

Dudrick, S.J., Wilmore, D.W., Var, H.M., et al. (1969). Can intravenous feeding as the sole means of nutrition support growth in the child and restore weight loss in an adult? *Ann Surg,* 6, 974–981.

Freedman, S.E., & Bosserman, G. (1993). Tunneled catheters. *Nursing Clinics of North America,* 28 (4), 851–858.

Fabian, B. (1995). Peripherally inserted central catheter exchange using a breakaway sheath: A new approach. *Journal of Intravenous Nursing,* 18 (2), 92–96.

Gahart, B.L., & Nazareno, A.R. (1999). *Intravenous Medications* (15th ed.). St. Louis: Mosby-Year Book.

Gray, H. (1998). *Anatomy, Descriptive and Surgical.* New York: Crown.

Hadaway, LC. (1998). Major thrombotic and nonthrombotic complications: loss of patency. *Journal of Intravenous Nursing,* 21 (5S), S143–S160.

Haire, W.D., Atkinson, J.B., & Stephens, L.C. (1994). Urokinase versus recombinant tissue plasminogen activator in thrombosed central venous catheters; a double-blinded, randomized trial. *ThrombHaemost,* 72, 543–547.

Holmes, K.R. (1998). Comparison of push-pull versus discard method from central venous catheters for blood testing. *Journal of Intravenous Nursing,* 21 (5), 282–285.

Intravenous Nurses Society (1997a). Position paper: Peripherally inserted central catheters. *Journal of Intravenous Nursing,* 20 (4), 172–174.

Intravenous Nurses Society (1997b). Position paper: Midline and midclavicular catheters. *Journal of Intravenous Nursing,* 20 (4), 175–178.

Intravenous Nurses Society. (2000). *Revised Standards of practice.* Philadelphia: Lippincott Williams & Wilkins.

Intravenous Nurses Society (1999). Peripherally inserted central catheter (PICC) education module. Cambridge: INS, Inc.

Jagger, J. (1999). Avoiding rebound injuries from Huber needles. *Nursing 99,* 99 (4), 74.

Josephson, D.L. (1999). *Intravenous Infusion Therapy for Nurses: Principles & Practice.* Albany: Delmar.

Krzywda, E.A. (1999). Predisposing factors, prevention, and management of central venous catheter occlusions. *Journal of Intravenous Nursing,* 22 (6S).

Larouere, E. (1999a). The art of accessing an implanted port. *Nursing 99,* 99 (5), 56–58.

Larouere, E. (1999b). Deaccessing an implanted port. *Nursing 99,* 99 (6), 60–61.

Macklin, D. (2000). Removing a PICC. *American Journal of Nursing,* 100 (1), 52–54.

Maki, D.G., & Mermel, L.A. (1998). Infections due to infusion therapy. In Bennett, J.V., & Brachman, P.S. (eds.). *Hospital Infections* (4th ed.). Philadelphia: Lippincott-Raven Publishers.

Marx. M. (1995). The management of difficult peripherally inserted central venous catheter line removal. *Journal of Intravenous Nursing,* 18 (5), 246–249.

Perrucca, R. (1995). Intravenous monitoring and catheter care. In Terry, J., Baranowski, L., Lonsway, R., & Hedrick, C. *Intravenous Therapy: Clinical Principles and Practice* (pp. 392–399). Philadelphia: W.B. Saunders.

Postgraduate Institute for Medicine (1999). *Management of Central Venous Catheter Occlusions: The Emerging Role of Alteplase.* Gardiner-Calwell SynerMed.

Sansivero, G. (1998). Venous anatomy and physiology. Considerations for vascular access device placement and function. *Journal of Intravenous Nursing, Supplement,* 21(55),S107–S113.

Weinstein, S.M. (2000). *Plumer's Principles and Practice of I.V. Therapy* (7th ed.). Philadelphia: J.B. Lippincott.

Wiener, E.S., & Albanese, C.T. (1998). Venous access in pediatric patients. *Journal of Intravenous Nursing. Supplment,* 21 (5S), S123–131.

ANSWERS TO CHAPTER 11

Pre-Test

1. d, **2.** c, **3.** b, **4.** a, **5.** e, **6.** a, **7.** e, **8.** a, **9.** d, **10.** d

Post-Test

1. d, **2.** d, **3.** c, **4.** b, **5.** b, **6.** c, **7.** d, **8.** c, **9.** b, **10.** c
11. a

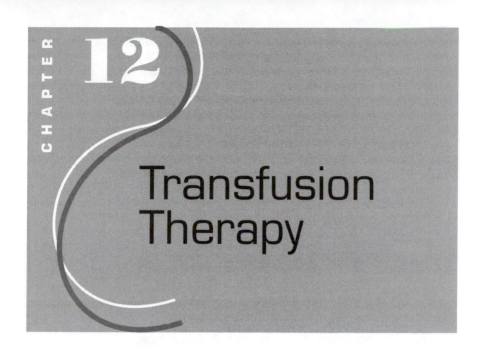

CHAPTER 12 Transfusion Therapy

Blood—a gift of life

Author Unknown

CHAPTER CONTENTS

LEARNING OBJECTIVES

Upon completion of this chapter, the reader will be able to:

1. Define the terms related to basic immunohematology and transfusion therapy.
2. Identify the antigens in the blood system.
3. Identify the universal red blood cell donor type.
4. Identify the location of antibodies in the blood system.
5. Identify the Rh antigens located on the red blood cells.
6. Identify the preservatives used in donor blood storage.
7. Summarize the tests used to screen donor blood.
8. Distinguish between homologous, autologous, and designated blood.
9. Describe each of the blood components.
10. List the indications for use of each blood component.
11. State the key points in the administration of red blood cells, platelets, granulocytes, fresh frozen plasma, and cryoprecipitate.
12. Describe the procedure for administration of blood components.
13. List the symptoms of hemolytic transfusion reaction, both acute and delayed.
14. State the signs and symptoms of febrile transfusion reaction and allergic transfusion reaction.
15. Differentiate between febrile and allergic transfusion reactions.
16. Use nursing process to deliver safe transfusion therapy.

GLOSSARY

ABO system Most important system determining compatibility; human blood groups that are inherited, groups determined according to which antigens are present on the surfaces of red blood cells, and which antibodies are present in the plasma

Agglutinin An antibody that causes particulate antigens, such as other cells, to adhere to one another, forming clumps

Agglutinogen An antigenic substance that stimulates the formation of a particular antibody

Allergic reaction Reaction from exposure to an antigen to which the person has become sensitized

Allogeneic Blood transfused to someone other than the donor

Alloimmunization Development of an immune response to alloantigens; occurs during pregnancy, blood transfusions, and organ transplantation

Antibody Protein produced by the immune system that destroys or inactivates a particular antigen

Antigen Any substance eliciting an immunologic response, such as the production of antibody specific for that substance

Autologous donation Blood donated before needed that is intended for use by the donor

Blood component Product made from a unit of whole blood such as platelet concentrate, red blood cells, fresh frozen plasma, cryoprecipitate

CPD Citrate-phosphate-dextrose; a preservative for collected blood

CPDA-1 Citrate-phosphate-dextrose-adenine; a preservative that extends the shelf life of stored blood to 35 days

Delayed transfusion reaction Adverse effect occurring after 48 hours and up to 180 days after transfusion

Designated donation Transfer of blood directly from one donor to a specified recipient

Febrile reaction Nonhemolytic reaction to antibodies formed against leukocytes

Hemoglobin Respiratory pigment of red blood cells having the reversible property of taking up oxygen or of releasing oxygen

Hemolysis Rupture of red blood cells, with the release of hemoglobin

Hemolytic transfusion reaction Blood transfusion reaction in which an antigen–antibody reaction in the recipient is caused by an incompatibility between red blood cell antigens and antibodies

HLA Human leukocyte antigen; used for tissue typing and relevant for transplant histocompatibility

Homologous donation Donation of blood by a volunteer donor whose blood structure is similar to the selected recipient

Hypothermia Abnormally low body temperature

Immunohematology Study of blood and blood reactions

Microaggregate Microscopic collection of particles such as platelets, leukocytes, and fibrin, which occurs in stored blood

Pheresis Derived from the Greek word "aphairesis," meaning "to take away"; used to denote the removal of blood, the separation into component parts, the retention of only the parts needed, and the return of the rest to the donor (e.g., removal of plasma is plasmapheresis)

Plasma Fluid portion of the blood, composed of a mixture of proteins in solution

Reaction The clinical symptoms that occur when a recipient responds negatively to substances in donor blood

Refractory Not responsive or readily yielding to treatment

Rh system Second most important system determining compatibility; Rh antigens are inherited and found on the surface of red blood cells; classified as positive or negative based on whether D antigen is present

Serum The cells and fibrinogen-free amber-colored fluid after blood or plasma clots

Thrombocytopenia Abnormally small number of platelets in the blood

PRE-TEST

1. The preservative CPDA-1 extends the life of collected cells to:
   - **a.** 25 days
   - **b.** 30 days
   - **c.** 35 days
   - **d.** 42 days
2. The universal RBC donor is:
   - **a.** A positive
   - **b.** O negative
   - **c.** AB positive
   - **d.** B negative
3. Transfusions are screened for all of the following **EXCEPT:**
   - **a.** Syphilis
   - **b.** HIV
   - **c.** Surface hepatitis B
   - **d.** Mononucleosis
   - **e.** Hepatitis C
4. The antigens in the blood system include all of the following **EXCEPT:**
   - **a.** ABO
   - **b.** Rh
   - **c.** HLA
   - **d.** IgM
5. The recommended infusion time for 1 U of RBCs is:
   - **a.** 1 hour
   - **b.** 2 hours
   - **c.** 4 hours
   - **d.** 6 hours
6. Nurses must check which of the following with another nurse before initiating a transfusion?
   - **a.** ABO and Rh
   - **b.** Patient name
   - **c.** Unit number
   - **d.** Expiration date
   - **e.** All of the above
7. The component FFP is used:
   - **a.** To increase levels of clotting factors
   - **b.** For patients who have developed HLA antibodies
   - **c.** To expand the plasma volume
   - **d.** All of the above
8. Cryoprecipitate is the component used to treat patients with:
   - **a.** Bleeding disorders related to factor VIII deficiency
   - **b.** Acute massive blood loss
   - **c.** Chronic anemia
   - **d.** Bleeding disorders related to factor IX deficiency

9. Platelets are used to provide:
   a. Protein
   b. Clotting factors
   c. RBCs
   d. Granulocytes

10. Which of the following is a symptoms of a febrile transfusion reaction?
   a. Itching
   b. Hives
   c. Rash
   d. Chills and fever

• • •

To ensure the delivery of safe transfusion therapy, nurses must possess a knowledge and understanding of the blood system as well as basic immunohematology. Nurses must also be knowledgeable about the theory and practical management of blood component therapy. The first part of this chapter presents fundamental concepts of immunohematology, blood grouping, and the criteria for donor blood, including homologous, designated, autologous, and donation. Fundamental concepts of blood component therapy, administration equipment, administration techniques for each blood component, and management of transfusion reactions are presented in the second part of the chapter.

BASIC IMMUNOHEMATOLOGY

Immunohematology is the science that deals with antigens of the blood and their antibodies. The antigens and antibodies are genetically inherited and determine each person's blood group. An **antigen** is a substance capable of stimulating the production of an antibody and then reacting with that antibody in a specific way. Antigens of the blood are called **agglutinogens.** Any substance that can elicit an immunologic response is an antigen, and they are located on the cell membrane. The three antigens on the red blood cells (RBCs) that cause problems and are routinely tested for are A, B, and Rh D. The human leukocyte antigen (HLA) is located on most cells in the body except mature erythrocytes. Antibodies are found in the **plasma** or **serum.**

ANTIGENS (AGGLUTINOGENS)

ABO System

The most important antigens in the blood are the surface antigens A and B, which are located on the RBC membranes in the ABO system (Table 12–1).

The name of the blood type is determined by the name of the antigen on the RBC. Individuals who have A antigen on the RBC membrane are

TABLE 12–1

ABO BLOOD GROUPING CHART

Blood Groupings	Recipient Antigens on RBCs	Antibodies Present in Plasma
A	A	Anti-B
B	B	Anti-A
AB	A and B	None
O	None	Anti-A and Anti-B

classified as group A; B antigens, group B; A and B surface antigens, group AB; and neither A or B antigens, group O. This **ABO system** was discovered in 1901 by Dr. Karl Landsteiner. (Table 12–2 provides an ABO compatibility chart.) Antigens are viewed as foreign substances when they enter the body (Cook, 1997a).

Unique to the ABO system is the development of antibody in the serum of persons who lack the corresponding antigen. This phenomenon occurs occasionally in other blood systems but appears to be ubiquitous within the ABO system. As a result, if antigen A is present on the RBC, then antibody to B (anti-B) is present in the serum. If antigens A and B are present, no antibody exists in serum; conversely, if no antigen is present, then both anti-A and anti-B are present in the serum. (Table 12–3 provides ABO compatibility for plasma.)

TABLE 12–2

ABO COMPATIBILITIES FOR PACKED RED BLOOD CELL COMPONENTS

Recipient	Donor Unit, First Choice	Donor Unit, Second Choice	Donor Unit, Third Choice
A+	A+	O+, A–	O–
B+	B+	O+, B–	O–
AB+	AB+	AB–, A+, B+	O+, A–, B–, O–
O+	O+	O–	—
A–	A–	O–	A+, O+
B–	B–	O–	B+, O+
AB–	AB–	A–, B–, O–	AB+, A+, B+, O+
O–	O–	O+	—

Note: The universal RBC donor is O negative; the universal recipient is AB positive.

TABLE 12–3

ABO COMPATIBILITY FOR FRESH FROZEN PLASMA

Recipient	Donor Unit
A	A or AB
B	B or AB
AB	AB
O	O, A, B, or AB

CULTURAL AND ETHNIC CONSIDERATIONS: BLOOD TYPES AND RH FACTOR

Blood groups differentiate people in certain racial groups. A prevalence for type O blood has been found among Native Americans, with some incidence of type A blood and virtually no incidence of type B blood. Almost equal incidences of types A, B, and O blood are found in Japanese and Chinese people with the AB blood type found in only about 10 percent of this population.

African American and European Americans have been found to have equal incidences of A, B, and O blood types, with predominate blood types of A and O (Giger & Davidhizar, 1999).

Persons with type O blood are at a greater risk for duodenal ulcers, and those with type A blood are more likely to develop cancer of the stomach (Jick et al., 1969).

The Rh-negative factor is most common in European Americans, much rarer in other racial groups, and absent in Eskimos (Giger & Davidhizar, 1999).

Rh System

After A and B, the most important RBC antigen is the D antigen, which was discovered in 1940 by Drs. Landsteiner and Wiener. The **Rh system** is so called because of its relationship to the substance in the RBCs of the Rhesus monkey. There are approximately 50 Rh-related antigens; the five principal antigens are D, C, E, c, and e. A person who has D antigen is classified as Rh positive; one lacking D is Rh negative. A total of 85 percent of the population is classified as D-Rh-positive (Vengelen-Tyler, 1999). There are no naturally occurring anti-D antibodies; however, D antibodies build up easily in D-negative recipients when stimulated with D-positive blood. Therefore, typing is done to ensure that D-negative recipients receive D-negative blood. Rh-negative recipients should receive Rh-negative whole blood, and any blood components that might contain RBCs should be Rh negative.

HLA System

The HLA antigen was originally identified on the leukocytes, but it has been established that **HLA** is present on most cells in the body. It is located on the surface of white blood cells (WBCs), platelets, and most tissue cells. HLA typing, or tissue typing, is important in patients with transplants or multiple transfusions and for paternity testing. The HLA system is very complex and is involved in immune regulation and cellular differentiation.

The HLA system is important in transfusion therapy because HLA antigens of the donor unit can induce **alloimmunization** in the recipient. This alloimmunization has been found to be a major factor in the onset of refractoriness to random donor platelet support. HLA incompatibility is a possible cause of hemolytic transfusion reactions, and HLA antibodies as well as granulocyte- and platelet-specific antibodies have been implicated in the development of nonhemolytic transfusion reactions.

Methods used to decrease HLA alloimmunization include HLA matching and leukocyte depletion of the donor unit (Vengelen-Tyler, 1999).

A standard unit of blood that has not been depleted of leukocytes contains 5 × 109 leukocytes. The American Association of Blood Banks (AABB) has designated that an RBC product may be labeled leukocyte-depleted if it retains 80 percent of the original RBC concentration but only 5 × 106 of leukocytes.

Blood may be depleted of leukocytes during three periods: (1) immediately after collection, (2) 6 to 24 hours after collection, and (3) at the time of infusion (Vengelen-Tyler, 1999).

The trend today is for pre-storage leukocyte depletion of packed RBCs and platelets. Early removal of leukocytes reduces the development of cytokines that appear to be implicated in many transfusion reactions.

Third-generation leukocyte-depleting filters used at the bedside remove all but an insignificant number of leukocytes from a unit of blood (Cook, 1995).

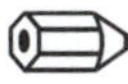

NOTE: Patients receiving multiple transfusions are at particular risk for developing complications related to leukocytes, such as sensitization to leukocyte antigens, nonhemolytic febrile reactions, transmission of leukocyte-mediated viruses, and graft-versus-host disease (Vengelen-Tyler, 1999).

ANTIBODIES (AGGLUTININS)

Antibodies within the blood system are proteins that react with a specific antigen. Antigens are **agglutinins** in that particulate antigens, such as other cells, adhere to one another in response to a specific antigen. The antibodies anti-A and anti-B are produced spontaneously in the plasma after birth and usually form in the first 3 months of life. An **antibody** has the same name as the antigen with which it reacts. For example, anti-A reacts to antigen A.

The naturally occurring antibodies, similar to those in the ABO system, are blood group antibodies that agglutinate erythrocytes containing corresponding antigens in a saline solution and are called saline antibodies. The naturally occurring antibody in the blood, which occurs within the inherited blood group, is from the class of antibodies called immunoglobulin mu (IgM). Complete antibodies are naturally occurring antibodies. Intravascular hemolysis may occur *in vivo* with naturally occurring antibodies (IgM).

Immunoglobulins or immune antibodies are a group of glycoproteins (i.e., complex molecules containing protein and sugar molecules) in the serum and tissues of mammals that possess antibody activity. Immunoglobulin molecules are divided into five categories. Some IgM antibodies, and all antibodies of the other four classes (IgG, IgA, IgD, and IgE) are produced by the immune system. These antibodies are produced by the immune system in response to previous exposure to the antigen via previous transfusion or pregnancy; they are not genetically inherited. When these antibodies meet with their corresponding antigen, the cells are affected but not destroyed in the intravascular system. The sensitized cells are removed intact by the reticuloendothelial system, primarily the spleen and liver (Cook, 1997).

OTHER BLOOD GROUP SYSTEMS

In addition to the ABO and Rh blood group antigens, more than 500 other antigens can be found on human RBCs (Vengelen-Tyler, 1999). There are 24 known systems associated with RBCs (Weir, 1995).

The following are the most common groups identified: ABO, Lewis, Rh, MNS, Kell, P, Duffy, Lutheran, and Kidd.

Corresponding antibodies to all but ABO and Rh systems are found so infrequently that they do not usually cause common problems in transfusion therapy.

TESTING OF DONOR BLOOD

At the time of donation, every unit of blood intended for homologous donation must undergo the following tests by the blood bank:

1. The ABO group must be determined by testing the RBCs with anti-A and anti-B serums and by testing the serum or plasma with A and B cells.
2. The Rh type must be determined with anti-D serum. Units that are D positive must be labeled as Rh positive.
3. Most blood banks test all donor blood for clinically significant antibodies. If all donors are not tested, then at least blood from donors with a history of previous transfusion or pregnancy should be tested for unexpected antibodies before the crossmatch.
4. All donor blood must be tested to detect transmissible disease. The blood component must not be used for transfusion unless the test results are nonreactive, negative, or within the normal range.
5. Each unit must be appropriately labeled. The label must include the following information: name of the component, type and amount of anticoagulant, volume of unit, required storage temperature, name and address of collecting facility, a reference to the circular of information, type of donor (i.e., volunteer, autologous, or paid), expiration date, and donor number (Fig. 12–1).

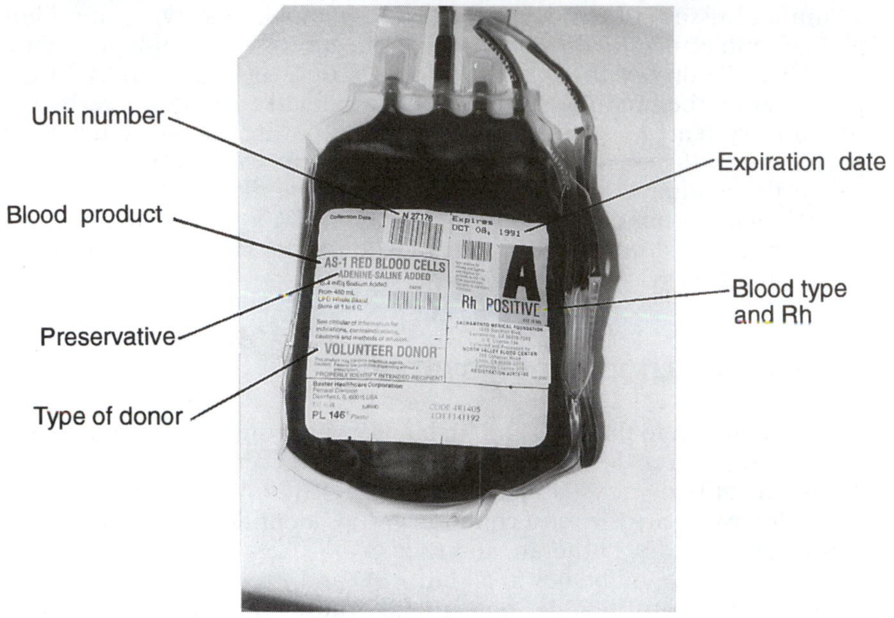

FIG. 12–1. Correct labeling of a unit of blood.

NOTE: The label should also include statements indicating "this product may transmit infectious agents" and "properly identify intended recipient."

6. The facility performing the compatibility testing must do ABO and Rh grouping confirmation tests on a sample obtained from the originally attached segment of all units of whole blood or RBCs (Vengelen-Tyler, 1999).

After blood is drawn from a donor, it is tested for ABO group (blood type) and Rh type (positive or negative), as well as for any unexpected RBC antibodies that may cause problems in the recipient. Screening tests are also performed for evidence of donor infection. The specific tests performed are:

- Hepatitis B surface antigen (HBsHg)
- Hepatitis B core antibody (anti-HBc)
- Hepatitis C virus antibody (anti-HCV)
- HIV-1 and HIV-2 antibody (anti–HIV-1 and anti–HTVL-II)
- HIV p24 antigen
- HTLV-I and HTLV-II antibody (anti–HTLV-I and HTLV-II)
- Serologic test for syphilis
- Nucleic acid amplification testing (NAT) (AABB, 9/99)

COMPATIBILITY TESTING

Recipients of transfusions must be tested for ABO and Rh grouping. In addition, antibody screening and compatibility testing must be performed. Previous exposure to an antigen by pregnancy or transfusion may have caused the recipient to develop an antibody against an antigen.

Compatibility testing is performed between the recipient's plasma and the donor's RBCs to ensure that the specific unit intended for transfusion to the recipient is not incompatible. Blood from the donor and recipient are mixed and incubated under a variety of conditions and suspending media. If the recipient's blood does not agglutinate the donor cells, compatibility is indicated. Blood bank personnel are responsible for providing serologically compatible blood for transfusion.

When testing is complete, transfusion therapy can begin. The blood bank has two objectives: (1) to prevent antigen–antibody reactions in the body and (2) to identify antibody that the recipient may have and to supply blood from a donation that lacks the corresponding antigen. The testing of donor blood and recipient blood is intended to prevent adverse effects of transfusion therapy.

BLOOD PRESERVATIVES

One donation of blood amounts to approximately 450 mL, and the volume of anticoagulant preservative is about 65 mL. There are several available RBC preservatives. Understanding of the RBC preservative is necessary because adverse reactions may occur in some patients as a result of chemicals in the anticoagulant preservative solution.

The solutions in the blood collection bag have a dual function: as anticoagulant and as RBC preservative. Citrate is used in all blood preservatives as an anticoagulant. Citrate binds with free calcium in the donor's plasma. Blood will not clot in the absence of free or ionized calcium. Citrate prevents coagulation by inhibiting the calcium-dependent steps of the coagulation cascade. Preservatives provide proper nutrients to maintain RBC viability, function, and metabolism. In addition, refrigeration at 1 to 6°C preserves RBCs and minimizes the proliferation of bacteria (Vengelen-Tyler, 1999).

In 1971, citrate-phosphate-dextrose (**CPD**) became a common preservative for blood. Phosphate is added to buffer the decrease in pH. The compound in the RBC that facilitates the transport of oxygen is 2,3-diphosphoglycerate (2,3-DPG). When the pH of the blood drops, there is a decrease in 2,3-DPG and therefore a lowering of the oxygen-carrying capacity of the blood. The 2,3-DPG levels remain higher in blood stored in CPD than in those with adenine-citrate-dextrose preservative. The expiration of RBCs preserved in CPD is 21 days stored at 1 to 6°C.

CPD-adenine (**CPDA-1**) was licensed in 1978. This preservative contains adenine, which helps the RBCs synthesize adenosine triphosphate (ATP) during storage. Cells have improved viability in this anticoagulant preservative because the energy requirements of the cell are better preserved than in ACD or plain CPD. This preservative lengthens the shelf life of the blood to 35 days at 1 to 6°C.

Newer additive solutions that contain CPDA-1 plus various preservative combinations of substances such as saline or mannitol are now available. These additives are used only with packed RBCs and extend their expiration to 42 days after the day of collection. Additives approved by the Food and Drug Administration (FDA) include AS-1 (ADSOL), AS-3 (Nutrice), and AS-5 (Optisol) (Vengelen-Tyler, 1999).

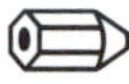

NOTE: RBCs prepared with AS-1, AS-3, and AS-5 have better flow rates and do not require dilution with saline.

Hypocalcemia is an adverse reaction that can occur when large amounts of citrated blood are infused in a person with impaired liver function.

BLOOD DONOR COLLECTION METHODS

HOMOLOGOUS

The term **homologous** donation describes transfusion of any blood component that was donated by someone other than the recipient. Most transfusions depend on homologous sources and are provided by volunteer donors.

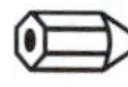

NOTE: Paid donor blood products are not transfused in the United States. The donor criteria are less limiting than with homologous blood. However, if homologous donation criteria are not followed, the unused units cannot cross over to the volunteer supply.

Guidelines for Homologous Donation

Donor selection for homologous collection is based on a limited physical examination and a medical history to determine the safety of the donated unit.

Strict criteria have been established for selection of prospective donors:

1. Brief health history, including illnesses, surgeries, drugs and medications, and immunization information
2. Screening for diseases
3. Stable vital signs
4. Age
5. Weight (smaller volumes should be drawn from donors weighing less than 110 lb)
6. No evidence of skin lesions at site of venipuncture
7. Adequate venous access for venipuncture
8. Donation of blood or plasma within the last 8 weeks
9. Hemoglobin and hematocrit of at least 12.5 g/dL and 38 percent in males and 12.0 g/dL and 36 percent in females

AUTOLOGOUS

Autologous donation is the collection, storage, and delivery of a recipient's own blood. This option is considered for patients who are likely to receive a transfusion during elective surgery. Patients may be able to donate their own blood before the operation. The use of **autologous** blood avoids the possibility of alloimmunization because it does not contain foreign RBCs, platelets, and leukocyte antigens. The risk of exposure and disease transmission is also eliminated. Because of this, the use of autologous blood is regarded as safer than homologous transfusion. However, risks associated with labeling and documentation are still present. The same precautions used for preparing and administering a homologous **blood component** must be observed.

Advantages include:

- Eliminates the risk of isoimmunization (sensitization to RBCs, platelet, and leukocyte antigens)
- Eliminates the risk of exposure to bloodborne infectious agents
- Expands the blood resources
- Reduces the need for homologous blood (decreases dependence on the volunteer donor supply)
- Provides an option for patients who find homologous transfusion unacceptable on religious grounds
- Has a physiologic pH and higher levels of 2,3-DPG than does banked blood; 2,3-DPG increases the oxygen-carrying capacity of **hemoglobin**
- Contains more viable RBCs than banked blood

Disadvantages include:

- Cost; a unit of predeposited autologous blood costs approximately $250 because of increased paperwork and special handling

Guidelines for Autologous Donation

Autologous transfusion can be accomplished through preoperative collection or from intraoperative or postoperative blood salvage. For preoperative collection, blood is collected into an anticoagulant preservative solution and stored. The 42-day shelf life of RBCs needs to be considered. If necessary, RBCs can be stored frozen. However, frozen storage is not routinely recommended because of the considerable expense and the limitations of some blood banks.

The criteria for patient selection for autologous donation is not as restrictive as with homologous donations. There are no age limits, and underweight patients can have proportionately smaller units withdrawn. Typically, autologous blood is not drawn more often than once a week. The last donation should be at least 72 hours and preferably 1 week before an operation to avoid hypovolemia during surgery. It is best to collect blood as far in advance of the intended date of surgery as is feasible. Except in special circumstances, the hemoglobin should be 11 g/dL and the hematocrit 33 percent or greater before each donation. Oral iron supplementation should be considered to replenish bone marrow iron reserves for autologous donors (AABB, 1999).

Types

There are four types of autologous blood donations currently in use: (1) predeposit or preoperative (PABD), (2) acute normovolemic hemodilution (ANH), (3) intraoperative blood salvage (IBS), and (4) postoperative blood salvage (PBS).

Predeposit or Preoperative Autologous Blood Donation

Predeposit or preoperative autologous blood donation is the collection and storage of the recipient's own blood for reinfusion during or after a later operation. This blood is held for use for elective surgery. Predeposit requires the approval of the donor recipient's physician and the blood bank physician (Oeltjen & Santrach, 1997).

Indication

- Elective surgical procedure with realistic possibility of transfusion

Typical uses

- Hip or knee replacement surgery
- Elective cardiac surgery
- Spinal fusion
- Elective major vascular surgery
- Heart–lung transplant

Contraindications

- Hemoglobin less than 11 g/dL
- Bacterial infection
- Severe aortic stenosis
- Unstable angina
- Severe left main coronary artery disease

Advantages

- No age limitations
- Less exclusionary donor criteria

Disadvantages

- Relatively costly
- Risk of clerical error

Acute Normovolemic Hemodilution

Acute normovolemic hemodilution involves the removal of whole blood from the patient, along with simultaneous replacement by a crystalloid solution, such as lactated Ringer's solution. This procedure takes place in the immediate preoperative period, either just before or just after the induction of anesthesia. The purpose of ANH is to decrease the loss of erythrocytes during surgery by decreasing the concentration of erythrocytes in the shed blood.

Indications

- Adequate preoperative hematocrit
- Anticipated intraoperative blood loss of more than 1 L

Typical uses

- Coronary artery bypass graft
- Major vascular surgery
- Spinal fusion
- Arteriovenous malformations

Contraindications

- Anemia
- Decreased renal function
- Significant coronary artery disease (CAD)
- Cerebrovascular disease
- Pulmonary disease
- Hepatic dysfunction

Advantage

- Practical means of obtaining fresh, whole blood

Disadvantages

- Increased potential for critical organ ischemia
- Lowest safe hemoglobin level in humans is unknown

Intraoperative Blood Salvage

Intraoperative blood salvage, or perioperative blood salvage or deposit, involves withdrawal of blood early in a procedure for use as a volume replacement later in the same procedure. Typically, two units of blood are collected early in the surgery. The collected volume is replaced with physiologic solution, and the units are then ready if volume replacement becomes necessary. The logic is that hemoglobin-rich blood is available for immediate reinfusion.

Indications

- Surgical procedure with anticipated major blood loss
- Patient unable to donate preoperatively

Typical uses

- Cardiac surgery
- Major vascular surgery

- Revision hip replacement
- Spinal fusion
- Liver transplant
- Arteriovenous malfunction resection
- Trauma

Contraindications

- Malignancy at operative site
- Bacterial contamination at operative site
- Use of microfibrillar collagen materials

Advantages

- May be acceptable to patients opposed to transfusions for religious reasons
- May eliminate need for allogeneic transfusion

Disadvantage

- Risk of air embolism

Postoperative Salvage

Postoperative salvage involves the salvage of blood from the surgical field in a single-use, self-contained reservoir for immediate return and reinfusion to the patient. This technique is used most often after cardiac surgeries and, recently, with orthopedic surgeries.

Indication

- Substantial bleeding in postoperative period

Typical uses

- Cardiac surgery
- Orthopedic surgery

Contraindication

- Same as IBS

Advantage

- May decrease allogeneic transfusion in some clinical settings

Disadvantages

- **Febrile reaction** to washed blood
- Cost increases if shed blood is washed

NOTE: Any autologous blood must be filtered during reinfusion to eliminate the possibility of microclots or debris being infused into the patient.

DESIGNATED

Designated donation refers to the donation of blood from selected friends or relatives of the patient. Most blood centers and hospitals provide this service. Designated donations have been requested more frequently because of the concern over the risk of transfusion-transmitted diseases. However, there is no evidence that designated donations are safer than blood provided by transfusion service (Vengelen-Tyler, 1999). Relatives or friends who may be members of a risk group may feel forced into donating and hesitate to identify themselves as a risk group member (Fig. 12–2).

Guidelines for Designated Donation

The selection and screening of designated donors are the same as for other homologous donors, except that the units collected are labeled for a specific recipient. The designated donor must pass all the history and screening tests required, and the unit must be compatible with the intended recipient (Vengelen-Tyler, 1999).

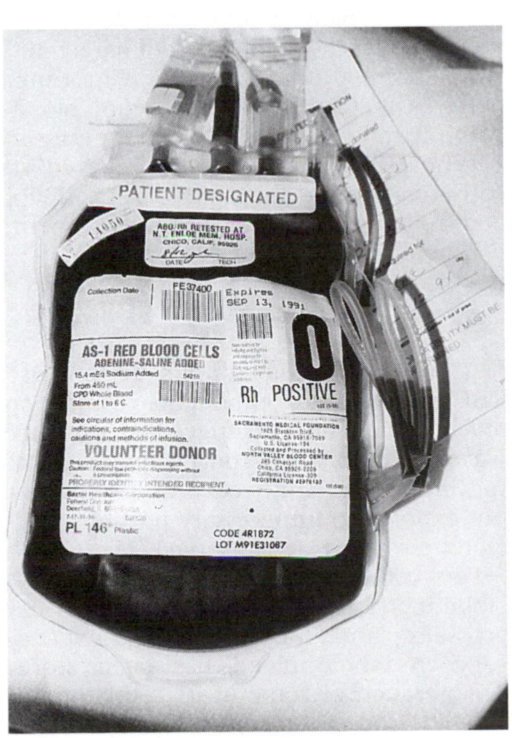

FIG. 12–2. Designated donor unit.

BLOOD COMPONENT THERAPY

Blood is the fluid tissue that circulates through the heart, arteries, capillaries, and veins. It supplies oxygen and food to the other tissues of the body and removes carbon dioxide and the waste products of metabolism from the tissues. Blood is a "liquid organ" with functions as extraordinary and unique as those of any other body organ. A total of 55 percent of blood is plasma (fluid); the remaining cellular portion (45%) is made up of solids: RBCs, WBCs, and platelets.

In the past decade, heightened awareness of the risks and benefits of transfusion therapy has dramatically affected transfusion practices. New methods of testing have lowered the risk of infection transmission; however, the association of blood product administration with virus activation, immunosuppression, increased tumor recurrence, and the increased incidence of bacterial infection has demanded serious consideration. As a result, the administration of **allogeneic** blood components is carefully evaluated. Autologous blood donations have increased substantially and, as an alternative to blood component administration, are evaluated and applied when appropriate.

WHOLE BLOOD

Whole blood is composed of RBCs, plasma, WBCs, and platelets. The volume of each unit is approximately 500 mL and consists of 200 mL of RBCs and 300 mL of plasma, with a minimum hemoglobin level of 38 percent. Advances in the use of blood components have made the administration of whole blood unnecessary.

Whole blood is never a "preferred" treatment, but is available for consideration. Fresh frozen plasma (FFP), packed RBCs, and crystalloid and colloids are preferred for treatment of massive hemorrhage over whole blood.

Uses

Most whole blood units are now used to prepare valuable separate RBC and plasma components to meet specific clinical needs. A whole blood unit can be centrifuged and separated into three components: RBCs, plasma, and platelet concentrates. By transfusing the patient with the specific component needed rather than with whole blood, the patient is not exposed to unnecessary portions of the blood product, and valuable blood resources are conserved (Fig. 12–3).

Few conditions require transfusion of whole blood. A unit of whole blood increases RBC mass, which provides oxygen-carrying capacity and provides plasma for blood volume expansion.

When whole blood has been stored for more than 24 hours, degeneration of some of its components occurs, resulting in nonviable platelets and granulocytes. In addition, levels of factor V and factor VIII decrease with storage. Therefore, a whole blood transfusion would not

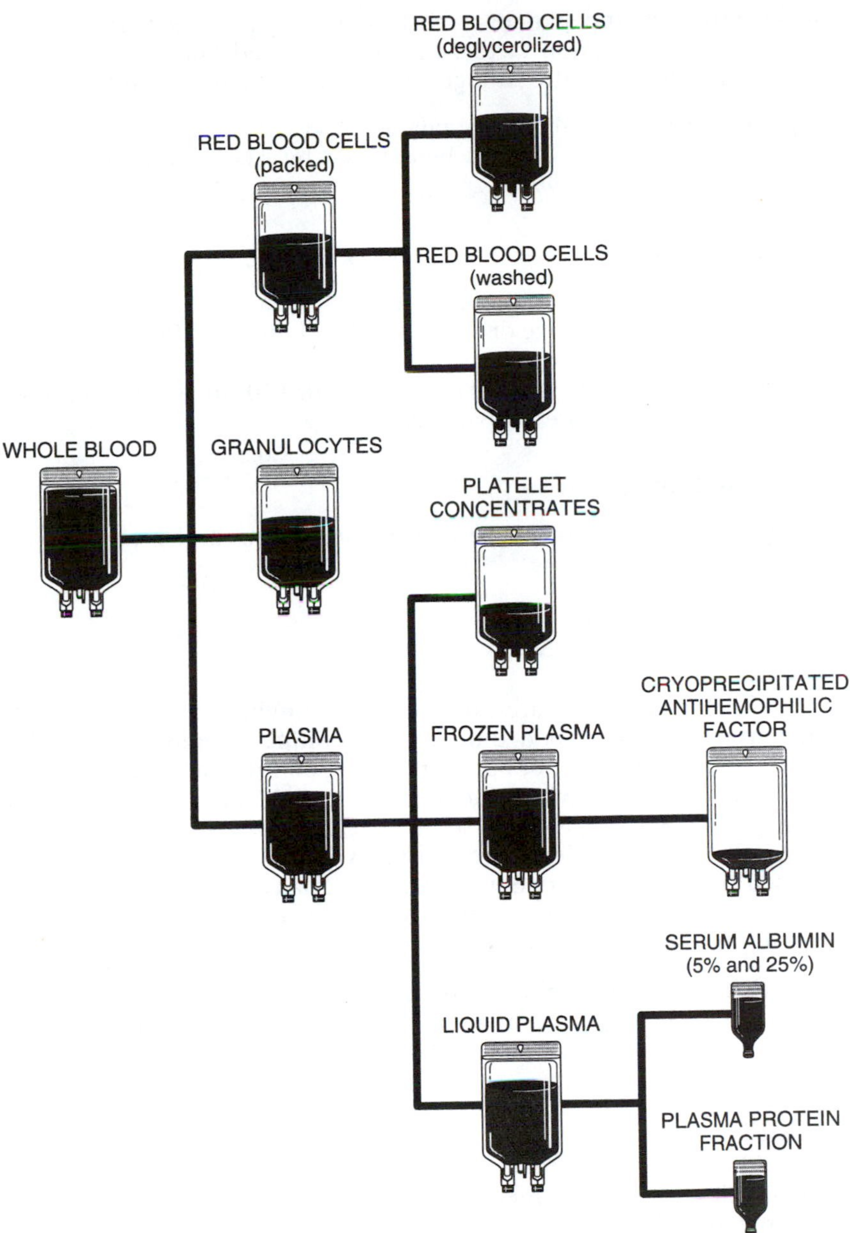

FIG. 12–3. Derivation of transfusible blood products.

provide a therapeutic platelet transfusion or replace several clotting factors. Stable coagulation factors II, VII, IX, X, and fibrinogen are well maintained throughout the storage period for whole blood units.

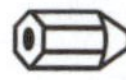
NOTE: In an adult, 1 U of whole blood increases the hemoglobin by about 1 g/dL or the hematocrit by about 3 to 4 percent (Vengelen-Tyler, 1999).

Administration

Amount: Volume of 500 mL
Cannula size: 20 gauge or larger preferred for rapid flow rates
Usual rate: 2 to 4 hours
Administration set: Straight or Y type with 170- to 260-micron filter or microaggregrate recipient set

Compatibility

Whole blood requires type and crossmatching and must be ABO identical.

RED BLOOD CELLS

Red blood cell units are prepared by removing 200 to 250 mL of plasma from a whole blood unit. The remaining packed RBC (PRBC) concentrate has a volume of approximately 300 mL. Each unit contains the same RBC mass as whole blood, as well as 20 to 30 percent of the original plasma, leukocytes, and some platelets. The advantages of RBCs over whole blood are decreased plasma volume in an RBC unit and decreased risk of circulatory overload. Another advantage is that because most of the plasma has been removed, less citrate, potassium, ammonia, and other metabolic byproducts are transfused.

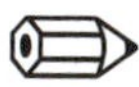
NOTE: In a normal adult patient, 1 U of RBCs should raise the hemoglobin level approximately 1 g/dL and the hematocrit 3 percent (Vengelen-Tyler, 1999).

Uses

Red blood cells are used to improve the oxygen-carrying capacity in patients with symptomatic anemia. The administration of RBCs should be considered only if improvement of the RBC count cannot be achieved by nutrition, drug therapy, or treatment of the underlying disease. A definitive hemoglobin and hematocrit threshold has not been established for when transfusion of RBCs is indicated or above which transfusion would be inappropriate. Criteria for transfusion are based on multiple variables, including hemoglobin and hematocrit levels, patient symptoms, amount and time frame of blood loss, and surgical procedures (Vengelen-Tyler, 1999). Patients with chronic anemia should undergo transfusion only if they are symptomatic owing to a decrease in oxygen-carrying capacity: they usually adjust to the lower hemoglobin level and should not be exposed to transfusion-associated risks unless necessary. Even if large volumes of blood are lost, other components (e.g., platelets and plasma coagulation factors) can be provided rather than using whole blood (Baranowski, 1993).

Administration

Administration of RBCs is used for an operative blood loss of more than 1200 mL. An operative blood loss of less than 1000 to 1200 mL can be replaced by crystalloid or colloid solutions rather than with RBCs (Vengelen-Tyler, 1999).

Transfuse RBCs:

- To increase oxygen-carrying capacity in anemic patient

Do not transfuse RBCs:

- For volume expansion
- In place of a hematinic
- To enhance wound healing
- To improve general well being (NIH, 1993)

Amount: 250 to 300 mL
Cannula size: 20 to 18 gauge preferred because the use of a 22-gauge cannula does not always allow free flow and may require an infusion pump
Usual rate: 1½ to 2 hours up to 4 hours
Administration set: Straight or Y type with 170- to 260-micron filter or microaggregate filter (Fig. 12–4.)

Compatibility

RBCs require typing and crossmatching before being transfused into a recipient.

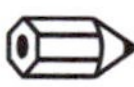

NOTE: The unit of PRBC does not have to be ABO identical, but it must be ABO compatible.

LEUKOCYTE-REDUCED RED BLOOD CELLS

A unit of whole blood contains more than 1 to 10 × 10^9 WBCs. Leukocyte-reduced blood is prepared by filtering blood with a special filter that removes WBCs by sieving and adherence mechanisms. Filtration may be done soon after collection (prestorage), after varying periods of storage in the laboratory, or at the bedside.

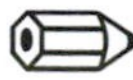

NOTE: Leukocyte-reduced blood must have a residual content of leukocytes $<5 \times 10^6$.

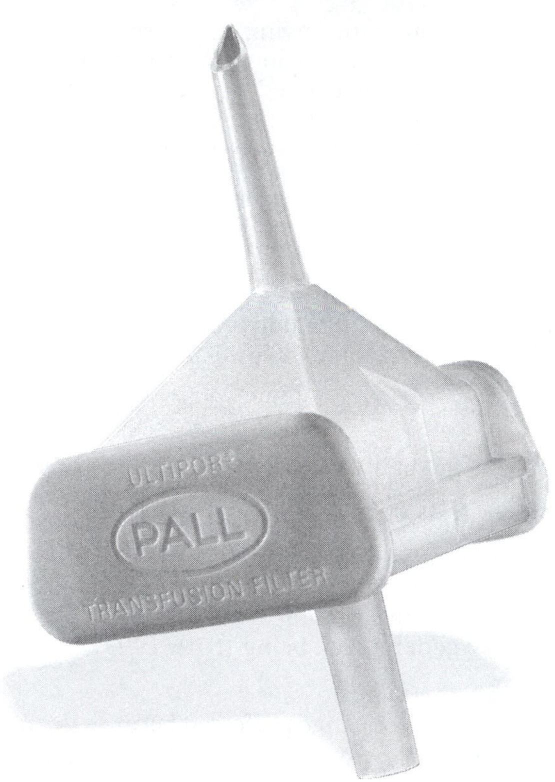

FIG. 12-4. Pall SQ40S microaggregate blood filter for red cell transfusion. (Courtesy Pall Medical, New York.)

The leukocyte-reduced component will have therapeutic efficacy equal to at least 85 percent of the original component (AABB, 1998).

Uses

Leukocyte-reduced components are indicated for the prevention of recurrent febrile, nonhemolytic transfusion reactions. These components may be beneficial in preventing HLA alloimmunization and in reducing transfusion-related immunomodulation.

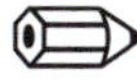 **NOTE:** Do not use leukocyte-reduced components to prevent graft-versus-host disease (AABB, 1998).

DEGLYCEROLIZED RED BLOOD CELLS

Deglycerolized RBCs are prepared to allow for freezing of cells for long-term storage to preserve rare units of RBCs and autologous donor units. The RBCs are frozen after removal of the plasma and glycerol (a cryoprotective agent) is added. The RBCs are stored at -65°C. Glycerol enters the cell and protects the cell from damage caused by cell dehydration and mechanical injury from ice formation. Before transfusion, glycerol is removed by washing to prevent osmotic **hemolysis.** This washing process also has the advantage of removing leukocytes, platelets, and plasma.

Uses

The uses and applications are the same as for washed cells.

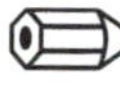 **NOTE:** Deglycerolization of RBCs extends storage to 10 years or more; a thawed unit is stored at 4°C and must be used within 24 hours (AABB, 1999).

REJUVENATED RED BLOOD CELLS

Red blood cells may be prepared from RBCs stored in CPD or CPDA-1 solutions. Addition of an FDA-approved solution containing inosine, phosphate, and adenine restores 2,3-DPG and ATP to levels approximating those of freshly drawn cells. The rejuvenation solution may be added at any time during the shelf life of the stored unit or up to 3 days after expiration. Rejuvenated RBCs may be stored at 1 to 6°C for up to 24 hours but must be washed before infusion to remove the inosine, which may be toxic (AABB, 1998).

GRANULOCYTES

Granulocyte concentrations are prepared by leukapheresis from a single donor. Each unit contains granulocytes and variable amounts of lymphocytes, platelets, and RBCs suspended in 200 to 300 mL of plasma.

Hydroxyethyl starch (HES) may be used as a sediment agent; if used, residual HES will be present in the final component. Pheresis should be administered as soon after collection as possible because of the well-documented possibility of deterioration of granulocyte function during short-term storage. If stored, it should be maintained at 20 to 24°C without agitation for no more than 24 hours (AABB, 1998).

Uses

Prophylactic use of granulocyte transfusion is of questionable therapeutic value, and this transfusion is given infrequently. Indications are limited, and the goals of therapy should be clearly defined (Vengelen-Tyler, 1999).

The use of granulocytes is indicated for patients with neutropenia who have been febrile for 24 to 48 hours and have evidence of significant infection that is unresponsive to appropriate antibiotic therapy or other modes of therapy. The patient should have a reasonable chance of recovering from the episode of neutropenia with an expected eventual chance for recovery of bone marrow function. Granulocyte transfusion has not proved effective in patients with localized infections or infections with agents other than bacteria. Septicemia should be documented by cultures to identify the infecting organism and sensitivities.

The patient is expected to experience chills, fever, and allergic reactions to the transfusion. These side effects can be managed with the use of diphenhydramine or meperidine, steroids, and nonaspirin antipyretics and by slowing the transfusion rate. The transfusion should not be discontinued unless severe respiratory distress occurs. The concentrate must be infused within 24 hours after collection; to achieve maximal clinical effect, it should be delivered as soon as possible (Vengelen-Tyler, 1999).

Administration

Amount: 300 to 400 mL suspended in 200 to 300 mL of plasma
Cannula size: 20 to 18 gauge preferred
Usual rate: 1 to 2 hours; slower if reaction occurs
Administration set: Straight or Y type with filter; microaggregate filter contraindicated

Compatibility

Donor blood must be ABO and Rh compatible because a unit of granulocytes is usually heavily contaminated with RBCs. There is no set standard regarding the amount or duration of granulocyte therapy, but generally transfusion therapy is delivered for at least 4 consecutive days.

PLATELETS

Platelets can be supplied as either random-donor concentrates or single-donor concentrates. Platelet concentrates (random donor) are prepared from individual units of whole blood by centrifugation. The platelets are stored at room temperature 20 to 24°C for 5 days with constant, gentle agitation to maintain the viability of the platelets. Platelets can be stored for up to 5 days, depending on the plastic formation of the storage bag. Single-donor platelet **pheresis** products are collected from a single donor, and all unneeded portions of the donor's blood are returned back to the donor. A single pheresis unit is equivalent to 6 to 8 U of random donor platelets (Fig. 12–5.)

The use of a single-donor unit has the obvious advantage of exposing the recipient to fewer donors and is ideal for treating patients who have developed HLA antibodies from previous transfusions and have become **refractory** (unresponsive) to random-donor platelets. HLA typing may

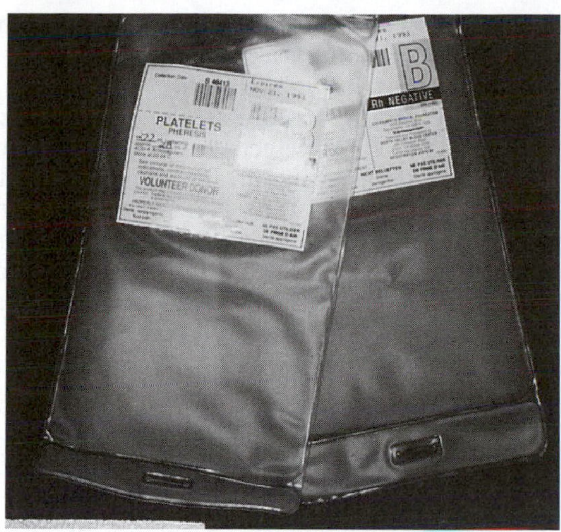

FIG. 12-5. Platelets.

be indicated when patients become refractory to platelets after multiple transfusions. Platelet crossmatch procedures are also being evaluated for their usefulness with refractory patients.

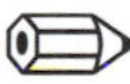 **NOTE:** One platelet concentrate should raise the recipient's platelet count 5000 to 10,000. The usual dose is 6 to 10 U random or 1 unit pheresis (Vengelen-Tyler, 1999).

Uses

Platelets are administered to control or prevent bleeding from platelet deficiencies resulting in **thrombocytopenia** or for the presence of functionally abnormal platelets. Indications for platelet transfusion include:

- Hemorrhage with platelet count less than 50,000/µL
- Surgery with platelet count less than 100,000/µL
- Nonbleeding patients with rapidly dropping counts, less than 15,000 to 20,000/µL
- Chemotherapy patients with a platelet count of 10,000/µL or less

Indications for platelet transfusion therapy should be based on the individual patient because patients do not carry the same risk of bleeding at all times. For example, many stable **thrombocytopenic** patients can tolerate platelet counts below 5000/μL with evidence of minor hemorrhage but without serious bleeding (Vengelen-Tyler, 1999).

Platelet transfusions at higher platelet counts may be required for patients with systemic bleeding and for those at high risk for bleeding because of additional coagulation defects, sepsis, or platelet dysfunctions related to medication or disease. Significant spontaneous bleeding with platelet counts above 20,000/μL is rare. Platelet transfusions are usually not effective in patients with conditions in which rapid platelet destruction occurs, such as those with idiopathic autoimmune thrombocytopenia purpura (ITP) and untreated disseminated intravascular coagulation (DIC). In patients with these conditions, platelet transfusions should be used only in the presence of active bleeding.

Administration

Transfuse platelets:

- To control or prevent bleeding associated with deficiencies in platelet number or function

Do NOT transfuse platelets:

- To patients with ITP (unless there is life-threatening bleeding)
- Prophylactically with massive blood transfusions
- Prophylactically after cardiopulmonary bypass

(NIH, 1993).

Transfusions may be repeated every 1 to 3 days. The platelets may be infused as rapidly as the patient tolerates, with infusion rates ranging from 1 to 2 mL/min up to 5 min/bag. Platelets should be delivered to infants by means of a syringe-type device and can be transfused at a rate of 1 mL/min.

The effectiveness of platelet transfusions may be altered if fever, infection, or active bleeding is present. To determine the effectiveness of a transfusion, platelet counts may be checked at 1 hour and 24 hours after transfusion. Poor platelet count recovery may also indicate that the patient may be refractory to random donor platelets.

Amount: 30 to 50 mL/U; usual dose 6 to 8 U
Cannula size: 20 to 22 gauge
Usual rate: 1 U in 5 to 10 minutes as tolerated
Filter: 170 micron
Administration set: Component syringe or Y drip set; tubing should be rubber free to prevent platelets from sticking; use saline as primer
Platelet concentrates may be pooled before administration or infused individually; after they are pooled, platelets should be transfused within 4 hours

Compatibility

Preferably, platelets should be ABO compatible; however, when ABO compatible platelets are unavailable, mismatched platelets may be given. Crossmatching is not required. Rh matching is also preferred but not required, especially with pheresed units that have very low RBC concentrations. Standard pretransfusion compatibility testing is not done for platelets.

FRESH FROZEN PLASMA

Fresh frozen plasma (FFP) is prepared from whole blood by separating and freezing the plasma within 8 hours of collection. FFP may be stored for up to 1 year at −18°C or lower. FFP stored at −65°C may be stored for up to 7 years. The volume of a typical unit is 200 to 250 mL. FFP does not provide platelets, and loss of factors V and VIII (i.e., the labile clotting factors) is minimal (Fig. 12–6).

Uses

Fresh frozen plasma is primarily used to provide replacement coagulation factors. It is indicated for patients with multiple coagulation factor deficiencies secondary to liver disease, DIC, and the dilutional coagulopathy resulting from massive volume load or volume replacement. FFP is indicated for patients with demonstrated factor deficiencies for which there is no coagulation concentrate available, such as deficiencies of factor V or XI. FFP may also be used for coumarin drug

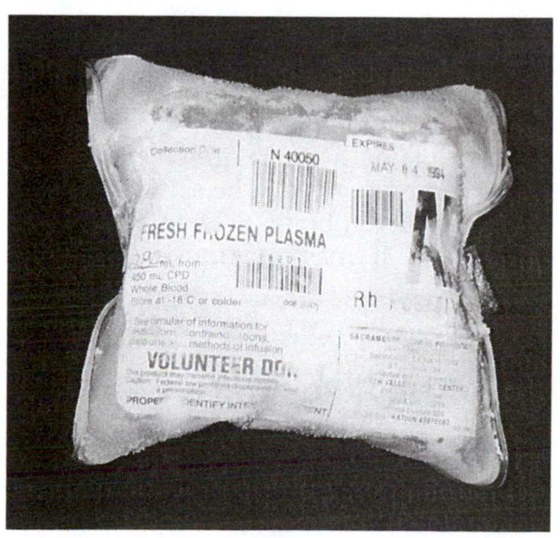

FIG. 12–6. Plasma.

reversal when time does not permit reversal by stopping the drug or administering vitamin K. Patients with other rare deficiencies, such as antithrombin III deficiency and thrombotic thrombocytopenia purpura, may also benefit from FFP.

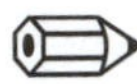

NOTE: FFP contains optimal levels of all plasma clotting factors, with approximately 200 U factor activity per bag and 200 to 400 mg fibrinogen per bag (AABB, 1999).

Administration

Before being transfused, FFP must be thawed in a 30 to 37°C water bath with gentle agitation or kneading. The thawing process takes up to 30 minutes, and the FFP should be transfused after thawing or within 6 hours. FFP must be delivered through a standard blood filter. It can be infused as fast as the patient tolerates or condition indicates. A rate of 4 to 10 mL/min has been suggested, and most units are generally completed within 1 to 2 hours.

Transfuse FFP:

- To increase the level of clotting factors in patient with a demonstrated deficiency

Do NOT transfuse FFP:

- For volume expansion
- As a nutritional supplement

Amount: 200 to 300 mL
Cannula size: 20 to 22 gauge
Usual rate: 1 to 2 hours
Administration set: Straight or Y type with filter

Compatibility

Compatibility testing is not required except to identify the recipient's ABO group to ensure that A or B antibodies present in the plasma are compatible with the recipient's RBCs. If the recipient's blood type is not known, group AB can be safely given. Rh matching is not required. The amount of antibody present in a single unit of FFP is not clinically important. If massive transfusion is anticipated, the significance may increase.

CRYOPRECIPITATE

Cryoprecipitate is the insoluble portion of plasma that remains as a white precipitate after FFP is thawed at 4°C under special conditions. The cold-insoluble precipitate is refrozen. Cryoprecipitate has a shelf life of 1 year and contains concentrated factor VIII: C; factor VIII: vWF (von Willebrand factor); fibrinogen; and factor XIII. It is the only concentrated source of fibrinogen.

The frozen component is thawed in a protective plastic overwrap in a water bath at 30 to 37°C up to 15 minutes. It should not be used if there is evidence of container breakage or thawing during storage.

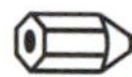 **NOTE:** Do not refreeze after thawing.

Uses

Cryoprecipitate is primarily used to control bleeding associated with a deficiency or defect in one of the coagulation factors. Its use is indicated for the treatment of hemophilia A, von Willebrand's disease, hypofibrinogenemia, factor VIII deficiency, and obstetric complications or other situations associated with consumption of fibrinogen, such as DIC.

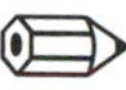 **NOTE:** Good patient management requires that the crypoprecipitated antihemophilic factor (AHF) treatment responses of factor VIII–deficient recipients be monitored with periodic plasma factor VIII: C assays (AABB, 1998).

Administration

Cryoprecipitate is thawed before being transfused and must be used within 6 hours. The inside of the bag should be rinsed with a small amount of saline to maximize recovery. Cryoprecipitate should be administered through a standard blood filter and, as with platelets administration sets, small priming volumes are recommended to decrease loss of the product in the set. The cryoprecipitate units are usually pooled to simplify administration. Cryoprecipitate should be transfused as rapidly as the patient can tolerate. Pooling of cryoprecipitate is not ubiquitously done.

Amount: 10 to 15 mL of diluent added to precipitate (3 to 5 mL) unit; usual dose 6 to 10 U
Cannula size: 20 to 22 gauge
Usual rate: As rapidly as possible; approximately 10 mL/min
Administration set: Component syringe or Y drip set

Compatibility

Compatibility testing is not done, but the cryoprecipitate should be ABO compatible with the patient's RBCs because a very small volume of plasma is present. If the patient's blood group is not known, group AB is preferred, but any group can be given in an emergency because the plasma volume is small. Rh matching is not required.

COLLOID VOLUME EXPANDERS

Products are available that do not require screening techniques. These products are colloid volume expanders. These include albumin, plasma protein fraction (PPF), dextran, and HES.

Normal human serum albumin is the most widely used colloid solution. It is heat treated for viral inactivation and to become free from hepatitis risk. PPF is also a hepatitis-free plasma derivative and is less expensive than albumin. Dextran is a branched polysaccharide available in low molecular weights: 40,000 (dextran 40) and 70,000 (dextran 70). It is dissolved in either 0.9 percent sodium chloride or 5 percent dextrose. Dextran's use as a volume expander is limited by two factors: (1) it can interfere with coagulation and platelet adhesion and (2) it has been associated with rare anaphylactic reactions (Phillips & Kuhn, 1999).

Hetastarch is an amylopectin derivative marketed in a 6 percent sodium chloride solution. Because of its structural similarity to glycogen, HES is less likely to cause anaphylaxis than dextran.

ALBUMIN AND PLASMA PROTEIN FRACTION

Albumin is a plasma protein that supplies 80 percent of plasma's osmotic activity and is the principal product of fractionation. Administered as PPF and as more purified albumin, albumin and PPF are derived from donor plasma, prepared by the cold alcohol fractionation process, and then subsequently heated. Both products do not transmit viral diseases because of the extended heating process. Normal serum albumin is composed of 96 percent albumin and 4 percent globulin and other proteins. It is available as a 5 or 25 percent solution. PPF is a similar product except that it is subjected to fewer purification steps in the fractionation process and contains about 83 percent albumin and 17 percent globulins. PPF is available only in a 5 percent solution.

Uses

Plasma protein fraction and 5 percent albumin are isotonic solutions and therefore are osmotically equivalent to an equal volume of plasma. They cause a plasma volume increase, are used interchangeably, and share the same clinical uses. Both are used primarily to increase plasma volume resulting from sudden loss of intravascular volume as seen in patients with hypovolemic shock from trauma or surgery. Their use may also be indicated in individual cases to support blood pressure during hypotensive episodes or induce diuresis in those with fluid overload to assist in fluid mobilization. The plasma derivatives lack clotting factors and other plasma proteins and therefore should not be considered plasma substitutes. Neither component will correct nutritional deficits or chronic hypoalbuminemia.

The 25 percent albumin is hypertonic and is five times more concentrated than 5 percent albumin. The 25 percent albumin is used to draw fluids out of tissues and body cavities into intravascular spaces. This solution must be given with caution. Principal uses for 25 percent albumin include plasma volume expansion, hypovolemic shock, burns, and prevention and treatment of patients with cerebral edema.

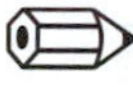

NOTE: Albumin 25 percent must not be used in dehydrated patients without supplemental fluids or in those at risk for circulatory overload.

Administration

Albumin and PPF are supplied in glass bottles. Depending on the brand, albumin in 5 percent concentrations is available as 50, 250, and 500 mL, and concentrations of 25 percent are supplied in units of 20, 50, and 100 mL. Manufacturers recommend that the solution be used within 4 hours of opening. Depending on the manufacturer, the solutions are sometimes supplied with an infusion set. Blood transfusion sets and filters are not required for infusion of albumin.

Albumin, 5 and 25 percent, may be given as rapidly as the patient tolerates for reduced blood volumes. When the blood volume is normal or only slightly reduced, rates of 2 to 4 mL/min have been suggested for 5 percent albumin, and 1 mL/min for 25 percent albumin. More caution is used when infusing PPF because hypotension may occur with a rate greater than 10 mL/min (AABB, 1999).

Amount: 5 percent solution: 250 mL; 25 percent solution: 50 to 100 mL
Cannula size: 20 to 22 gauge
Usual rate: 5 percent solution: 2 to 4 mL/min; 25 percent solution: 1 mL/min
Administration set: Comes with administration set in package

Compatibility

ABO or Rh matching and compatibility testing are not necessary for these components because antigens and antibodies are not present in these products.

A summary of blood components is listed in Table 12–4.

WEB SITES:
National Institute of Health: *www.nih.gov*
FDA: *www.fda.gov/ola/plasma*
American Association of Blood Banks: *www.aabb.org*
Others: ______________________________

TABLE 12–4

SUMMARY OF BLOOD COMPONENTS

Blood Component	Volume	Action and Use	Infusion Guide	Special Considerations
RBCs	250 to 350 mL	Improved oxygen-carrying capacity in patient with symptomatic anemia, aplastic anemia, bone marrow failure caused by malignancy, or chemotherapy	0.9% sodium chloride primer; transfuse in 4 hours, use standard 170 micron Y administration set Recommend leukocyte reduction filter	AB and Rh compatible; 1 U raises the hemoglobin 1 g and hematocrit 3 to 4%
Irradiated RBCs	200 to 250 mL	Prevent GFHD in immunocompromised patients	Same as for RBCs	Same as for RBCs
Deglycerolized RBCs (frozen)	200 to 250 mL	Prolonged storage of blood for rare blood types and autologous donations; minimizes allergic reactions	Same as for whole blood; infuse within 4 hours	Must be used within 24 hours of being thawed and deglycerolized
Granulocytes (leukapheresis)	300 to 400 mL Note: Suspended in 200 to 250 mL of plasma	For neutropenia, fever, or significant infection unresponsive to antibiotics	Usually administered for 4 consecutive days Standard blood filter; administer slowly over 2 to 4 hours as soon as collected or at least within 24 hours	ABO-/Rh-compatible; reactions common Check vital signs every 15 min Note: Febrile reactions occur in about two thirds of patients; chills, fever, and allergic reactions common Requires premedication to control reactions

Platelets, random donor	50 to 70 mL/U Usual dose: 6 to 10 U	Control or prevent bleeding associated with platelet deficiencies	Administer as rapidly as patient can tolerate: 1 U/10 min or less Use blood filter, syringe push, or standard Y administration set; leukocyte depletion filter for platelets as ordered Note: RBC leukocyte filters cannot be used with platelets	1 U increases platelet count of 70-kg adult by 5000/gmL Infuse individually or may be pooled; requires 20 minutes' pooling time by laboratory; ABO/Rh preferred but not necessary Prophylactic medication with antihistamines; antipyretics may be needed to decrease the incidence of chills, fever, and allergic reactions
Platelets, pheresis	Equivalent to 6 U from random donors	Same as for random donor; consider for patients anticipated to receive multiple long-term transfusions to limit exposure to multiple donors and reduce incidence of refractoriness	Same as for random-donor platelets	Same as for random-donor platelets
FFP	200 to 250 mL	Replacement of clotting factors in patients with a demonstrated deficiency or for single-factor deficiency when concentrate not available	Storage is at 18°C for 1 year Standard blood filter; may be infused rapidly: 20 mL over 3 minutes or more slowly within 4 hours	Does not provide platelets 1 U (200 U) raises the level of clotting factor 2 to 3%; requires 20 minutes' thawing time by laboratory Must be AB compatible

(Continued)

TABLE 12–4

SUMMARY OF BLOOD COMPONENTS *(Continued)*

Blood Component	Volume	Action and Use	Infusion Guide	Special Considerations
Cryoprecipitate	Each unit contains factor VIII, vWF, factor XIII, fibrinogen 15 mL plasma (5 to 10 mL U). Usual order is for 6 to 10 U	Controls bleeding associated with deficiency in coagulation factors; treatment of patients with hemophilia A, von Willebrand's disease, hypofibrinogenemia, factor VIII deficiency, DIC associated with obstetric complications	Standard blood filter; administer as fast as patient tolerates	ABO compatible with patient's RBCs; if blood group unknown, use AB blood; Rh matching not required Infuse within 6 hours of thawing; saline may be added to bag to facilitate recovery of product
Albumin (5% =12.5 g/250 mL; 25% =12.5 g/50 mL)	5% solution is in concentration of 250 mL or 500 mL; 25% solution is in 50 to 100 mL concentration	Plasma volume expander For hypovolemic shock Supports blood pressure during hypotensive episodes; induces diuresis in fluid overload	May be administered as rapidly as tolerated for reduced blood volume Normal rates: 2 to 4 mL/min for 5% solution; 1 mL/min for 25% solution Supplied in glass bottles with tubing for administration	25% albumin is hypertonic and is five times more concentrated than 5% solutions Give with extreme caution; can cause circulatory overload No type and crossmatching necessary; store at room temperature
Plasma protein fraction	Glass bottle with tubing 250 mL	Same as for albumin	Equivalent to 5% albumin	Has fewer purification steps than albumin; no type and crossmatching necessary; has high sodium content

ALTERNATIVE PHARMACOLOGIC THERAPIES

Alternatives for homologous blood continue. This issue has been addressed by alternative therapies to blood components, such as hematopoietic growth factor erythropoietin and desmopressin acetate (DDAVP). Erythropoietin is used for managing chronic anemia in dialysis patients. DDAVP is a synthetic analogue of l-arginine vasopressin and is used for increasing factor VIII and vWF and for managing patients with hemorrhagic disorders related to thrombocytopenia. Theses drugs decrease blood loss and the risk of bleeding, resulting in a reduced need for blood components (Baranowski, 1993).

BLOOD SUBSTITUTES

Efforts continue in the search to develop a practical RBC substitute. Several products continue to be evaluated for their ability to serve as oxygen carriers as a substitute for RBCs. One is a synthetic material, a perfluorocarbon emulsion, that was found to not carry enough oxygen under practical conditions (Baranowski, 1993). Other preparations being developed include intramolecular cross-linked or polymerized hemoglobin and products containing hemoglobin encapsulated in phospholipid liposomes (Pisiotto, 1989). Recombinant human hemoglobin is a cell-free hemoglobin-based blood substitute being investigated for perioperative blood replacement.

The three products currently under development as synthetic blood include Fluorovent, Oxycyte, and an implanted glucose sensor. These products are based on perfluorocarbon and biosensor technology (Synthetic Blood Internation, Inc, 1999).

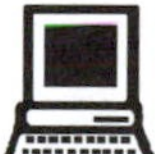

WEB SITES:
Synthetic Blood International, Inc. *www.sybd@siscom.net*
Others: ______________________________

ADMINISTRATION OF BLOOD COMPONENTS

The procedure for obtaining a blood component from a hospital blood bank varies from institution to institution. Regardless of the specific institutional procedure, certain essential guidelines must be followed (Table 12–5).

INS STANDARDS Nurses are responsible for blood product inspection; verification of patent identification, product and expiration date; confirmation of compatibility between recipient and donor; confirmation of informed patient consent; patient education; monitoring during and after administration; identification of immediate and delayed reactions; accountability for initiating appropriate interventions; written documenta-

TABLE 12–5

STEPS IN THE ADMINISTRATION OF A BLOOD COMPONENT

Step 1: Verifying the physician's order
Step 2: Blood typing and crossmatching the recipient
Step 3: Selecting and preparing the equipment
Step 4: Preparing the patient
Step 5: Obtaining blood product from the blood bank
Step 6: Preparing for administration
Step 7: Initiating transfusion
Step 8: Monitoring the transfusion
Step 9: Discontinuing transfusion

tion; communication of pertinent data to physicians and other healthcare providers involved in patient care; adherence to aseptic technique and standard precautions (INS, 2000, 75).

STEP 1: VERIFYING THE PHYSICIAN'S ORDER

A physician's order for the blood component is required. The order should specify which component to transfuse and the duration of the transfusion (up to 4 hours). When transfusing multiple types of components, the order should specify the sequence in which they are to be transfused and should specify any required modifications to the component (e.g., leukocyte filtration, irradiation, washing, HLA matching). Orders must specify premedications that are to be given before transfusion.

STEP 2: BLOOD TYPING AND CROSSMATCHING THE RECIPIENT

ABO forward typing is the process in which RBCs are mixed with a known antibody (anti-A or anti-B). This process identifies the antigens present in the RBCs by visually apparent agglutination of the cells when the antibody combines with its corresponding antigen.

ABO reverse typing is the testing of serum for the presence of predicted ABO antibodies by adding RBCs of a known ABO type to it.

Rh typing is accomplished by testing the RBCs against anti-D serum. If agglutination occurs, the RBCs possess the D antigen and the blood is Rh positive. If no agglutination is apparent, the RBCs must be tested further to rule out the presence of the weakly expressed D antigen called weak D (formerly referred to as D). This antigen can be identified most reliably by indirect antiglobulin testing (IAT) after incubating the RBCs with anti-D sera. RBCs that possess the weak D are given to Rh-positive recipients.

STEP 3: SELECTING AND PREPARING THE EQUIPMENT

Selecting the proper equipment involves selecting the cannula and solution selection and obtaining administration sets, special filters, blood warmers, and electronic monitoring devices.

Cannula

An I.V. line should be started according to institution protocol, using the gauge size recommended for the component to be administered. Usually an 18- or 20-gauge catheter is used to provide adequate flow rates. Free flow through a 22-gauge catheter is sometimes difficult with RBC units and may require the use of a pump. A 22-gauge catheter is appropriate for delivering plasma products. After deciding to use a pump, the nurse should make sure that flow is not hindered because of the cannula size or condition (e.g., kinked).

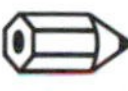

NOTES: Forcing blood through a tiny or damaged catheter may cause lysis of the cells.

If the patient requires medication or solution administration while the blood component is being administered, a second I.V. site should be initiated.

Solution

INS STANDARDS The use of 0.9 percent sodium chloride in transfusion therapy should be established in policies and procedures (INS, 2000, 75).

The use of dextrose in water can cause RBC hemolysis, and lactated Ringer's solution is not recommended because it contains enough ionized calcium to overcome the anticoagulant effect of CPDA-1 and allows small clots to develop.

Administration Sets

Blood administration sets are available as a two-lead Y-type tubing or as single-lead tubing. Y-type administration sets allow for infusion of 0.9 percent sodium chloride before and after each blood component. A Y-type set also allows for dilution of RBCs that are too viscous to be transfused at an appropriate rate. Platelets and cryoprecipitate should be infused through a filter similar to the standard blood filter but with a smaller drip chamber and shorter tubing so that less priming volume is needed. A syringe device designed specifically for platelets, and cryoprecipitate may also be used to administer these products.

Blood administration sets come with an inline filter. Most routine blood filters have a pore size of 170 microns designed to remove the debris that accumulates in stored blood.

INS STANDARDS Blood and blood components should be filtered. The minimum pore size of a standard blood filter is 170 microns (INS, 2000, 75).

It is necessary to fill the filter chamber completely to use all the surface area. One filter can usually be used for 2 to 4 U, depending on the manufacturer, the type of filter, the type of blood product, and the age of the cells. As debris in the filter accumulates, the rate of flow through the filter is slowed. In addition, because of the hazard of hemolysis and bacterial contamination, the filter should not be left hanging in place for extended periods and then reused.

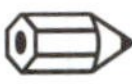 **NOTE:** The maximum time for use of a blood filter is 4 hours.

Special Filters

Microaggregate filters and leukocyte-depleting filters are also available. These filters are designed to be added to a standard administration set or come already incorporated into the tubing. **Microaggregate** filters are designed to remove 20- to 80-micron particles, filtering out the microaggregates that develop in stored blood. Microaggregates consist primarily of degenerated platelets, leukocytes, and strands of fibrin. Leukocyte-depleting filters are used for the delivery of RBCs and platelets (see Fig. 12–7).

 **INS STANDARDS** The use of microaggregate blood filters is recommended in the administration of blood products that have been stored for 5 or more days when administering multiple units (three or more) (INS, 2000, 75).

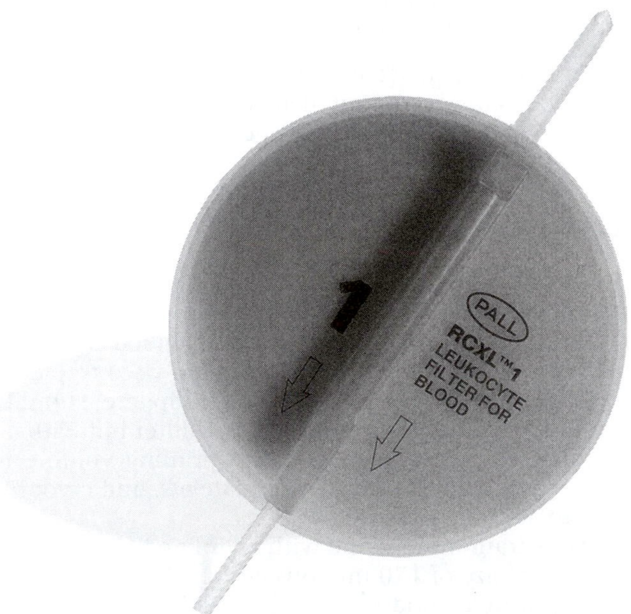

FIG. 12–7. Pall RCXL™1 leukocyte reduction filter for red cell transfusion. (Courtesy of Pall Medical, New York.)

The filters may be used for leukocyte depletion after blood collection in the blood bank or at the time of administration. HLA immunization (alloimmunization) is directly linked to the number of leukocytes present in a blood product (Cook, 1995). These filters are capable of removing more than 99.9 percent of the leukocytes present in the unit. These new-generation filters were developed in response to data supporting clinical benefits associated with the administration of leukocyte-poor blood products. The benefits include prevention of nonhemolytic transfusion reactions, HLA alloimmunization, and leukocyte-mediated viral transmission. These filters are more expensive than the standard blood filter and therefore are generally used only per physician order. When using microaggregate or leukocyte-removal filters, follow manufacturer recommendations regarding the number of units that can be filtered through one filter.

INS STANDARDS Consideration may be given to the use of leukocyte-depleting filters for patients with a history of severe febrile transfusion reactions (INS, 2000, 75).

Blood Warmers

Specific equipment is also available to warm blood if needed. Most transfusions do not require the use of a blood warmer. Warming of blood toward body temperature is indicated for rapid or massive transfusions, in neonatal exchange transfusions, and for patients with potent cold agglutinins.

The manufacturer's guidelines should be adhered to when using any of the many types of blood and fluid warmers. The temperature control should not warm the blood or fluid above 42°C (AABB, 1998).

INS STANDARDS Consideration should be given to the use of blood warmers for massive-rapid transfusions, exchange transfusions, and patients with clinically significant cold agglutinins (INS, 2000, 75).

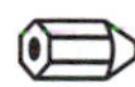

NOTE: Only temperature devices specifically designed to warm blood should be used. Blood components should not be placed in microwave ovens because damage to RBCs may occur. Do not use hot water baths, either.

Electronic Monitoring Devices

Some transfusions may require an electronic monitoring device to control the blood flow. Only pumps designed for the infusion of whole blood and RBCs may be used because other types of infusion pumps may cause hemolysis. Pumps require the use of special tubing and filters. Little if any increased hemolysis occurs secondary to the use of most infusion pumps. A pump's manufacturer should be consulted for detailed information on the pump's suitability for transfusing blood components.

A pressure bag is a commonly used device for increasing flow rates during transfusion, usually in emergencies or during surgery. This device has a sleeve into which the blood bag is inserted, and the sleeve is inflated by filling it with air from a pressure manometer. As the unit of blood empties, the pressure of the sleeve decreases; therefore, it should be observed frequently and reinflated when necessary. (See Chapter 6 for further information and an illustration of blood administration equipment.)

STEP 4: PREPARING THE PATIENT

Patient preparation begins when the transfusion of a blood component is anticipated. Urgency factors related to the transfusion may affect the amount of time available to prepare the patient for the transfusion. The steps of the nursing process are activated, including assessment and the establishment of new goals and interventions related to the transfusion.

The patient's and the patient's family's understanding of the need for blood, the procedure, and related concerns need to be assessed. Concerns are typically expressed regarding the risks of disease transmission; these need to be addressed.

NOTE: As required by institution-specific protocols, informed consents should be done and a written consent form signed.

The patient should be instructed regarding the length of time for the procedure and the need for the monitoring of his or her physical condition and vital signs. Signs and symptoms that may be associated with a complication of the component to be given should be explained to the patient and his or her family. It is not necessary to offer graphic explanations regarding symptoms; rather, the patient should be asked to report any different sensations after the transfusion has been started along with brief descriptions of possible symptoms. Because transfusions typically take several hours, preparation also includes making the patient physically comfortable.

The final step of patient preparation includes a thorough assessment of the patient. Baseline vital signs should be taken. If the vital signs are abnormal, consult with the physician before initiating the transfusion. Premedication with diuretics, antihistamines, or antipyretics may be necessary to help keep the vital signs at an acceptable level. The patient should also be questioned regarding any symptoms he or she may be experiencing that could be confused with a transfusion reaction.

NOTE: The patient teaching and assessment should be documented in the chart.

STEP 5: OBTAINING BLOOD PRODUCT FROM THE BLOOD BANK

As a rule, except in emergency situations, if blood is obtained from an onsite blood bank, only one product will be issued at a time and must be initiated within 30 minutes or returned to blood bank for proper storage. The blood component should not be obtained until the patient is ready to receive the component. If blood is obtained from an offsite blood bank, multiple units may be issued at one time. These units will be packaged to provide optimum storage conditions, and time limits for safe initiate will be detailed by the blood bank.

No unit of blood is to be placed in a refrigerator after leaving the blood bank. Most refrigerators cannot assure the rigid temperature controls required to prevent storage lesions. If the transfusion will be initiated within 30 minutes, the blood should be left at room temperature. If a longer period of time will pass (for alternate sites), the blood should be continued to be stored in the container in which it was sent.

NOTE: Refrigerators on the units may not be used to store blood products.

Proper identification of the blood component and the recipient are essential. Several items must always be verified and recorded before the transfusion is initiated.

- The physician's order should always be verified before the component is picked up.
- When the blood is issued, verification should include the name and identification number of the recipient, which must be recorded on the blood request form.
- The nurse should verify that the transfusion has not already been completed.

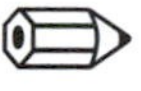

NOTE: The transfusion form becomes part of the patient's permanent record.

- The notation of ABO group and Rh type must be the same on the primary blood bag label as on the transfusion form. This information is to be recorded on the attached compatibility tag or label.
- The donor number must be identically recorded on the label of the blood bag, the transfusion form, and the attached compatibility tag.
- The color, appearance, and expiration date of the component must be checked.
- The name of the person issuing the blood, the name of the person to whom the blood is issued, and the date and time of issue must be recorded. Often this is in a book in the laboratory.

STEP 6: PREPARING FOR ADMINISTRATION

Before obtaining the blood component (Step 4), the correct tubing, 0.9 percent sodium chloride, and appropriate catheter should be in place. It is vitally important that the site be checked to ensure that the I.V. line is patent.

Baseline vital signs, including the patient's temperature, blood pressure, pulse, and respirations, should be obtained. The patient should also be

BLOOD TRANSFUSION RECORD

Resident's name: ____________________ ID #: __________

Transfusion visit Date: ________ Start time: ________ Completion time: ________ Nurse: ________

Blood component: Unit # ____________ ABO type ________ Rh ________ Exp. date ________

Unit # ____________ ABO type ________ Rh ________ Exp. date ________

Component: ☐ Intact ☐ not intact Transport Temp: At Blood Bank ____ Time ______ At infusion site ____ Time ______

Unit(s) match order: ☐ Yes ☐ No ____________________

Unit(s) match Blood Bank tag: ☐ Yes ☐ No ____________________

Unit(s) match resident identification band: ☐ Yes ☐ No ____________________

Identification band on resident's wrist or ankle: ☐ Yes ☐ No ____________________

Pre-Medication ☐ Yes ☐ No	Drug	Dose	Route	Time
	________	____	____	____
	________	____	____	____

Anaphylaxis kit present: ☐ Yes Exp. Date ________ ☐ No Explain ____________

Transfusion start: Unit #	Time	Unit #	Time
________	____	________	____
________	____	________	____

Vital signs (15 minute intervals recommended up to 30 minutes post-transfusion)

Time	BP	Temp	Pulse	Resp	Observations

Symptom	Pre-transfusion		During/Post	Time	Observation/Treatment
Fever	☐ Yes	☐ No	☐ Yes	____	________
Chills	☐ Yes	☐ No	☐ Yes	____	________
Hives/rash	☐ Yes	☐ No	☐ Yes	____	________
Itching	☐ Yes	☐ No	☐ Yes	____	________
Dyspnea/SOB	☐ Yes	☐ No	☐ Yes	____	________
Chest pain	☐ Yes	☐ No	☐ Yes	____	________
Hypotension	☐ Yes	☐ No	☐ Yes	____	________
Tachycardia	☐ Yes	☐ No	☐ Yes	____	________
Bradycardia	☐ Yes	☐ No	☐ Yes	____	________
Other	☐ Yes	☐ No	☐ Yes		________

Nurse Signature: ____________________ Date/Time: ________

Post transfusion follow-up Resident's response: ☐ Tolerated without complications ☐ Post-transfusion reaction noted

Remarks: ____________________

☐ Lab tests drawn	Date	Time	Test	Result
	____	____	____	____
	____	____	____	____
	____	____	____	____

FIG. 12–8. Transfusion record. (Courtesy Lynda Cook, CRNI and Linda Timmons, CRNI.)

assessed for any symptoms that could later be confused as a transfusion reaction (e.g., rash, fever, shortness of breath, lower back pain). A transfusion record and report form are helpful for recording component specifics, vital signs, administration specifics, and reactions (Fig. 12–8).

At the time of infusion, verification should include checking the component against the physician's order. The blood component should be verified with another registered nurse or a state-certified licensed vocational or practical nurse or physician.

Compare donor numbers and the ABO group and Rh type on the transfusion record with the information on the blood component. The information on the label and compatibility tag should be identical.

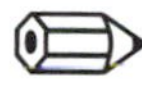 **NOTE:** It is helpful if one nurse reads the information for verification to the other nurse; errors can be made if both nurses look at the tags together.

Check the expiration date and time.

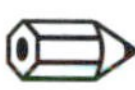 **NOTE:** Unless the exact time is given, the component expires at midnight on the expiration date.

At the bedside, compare the patient's full name and hospital identification number on the patient's identification wristband with the patient name and number that is on the form attached to the blood component.

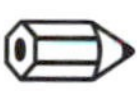 **NOTE:** Watch for any discrepancies during any part of the identification process; the transfusion should not be initiated until the blood bank is notified and any discrepancies are resolved.

The patient's wristband must be attached to the recipient, not lying on bedside table or attached to the bed rail!

STEP 7: INITIATING TRANSFUSION

To administer whole blood or RBCs, spike the blood container with the Y set and hang it up. Turn off the 0.9 percent sodium chloride and turn on the blood component. It is recommended that transfusions of RBCs be started at 5 mL/min for the first 15 minutes of the transfusion (AABB, 1998). If the patient shows signs or symptoms of an adverse reaction, the transfusion can be stopped immediately and only a small amount of blood product will have been infused. After the first 15 minutes has safely passed, the rate of flow can be increased to complete the transfusion within the amount of time indicated by the physician or by policy. The rate of infusion should be based on the patient's blood volume, hemodynamic condition, and cardiac status. Gloves should be worn to handle blood products (Fig. 12–9).

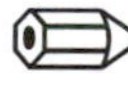 **NOTE:** Blood should be infused within a 4-hour period (AABB, 1998). When a longer transfusion time is clinically indicated, the unit may be divided by the blood bank and the portion not being transfused can be properly refrigerated.

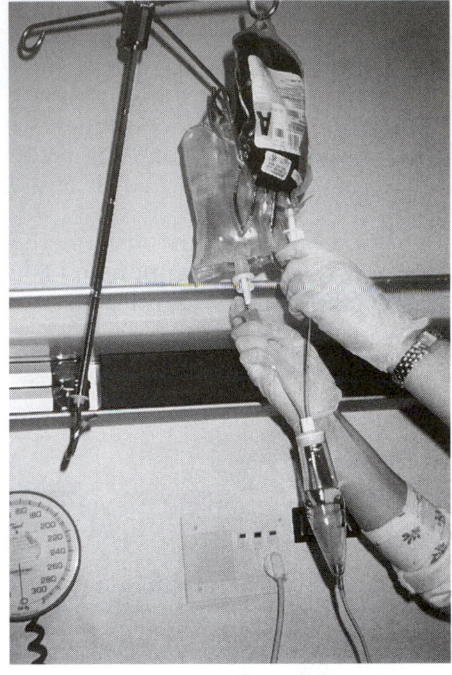

FIG. 12-9. Hanging PRBCs with Y administration set. Always wear gloves when handling blood products.

STEP 8: MONITORING THE TRANSFUSION

The patient's vital signs should be monitored at the end of the first 15 minutes and then periodically throughout the transfusion. Careful observation of the patient during and after a blood transfusion is necessary to provide a more reliable assessment. Vital signs must be recorded before and after the transfusion (AABB, 1998).

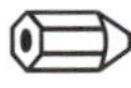 **NOTE:** Patients should be monitored for 15 minutes after initiation of a blood component (INS, 2000, 75).

Patient education is required for conscious patients. They should be instructed to call if any unusual symptoms or sensations occur during a transfusion.

A Note on Medications

Drugs should never be mixed with the blood component to be administered. One reason is the indeterminate effect the medication may have on the blood component. Also, if a reaction occurs, it would be difficult to ascertain whether it was the drug or the blood component that was responsible for the adverse effect. Another reason is that if the transfusion needs to be interrupted, it would be impossible to calculate the amount of drug that the patient received. If a patient requires I.V. medications during the course of the transfusion, a separate I.V. site should be started for the blood.

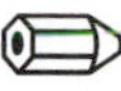

NOTE: Absolutely no medications or solutions other than 0.9 percent sodium chloride shall be added to blood or blood components (INS, 2000, 75; Vengelen-Tyler, 1999).

STEP 9: DISCONTINUING TRANSFUSION

When the transfusion is complete, flush the tubing with 0.9 percent sodium chloride (except when using leukocyte filters). Because of the sodium and chloride content, a minimal amount should be used to complete the transfusion. At this point, another unit may be infused, the unit and line may be discontinued, the line can be capped with a PRN adaptor, or a new infusion line and solution container may be administered.

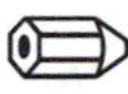

NOTE: Do not save previous solutions and tubing, which were interrupted to give the blood component; they are considered contaminated. Restart with a fresh set and solution (Walker, 1993).

When the unit of blood has been infused, the time, volume given, and patient's condition should be documented. Some transfusion service departments require that a copy of the completed transfusion form be returned to them. Returning the blood component after an uncomplicated transfusion is not required in all facilities. If disposal is allowed on the unit, use hospital standards in disposing the blood bag in contaminated trash.

COMPLICATIONS ASSOCIATED WITH BLOOD COMPONENT THERAPY

Despite its numerous and obvious benefits, there are also complications associated with blood component therapy. The administration of any blood component carries with it the potential of adverse reactions. Most reactions are caused by biologic aspects of blood; however, nonimmune reactions can occur and may be linked to the collection, preparation, or administration of the blood.

INS STANDARDS Standards of Practice (2000, 75) dictate that a transfusion reaction requires immediate intervention. Interventions include but are not limited to:
Terminating the transfusion
Maintaining patency of the cannula with 0.9 percent sodium chloride
Notifying the physician and hospital blood bank or transfusion services
Implementing other interventions as indicated

BIOLOGIC (IMMUNE) REACTIONS

Acute Hemolytic Reactions

Hemolytic transfusion reactions may be acute or delayed. The most serious and potentially life-threatening reaction is acute **hemolytic transfusion reaction.** This reaction, according to Association of Blood

Banks, occurs in 1 in 600,000 transfusions. This type of reaction occurs after infusion of incompatible RBCs. There are two types of RBC destruction. First, intravascular hemolysis, in which the RBCs are destroyed with hemolysis directly in the bloodstream, is usually seen with ABO-incompatible RBCs. Second, extravascular hemolysis, in which the cells are coated with the antibody and subsequently removed by the reticuloendothelial system, is seen in Rh incompatibility. These incompatibilities may lead to an activation of the coagulation system and release of vasoactive enzymes, which can result in vasomotor instability, cardiorespiratory collapse, or DIC. Intravascular hemolysis is the most serious and is usually fatal (National Blood Resource Group, 1991).

Incompatibilities involving other RBC antigens and IgG antibodies can result in fever, anemia, hyperbilirubinemia, and a positive direct antibody test result. The severity of the reaction can be dose related but can occur with less than 30 mL of blood administered. Most hemolytic reactions are a result of clerical errors, such as incorrect labeling of the blood specimen or errors in identifying the recipient.

Signs and Symptoms

The first symptoms include a burning sensation along the vein in which the blood is being infused. This symptom is quickly followed by lumbar pain, flank pain, flushing of the face, and chest pain.

If infusion is allowed to continue, symptoms include fever, chills, hemoglobinemia, oozing of blood at the injection site, shock, and DIC.

Interventions

Stop the transfusion. Disconnect the tubing from the I.V. catheter and infuse fresh saline not contaminated by the blood.

NOTE: In acute hemolytic transfusion reaction, you must not give the recipient another drop of donor blood.

Notify the physician and blood bank or transfusion service *immediately.* Monitor vital signs and maintain intravascular volume with fluids to prevent renal constriction. In addition, diuretics, mannitol, and dopamine can support the renal and vascular systems. This is an emergency situation. The patient's respiratory status may have to be supported.

Prevention

Extreme care during the entire identification process is the first step in prevention. The transfusion must be started slowly, and nurses must remain with the patient during the first 5 to 15 minutes of the transfusion.

Delayed Hemolytic Reaction

Delayed transfusion reaction is a result of RBC antigen incompatibility other than the ABO group. Rapid production of RBC antibody occurs shortly after transfusion of the corresponding antigen as a result of sensitization during previous transfusions or pregnancies. Destruction of the transfused RBCs gradually occurs over 2 or more days or up to several weeks after the transfusion. Most reactions of this type go unnoticed and are common.

Signs and Symptoms

A decrease in hemoglobin and hematocrit levels, persistent low-grade fever, malaise, and indirect hyperbilirubinemia are symptoms that occur with delayed transfusion reaction.

Interventions

No acute treatment is usually required. Monitor hematocrit level, renal function, and coagulation profile routinely for all patients receiving transfusions. Notify physician and transfusion services if delayed reaction is suspected.

Prevention

Avoid clerical errors.

Nonhemolytic Febrile Reactions

Nonhemolytic febrile reactions are defined as a temperature rise of 1°C or more occurring in association with transfusion and not having any other explanation. These are usually reactions to antibodies directed against leukocytes or platelets. Febrile reactions occur in only 1 percent of transfusions; repeat reactions are uncommon. These reactions can occur immediately or within 1 to 2 hours after transfusion is completed. Fever is the symptom associated with this type of transfusion reaction.

Signs and Symptoms

Signs and symptoms of a nonhemolytic febrile reaction are fever, chills, headache, nausea and vomiting, hypotension, chest pain, dyspnea and nonproductive cough, and malaise.

Interventions

Stop the transfusion. Keep the vein open with normal saline and notify the physician. Monitor vital signs. The physician might order antipyretic agents.

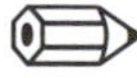

NOTE: In a nonhemolytic febrile reaction, you may turn off the blood and turn on the sodium chloride primer and infuse slowly. Do not take down the blood until notified by the physician; leave the blood hanging but clamp the Y connector to the blood unit.

Prevention

This type of reaction can be prevented or reduced by the use of leukocyte-reduced blood components. HLA compatible products may also be indicated.

Allergic Reactions

In its mild form, **allergic reactions** constitute the second most common type of reaction and are probably caused by antibodies against plasma proteins. The patient may experience mild localized urticaria or full systemic anaphylactic reaction. This can occur immediately or within 1 hour after infusion. Most reactions are mild and respond to antihistamines.

Signs and Symptoms

Signs and symptoms of allergic reactions include itching, hives (local erythema), rash, urticaria, runny eyes, anxiety, dyspnea, wheezing, decreased blood pressure, shock, gastrointestinal distress, and cardiac arrest and death.

Interventions

Stop the transfusion. Keep the vein open with normal saline. Notify the physician. Monitor the vital signs. For mild reaction, administer antihistamines per physician order and continue transfusion if symptoms subside. For severe anaphylactic reactions, administer epinephrine, steroids, and dopamine, and maintain intravascular volume with fluids as ordered by the physician.

Prevention

For mild reactions, the patient may receive antihistamines, such as diphenhydramine (Benadryl), before the transfusion. Transfuse patients who have a history of anaphylaxis with IgA-deficient blood products, washed RBCs, or deglycerolized RBCs. With mild reaction, the transfusion may be continued after antihistamines are administered and the symptoms have subsided. Severe reactions may require discontinuation of the transfusion and drug therapy to support the vascular system.

Alloimmunization and Refractoriness

Alloimmunization is defined as stimulation of antibody development by foreign blood cell antigens. The reaction is delayed and occurs after multiple transfusions. The offending agent can be leukocytes or RBCs.

Alloimmunization directed against RBC antigens creates a more serious issue. The risk, however is low: 1.0 to 1.4 percent per unit. After an offending antibody has been recognized, RBC products should be screened for the offending antigen. These units may be labeled "this unit negative for. . ." to indicate the absence of the offending agent.

Refractoriness is a state in which there is not a reasonable increase in the recipient's platelet count after transfusion. Refractoriness may result from immunization to HLA or to other platelet-specific antigens.

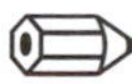 **NOTE:** Recipients who are in a refractory state will benefit if future transfusions are with HLA-specific platelets (Cook, 1997a).

Graft-Versus-Host Disease

A delayed reaction commonly associated with allogenic bone marrow transplant is graft-versus-host disease (GVHD). It may occur rarely as a result of blood transfusions. Signs and symptoms include fever, rash, hepatitis, diarrhea, bone marrow suppression, and overwhelming infection.

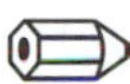 **NOTE:** Immunoincompetent recipients are at risk.

In transfusions, acquired GVHD (TA-GVHD) morbidity is 75 to 90 percent compared with 10 to 15 percent after bone marrow transplantation (Cook, 1997a).

Irradiation of blood products renders 85 to 95 percent of the lymphocytes incapable of replication but does not affect the function of the cell. Even after irradiation, the WBCs are capable of mounting a leukocyte reaction. To prevent alloimmunization, use a leukocyte-reducing filter (Cook, 1997a).

NONIMMUNE REACTIONS

Circulatory Overload

The rapid administration of any blood product can lead to circulatory overload. RBC products, plasma products and albumin 25 percent are the blood components most commonly associated with overload. Patients at risk for circulatory overload are those of small stature, infants and young children, and frail and elderly individuals. Individuals with compromised cardiac or pulmonary function are also at risk (Cook, 1997b).

Signs and Symptoms

Dyspnea, engorged neck veins, congestive heart failure, and pulmonary edema.

Interventions

Stop the transfusion. Elevate the patient's head of the bed and notify the physician. Administer diuretics if necessary.

Prevention

Minimize the risk of overload by using RBCs instead of whole blood, infusion at a reduced rate for the high-risk patient, and administering a diuretic when beginning the transfusion in select recipients. Circulatory overload is the easiest reaction to prevent. Monitor vital signs throughout the transfusion.

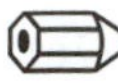

NOTE: Recommendations are to administer blood at a rate not to exceed 2 to 4 mL/kg body weight/h, which is about 2 h/U (Cook, 1997b).

Potassium Toxicity (Hyperkalemia)

Potassium toxicity is a rare complication. As the blood ages during storage, potassium is released from the cells into the plasma during RBC lysis. When RBCs have been stored at 1 to 6°C, biochemical changes, known as storage lesions, develop. During the first few weeks of storage, extracellular potassium in the unit may increase by as much as 1 mEq daily (AABB, 1999). As a result of this storage lesion, the recipient receives excessive potassium. Single unit transfusion is generally not a problem, but individuals who receive multiple units of aged blood may experience this reactions.

Signs and Symptoms

Signs and symptoms of potassium toxicity include immediate onset of hyperkalemia; slow, irregular heartbeat; nausea; muscle weakness; and electrocardiographic changes.

Interventions

The goal is to remove the excess potassium. The concurrent administration of insulin and hypertonic dextrose provides a hypokalemic action, which may be effective for 4 to 6 hours. (Refer to Chapter 4 for further treatment modalities for patients with hyperkalemia.)

Prevention

Use fresh blood.

Hypothermia

When large volumes of blood are administered, hypothermia can occur owing to the consistently cool temperature of the blood. This risk brings about decreased temperature and chills. The treatment is to warm the patient with blankets. Use of a blood warmer during transfusions can be helpful to minimize this risk.

Hypocalcemia

A reaction to toxic proportions of citrate, which is used as a preservative in blood, can cause hypocalcemia. The citrate ion can combine with the recipient's serum calcium, causing a calcium deficiency, or normal citrate metabolism is hindered by the presence of liver disease.

Signs and Symptoms

Signs and symptoms of hypocalcemia include a tingling sensation in the fingers, muscle cramps, hypotension, and tetany. Calcium levels should be carefully monitored in patients with liver disease. The use of washed RBCs helps to prevent this risk.

Prevention

Administer calcium gluconate as CaCl as indicated.

Bacterial Contamination

Bacterial contamination of blood may occur at any time during donation or processing of a unit. Two types of organisms are implicated in contamination: warmth-loving organisms such as *Salmonella* spp. and *Staphylococcus* spp., and cold-loving organisms such as *Pseudomonas* spp., *Citrobacter* spp., *Escherichia coli*, and *Yersinia enterocolitica*.

It is difficult to eliminate contaminated units based on visual inspection. However, RBCs that are severely contaminated may have a purplish hue; unsuspended supernatant may be pink, which indicates hemolysis.

Signs and Symptoms

The recipient may not exhibit symptoms until the transfusion has been completed. Fatality from transfusion-induced septicemia is estimated at 50 to 80 percent (Cook, 1997b). Septic shock is characterized by sudden high fever, marked hypotension, and cardiovascular collapse in an apparently "well" individual. Multiorgan system failure is caused by endotoxic poisoning.

Interventions

The aim is to identify the causative organism and support the patient's blood pressure, pulse, and respirations. Infusion of broad-spectrum antibiotics should be started immediately.

Prevention

Disposable equipment has greatly reduced bacterial contamination. Using a strict sterile technique at the time of harvest and during the processing of components is essential. The AABB standards require that

RBCs be infused within 4 hours to reduce the potential of bacterial growth. A unit of blood that reaches 10°C and is not transfused has increased potential for bacterial growth.

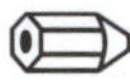 **NOTE:** If slower rates are required, the unit may be split and alloquints may be transfused. Blood should be warmed only as it passes through the administration set; warming the entire unit at one time may increase the chance of microbial growth.

Transmission of Infectious Disease

Despite dynamic advances in blood banking and transfusion medicine, there are still risks to blood component therapy. Patients should be told of alternatives to transfusion, including risks to the patient if transfusion is not undertaken. Furthermore, patients need to know about the blood center's autologous transfusion and patient-designated donor programs, without an implication that there is added safety to the latter.

Interview screening is performed to eliminate donors who may be suspected of carrying transmittable diseases. Donor selection is further safeguarded by the refusal of collection agencies to seek volunteers in areas suspected of having a high percentage of infected populations. These include prisons, homes for the mentally retarded, and groups or institutions that are known to contain homosexuals tend to include a large number who have hepatitis, HIV, and other transmittable diseases. Paid blood donors have a much higher percentage of testing positive for infectious disease; therefore, the paid commercial blood source was eliminated from the United States in 1978 (AABB, 1999). (Table 12–6 provides the incidence of transfusion-acquired infections.)

Viral hepatitis is still a serious risk of transfusion. With the current screening procedures, a recipient's chance is 1 in 200,000 that a pint of blood may result in non-A or non-B viral hepatitis. Currently the risk of a transfusion-associated HIV infection is remote; it is no more than 1 in 825,000.

TABLE 12–6

RISKS OF TRANSFUSION THERAPY

Disease	Risk Factor
Hepatitis C	1:3,300
HTLV-I/II	1:50,000
Hepatitis B	1:200,000
HIV	1:825,000
CMV, malaria, and other rare diseases	1:1,000,000

NURSING PLAN OF CARE

DELIVERY OF BLOOD COMPONENT THERAPY

Focus Assessment

Subjective

- Interview regarding understanding of need for blood component.
- Determine patient's understanding of options: autologous, homologous, and directed donations.

Objective

- Assessment of vital signs (blood pressure, pulse, respiration, temperature)
- Assessment of renal and cardiovascular systems
- Assessment and evaluation of I.V. site before administration of blood component
- Assessment of body weight
- Assessment of level of consciousness
- Review laboratory test
- Current intake and output

Patient Outcome Criteria

The patient will:

- Receive blood product without untoward effect or complications
- Display improvement of hemodynamic parameters and urine output of 1/2 m/kg/h
- Verbalize an understanding of the reasons for the use of the blood component
- Verbalize an awareness of anxiety

Nursing Diagnoses

- Anxiety (mild, moderate, severe) related to threat to or change in health status; misconceptions regarding therapy
- Decreased cardiac output related to sepsis, contamination
- Fear related to homologous blood transfusion and the transmission of disease; fear of needles
- Hyperthermia related to increased metabolic rate, illness, dehydration
- Hypothermia related to exposure to cool or cold blood
- Impaired physical mobility related to pain or discomfort resulting from placement and maintenance of I.V. catheter
- Impaired skin integrity related to I.V. catheter, irritating I.V. solution, inflammation, infection, infiltration
- Impaired tissue integrity related to altered circulation, fluid deficit or excess, irritating solution, inflammation, infection, infiltration
- Impaired gas exchange related to ventilation perfusion imbalance, decreased oxygen-carrying capacity of the blood

(continued)

(continued)

- Knowledge deficit related to purpose of blood component therapy; signs and symptoms of complications
- Risk for infection related to broken skin or traumatized tissue

Nursing Management

1. Verify the physician's orders.
2. Obtain the patient's informed consent.
3. Monitor the patient's immunologic status.
4. Verify that the blood product matches the patient's blood type.
5. Administer blood products as appropriate.
6. Prime the administration system with 0.9 percent sodium chloride.
7. Prepare an I.V. pump as indicated.
8. Perform venipuncture using the appropriate technique.
9. Monitor the I.V. site for signs and symptoms of infiltration, phlebitis, and local infection.
10. Monitor vital signs.
11. Monitor for fluid overload and physical reactions.
12. Monitor and regulate flow rate during infusion.
13. Refrain from rapidly administering lagging blood products.
14. Refrain from administering I.V. medication into blood or blood product lines.
15. Change administration set if clogging of the filter occurs.
16. Administer sodium chloride to clear the line after transfusion is complete.
17. Document the timeframe of transfusion and volume infused.
18. Stop the transfusion if blood reaction occurs and keep veins open with 0.9 percent sodium chloride.
19. Obtain the first voided urine specimen after a transfusion reaction.
20. Coordinate the return of the blood container to the laboratory after a blood reaction.
21. Notify the laboratory immediately in the event of a blood reaction.
22. Maintain standard precautions.
23. Evaluate the effect of transfusion on laboratory test within 24 hours.

PATIENT EDUCATION

- Inform about signs and symptoms of transfusion reactions.
- Instruct on the need and physiologic benefit of blood product.
- Inform on options: autologous, homologous, or designated donation.
- Instruct on current statistics on transfusion risks.

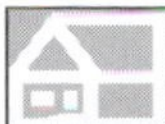

HOME CARE ISSUES

Transfusion services can be delivered safely and efficiently in the home setting. This is an appropriate alternative for patients who require frequent transfusions but for whom hospitalization is not otherwise indicated. Usually the patient has physical limitations that make travel outside the home difficult (Grace & Tomaselli, 1995). For non-homebound patients who require transfusions, administration in an outpatient infusion clinic may be a more cost-effective alternative.

Guidelines and standards need to be set with the patient's best interest in mind. The AABB is creating standards for the home transfusion procedure, and the INS standards should be considered in the formulation of home transfusion therapy. Transfusions in the home setting include packed RBCs, modified RBCs, platelets, cryoprecipitate, plasma, plasma derivatives, and factor VIII concentrate.

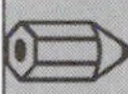

NOTE: Whole blood is not an alternative in the home setting

Guidelines for Home Transfusion Therapy

1. Written physician's order is required.
2. The patient should be:
   - In stable cardiopulmonary status and medical condition
   - Alert, cooperative, and able to respond appropriately to body reactions and communicate information to the nurse
3. The following also must be evaluated:
   - Conducive home environment
   - Capable adult present during transfusion
   - Telephone access available
   - Ready access to emergency medical service and primary physician during transfusion (Grace & Tomaselli, 1995)
4. Blood components should be transported to the home setting using blood bank standards.
5. Proper blood and patient identification must be carried out.
6. Baseline assessments should be made according to INS Standards for monitoring the infusion.
7. Appropriate blood filter should be used.
8. Electromechanical devices may be used, but the product information should be checked to ensure that the pump is indicated for transfusion delivery and will not cause hemolysis of RBCs.
9. Use only 0.9 percent sodium chloride solutions to prime the administration set.
10. The nurse administering the transfusion must remain in the home setting throughout the transfusion and for an appropriate time after transfusion to check for complications.

(continued)

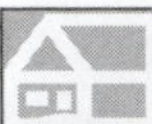

HOME CARE ISSUES ***(continued)***

11. Blood warming should not be considered for home transfusion because no more than 2 U of blood should be administered at one time in the home setting. Patients with cold agglutinins are not appropriate candidates.
12. A biohazard bag should be brought to the home and all contaminated equipment disposed of according to state regulations.
13. The physician must be immediately available at all times for telephone consultation.
14. Post-transfusion instructions should be left; these include but are not limited to:
    - Emergency telephone numbers
    - Information regarding signs and symptoms of delayed reactions
    - Schedule of the post-transfusion assessment visit
15. Notify the physician of the transfusion completion and the patient's response to therapy.
16. Documentation must include, but not be limited to:
    - Type of I.V. solution and time started
    - Type of blood product
    - Vital signs, skin condition, and appearance
    - Any patient symptoms or complaints
    - The time blood product is discontinued
    - Volume infused
    - Reason for discontinuing the transfusion if done before completion of the infusion
    - Patient reactions to the procedure

KEY POINTS

- Immunohematology is the science that deals with antigens of the blood and their antibodies.
- Blood groups are based on the antigens present on the cell surface of RBCs. The two major antigen groups are the ABO and Rh systems. Every human being has two genotypes that, when paired, determine one of four blood types (A, B, AB, or O).
- The universal RBC donor is O negative; the universal plasma donor is AB.
- The majority of people (85%) have the Rh antigen D, making them Rh positive. Those without the antigen D are Rh negative.
- ABO incompatibility is the major cause of fatal transfusion reactions.
- The most common preservatives added to blood to extend the shelf life are CPDA-1 (35 days) ADSOL (42 days).
- Blood donor collection methods include:
  - Homologous: Blood donated by someone other than the intended recipient (allogeneic)
  - Autologous: Recipient's own blood; collected in one of four ways: preoperative blood salvage, intraoperative blood salvage, ANH, postoperative blood salvage
  - Designated (directed) blood donated from selected friends or relatives of the recipient
- Blood product transfusions are indicated for:
  - Maintenance of oxygen-carrying capacity of the blood
  - Replacement of clotting factors
  - Replacement of vascular volume
- Governmental agencies (i.e., the AABB, INS, and FDA) set standards for responsibilities of nurses in the safe administration of blood products.
- Biologic (immune) reactions include acute hemolytic transfusion reactions, delayed transfusion reactions, nonhemolytic febrile reactions, allergic reactions, GVHD reactions, and alloimmunization and refractoriness.
- Nonimmune complications associated with transfusion therapy include circulatory overload, potassium toxicity, hypothermia, hypocalcemia, bacterial contamination, and infectious disease transmission.
- Key steps in the procedure to delivery blood transfusion are:
  - Verify physician's order
  - Type and crossmatch
  - Equipment selection and preparation
  - Patient preparation
  - Obtain blood from blood bank
  - Prepare for administration
  - Initiate the transfusion
  - Monitor the transfusion
  - Discontinue the transfusion

CHAPTER ACTIVITIES

COMPETENCY CRITERIA: Blood Administration
COMPETENCY STATEMENT: Competent I.V. nurses will demonstrate safe delivery of blood components.
Note: The cognitive (knowledge) information that is embedded within this performance-based competency includes knowledge of immunohematology.
This competency *links* to infection control, initiation of peripheral I.V. therapy, and equipment integrity.

Performance	**Skilled**	**Needs Education**
Critical Action Statements		
1. Verifies physician written order for administration of blood component		
2. Selects appropriate equipment for transfusion A. Y set administration set B. 0.9 percent sodium chloride		
3. Prepares patient for transfusion A. Explains procedure to patient B. Reviews laboratory data: Hgb, Hct, platelet counts C. Assesses lungs and kidney function D. Obtains baseline vital signs		
4. Verifies patent I.V. access before obtaining blood from blood bank		
5. Obtains blood product from blood bank A. Verifies component with blood bank: ABO and Rh Unit number Expiration date Collect blood component Patient identification number		

(continued)

(continued)

Performance	Skilled	Needs Education
Critical Action Statements		
6. Prepares for administration of blood component A. Verifies blood component with another nurse ABO and Rh Unit number Expiration date Collect blood component Patient identification number B. Primes Y set with 0.9 percent sodium chloride C. Obtains vital signs and records on flow sheet		
7. Initiates transfusion A. Starts infusion at site B. Stays with patient first 5 minutes		
8. Monitors transfusion A. Takes vital signs and observes patient throughout transfusion B. Reports any adverse effects		
9. Disposes of blood component bag in appropriate biohazard container		
10. Documents procedure		

EVALUATION CRITERIA

1. Validation of transfusion procedure with preceptor.

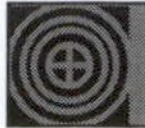

CRITICAL THINKING ACTIVITY

1. A friend wants to know if she can donate blood to be directly designated for her father. What do you tell her?

2. While you are caring for a patient who is to receive a unit of RBCs, the patient expresses a fear of contracting AIDS from the transfusion. What do you tell the patient? Are there risks?

3. As a new graduate, what resources are available to you for providing patient teaching related to the donation of blood?

4. Review the policy and procedure for blood transfusion at the facility at which you work. Does the policy designate who should pick up the blood from the laboratory? Is the procedure clear about how to check out blood from the laboratory and how to administer the component safely?

5. If you were unclear on how to administer cryoprecipitate, what would you do?

6. Your patient develops an increase in temperature during a transfusion of RBCs, his pulse rate is 120, and he is slightly short of breath. You discover baseline vital signs had not been taken, as you directed a nurse's aide to do before administering the transfusion. What would you do? Also, who is at fault?

7. At the beginning of your shift, you check on a unit of blood that had been hung before your shift. The unit of RBCs is infusing slowly, with approximately 100 mL left. You agitate the bag slightly and discover a pinhole at the top of the bag. What do you do?

POST-TEST

1. All the following statements related to the HLA system are true **EXCEPT:**
   a. HLA is located on the surface of WBCs.
   b. Alloimmunization to HLA antigens is a factor in refractoriness to platelets.
   c. The use of blood typing and crossmatching reduces the alloimmunization to the HLA antigen.
   d. The use of leukocyte-depleted blood can reduce the sensitization to HLA antigens.
2. Antibodies are found in:
   a. RBCs
   b. WBCs
   c. Plasma
   d. Antigens
3. Previous exposure to an antigen by pregnancy or previous transfusion may cause the patient to develop:
   a. An antibody to the antigen
   b. More antigens
   c. Alloimmunization to the antibody
   d. A tolerance to the transfusion
4. A chemical added to donor units to preserve the blood is:
   a. Sodium heparin
   b. Sodium citrate
   c. Sodium phosphate
   d. Dextrose aluminum
5. Blood bank testing for donor blood includes tests for the following diseases **EXCEPT:**
   a. HbsAg
   b. Anti–HIV-1
   c. Anti–HTLV-1
   d. EBV (Epstein-Barr virus)
6. Indications for platelet transfusion include:
   a. Hemorrhage with a platelet count less than 50,000
   b. Nonbleeding patients with a platelet count of 80,000
   c. Preoperative patient with a platelet count of 150,000
7. The nursing intervention for an acute hemolytic reaction would be to:
   a. Slow the transfusion and call the physician.
   b. Stop the transfusion and turn on the saline side of the administration set.
   c. Stop the transfusion, disconnect the tubing from the I.V. catheter, and initiate new saline and tubing to keep the vein open.
8. The component albumin 25 percent is hypertonic. Caution should be used by nurses when infusing 25 percent albumin because this product can:
   a. Cause circulatory overload
   b. Cause clotting disorders
   c. Increase RBC hemoglobin
   d. Lower the blood pressure

9. Nurses must check all of the following with another nurse before initiating a unit of blood EXCEPT:
   a. ABO and Rh
   b. Patient name
   c. Unit number
   d. Expiration date
   e. Preservative
10. The universal recipient is a person with blood type
   a. A positive
   b. AB positive
   c. O negative
   d. AB negative

REFERENCES

American Association of Blood Banks. (1999). *Standards for Blood Banks and Transfusion Services* (19th ed.). American Association of Blood Banks, Bethesda, Maryland.

American Association of Blood Banks. (1999). Facts about blood. Internet. Available: www.aabb.org/docs/facts.html 9/99.

American Association of Blood Banks. (1998). *Circular of Information for the Use of Human Blood and Blood Components,* Sacramento: AABB OP1594 ARC 1751.

Baranowski, L. (1993). Current trends in blood component therapy: The evolution of safer, more effective product. *Journal of Intravenous Therapy,* 15 (3), 136–149.

Cook, L.S. (1995). An overview of leukocyte depletion in blood transfusion. *Journal of Intravenous Therapy,* 18 (1), 11–15.

Cook, L.S. (1997a). Blood transfusion reactions involving an immune response. *Journal of Intravenous Nursing,* 20 (1) 5–13.

Cook, L.S. (1997b). Nonimmune transfusion reactions: When type and cross match aren't enough. *Journal of Intravenous Nursing,* 20 (1) 15–22.

Friedman, M.M. (1997). Risk management strategies for home transfusion therapy. *Journal of Intravenous Nursing,* 20 (4), 179–187.

Giger, J.N., & Davidhizar, R.E. (1999). *Transcultural Nursing: Assessment and Intervention.* St. Louis: Mosby, 140.

Gridley, J.H. (1986). Blood component therapy. *Trauma Quarterly,* 2 (3), 45–54.

Hadaway, L. (1999). Understanding leukocyte reduction in blood transfusions. *Nursing 99,* 29 (10), 74.

Harovas, J., & Anthony, H. (1993). Your guide to trouble-free transfusions. *RN,* 93 (1), 28–35.

Intravenous Nursing Society. (2000). Revised Standards of practice. *Journal of Intravenous Nursing Supplement.* Philadelphia: Lippincott Williams & Wilkins.

Jick, H., Slone, D., Westerhom, B., et al. (1969). Venous thromboembolic disease and ABO blood type. *Lancet,* 1, 539–542.

National Institute of Health. (1993). Transfusion alert: Indications for use of red blood cells, platelets and fresh frozen plasma. No. 93–2974a. Bethesda, MD: U.S. Department of Health and Human Services.

Oeltjen, A.M., & Santrach, P.J. (1997). Autologous transfusion techniques. *Journal of Intravenous Nursing,* 20 (6), 305–310.

Phillips, L.D., & Kuhn, M. (1999). *Manual of IV Medications* (2nd ed.). Philadelphia: Lippincott-Raven Publishers.

Raife, T.J. (1997). Adverse effects of transfusion caused by leukocytes. *Journal of Intravenous Nursing,* 20 (5); 238–244.

Synthetic Blood International. (1999). Product information. Internet Available www.sybd.com/Synthetic.html February 26, 2000.

Vengelen-Tyler (1999). *American Association of Blood Banks Technical Manual* (13th ed.). Bethesda, Maryland: American Association of Blood Banks.

Weir, J. (1995). Blood component therapy. In Terry, J., Baranowski, L., Lonsway, R., & Hedrick, C. (eds.). *Intravenous Therapy: Clinical Principles and Practices.* Philadelphia: W.B. Saunders, 165–187.

ANSWERS TO CHAPTER 12

Pre-Test

1. c, **2.** b, **3.** d, **4.** d, **5.** c, **6.** e, **7.** c, **8.** a, **9.** b, **10.** d

Post-Test

1. c, **2.** c, **3.** a, **4.** b, **5.** d, **6.** a, **7.** c, **8.** a, **9.** e, **10.** b

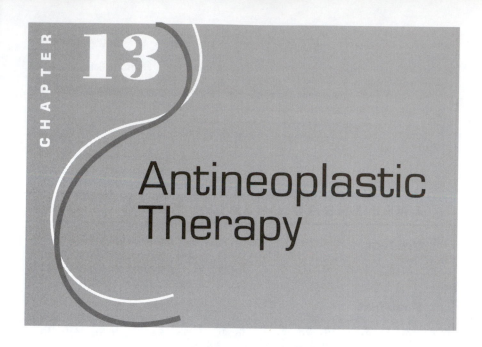

CHAPTER 13 Antineoplastic Therapy

These seasons of surviving are like the changing seasons of the year. We delight in the fragrant smell of spring, bask in the hot days of summer, then welcome the cool, crisp days of fall.

Lest we get too used to it all, the frosty chill of winter is upon us, and when we despair of ever seeing those spring daffodils, violets and tulips again, up they blossom once again to delight us, only in a different way.

Enduring seasons in survival give us renewed opportunities to learn more clearly the meaning of living and dying.

Karen Hassey Dow, RN, MS, Cancer Survivor

CHAPTER CONTENTS

LEARNING OBJECTIVES

Upon completion of this chapter, the reader will be able to:

1. Define terminology related to administration of antineoplastic agents.
2. Discuss the principles of cellular kinetics.
3. Identify the phases of the cell cycle.
4. Identify the goals of cancer antineoplastic therapy.
5. Define the terms "cell cycle specific" and "cell cycle nonspecific."
6. Identify the role of the clinician in administration of chemotherapy.
7. State the action, drug specificity, and major side effects and specific nursing interventions with alkylating agents, antimetabolites, vinca alkaloids, hormones and hormone antagonists, and biologic response modifiers.
8. State specific nursing interventions that are useful in helping patients deal with alopecia.
9. List the medications available for treating patients with nausea and vomiting.
10. Identify the general procedure for extravasation.
11. Identify agents available for oral care of patients receiving chemotherapy to prevent and treat stomatitis.
12. Identify the major toxicities that can occur with antineoplastic therapy.
13. Identify the common routes used for antineoplastic therapy.
14. Use the nursing process in planning care for a patient receiving antineoplastic therapy.
15. List the key areas of patient education for patients receiving chemotherapy.

GLOSSARY

Adjuvant Addition to primary treatment

AGC Absolute granulocyte count

Alopecia Loss of hair (scalp, facial, axillary, pubic, and body)

Antineoplastic Medication used for the treatment of patients with cancer

Biologic response modifiers Agents that mimic, stimulate, enhance, inhibit, or alter the modifiers hosts responses to cancer

BSA Body surface area

Cellular kinetics Study of mechanisms and rates of cellular changes; provides the basis for an understanding of the action and side effects of anticancer agents

Chemotherapy Treatment of disease with chemical reagents that have a specific and toxic effect on the disease-causing microorganisms

Curative Successful treatment of a disease

Cytomodulatory Biotherapy agents that cause recognition of tumor-associated antigens

Cytotoxic The degree to which an agent possesses a specific destructive action on certain cells or the possession of such action; antineoplastic agents that selectively kill dividing cells

Desquamation Shedding of the epidermis

Extravasation Leakage of a vesicant or irritant drug into the subcutaneous tissue that is capable of causing pain, necrosis, or sloughing of tissue

Integumentary Cutaneous; dermal

Intraperitoneal (IP) Within the peritoneal cavity

Intraventricular: Within a ventricle

Irritant: A cancer chemotherapeutic agent capable of producing venous pain at the site and along the vein, with or without an inflammatory reaction

Leukopenia Any situation in which the total number of leukocytes in the circulating blood is less than normal, the limit of which is generally regarded as 5000 cells/mm^3

Mitosis Indirect cell division involving indirect nuclear division and division of the cell body; the process by which all somatic cells of multicellular organisms multiply

Myelosuppression Decrease in function of bone marrow resulting in decrease in fully functioning blood cells

Nadir count Point at which the blood counts are the lowest; usually 7 to 14 days after the first day of chemotherapy

Neutropenia Diminished number of neutrophils in the blood

Nonstem cells Cells that differentiate

Oncologist Physician involved in the study and treatment of tumors

Palliative Use of procedures to promote client comfort and quality of life without the goal of cure of disease

Peripheral neuropathy: Dysfunction of postganglionic nerves ranging from paresthesia to paralysis
Pruritus: Itching
Stem cells Mother cells having the capacity for both replication and differentiation
Thrombocytopenia A condition in which there is an abnormally small number of platelets in the circulating blood
Vesicant A drug capable of causing or forming a blister or causing tissue necrosis upon skin contact

PRE-TEST

1. Which of the following antineoplastic agent classifications is cell cycle dependent?
   - a. Folic acid analogues
   - b. Nitrogen mustards
   - c. Nitrosoureas
   - d. Platinum complexes
2. When a patient is receiving a chemotherapeutic agent that is nephrotoxic, which laboratory value should the nurse monitor?
   - a. Alkaline phosphatase
   - b. BUN/creatinine
   - c. Uric acid
   - d. Serum sodium
3. A drug commonly prescribed on a scheduled basis before and after chemotherapy to prevent nausea and vomiting is:
   - a. Diazepam
   - b. Haloperidol
   - c. Ondansetron
   - d. Ranitidine
4. Before administration of an antimetabolite antineoplastic agent, it is important that the patient:
   - a. Has antiemetic medication
   - b. Is well hydrated
   - c. Receives an antacid
   - d. Receives a sedative
5. Agents given to increase hematopoiesis are:
   - a. Colony-stimulating factors
   - b. Interferons
   - c. Interleukins
   - d. Monoclonal antibodies
6. Agents given to enhance the body's immune system are:
   - a. Antiestrogenic compounds
   - b. Biologic response modifiers
   - c. Hormones
   - d. Alkylating agents
7. A patient receiving paclitaxel who has symptoms of peripheral neuropathy is most likely to be:
   - a. Cardiotoxic
   - b. Neurotoxic
   - c. Nephrotoxic
   - d. Hepatotoxic
8. A vesicant antineoplastic agent is infusing and the nurse checks the infusion and suspects infiltration. The first nursing action would be to:
   - a. Remove the cannula
   - b. Photograph the suspected site

c. Apply warm compresses and continue administering the medication
d. Stop administering the medication

9. The protocol for holding the antineoplastic agent until discussion with the physician would be when the patient presents with a white blood cell count of:
   a. 6000/µL
   b. 5000/µL
   c. 4000/µL
   d. Below 3000/µL
10. All the following are common nursing diagnoses associated with delivery of chemotherapeutic agents **EXCEPT:**
   a. Altered nutrition
   b. Altered oral mucous membrane
   c. Fatigue
   d. Alteration in urinary elimination
11. A patient considered neutropenic from bone marrow suppression is at risk for:
   a. Dehydration
   b. Infection
   c. Seizures
   d. Disseminated intravascular coagulation

● ● ●

Nurses participating in administration of antineoplastic agents have a tremendous responsibility. This chapter emphasizes nurses' roles in understanding cellular kinetics, pharmacology of antineoplastic agents, routes of administration, and common side effects of chemotherapy.

INS STANDARDS The nurse's responsibilities for administering antineoplastic therapy include knowledge of disease process, drug classifications, pharmacologic indications, actions, side effects, adverse reactions, method of administration, rate of delivery, treatment goal, and drug properties (e.g., vesicant, nonvesicant, and irritant.) (INS, 2000, 70)

THE ROLE OF THE CLINICIAN

Administering **antineoplastic** agents and caring for patients with cancer require specific educational preparation and practical experience. The Oncology Nursing Society (ONS) has developed credentialing for oncology nurses.

Nurses practicing in this specialty area are required to be knowledgeable about the biology of cancer, the pharmacology and principles of cancer **chemotherapy,** specific antineoplastic agents, major principles governing the administration of chemotherapy, and patient assessment and management (Weinstein, 1997).

PATIENT ASSESSMENT AND HISTORY

Assessment begins by first determining the patient's knowledge base of the classification of their cancer and the symptoms and course of the disease. This is the first step in gathering a history from the client. The information gathered provides a framework for patient education. The history should also include the patient's past medical history; previous organ impairment; or any secondary diagnosis that might influence the toxicities, side effects, and treatment modalities. A record of the total chemotherapeutic agents administered, doses, and any radiation (number of rads) is necessary to complete a cancer history (Table 13–1).

Physical assessment includes the patient's laboratory and diagnostic imaging studies, nutritional status, and psychosocial and spiritual states. Appropriate nursing interventions are based on a complete history and physical assessment.

TREATMENT OBJECTIVES

The role of the clinician also includes an understanding of treatment goals and their rationale. The treatment goal of chemotherapy depends on the situation. Chemotherapy can be **curative** when given as primary treatment. The therapeutic goal is also curative when chemotherapy is given as an adjuvant for tumors. Knowledge of the chemotherapy

TABLE 13–1

ONCOLOGY PATIENT ASSESSMENT

Interview
- Cancer history
- Knowledge of classification of cancer
- Symptoms
- Course of disease
- Past medical history
- Previous organ impairment
- Secondary diagnosis

Physical assessment
Nutritional status
Laboratory tests
Diagnostic imaging studies:
- Computed tomography
- Magnetic resonance imaging
- Radiography

Psychological state
Spiritual state

treatment, long- and short-term side effects, symptom management, and lifestyle effects are important because two out of three cancer patients are candidates for chemotherapy at some point in their disease process.

Chemotherapy can also be given to control the disease when cure is not realistic. The goal of **palliative** treatment is pain control. Chemotherapy can decrease pain caused by a tumor by relieving pressure on nerves, decreasing lymphatic congestion, and relieving organ obstruction (Doyle, 1995).

There are few absolute rules related to antineoplastic therapy; however, there are certain basic considerations in chemotherapy treatment:

1. The smaller the tumor burden, the easier the patient is to treat.
2. Surgical debulking decreases the tumor burden and recruits resting malignant cells to start dividing, thereby increasing the sensitivity to chemotherapy.
3. The higher the chemotherapy dose, the better the chance for a tumor response.
4. Doses of chemotherapeutic agents are altered based on the degree of toxicity that the patient experiences.
5. The therapeutic margin is the difference between the dose producing the desired benefit and the dose resulting in unacceptable toxicity.
6. The therapeutic margin of antineoplastic agents is narrow compared with that of other types of drugs.
7. If the efficacy of the chemotherapeutic agents can be increased, there is better tumor response with a lower chemotherapy dose.

WEB SITES:
Oncology Nursing Society (ONS): *www.ons.org*
CancerNet: *www.cancernet.nci.nih.gov*
Cancer Treatment Centers of America: *www.cancercenter.com/home*
Oncology Online Journals: *www.cancerlink.s.usa.com/professional/journal*
American Cancer Society: *www.cancer.org*
Harvard Center for Cancer Prevention: *www.hsph.harvard.edu/organizations/canprevent/index.html*
National Cancer Institute's CancerNet Cancer Information: *http://cancernet.nci.nih.gov*
American Society of Clinical Oncology: *www.asco.org*
Others: ______________________________

CELLULAR KINETICS

Cellular kinetics is the study of mechanisms and rates of cellular changes. This study is becoming increasingly more useful in planning treatment regimens and scheduling drug administration. Chemotherapy exerts a cytotoxic action by interfering with the reproductive cell cycle. Cancer cells are the intended target of treatment; however, **cytotoxic** action also affects normal cells.

CELL CYCLE

Antineoplastic agents act primarily on proliferating cells; therefore, it is important to examine the cell cycle and the growth of normal and malignant cells to understand the rationale for and effects of drug therapy (Fig. 13–1).

Five phases complete the cell growth cycle: G_0, G_1, S, G_2, and M. The letter "G" refers to gap phases or periods when cells are preparing for a more active phase of reproduction (Moran, 2000). Some cells move out of the cell cycle after **mitosis** into G_0, becoming resting and nondividing cells. Other cells enter the first phase, G_1, which is the period between mitosis and the beginning of deoxyribonucleic acid (DNA) synthesis when active ribonucleic acid (RNA) and protein synthesis occurs.

The G_1 phase is the most variable of all phases, and its length influences the rate of cell proliferation. The G_1 phase is called the first growth phase, and it is characterized by the production of RNA, enzymes, and proteins, all of which are essential in later cycles. Whereas cells that are growing slowly have many cells in the G_1 phase, cells that are growing rapidly have few cells in the G_1 phase.

The cells then emerge from the G_1 phase and enter the S phase, in which enzymes necessary for DNA synthesis increase in activity. Called the synthesis phase, the predominant event in this phase is the creation of DNA, the genetic code of all information needed for cell life. At the end of the S phase, the cell contains twice the original amount of DNA in

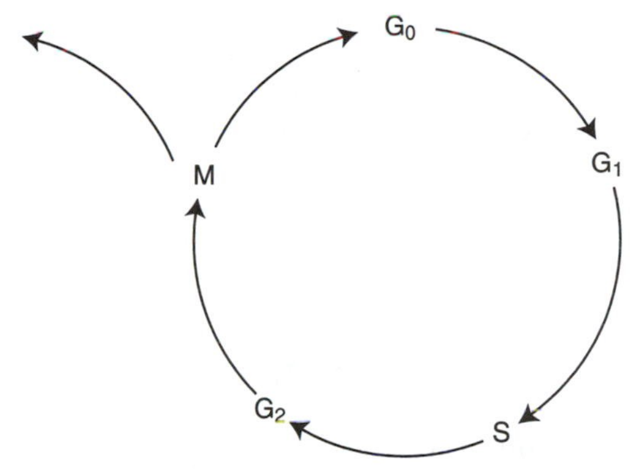

G_0	Nonproliferative resting phase
G_1	Presynthetic stage
S	Synthesis of DNA
G_2	Interval after synthesis of DNA
M	Mitosis (G_2 cell divides into two cells)

FIG. 13–1. Cell cycle.

preparation for the creation of new daughter cells. The duration of this phase ranges from 10 to 20 hours (Moran, 2000).

After the S phase, a resting period called G_2 occurs. During this phase, the RNA and protein necessary for mitosis are synthesized. This phase extends from the end of DNA synthesis to the beginning of mitosis.

The last phase of the cell cycle is the M phase, in which mitosis takes place. This is a brief phase, lasting only about 1 half hour to 1 hour, in which cell division occurs. The formation of the spindle, separation of chromosomes, and the division of the cell into two cells occur, creating a new daughter cell. After mitosis, the cell may resume the cycle at G_1 or move into a dormant state in G_0.

The phases of the cell cycle relate to the delivery of antineoplastic agents for specific types of cancer. Most agents kill only cells that are actively reproducing, leaving relatively unaffected the cells that are in the G_0 or resting phase. If a tumor mass consists of a large percentage of cells in G_0 at the time of chemotherapy exposure, there will be much less cell kill than would occur in a tumor with a high percentage of cells actively reproducing (Ingwersen, 1996). The concept of cells in cycle versus resting is essential to understanding tumor growth patterns, or tumor kinetics (Moran, 2000).

TUMOR KINETICS

In both normal and malignant tissues, three different cell populations affect growth: cycling cells, nondividing cells, and resting cells called G_0 cells. The cells that are dividing continuously are the *cycling cells*. The group of cells that divide for a time and then complete their life cycle without dividing again are called *nondividing cells*. The third group is made up of G_0, or resting cells, which leave the cell cycle and remain dormant until conditions stimulate them to reenter the cell cycle and divide. Cycling cells and G_0, or resting cells, are further divided into **stem cells** and nonstem cells. Stem cells replenish the stem cell pool, and **nonstem cells** differentiate and enter the maturing groups of cells. As long as G_0 stem cells remain, a damaged cell population can be renewed.

GROWTH FRACTION

Four interrelated factors must be considered during the assessment of normal or tumor cells: the cell cycle time, growth fraction, total number of cells in the population, and rate of cell loss (Skeel, 1999). The first factor, the cell cycle time, is the amount of time required for the cell to move from one mitosis to the next. Second, the growth fraction is the percentage of cycling cells in the entire cell population. The third factor is the total number of cells in the population determined at some point in time, which indicates how advanced the cancer is and provides a basis for growth measurement. As the total number of cells increases, so does the number of resistant cells. The fourth factor is the rate of cell loss or the number of cells that die or leave the cell population. Growth depends on the number of cells produced and the number of cells that die. Rate of growth depends on the cell cycle time, the growth fraction, and the rate of cell loss.

DOUBLING TIME

In tumor growth, there is a theory that as the tissue mass increases in size, the doubling time slows. Another factor that affects tumor growth is the decrease in nutrients available for each cell as the total mass increases and blood supply is outgrown. It has been found that some normal cells cycle faster than tumor cells in human beings. Overall, tumor cell cycling times range from 24 to 120 hours. The doubling time of most tumor cells ranges from 5 days to 2 years, with a mean of 1 to 3 months (Moran, 2000). This longer doubling time is caused by several factors. First, the growth fraction of human tumors varies from 0 to 100 percent. Second, many tumor cells die spontaneously. Spontaneous death occurs from inadequate nutrition, cumulative genetic damage in tumor cells, and cell differentiation into nondividing cells.

CELL KILL HYPOTHESIS

The goal of modern chemotherapy is to prevent cancer cells from multiplying, invading, metastasizing, and ultimately killing the host (Skeel, 1999). Most active cytotoxic agents are selectively toxic to rapidly proliferating cells; many G_0 or resting cells remain untouched. Resting stem cells can regenerate the tumor cell population. The tumor mass increases in size, and the cells cycle at a slower rate; therefore, the growth fraction decreases and the cytotoxic effects of the drug diminish. The drugs are not only specific to cancer cells but are also toxic to normal proliferating cells. Normal cells most affected by chemotherapeutic drugs include hematopoietic or bone marrow cells, gastrointestinal (GI) epithelial cells, hair follicle cells, germinal cells, and embryonic cells.

The ability of antineoplastic agents to kill tumor cells comes from research showing that these drugs kill tumor cells according to first-order kinetics. Certain drug doses destroy a constant fraction of tumor cells in the body, rather than a constant number of cells. Also, these drugs follow an exponential, or "log-kill," model. Therefore, cell kill may be expressed as a log-kill of two, meaning that the body's tumor burdens decreased from 108 to 106 cells (from 100,000,000 to 1,000,000). The maximum cell kill from a single drug dose has been found to be 2 to 5 logs. Treatment must be repeated many times to decrease the number of tumor cells in the body. Because a single dose always kills a fraction of the tumor cells, this hypothesis suggests that chemotherapy can never destroy all malignant cells in the body (Skeel, 1999).

The second hypothesis proposes that cell kill caused by antineoplastic drugs is related to the relative growth fraction of the tumor at the time of treatment. Thus, the greatest tumor cell kill occurs when the growth fraction is greatest. The growth fraction is greatest when tumors are of intermediate size; the growth fraction is less when they are very small or very large (ONS, 1999).

The biologic control of normal cells and tumor growth at the modular level has not yet led to improved therapy for patients with cancer; however, it has helped to explain differences in response among populations of patients. Further work in this area may provide a powerful selective means of controlling neoplastic cell growth and lead to effective cancer treatment in the next decade. This is further discussed under Biologic Control Modifiers.

DRUG RESISTANCE

Resistance to antineoplastic therapy is a combined characteristic whereby the drug is ineffective in controlling the tumor without excessive toxicity. Factors that influence resistance include the specific drug, the specific tumor, and the specific host.

The first dose of a drug is usually very effective in treating tumor cells, but successive doses at times decreases the effectiveness until no effect is seen. Many malignant cells develop drug resistance. There appears to be a similarity between cancer cell resistance to drugs and bacterial resistance to antibiotics. Thus, similar approaches such as large initial doses, combination drugs, alternating combinations of drugs, and earliest possible treatment of disease are used to overcome resistance and eventual tumor recurrence (ONS, 1999).

Cell resistance to antineoplastic drugs can be natural or acquired. Natural resistance results from the initial unresponsiveness of a tumor to a given drug. Acquired resistance is the unresponsiveness that emerges after initially successful treatment (Skeel, 1999).

CULTURAL AND ETHNIC CONSIDERATIONS: CANCER

Cancers of the stomach, esophagus, and liver occur more frequently among Japanese-Americans than among their European-American counterparts. It is believed that eating dried, salted fish is a predisposing factor

In Haiti, cervical cancer accounts for 39 percent of all cancers and is related to poor feminine hygiene, having multiple sexual partners, and failure to have Pap smears. GI cancer is related to poor nutrition and low vitamin intake.

Certain cancers are more frequent in certain groups of Jewish people. For example, stomach cancer is more prevalent among Jews from Europe and the United States. Breast cancer is the most frequent cancer for all Jewish women groups except those from Iran. Studies indicate that Ashkenazi Jewish women have a high incidence of specific mutations of *BRAC1* and *BRAC2.* These changes have been associated with an increase in breast and ovarian cancer. Cancer of the cervix has been historically lower in Jewish women than those who are not Jewish.

Because of accumulated genetic damage caused by the Chernobyl nuclear power plant accident, Russians have a 250 percent higher rate of certain cancers than Americans (Giger & Davidhizar, 1999).

ANTINEOPLASTIC AGENTS

The goal of antineoplastic therapy is total cell kill by selective toxicity. Several principles make this goal difficult to achieve. First, the presence of a single malignant cell may yield sufficient daughter cells to kill the human host. The second factor is the negligible contribution of host immune mechanisms and defenses in augmenting therapy. Administering **chemotherapy** in combination or sequences is a way of dealing with the residual body burden of tumor cells. Other methods include reductive, adjuvant, and intermittent therapy.

CLASSIFICATIONS

Antineoplastic agents are classified according to the cell life cycle. This classification has two categories: (1) cell cycle phase–specific (CCPS) agents and (2) cell cycle phase–nonspecific (CCPN) agents.

TABLE 13–2

CELL CYCLE PHASE–SPECIFIC AGENTS

Phase	Agents
G_1	L-asparaginase, prednisone
S	Cytarabine, 5-fluorouracil (5-FU), hydroxyurea, methotrexate, thioguaine
G_2	Bleomycin, etoposide
M	Vinblastine, vincristine, vindesine, paclitaxel

Cell cycle phase–specific agents kill cells that are actively in cycle, anywhere from G_1 through M. This category additionally is divided into groups that affect specific phases of the cell cycle (Table 13–2). The key to CCPS agents lies in timing. Many CCPS regimens employ small divided doses given at repeated intervals or by continuous infusion in an attempt to expose cells during a vulnerable phase. These regimens exploit the fact that 20 percent of reproducing cells are in the S phase at any give time (Moran, 2000).

Agents that are CCPN do not depend on cells' being in a specific phase; rather, they are effective throughout the reproductive cycle and, to a certain extent, in the resting phase. CCPN agents disrupt DNA synthesis in a variety of ways. Cellular contents become unbalanced and the cell dies when it tries to divide. The CCPN drugs do not rely on cycle phase to be effective (Moran, 2000).

The chemical structure also provides a category by which the drugs can be classified; these are alkylating agents, antimetabolites, natural products, hormones and hormone antagonists, and biologic response modifiers.

Chemotherapeutic agents can also be classified according to their potential to cause local tissue reactions. The potential for alteration in skin and tissue integrity ranges from transient local discomfort during administration to severe tissue necrosis. Classification includes **irritants** and **vesicants** (ONS, 1999).

COMBINATION CHEMOTHERAPY

Combination regimens are the mainstay today of cancer chemotherapy, and new combinations of old drugs continue to emerge along with the incorporation of new drugs into regimens. The decisions to use multidrug regimens is based on cell biology (Moran, 2000):

1. One or more drugs in the regimen should have at least some cytotoxicity against the target tumor cell.
2. Each drug should have a different mechanism of action to exploit different events occurring in the cell cycle.

3. Each drug should have different potential side effects from the other drugs or at least exert similar side effects at a different time. An example is the MOPP regimen for treating Hodgkin's disease: mechlorethamine, oncovin, procarbazine, and prednisone (Ingwersen, 1996).

REDUCTIVE THERAPY

Reductive therapy decreases the body burden of cancer cells before chemotherapy through surgery, radiotherapy, or other therapy.

ADJUVANT CHEMOTHERAPY

Adjuvant chemotherapy is the administration of chemotherapy to destroy micrometastasis and to prevent secondary tumors after the removal or destruction of a primary tumor. This therapy is aimed at reducing residual tumor burden to levels more likely handled by the host's immunologic mechanisms.

INTERMITTENT THERAPY

The timing of chemotherapy doses can be critical. Intermittent high-dose (pulse) therapy with CCPS and CCPN agents gives better therapeutic results with less toxic side effects than more frequent divided doses. Timing drug dose in relation to another drug can allow for cell synchronization to yield greater cell kill (Moraca-Sawicki, 1998).

CHEMOTHERAPY DOSING

Dose Calculations Using Body Surface Area

Doses of antineoplastic agents used in chemotherapy are calculated according to body surface area (**BSA**). Clinical trials have provided a formula to determine the amount of each drug to be used in a particular regimen.

A nomogram chart is used to calculate the log of the height and weight. Many institutions have computers that are programmed to determine the BSA. The **oncologist** uses weight changes to determine whether an adjustment in the total dosage is necessary to avoid overdosing or underdosing the patient.

The basic formula for determining the chemotherapy dosage is:

$$\text{BSA} \times \text{mg/m}^2 = \text{total dose}$$

NOTE: It is important to weigh the patient before each course of chemotherapy and it is important to note whether the BSA was determined from ideal body weight or actual weight.

Dose Calculations Using the Clavert Formula

Another formula that attempts to individualize the dose of a drug so that optimal therapeutic response is achieved without toxic effects is use of the Clavert formula. The Clavert formula makes it possible to individualize the carboplatin dose in order to obtain a maximally effective dose with tolerable side effects (Groenwald & Goodman, 1999).

Carboplatin dose (mg) =
Target AUC (area under the curve) × (GFR [glomerular filtration rate] + 25)

CLASSES OF DRUGS

Chemotherapeutic agents are divided into several classes. For two of the classes (e.g., alkylating agents and antimetabolites), the names indicate the mechanism of cytotoxic action. The hormonal agents refer to the physiologic type of drug, and the natural products reflect the source of the drugs. **Biologic response modifiers** mimic, stimulate, enhance, inhibit, or otherwise alter the host responses to the cancer (Skeel, 1999). Table 13–3 presents commonly prescribed chemotherapeutic agents.

Alkylating Agents

Alkylating agents were derived from the sulfur mustard gases used in World War I and II (Moraca-Sawicki, 1998). These agents are a diverse group of chemical compounds capable of forming molecular bonds with nucleic acids, proteins, and many molecules of low molecular weight. The basis for their therapeutic use against cancers is the process of alkylation by which they cause interstrand and intrastrand cross-linkages in DNA, thereby blocking replication.

The alkylating agents are cell cycle independent because they act on cells at any phase of the cycle. Most of the agents in this group are considered polyfunctional alkylating agents because they contain more than one alkylating group. The nitrosoureas are unique under the class of alkylating agents with respect to being non–cross-resistant with other alkylating agents, being highly lipid soluble, and having delayed myelosuppressive effects. These agents can cross the blood–brain barrier (BBB).

The alkylating agents used as antineoplastic agents are nitrogen mustards, ethylenimines, alkyl sulfonate, nitrosoureas, triazine, and metal salts.

Alkylating agents can cause serious adverse reactions. Major side effects include toxicities to the hematopoietic, GI, and reproductive systems. In addition, all alkylating agents can be carcinogenic. These agents as a class share common side effects of alopecia, bone marrow depression, nausea and vomiting, and diarrhea.

Key Nursing Interventions and Assessment

1. Monitor I.V. sites for infiltration; many alkylating agents cause tissue necrosis with infiltration.

TABLE 13–3

CHEMOTHERAPEUTIC AGENTS

Alkylating Agents	Chlorambucil Carmustine Cyclophosphamide Lomustine Ifosfamide Streptozocin Mechlorethamine Dacarbazine Melphalan Cisplatin Thiotepa (triethylenethriophosphoramide) Carboplatin Busulfan Iproplatin*
Antimetabolite Agents	Methotrexate Azacitidine Mercaptopurine Thioguanine Cytarabine Pentostatin Floxuridine Cladribine Fluorouracil Fludarabine Hexamethylmelamine*
Miotic Inhibitors	Vinblastine Paclitaxel (Taxol) Vincristine Docetaxel Vindesine Etoposide Vinorelbine Teniposide
Antineoplastic Antibiotics	Anthracycline Antibiotics ● Daunorubicin ● Doxorubicin ● Idarubicin ● Aclacinomycin A Other Antibiotics ● Bleomycin ● Plicamycin ● Mitomycin ● Mitoxantrone hydrochloride

(Continued)

TABLE 13–3

CHEMOTHERAPEUTIC AGENTS *(Continued)*

Hormones and Hormone Antagonists	Androgens ● Fluoxymesterone Corticosteroids ● Prednisone ● Dexamethasone Estrogens ● Diethylstilbestrol Progestins ● Megestrol acetate ● Medroxyprogesterone acetate Estrogen antagonists ● Tamoxifen
Miscellaneous Agents	Hydroxyurea Paclitaxel Docetaxel Procarbazine L-Asparaginase

*Investigational.

2. Monitor complete blood count (CBC) and platelets and liver enzymes.
3. Administer antiemetic agents.
4. Assess respiratory status and blood pressure with cyclophosphamide and carmustine; monitor for hypotension with busulfan melphalan.
5. Prehydrate for cisplatin and carboplatin.
6. Assess oral cavity for stomatitis.

Antimetabolites

The antimetabolites are a group of low molecular weight compounds that exert their effect because of similarity to naturally occurring metabolites involved in nucleic acid synthesis. This class includes the folic acid antagonists, pyrimidine antagonists, purine antagonists, and immunosuppressant azathioprine (Imuran).

They are structurally similar to vitamins, coenzymes, or normal cell products needed for growth and division of both normal and neoplastic cells. They interfere with the metabolic pathways of dividing cells and exert their greatest effect in the S phase of the cell cycle. A drug-induced blockage of DNA synthesis occurs when the antimetabolic agent, rather than the necessary nutrient or enzyme, is taken into the cell. This is the major cause of cell death from antimetabolite therapy (Moraca-Sawicki, 1998).

Folic Acid Analogues

Folic acid and its derivatives are critical for the metabolism of proliferating cells. These drugs are potentially nephrotoxic. Methotrexate is an example of a folic acid analog. Side effects include pancytopenia, GI toxicity, skin rash, headache, hepatotoxicity, and pulmonary toxic effects. Methotrexate is used as an immunosuppressive agent to prevent graft-versus-host disease after allogeneic bone marrow transplantation.

Pyrimidine Analogues

These agents inhibit critical enzymes necessary for nucleic acid synthesis and may become incorporated into the DNA and RNA. Common side effects with pyrimidine agents include GI disturbances, cardiac toxicity, and ataxia.

Purine Analogues

Purine agents interfere with normal purine interconversions and thus with DNA and RNA synthesis. These agents can cause bone marrow suppression, hyperuricemia, and acute hepatic toxicity.

The common side effects of antimetabolites are **myelosuppression** and GI disturbances. Other side effects are **stomatitis,** esophagitis, elevation in liver function test results, photosensitivity, and severe nausea and vomiting.

Key Nursing Interventions and Assessment

1. Assess oral mucosa for stomatitis.
2. Monitor CBC, platelets, and liver and renal enzymes.
3. Stop drug if white blood cell (WBC) count drops below 3000/μL.
4. Administer antiemetics, especially with cytarabine and mercaptopurine.
5. High-dose methotrexate requires leucovorin rescue.

Miotic Inhibitors

The natural products (miotic inhibitors) include vinca alkaloids, antibiotics, and enzymes. Their modes of action differ significantly. These products are unlike the alkylating and antimetabolite agents, which are classified by their modes of action. Natural products are classified together because their sources are naturally occurring. Although they are classified together, their modes of action differ significantly (Moraca-Sawicki, 1998).

Vinca Alkaloids

The vinca alkaloids (i.e., vinblastine, vincristine, vinorelbine, and vindesine) are derivatives of the plant vinca rosea (periwinkle). These agents are CCSP, active only when the cell is in the mitotic (M) phase of division. Vinca alkaloids interfere with the microtubule assembly in the mitotic spindle formation.

Adverse effects common with use of the plant alkaloids are numbness and tingling of the extremities, loss of deep tendon reflexes, and ataxia. Vinca alkaloids can produce tissue necrosis if I.V. infusions containing these agents are allowed to extravasate.

Antineoplastic Antibiotics

Anthracycline Antibiotics

Anthracycline agents are derived from fermented products of different *Streptomyces* spp. They are called anthracyclines because the anthracycline portion of their molecules produces the antineoplastic effect. These drugs act by reacting with DNA to form complexes that block DNA-directed RNA and DNA transcription. Current evidence suggests that both drugs are probably effective during all phases of the cell cycle and are therefore CCPN agents.

The major side effects are leukopenia, thrombocytopenia, cardiac toxicity, arrhythmias, cardiomyopathy, nausea, vomiting, stomatitis, skin hyperpigmentation, hepatotoxicity, and enhancement of cyclophosphamide-induced bladder injury. Some agents in this class can cause tissue necrosis if infiltration into subcutaneous tissues occurs (Moraca-Sawicki, 1998).

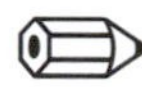

NOTE: The drug dextrazoxane (Zinecard) can now be used after doxorubicin to protect the heart from cardiotoxicity. It is not advised to use dextrazoxane for preventing cardiotoxicity at this time.

Other Antibiotics

Other antibiotics are CCPS that have their action on the G2 and mitosis phases of the cell cycle. These antibiotics are useful in treating patients with a variety of cancers. These agents are often used in combination with other antineoplastic agents. Examples of this classification include bleomycin, plicamycin, mitomycin, and mitoxantrone hydrochloride.

The major side effects are similar to those of the anthracycline antibiotics: myelosuppression and cardiac problems.

Hormones and Hormone Antagonists

The hormones and hormone antagonists include steroidal estrogens, progestins, androgens, corticosteroids and their synthetic derivatives, nonsteroidal synthetic compounds with steroid or steroid antagonist activity hypothalamic-pituitary analogues, and thyroid hormones. Each agent has diverse effects.

Androgens

Androgens exert their antineoplastic effect by altering pituitary function or directly affecting the neoplastic cells.

Nausea, vomiting, anorexia, myalgia, fluid retention, libido changes, and sterilization can result from use of androgens. Synthetic substances exert little or no masculinizing effects.

Corticosteroids

Corticosteroids can cause lysis of lymphoid tumors that are rich in specific cytoplasmic receptors and may have other indirect effects as well. Anti-inflammatory effects help reduce the sequelae of neoplastic activity and nausea and help to reduce cerebral edema secondary to cranial tumor growth or radiation.

Corticosteroids can cause muscle weakness, diarrhea, nausea, increased appetite, euphoria, pancreatitis, and thrombophlebitis. Changes in body fat distribution, increased risk of infection, potassium loss, and, rarely, psychosis may also result.

Estrogens

Estrogens suppress testosterone production in males and alter breast cancer cell response to prolactin. Headache, nausea, weight changes, thromboembolism, and feminization in males can result from use of estrogens.

Progestins

Progestins act directly at the level of the malignant cell receptor to promote differentiation. Edema, pulmonary embolism, breast tenderness, hyperglycemia, and increased appetite can result from use of progestins.

Estrogen Antagonist

Estrogen antagonist acts by competing with estrogen for binding on the cytosol estrogen receptor protein in cancer cells and affects the natural growth factors.

Anorexia, nausea, vaginal discharge, bleeding, hot flashes, and a temporary drop in WBCs can result from the use of estrogen protagonist.

Key Nursing Interventions and Assessment

1. Assess for mood swings and changes in psychological state.
2. Monitor electrolytes in those taking steroids.
3. Monitor blood pressure.
4. Assess males for signs of feminization with estrogens.
5. Assess for signs of phlebitis at I.V. site.
6. Assess females for masculinizing effects with androgens.

7. Encourage low salt diet.
8. Monitor weight.

Miscellaneous Agents

Miscellaneous agents include L-asparaginase, paclitaxel, docetaxel, procarbazine, and hydroxyurea.

L-Asparaginase

The agent L-asparaginase represents a unique development in the field of cancer chemotherapy. This enzyme was first isolated from *Escherichia coli* and is primarily used in the treatment of patients with acute lymphoblastic leukemia.

Asparaginase destroys the amino acid asparagine, which is needed for protein synthesis, and thus leads to cell death. Many normal cells are not sensitive to the effects of this drug enzyme because they can synthesize their own supply of asparagine, which tumor cells cannot do. Antitumor effects of this drug are primarily in the G_1 phase of the cell cycle.

Because L-asparaginase is a foreign protein, it can produce hypersensitivity and anaphylactic reactions. Fever, anorexia, nausea, and vomiting all are signs of acute toxic reaction. Elevated blood urea nitrogen (BUN) and ammonia levels can result from the enzyme action of this agent. Liver function is often impaired and can increase the toxicity of other drugs.

Paclitaxel and Docetaxel

Paclitaxel is obtained from the bark of the yew tree, and taxotere is obtained from the tree's needles. Both agents are used to treat recurrent patients with ovarian carcinoma.

Paclitaxel is a novel antimicrotubule agent. Its action inhibits the normal dynamic reorganization of the microtubule network essential for vital interphase and miotic cellular functions. This agent is more active in patients who have not received previous chemotherapy (Gahart & Nazareno, 1999).

Severe hypersensitivity reactions, flushing, myalgia, arthralgia, nausea, vomiting, alopecia, bone marrow depression, and cardiovascular symptoms (including bradycardia) (Kuhn, 1998) may occur with its use.

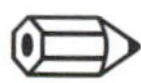

NOTE: Standard pretreatment options include (1) dexamethasone 20 mg I.V. or orally 12 hours and 6 hours before treatment or (2) diphenhydramine 50 mg orally and cimetidine or ranitidine 30 to 60 minutes before paclitaxel.

Procarbazine

This agent, although it is not an antibiotic, acts in a similar manner. This agent has a plasma half-life of only 7 minutes. Its greatest clinical use is as a component of the MOPP regimen in the treatment of patients with Hodgkin's disease.

Hydroxyurea

This agent acts as an antimetabolite, but it cannot be assigned to any of the previous subgroups. Hydroxyurea inhibits DNA synthesis through its action on the enzyme ribonucleotide diphosphate reductase and acts specifically in the S phase of the cell cycle (Kuhn, 1998).

Bone marrow depression is the major toxic effect and subsides rapidly after drug is discontinued several days. Other major side effects include GI disturbances; mild dermatologic reactions; and, rarely, stomatitis, alopecia, and neurologic manifestations.

Key Nursing Interventions and Assessment

1. Monitor patient closely during infusion for possible hypersensitivity reaction.
2. Premedicate with dexamethasone, diphenhydramine, or cimetidine before administering paclitaxel.
3. Assess oral mucosa.
4. Assess infusion site frequently for infiltration; avoid extravasation.
5. Monitor CBC and platelets, cardiac enzymes, and electrocardiogram (ECG).
6. Make neurologic assessment to monitor for deviation and severity of peripheral neuropathy.
7. Administer antiemetics.
8. Monitor renal function.

Biologic Response Modifiers

The term **biologic therapy** describes a variety of agents and therapeutic approaches derived from the biology of the immune system, the nature of tumor cells, and the relation between them (Parkinson, 1995). The goals of biologic response modifying agents are to (1) stimulate immunocompetence by active or passive means, (2) promote tumor-specific immunity, and (3) serve as an adjunct to other treatments to produce tumor regression.

No clear classification system of biotherapeutic agents exists because many are pleomorphic, having multiple immunologic activities against tumors. Early attempts to classify agents used the active and passive delineations typical of vaccines; however, these are not an accurate reflection of the activities of biologic agents used as antineoplastic therapy. Currently, clinicians group agents as (1) antitumor, (2) adoptive, (3) restorative, (4) **cytomodulatory,** and (5) gene manipulative (ONS, 1999; Table 13–4).

Antitumor Biotherapy

Antitumor biotherapy uses agents that combine active and passive mechanisms to enhance or stimulate the nonspecific and specific host tumor immune responses of the individual. Antitumor biotherapeutic

TABLE 13–4

BIOLOGIC RESPONSE MODIFIERS

Antitumor Cytokines
Interferon alpha-2a (Roferon-a)
Interferon alpha-2b (Intron-a)
Interferon alpha-n1 (Wellferon)
Interferon alpha-n3 (Alferon N)
Interferon beta (Betaseron)
Interferon gamma (Actimmune)
Aldesleukin (Proleukin)
Monoclonal Antibodies
Satumomab penditide (OncoScint)
Traztuzumab (Herceptin)
Rituximab (Rituxan)
Colony-stimulating Factors
Epoetin alfa (Epogen, EPO)
Granulocyte colony-stimulating factor (filgrastim [Neupogen])
Granulocyte macrophage colony-stimulating factor (sargramostim [Leukine])
Opreluekin (Neumega)
Cytomodulatory Agents
Levamisole hydrochloride (Ergamisol)

agents include cytokines, vaccines, and monoclonal antibodies (Moraca-Sawicki, 1998).

Cytokines are a general classification of cellular proteins that are produced and secreted in response to stimuli by the immune system. Their two main functions are to regulate and differentiate cell growth and to augment cell activities. This class includes the interferons, interleukins, and colony-stimulating factors. More than 25 cytokines have been isolated (Coleman, 1998).

Antibodies binding to tumor-associated cell surface antigens can result in the destruction of tumor cells through a number of possible mechanisms, such as activation of complement and antibody-dependent, cell-mediated cytotoxicity. These antibodies may be useful as means of targeting cytotoxic radioisotopes, toxins, or drugs to tumors. Monoclonal antibody technology has made important contributions to cancer medicine.

Adoptive Biotherapy

Adoptive biotherapy is based on the assumption that tumor-associated antigens exist that can elicit an autologous antitumor response in the host (patient). Clinical trials using the patient's own genetically altered tumor cells are called tumor infiltrating lymphocytes (TILs) (Moraca-Sawicki, 1998).

Restorative Biotherapy

Restorative biotherapy uses agents that increase the patient's immune response, especially the number of mature, functioning leukocytes. Agents that augment the patient's immune system in this manner are called immunologic stimulants or hematopoietic growth factors.

This category of agents includes natural products such as cyclosporine and tacrolimus used as immunosuppressive agents after solid organ transplantation. These agents exert a variety of immunoproliferative or immunomodulatory functions that are thought to enhance the patient's existing immune defenses. Anticancer agents classed as cytomodulatory include levamisole hydrochloride and retinoids (Moraca-Sawicki, 1998).

Gene Manipulative Biotherapy

Human gene therapy involves a biologic technique to insert a functioning gene into a patient's cells to reverse a defective gene or add functions to an existing cell. Gene therapy has been used investigationally to correct enzyme deficiencies or augment intrinsic antitumor immune responses. This technology is not yet able to remove dysfunctional genes or limit the overproduction of biologic substances (Moraca-Sawicki, 1998).

Toxicities of Biologic Response Therapy

The toxicities of biologic agents are related to doses and schedules. Administration of interferons on a daily basis is associated with systemic symptoms, fever, fatigue, and myalgia. The toxicities associated with IL-2 are dose dependent and involve significant cardiovascular complications, including hypotension and the development of capillary leak syndrome. Also, with IL-2, some patients develop an erythematous rash that may progress to **desquamation** (Moraca-Sawicki, 1998).

Key Nursing Interventions and Assessment

1. Assess emotional status.
2. Assess for flu-like symptoms.
3. Assess CBC, differential, platelets, electrolytes, and liver function before initiating therapy.
4. Assess for presence of infection.
5. Assess cardiac and pulmonary function.

COMMON SIDE EFFECTS OF CHEMOTHERAPY

Common side effects associated with chemotherapy include short-term complications, acute side effects, and toxicities (Table 13–5).

TABLE 13–5

COMMON SIDE EFFECTS OF CHEMOTHERAPY

- Short-Term Complications
  - Venous fragility
  - Alopecia
  - Diarrhea
  - Altered nutritional status
  - Anorexia or taste alteration
  - Fatigue
- Acute Side Effects
  - Hypersensitivity or anaphylaxis
  - Extravasation
  - Stomatitis and mucositis
  - Nausea and vomiting
  - Myelosuppression
  - Toxicities
    - Cardiac
    - Neurologic
    - Renal
- Pulmonary

INS STANDARDS Because of the high level of toxicity associated with the administration of antineoplastic agents, a physician or registered nurse who administers these agents and monitors the patients receiving these therapies must possess specialized knowledge and skills (INS, 2000, 70).

SHORT-TERM COMPLICATIONS

Venous Fragility

Fragile veins are present in elderly, poorly nourished, and debilitated patients. However, all patients receiving cytotoxic agents have an increased risk of vein fragility. If a patient has fragile veins, the nurse should attempt to cannulate the vein without the use of a tourniquet (Weinstein, 1997).

It is imperative that patients with fragile veins be assessed carefully before a cannula is placed for delivering chemotherapy. Such patients are at higher risk for developing irritation from antineoplastic agents. Patients receiving corticosteroid therapy have increased vascular fragility, and bleeding and bruising can occur around their I.V. sites. Patients receiving chemotherapy and radiation therapy may have thrombocytopenia and therefore depression of platelet production, which increases vascular fragility (Smith, 1995).

Alopecia

The hair follicles are a group of rapidly dividing normal cells that are affected by the nonspecific action of some chemotherapeutic drugs. Chemotherapy-induced hair loss (**alopecia**) is reported to occur by two mechanisms, depending on the drug and dosage received. Atrophy of the hair bulb occurs from drug insult, and the hair falls out spontaneously or in response to a mechanical action such as combing. If the insult is minimal, a marked constriction of the hair shaft occurs, and the hair breaks off (ONS, 1999).

The hair loss from chemotherapy, which often occurs 2 to 3 weeks after chemotherapy, is usually temporary, and hair growth returns in about 1 to 2 months after treatment is completed. The new hair may have a different texture or color than its pretreatment characteristics (Tipton & Skeel, 1999).

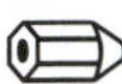 **NOTE:** Patient education should include information about the loss of body hair in addition to the loss of scalp hair.

Key Nursing Interventions for Alopecia

1. Provide information about hair loss.
2. Provide information about hair and scalp care.
3. Provide information about when to expect hair loss.
4. Provide information about obtaining a wig if the patient desires. Some sources recommend that patients purchase a wig after therapy because of weight loss and the possibility of poor fit if purchased before therapy.
5. Recommend keeping hair cut short because it is easier to manage.
6. Protect the scalp from sun and cold (ONS, 1999).

Diarrhea

Diarrhea and abdominal cramping most often result from antimetabolites. There are many possible causes of diarrhea, such as *Clostridium difficile* infection, other intestinal infections, malabsorption syndrome, cancer-related treatments of chemotherapy, and radiation and biologic therapy (Doyle, 1995). Diarrhea can lead to discomfort, severe electrolyte abnormalities, altered social life, and poor quality of life.

The treatment of patients with diarrhea is often symptomatic and usually requires no alteration in cancer therapy. Diarrhea can be a dose-limiting factor with 5-fluorouracil (5-FU). Agents that decrease bowel motility should not be used for longer than 24 hours unless significant infections have been excluded. Medications commonly used to treat patients with diarrhea are loperamide hydrochloride and diphenoxylate hydrochloride with atropine sulfate (Table 13–6).

TABLE 13-6

PHARMACOLOGIC MANAGEMENT OF PATIENTS WITH DIARRHEA

Agent	Recommendations
Loperamide (Imodium)	Two capsules (4 mg) orally every 4 hours initially; then add one capsule (2 mg) after each loose stool; do not exceed 16 capsules per day
Kaopectate	30 to 60 mL orally after each loose stool
Diphenoxylate and atropine (Lomotil)	1 to 2 tablets orally every 4 hours as needed; should not exceed 8 tablets per day
Paregoric	1 tsp orally 4 × per day
Octreotide	May be useful for 5-FU-induced diarrhea Dose is 0.05 to 0.1 mg subcutaneously 3 times per day

Key Nursing Interventions for Diarrhea

1. Educate patients on the importance of early intervention to avoid complications related to diarrhea.
2. Tell patients to increase intake of constipating foods such as cheese and eggs; use caution with dairy products; and eat food high in pectin, bulk, and fiber to help slow down peristalsis.
3. Educate patients to avoid spicy, fatty, and greasy foods. Other items to avoid ingesting include raw fruits and vegetables, nuts, caffeine, seeds, popcorn, and alcohol.
4. Establish a baseline history of usual elimination patterns.

Constipation

Managing the constipation of patients with cancer is not the same as that for medical surgical patients. Enemas should be used with caution in myelosuppressed patients because enemas can be irritating to the mucous membranes and cause microscopic tears that can result in additional complications. In patients with low platelet counts, bleeding can occur; in patients with neutropenia, infection can result.

There are many causes of constipation; along with specific chemotherapeutic agents, narcotics, dietary deficiencies, and tumor involvement can result in intrinsic or extrinsic compression. Interventions depend on the underlying cause.

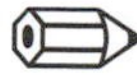

NOTE: Patients taking narcotics and those receiving vincristine or vinblastine require prophylactic stool softeners.

Key Nursing Interventions for Constipation

1. Unless contraindicated, the patient should drink 2 to 3 L of fluids per day.
2. Advise the patient to avoid foods known to be constipating (e.g., cheeses, eggs, refined starches, chocolate, candy).
3. Advise the patient to eat at the same times each day.
4. Encourage the patient to respond to the urge to defecate immediately and not wait.
5. Use stool softeners, laxatives, cathartics, and lubricants when appropriate; bulk laxatives keep the stool soft and have been found to be gentle (Tipton & Skeel, 1999).

Altered Nutritional Status

Malnutrition is reported to occur in 50 to 80 percent of patients with advanced disease. Nutritional management of patients with cancer involves early intervention using a supportive healthcare team. Patients with cancer often experience progressive loss of appetite and sometimes severe malnutrition. This side effect can be a result of therapy or a direct effect of the cancer. Malnutrition can result in a poorer response to therapy, an increased incidence of infections, and an overall worsening of the patient's well being (Tipton & Skeel, 1999).

Key Nursing Interventions for Altered Nutritional Status

1. Nutritional assessment: Diet history, nutritional intake, anthropometric measurements, laboratory tests for anemia and serum albumin.
2. Nutritional intervention: Diet, symptomatic treatment of nausea and vomiting, stomatitis and other GI effects of chemotherapy, and supplemental nutrition, which can include creative high-protein and calorie supplements, enteral nutrition, or total parenteral nutrition.
3. Pharmacologic interventions: Pharmacologic appetite stimulation promotes increased weight gain in some patients and decreased rate of weight loss in others. Currently being investigated to increase appetite are megestrol acetate 40 to 80 mg four times per day, cyproheptadine 8 mg three times per day, hydrazine sulfate, and pentoxifylline (Tipton & Skeel, 1999).

Anorexia and Alteration in Taste

Many treatments that patients receive result in taste alterations. Familiar foods may taste different when the gustatory sense is impaired. Patients receiving cisplatin, cyclophosphamide, or vincristine frequently complain that nothing tastes right. Some patients experience a bitter or metallic taste.

Key Nursing Interventions for Anorexia and Alterations in Taste

1. Serve foods on glass dishes.
2. Use plastic utensils rather than metal.
3. Use good oral hygiene before meals.
4. Arrange foods attractively on the plate.
5. Provide pleasant, relaxed environment for eating meals.
6. Use pleasant odors, such as cloves.
7. Avoid noxious odors.
8. Serve cold rather than hot foods.
9. Provide small, frequent meals.
10. Administer antiemetic agents before meals.
11. Add salt or sugar to foods to increase palatability (Doyle, 1995)

Fatigue

Approximately 78 percent of cancer patients suffer from debilitating fatigue caused by chemotherapy or radiation therapy. In a nationwide survey, 61 percent said that fatigue was the most debilitating side effect (*Nursing 97*).

Key Nursing Interventions for Fatigue

1. Encourage patient to eat small meals and snacks throughout the day.
2. Encourage patient to take short walks and exercise lightly.
3. Encourage patient to keep a diary of fatigue symptoms, including when they are least and most tolerable.
4. Have patient plan activities to coincide with times when energy level is highest.
5. Have patient take short naps or breaks between activities.
6. Some patients might benefit from antidepressants, antianxiety medications, or psychological counseling (*Nursing 97*).

ACUTE REACTIONS

Hypersensitivity and Anaphylaxis

Some chemotherapeutic agents have a potential for causing hypersensitivity with or without an anaphylactic response. Nurses should be knowledgeable about chemotherapy and which agents are prone to evoke hypersensitivity. An allergy history should be documented. The following are agents for which hypersensitivity reactions may occur:

- Mechlorethamine (topical)
- Mephalan (I.V.)
- Arthracycline antibiotics

- L-asparaginase
- Bleomycin
- Cisplatin
- Mechlorethamine (topical)
- Mephalan (I.V.)
- Paclitaxel
- Procarbazine
- Teniposide

If a drug is known to cause hypersensitivity reactions, a test dose should be administered. A patient also can be premedicated prophylactically with corticosteroids, histamine antagonists, or both to prevent reactions. Emergency equipment should be immediately accessible, including oxygen, AMBU respiratory assist bag, intubation equipment, and medications (e.g., epinephrine, 1:10,000 solution; diphenhydramine [Benadryl] 25 to 50 mg; methylprednisolone [Solu-Medrol], 30 to 60 mg; hydrocortisone [Solu-Cortef], 100 to 500 mg; dexamethasone, 10 to 20 mg; aminophylline; and dopamine) (Tipton & Skeel, 1999).

Extravasation

Extravasation of a vesicant agent is a major complication of an antineoplastic drug administration. As the vesicant escapes the vein, the patient may experience a burning sensation at the insertion site, redness, or swelling. In the days to weeks that follow, the site may become reddened, firm, and necrotic, leading to infection, prolonged illness, and functional as well as cosmetic problems (Tipton & Skeel, 1999). Irritant drugs cause inflammation or pain at the site of insertion.

Commonly used vesicant agents include:

- Plicamycin (Mithramycin, Mithracin)
- Mechlorethamine (nitrogen mustard)
- Dactinomycin (Actinomycin D)
- Daunorubicin (Daunomycin)
- Doxorubicin (Adriamycin)
- Idarubicin (Idamycin)
- Plicamycin (Mithramycin, Mithracin)
- Mitomycin (Mutamycin)
- Mechlorethamine (nitrogen mustard)
- Vinblastine (Velban)
- Vincristine (Oncovin)
- Vindesine (Eldisine)
- Vinorelbine (Navelbine)

Irritant agents include:

- Carmustine (BCNUO)
- Mitoxantrone (Novantrone)
- Carmustine (BCNUO)
- Dacarbazine (DTIC)

- Etoposide (VP-16)
- Mitoxantrone (Novantrone)
- Paclitaxel (Taxol)
- Teniposide (VM-26)

Large extravasations of concentrated solutions of cisplatin and 5-FU may be considered irritants (Tipton & Skeel, 1999; see Chapter 8).

INS STANDARDS Decreasing exravasation and associated complications requires technical expertise in cannula placement and immediate recognition of drug extravasation (INS, 2000, 70).

The management of patients with extravasated vesicants is controversial, with disagreements in the literature on antidotes. Table 13–7 provides the general procedure for patients with suspected extravasation.

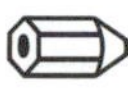

NOTE: The most effective management of extravasation is prevention.

A complaint of pain or burning should be considered a symptom of extravasation until proven otherwise. Extravasation kits with the necessary drug antidotes and supplies are helpful (Table 13–8).

INS STANDARDS Extravasation protocols for vesicants should be established in policies and procedures and administered when a vesicant infiltrates (INS, 2000, 61).

After extravasation of a vesicant agent occurs, the extremity should not be used for subsequent cannula placement, and alternative interventions should be explored (INS, 2000, 61).

TABLE 13–7

GENERAL PROCEDURE FOR EXTRAVASATION

1. Stop administration of chemotherapeutic agent.
2. Leave needle in place and immobilize the extremity.
3. Aspirate any residual drug left in the tubing, the needle, or the suspected extravasation site; infiltrate the antidote, if ordered.
4. Remove the needle.
5. Avoid applying pressure to the extravasation site.
6. Inject appropriate antidote drug for the specific chemotherapy drug that extravasated.
7. Photograph the suspected area.
8. Apply warm or cold compresses as indicated.
9. Elevate the arm.
10. Notify the physician.
11. Document the condition of site and treatment of extravasation thoroughly.

TABLE 13-8

RECOMMENDED EXTRAVASATION KIT CONTENTS

3-mL disposable syringe
5-mL disposable syringe
10-mL disposable syringe
1-mL disposable tuberculin syringe
Several disposable needles: 25-gauge; 5/8 inch (need separate one for each subcutaneous injection)
Luer-Lok caps
Alcohol wipes
Cold and warm packs
Sterile surgical latex gloves
Sterile water for injection in 10-mL vial
Hyaluronidase 150 U/vial
Sodium thiosulfate (25%) for 50-mL vial
Other antidotes per protocol

Source: Angel, 1995.

Stomatitis and Mucositis

The oral mucosa is vulnerable to the effects of chemotherapy. The likelihood of developing stomatitis from a drug depends on the agent, the dose, and the schedule of administration. Continuous rather than intermittent administration is more likely to cause stomatitis with antimetabolites (Tipton & Skeel, 1995).

Specific antineoplastic agents that may cause stomatitis include plant alkaloids (vincristine, vinblastine, etoposide), antimetabolites (methotrexate, 5-FU, cytarabine), antitumor antibiotics (doxorubicin, dactinomycin, mitoxantrone, mitomycin, bleomycin), miscellaneous agents (hydroxyurea), and biologic agents (interleukins, lymphokine-activated killer [LAK] cell therapy).

It is important to implement good oral hygiene before initiating chemotherapy. The primary goal is prevention; however, when oral complications develop, the focus of care should be treatment of symptoms and continued good oral care. Patients with poor dental hygiene are more likely to develop stomatitis. Predisposing factors for stomatitis include poor oral hygiene, poor nutritional status, head and neck radiation, concurrent corticosteroid therapy, and high doses of chemotherapy (Doyle, 1995).

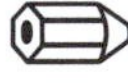

NOTE: Commercial mouthwashes and lemon glycerin swabs are not recommended for use because of their irritating and drying effects (Tipton & Skeel, 1999).

Key Nursing Interventions for Mouth Care

1. Examine mouth at least once daily and report changes.
2. Keep mouth clean and moist (Table 13–9).
3. Gently massage gums, tongue, and top of mouth.

TABLE 13–9

AGENTS FOR ORAL CARE

Oral Agents	Effects
Cleansing Agents	
Normal saline solution (½ tsp salt in 8 oz of water)	Economical, nondamaging
1.5% Hydrogen peroxide (one part to three parts) or flavored 1.5% hydrogen peroxide (Peroxamint)	Dilute tap water; germicidal debriding
Sodium bicarbonate	Nonirritating, neutralizing acid in mouth
Lubricating Agents	
Saliva substitutes	Decrease dryness, similar to human saliva
Water- or oil-based lubricants	Useful emollient; oil-based lubricants should not be used in mouth owing to danger of aspiration
Analgesic Agents	
Healing or Coating Agents	
Sucralfate	Binds to mucosa; forms protective coating
Vitamin E	Protection to mucosa has healing properties
Antacids	Enhance comfort; coat mucosa
Allopurinol	Decrease intensity of mucositis
Topical Anesthetics	
Lidocaine viscous	Transient pain relief; absorbed systematically
Diclonime	Transient pain relief; minimal systemic absorption
Benzocaine	Transient pain relief; minimal systemic absorption
Systemic Analgesics	
Narcotic analgesics	Take before meals and as needed

4. Do not floss when platelet count is low.
5. Keep dentures in only during meals.
6. Keep lips and inside of mouth coated with water-based mouth moisturizer.
7. If mouth is dry, drink water and other fluids frequently.
8. Chew sugarless gum or suck on sugarless hard candy.
9. Avoid irritating foods, alcohol and tobacco.
10. Use benzocaine or xylocaine before meals for anesthetic effects. Take pain medication 1.5 to 2 hours before meals.
11. Encourage a well-balanced diet (Groenwald & Goodman, 1997).

Nausea and Vomiting

Over the past 10 years, there have been many improvements in the prevention and control of nausea and vomiting in patients undergoing chemotherapy. Nausea and vomiting are major complications of chemotherapy administration. For many patients, nausea and vomiting are the most distressing symptoms that interfere with their quality of life. Studies have shown that approximately 70 percent of all cancer patients receiving chemotherapy experience nausea and vomiting. Uncontrolled nausea and vomiting can lead to severe fatigue and discomfort, fluid and electrolyte imbalances, nutritional problems, and gastroesophageal tears, and it may affect patient compliance with therapy.

Patients with a history of motion sickness or morning sickness are more prone to chemotherapy-induced nausea and vomiting. Previous exposure to chemotherapy may stimulate anticipatory nausea and vomiting, especially in younger women. Entering the outpatient waiting room or hearing the sound of an I.V. pole may result in the patient's experiencing nausea. Multiple assessment scales have been used to measure nausea. Because of the subjective element, measurement is not always clear cut (Doyle, 1995). The goal of therapy is to prevent the three phases of nausea and vomiting: (1) anticipatory (occurring before treatment), (2) acute (occurring the first 24 hours after treatment), and (3) delayed (occurring more than 24 hours after treatment).

Key Nursing Interventions for Nausea and Vomiting

1. Interventions such as ingesting hard candy and sour or tart foods such as lemons are helpful in controlling nausea.
2. Avoiding fatty foods and foods with strong odor can decrease nausea and vomiting.
3. Acupressure in the form of bracelets positioned on the wrist over the acupressure point that controls nausea is a noninvasive, nontoxic intervention and is helpful for the patient who is only slightly nauseated or who is reluctant to take antiemetics.
4. Pharmacologic interventions include administration of antiemetics such as anticholinergics, antihistamines, barbiturates, benzodiazepines, benzoquinolizines, butyrophenones, cannabinoids,

phenothiazines, corticosteroids, and substituted benzamides (Table 13–10).

Most of these antiemetics cause sedation or extrapyramidal symptoms. A new class of antiemetics that is selective for serotonin antagonist receptors, ondansetron (Zofran), given orally or I.V., has demonstrated its efficacy in alleviating nausea and vomiting without the undesirable side effects of extrapyramidal symptoms.

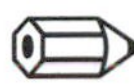

NOTE: Ondansetron (Zofran), I.V. or oral, is used frequently to control nausea.

Myelosuppression

Myelosuppression is the most common dose-limiting factor in the administration of antineoplastic therapy. All antineoplastic agents have some effect on blood counts, but certain drugs or dose escalations can result in severe myelosuppression. Doses of chemotherapeutic agents are escalated until myelosuppression is achieved. Patients at risk for prolonged myelosuppression include elderly patients with aplastic marrow, patients with bone marrow involvement, patients with previous radiation to the flat bones, patients heavily pretreated with chemotherapy, and patients with neoplastic infiltrates.

Neutropenia

Neutropenia (diminished number of neutrophils in the blood) predisposes patients to infection, and an absolute granulocyte count (**AGC**) of 1500 to 2000/μL puts patients at a moderate risk for infection. An AGC lower than 500/μL places the patient at a severe risk for infection. Such patients should be started on broad-spectrum antibiotics within 12 hours of a decrease in WBC count. **Leukopenia** is a drop in WBC count below 5000/μL. In patients with neutropenia, the only sign of infection may be an elevated temperature.

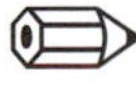

NOTE: Antipyretic agents should be used with caution in patients with leukopenia so as not to mask infection.

Although major medical advances have resulted in an improved survival rate, serious infections continue to place immunocompromised patients at risk. Infection, together with neutropenia, is regarded as an emergency situation. Precautions are usually initiated when the patient's AGC is lower than 1000/ μL.

The AGC can be calculated with the following formula.

$$\text{AGC} = \text{total WBC} \times (\text{\% of segs} + \text{\% of bands})$$

Key Nursing Interventions for Neutropenia

1. Place the patient in a private room with the door closed at all times.
2. Place "Neutropenic Precaution" sign on door.

TABLE 13–10

ANTIEMETICS COMMONLY USED FOR THE PREVENTION AND TREATMENT OF CHEMOTHERAPY-INDUCED NAUSEA AND VOMITING

Agent	Route	Dosage (Adult)	Comments
Phenothiazines			
Prochlorperazine (Compazine)	PO I.V. IM PR	PO/I.V. (slow): 10 mg q 4–6 h IM: 15–30 mg q 12 h PR: 2–10 mg q 8–12 h	Some extrapyramidal reactions; potential for severe postural hypotension when the agent is given I.V.; closely observe the patient and assist when he or she is getting out of bed or sitting up
Thiethylperazine (Torecan)	PO PR IM	PO/PR: 10 mg q 4–6 h IM: 2 mg q 4–6 h	Some extrapyramidal reactions
Trimethobenzamide (Tigan)	PO IM PR	PO: 250 mg q 4–6 h IM/PR: 200 mg q 4–6 h	Some extrapyramidal reactions
Butyrophenones			
Haloperidol (Haldol)	IM PO	IM/PO: 2–5 mg q 2–4 h	Some extrapyramidal reactions
Metoclopramide (Reglan)	PO I.V.	PO: 10–40 mg q 6 h I.V.: over 20 minutes 1–2 mg/kg at 2-hour intervals	Extrapyramidal reactions common, particularly at higher doses; worse in younger patients; diarrhea may occur

Benzodiazepine			
Lorazepam (Ativan)	PO I.V.	PO: 1–2 mg q 4–6 h I.V.: 2 mg 30 min before chemotherapy; may be repeated q 4 h prn	Sedation frequent; patients advised not to drive for 24 hours after taking
Corticosteroid			
Dexamethasone (Decadron)	PO I.V.	PO: 4–8 mg q 4 h I.V.: 4–20 mg q 4–6 h	Similar to ondansetron, for highly emetogenic therapy Potential agitation, delirium
Serotonin (5HT3) Antagonists			
Ondansetron (Zofran)	I.V. PO	I.V.: 8–32 mg × 1 or 0. 15 mg/kg q 4 h × 3 PO: 8 mg q 8 h	For highly emetogenic therapy; may be a mild headache and mild transient transaminase elevations; lower doses effective for less emetogenic regimens
Granisetron (Kytril)	I.V. PO	I.V.: 10 u/kg × 1 PO: 2 mg before or 1 mg q 12 h	Similar to ondansetron, for highly emetogenic therapy
Dolasetron (Anzemet)	I.V. PO	100 mg before chemotherapy, either PO or I.V.	Similar to ondansetron
Cannabinoid			
Dronabinol (Marinol)	PO	2.5–10.0 mg PO q 4–6 h	May be habit forming; is a controlled substance; causes sedation

3. Place the patient on a low microbial neutropenic diet (i.e., serve only cooked food; avoid unpaired fresh fruits, raw vegetables, and garnishes).
4. Upon entering and leaving the patient's room, all persons must consistently and thoroughly wash hands.
5. Prohibit patient contact by staff and visitors with transmissible illness.
6. Avoid contact with persons who have recently been vaccinated with live or attenuated virus vaccines.
7. Avoid exposure to stagnant water (e.g., denture cups, soap dishes, flower vases, water pitchers, respiratory equipment, and irrigation containers); stagnant water provides medium for *Pseudomonas aeruginosa*.
8. Prohibit fresh flowers, plants, or fresh fruit baskets (soil is source of *Staphylococcus marcescens*).
9. Assess patient's oral mucosa every 12 hours for stomatitis and his or her skin for infection breakdown, lesions, and rashes.
10. Prevent rectal trauma by avoiding the use of rectal temperatures, suppositories, and enemas.
11. Assess for changes in neurologic function every 4 hours; central nervous system (CNS) changes are often the first indicators of sepsis.
12. Avoid insertion of indwelling urinary catheters.
13. Assess the I.V. site at least once per shift for signs of phlebitis.
14. Monitor the patient's vital signs every 4 hours around the clock.
15. Use strict sterile technique when performing invasive procedures.

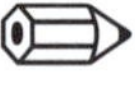

NOTE: Notify the physician immediately of any indicators of impending infection; sepsis progresses rapidly in immunocompromised patients.

Thrombocytopenia

A normal platelet count ranges from 150,000 to 450,000/µL. When the count is below 100,000/µL, there is a concern for the potential of bleeding. Values of 20,000 to 30,000/µL warrant closer watching. Presenting signs of a problem include bleeding gums, petechiae, nosebleeds, and multiple bruises. If the platelet count is lower than 20,000/µL, spontaneous frank bleeding can occur.

Thrombocytopenia places a patient at risk for CNS and GI bleeding. The use of platelet transfusions for nonbleeding patients is controversial. Some authorities recommend holding transfusions until the patient shows signs of bleeding, but others transfuse a patient when the platelet count is lower than 20,000/µL. Interventions include protecting the patient from unnecessary bleeding risks (Smith & Khan, 1999).

If thrombocytopenia is lower than 100,000/µL, consider:

- Bone marrow failure
- Increased consumption of platelets
- Splenic pooling of platelets (Smith & Khan, 1999)

Key Nursing Interventions for Thrombocytopenia

1. Encourage shaving with an electric razor.
2. Advise the patient to avoid using tampons.
3. Advise the patient to avoid hazardous activity that may cause injury (e.g., contact sports and working with sharp instruments).
4. Avoid invasive procedures such as enemas and taking rectal temperatures.
5. Avoid using aspirin-containing products and products with ibuprofen and indomethacin.

Anemia

A patient is considered anemic if his or her hemoglobin level is lower than 8 g/dL. Anemic patients may be asymptomatic or may present with headache, dizziness, lightheadedness, shortness of breath, fatigue, pallor, hypothermia, and pale nailbeds and conjunctiva.

When fatigue is a factor, patients should be instructed to plan rest periods around activities. Weekly CBCs are needed to adjust the dosage of a chemotherapeutic agent, depending on the nadir. The **nadir count** is usually the point at which the blood counts are the lowest; this is usually 7 to 14 days after the first day of chemotherapy (but is drug-specific). Refer to individual drug literature for specific information on the nadirs of chemotherapeutic drugs (Phillips & Kuhn, 1999).

It is important to obtain blood counts just before administering chemotherapy because of bone marrow depression. That is, chemotherapy affects the stem cells in the bone marrow, which are rapidly dividing, rather than the cells in the circulation, which have reached maturity. Most protocols require the WBC count to be at least 3000/µL with an AGC of 1500/µL (Doyle, 1995).

TOXICITIES

Neurotoxicity

Neurotoxicity can be an acute or chronic encephalopathy of the CNS or a peripheral degeneration. **Peripheral neuropathy** can cause considerable sensory and motor disability. The most common agents that cause neurotoxicity are paclitaxel (Taxol), cisplatin, carboplatin, and vinca alkaloids.

Patients usually complain of numbness and tingling of the hands and feet as beginning symptoms. As toxicity increases, patients complain of muscle pain, weakness, and disturbances in depth perception. Other symptoms are decreased sensation, constipation, and paralytic ileus. The symptoms, depending on severity, usually disappear in a few weeks (Tipton & Skeel, 1999).

Because of the decreased sensation, a patient with neurotoxicity in his or her family must be aware of safety issues. The decrease in sensation causes concern for caution with temperature changes (e.g., hot water, heating pads, electric blankets, hot stoves, and radiators). Exposure to cold is also a concern because these patients are less likely to realize the severity of the temperature.

Cardiac Toxicity (Congestive Cardiomyopathy)

The anthracyclines, especially doxorubicin or daunorubicin, can cause cardiotoxicity. The lifetime dose of anthracyclines is 550 mg/m^2. Certain other chemotherapeutic agents, such as paclitaxel, mitoxantrone, idarubicin, cyclophosphamide, 5-FU, and 5-FU deoxyribonucleoside (FUDR), have also shown potential for cardiac toxicity. Early signs of cardiotoxicity include decrease in voltage of QRS complex and nonspecific ST- or T-wave change. The heart muscle becomes weakened, resulting in a decreased cardiac output with progression to congestive heart failure. These symptoms are difficult to diagnose. Frequent ECG monitoring to detect changes in the voltage of the QRS helps to identify early signs of toxicity. A baseline MUGA scan or an echocardiogram with an ejection fraction before administration of the known cardiotoxic chemotherapeutic agent and then repeat these tests at the halfway point of the total accumulated lifetime dose of drug assists in monitoring for cardiac toxicities.

Risk factors for cardiac damage are hypertension, arteriosclerosis, coronary artery disease, and previous radiation to mediastinum.

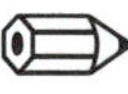

NOTE: Because of the large number of women with breast cancer who are treated with doxorubicin as part of an adjuvant chemotherapy regimen, this group is of special concern and warrants ongoing clinical follow-up (Skeel & Ganz, 1999).

Dexrazoxane (Zinecard) for injection is being used as a cardioprotective agent after administration of cumulative doses of doxorubicin. Because this drug is always given with cytotoxic drugs, patients should be monitored closely. Dextrazoxane may add to the myelosuppression caused by chemotherapeutic agents and should not be used with chemotherapy regimens that do not contain an anthracycline (Pharmacia, 1995).

Pulmonary Toxicity

Toxicity to the pulmonary tissue damages the endothelial cells of the lung and results in pneumonitis and interstitial fibrosis. The agents that predispose patients to pulmonary toxicity are bleomycin in doses exceeding 250 U/m^2 or 400 U total dose and carmustine in total doses of 1500 mg/m^2. Other antineoplastic agents known to be responsible for pulmonary toxicity are mitomycin, methotrexate, melphalan, procarbazine, and busulfan. Some combination therapies can increase the risk of pulmonary toxicity.

Symptoms of pulmonary toxicity include dry, hacking cough; complaints of dyspnea; and crackles in the lungs upon auscultation. Patients at risk for this complication include those who smoke and those with previous pulmonary conditions. The evaluation of high-risk patients involves a pulmonary function test. The chemotherapeutic drug should be discontinued at the first sign of this complication. Corticosteroids have been used in the treatment of symptomatic relief of pulmonary toxicity (Skeel & Ganz, 1999).

Renal Toxicity

Renal toxicity is an elevation of the BUN and creatinine levels. Agents that cause renal damage are cisplatin, methotrexate, mitomycin, and carboplatin.

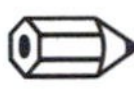

NOTE: Renal toxicity is a life-threatening complication. The risk of renal compromise versus renal toxic agents that could produce a meaningful tumor response must be weighed carefully. Vigorous hydration is required before administering agents that are nephrotoxic.

Hypertonic sodium chloride solution helps to maintain a high renal flow. Mannitol and furosemide (Lasix) may be ordered in an effort to flush the kidneys. Accurate intake and output as well as frequent weights must be recorded.

The risk of **hyperuricemia** from tumor lysis syndrome is another factor that needs to be considered when administering nephrotoxic drugs. Alkalizing the urine prevents the precipitation of uric acid crystals, and the administration of allopurinol helps to prevent their formation. Prophylactic measures begin 12 to 24 hours before chemotherapy.

CHEMOTHERAPY: ROUTES OF ADMINISTRATION

Chemotherapy is administered by a variety of routes. The route chosen is an important variable in optimal drug delivery within the body, in minimizing side effects, and in maintaining the person's level of functioning. The oral route is used for drugs that are well absorbed and nonirritating to the GI tract (Table 13–11).

SYSTEMIC ROUTES

Intravenous Route

The I.V. route is the most common route of chemotherapy administration, and it has two advantages. First, the I.V. route quickly achieves a therapeutic blood level. Second, most chemotherapeutic agents are not absorbed in the GI tract, making the I.V. route more desirable. The subcutaneous and intramuscular routes, used commonly for delivery of other drugs, have limitations with anticancer drug therapy because of the chemotherapeutic drug's irritation of the tissues. Other methods are used that eliminate or reduce tissue irritation.

TABLE 13-11

METHODS OF DELIVERING ANTINEOPLASTIC AGENTS

Systemic Routes
- I.V.
- Indwelling silastic catheters
- Peripherally inserted central lines
- Implanted ports
- Intrathecal

Regional Routes
- Intra-arterial
- Intraperitoneal
- Cerebrospinal reservoirs

Intrathecal Route

Other routes are used when the delivery of a drug is required to pass the BBB. The intrathecal route allows the drugs to be given directly into the cerebrospinal fluid (CSF). Methotrexate and cytosine arabinoside are most commonly given by this route in treating patients with CNS leukemia and carcinomatosis meningitis (see Chapter 10).

REGIONAL ROUTES

Systemic delivery of chemotherapy is most commonly done by the I.V. route; some tumors respond better to local exposure to antineoplastics. An advantage to regional delivery of chemotherapy is that they can "bathe" the affected body cavity or organ without systemically imposing toxic effects.

Intra-arterial Route

Chemotherapy administered through the intra-arterial route allows for high concentrations of antineoplastic agents to be delivered directly into tumor sites by means of arterial catheters or devices. A temporary catheter is placed via percutaneous angiography for carotid, brachial, femoral, or specific limb artery for short-term therapies (from hours to 5 days). This therapy is repeated by means of a new catheter insertion each time for 3 to 6 months of therapy.

An implantable arterial port is placed subcutaneously near the tumor site over a bony surface and sutured in place; the catheter is then threaded into the tumor artery site. The Infusaid Pump (Infusaid Corporation, Norwood, MA) is the most common totally implantable drug-delivery system. The port is accessed via a noncoring needle, covered with a transparent dressing, and connected to a heparinized saline solution via an infusion pump.

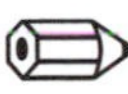 **NOTE:** Implantable arterial ports must be flushed with heparin weekly to maintain catheter patency if a continuous infusion solution is not being administered.

Key Points in Nursing Care of Intra-arterial Infusions

1. Intra-arterial drug infusion requires astute clinical observations and interventions.
2. Percutaneous arterial catheters have the potential for restricting tissue perfusion.
3. The insertion site and the affected extremity should be observed every 2 to 4 hours.
4. Monitor vital signs.
5. Femoral catheter placement requires bedrest with log rolling to maintain catheter alignment.
6. Brachial catheter placement requires immobilizing the affected extremity.
7. All chemotherapy supplies should have Luer lock connections, and infusion pumps may require a higher psi (pounds per square inch) setting to overcome arterial flow resistance (ONS, 1999).

Intraperitoneal Route

Intracavitary drug administration instills drugs directly into body cavities, such as the bladder, peritoneum, pleura, and pericardium. This technique is used most frequently to control malignant effusions, but it is also used for those with localized malignancies (ONS, 1999). Infusions via the **intraperitoneal** route (IP) involve the administration of therapeutic agents directly into the peritoneal cavity (Fig. 13–2).

The purpose of IP therapy is to increase the concentration of the antineoplastic agent at the tumor site (in this case, the peritoneal cavity) to enhance its penetration and cell kill while limiting systemic effects. The peritoneal cavity acts as a reservoir for the drug. The goal is to decrease systemic toxic effects and increase the antitumor action of the antineoplastic agent. Chemotherapeutic agents that are delivered via the IP route include cisplatin, carboplatin, cytosine arabinoside, mitoxantrone, calcium folinate, doxorubicin, and 5-FU.

Key Points in Nursing Care of Intraperitoneal Infusions

1. Follow the procedure for intraperitoneal therapy (Procedure 13–1).
2. Assess for complications associated with IP therapy:
   - A. Pain
   - B. Subcutaneous leakage
   - C. Hematoma or bleeding (rare)
   - D. Local infection
   - E. Catheter dislodgement
   - F. Obstruction
   - G. Rotation
   - H. Colon perforation (Topuz & Aydiner, 1997).

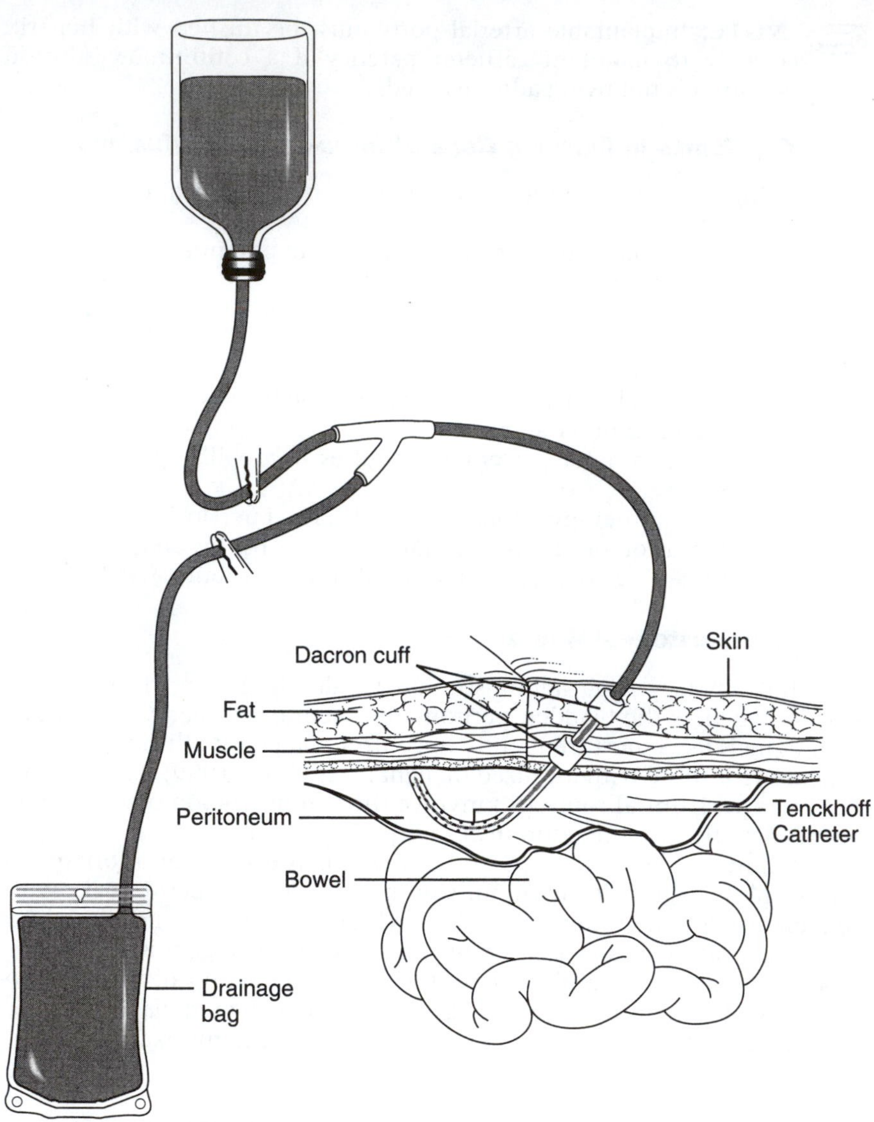

FIG. 13–2. Intraperitoneal infusion via a Tenckhoff catheter directly into the peritoneal cavity.

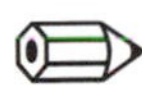

NOTE: For IP administration to be effective, the patient must have limited intra-abdominal adhesions.

3. The disease must be limited to the body region in which the antineoplastic agent is administered.
4. Nursing staff must be well prepared to care for an IP catheter.
5. The nurse and family must be familiar with the therapeutic effects of antineoplastic agents.
6. Advantages include:
   A. When not in use, the IP device is invisible, enhancing a positive body image.
   B. There is no catheter site care.
   C. Cytotoxic drugs are administered directly to the tumor area.
7. Disadvantages include:
   A. It can be difficult to locate and access the port.
   B. Catheter infections can occur.
   C. Build-up of fibrin sheath can occur on the distal catheter tip
   D. Abdominal adhesions can cause spaces in the cavity, preventing the flow of the infusion.

PROCEDURE 13–1: INTRAPERITONEAL THERAPY

Equipment Needed:

- Sterile gloves, mask, and gown
- Gauze pads
- Transparent semipermeable membrane (TSM) dressing
- Warmed infusate
- Povidone-iodine
- Drainage bag
- Y-type dialysis administration set
- Large-gauge noncoring needle (if using a port)

Instructions to Patients:

Inform patient that a peritoneal dialysis catheter or port is placed to provide access to the peritoneal cavity for instillation of medication. Explain to patient the need to measure abdominal girth and obtain weight before procedure.

Procedure:
Pretreatment and Site Care

1. Maintain strict sterile technique; wash hands with antimicrobial solution before handling system.
2. Verify the drug order and normal serum electrolyte levels.
3. Ensure that I.V. therapy is proceeding as ordered.
4. Assess the area around the catheter or port for redness, edema, warmth, or tenderness.
5. Organize materials and don gloves (and gown if desired).

(continued)

(continued)

6. Anesthetize the skin surface before access with 2 percent xylocaine, Emla Cream, or ice.
7. Access implanted port using aseptic technique with a large-gauge, noncoring, 90-degree needle of appropriate length (usually 1 to 15 in).
8. Flush the catheter with 10 to 20 mL of nonbacteriostatic sterile saline; catheter should flush easily.
9. Administer antiemetics if ordered.

Drug Administration

10. Initiate chemotherapeutic agent.
11. Position patient comfortably in a semi-Fowler's position
12. Open the clamp on the tubing and infuse the warmed IP chemotherapy at the prescribed rate (usually over 30 min to several hours).
13. Stop infusion immediately if severe pain is experienced and check for catheter migration.
14. Slow the rate of infusion if the patient experiences shortness of breath or discomfort.
15. Administer analgesics as prescribed.
16. Apply blankets if patient feels chilly.
17. Close the clamp on the tubing when the infusion is complete and encourage repositioning from side to side every 15 minutes during the indwelling time (usually 2 to 4 hours).
18. Monitor the patient's comfort levels.
19. After the prescribed indwelling time, open the clamp to the drainage bag and allow the solution to drain.
20. Recognize that the volume of drained fluid may be less than that infused and reassure the patient that the fluid will be reabsorbed and metabolized.
21. Clamp tubing on the drainage bag after the fluid has drained (usually 30 min to 2 hours) and send specimen, properly labeled as cytotoxic, to cytology or dispose of in proper hazardous waste container.

Postadministration Care

22. Flush the catheter or port with nonbacteriostatic sterile saline; if using a port, follow with heparinized saline.
23. Secure the site using the standard technique (e.g., cap and secure the catheter or remove the needle from the port and cover the site with a small dressing, if necessary).
24. Establish I.V. fluids as prescribed or discontinue I.V. needle.
25. Assess the patient's status; ensure his or her ability to perform self-care, if appropriate.

Documentation

26. Document in the medical record (Groenwald & Goodman, 1997).

Cerebrospinal Fluid Reservoirs

Intraventricular chemotherapy allows for the administration of antineoplastic agents into the CSF via an Ommaya reservoir (Baxter, Illinois) (Fig. 13–3) A physician must place the ventricular reservoir. The

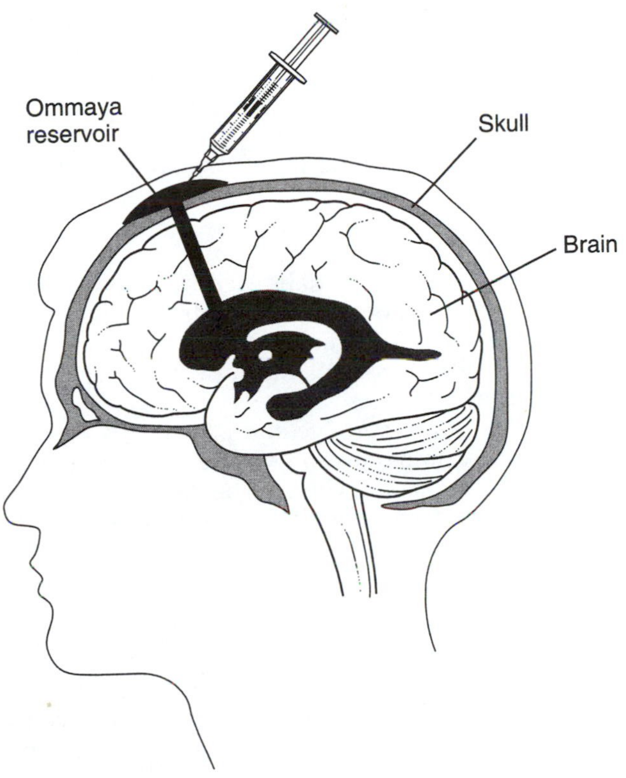

FIG. 13–3. The Ommaya reservoir. Intraventricular chemotherapy administration (Source: Otto, S.E. [1995]. Advanced concepts in chemotherapy drug delivery regional therapy. *Journal of Intravenous Nursing, 18(4),* 170–176, with permission.)

nurse administering medications into the reservoir must follow the Nurse Practice Act for the state in which he or she practices. An Ommaya reservoir is a silicone rubber device that is implanted surgically under the scalp and provides access to CSF through a burr hole in the skull. Drugs are injected into the reservoir with a hypodermic syringe, and then the domed reservoir is depressed manually to mix drug with the CSF.

Key Points in Nursing Care of the Delivery of Chemotherapy via a Ventricular Reservoir

1. The patient should be taught the purpose of the reservoir.
2. When accessing the ventricular reservoir, wear sterile gloves and a mask.
3. Use only preservative-free medications.
4. Aspirate to check placement before drug delivery; CSF should be present.

5. Withdrawal of CSF for diagnostic purpose is a medical act.
6. Advantages include:
   A. Well tolerated
   B. Eliminates need for multiple lumbar punctures
7. Disadvantages include:
   A. Increased risk of infection to the spinal cord and brain

Infusion Pumps

Infusion pumps have been widely used in chemotherapy administration to provide continuous or intermittent drug delivery. These pumps are essential in intra-arterial administration, in which the drug must be given against arterial pressure, but they are used in delivery of antineoplastic agents by all routes.

Pumps are available as nonportable and portable. Nonportable pumps are usually designed to clamp onto an I.V. pole and are quite bulky; these are used in hospital or outpatient clinics. The compact, battery-operated, portable pumps have enabled individuals to receive continuous chemotherapy on an outpatient or home care basis.

AGE-RELATED CONSIDERATIONS: PEDIATRIC ONCOLOGY

Cancer is the primary cause of death from disease in children who are between 1 and 14 years old (Parker, 1996). Pediatric oncology as a nursing specialty has grown rapidly during the past 20 years.

The Children's Cancer Group (CCG) was founded in 1955. It is a cooperative research group that has developed criteria, policies, and procedures to ensure that cooperative clinical trails are conducted uniformly at all participating institutions and to permit the pooling of data from all patients.

The diagnosis of pediatric cancer involves many members of the healthcare team. New techniques to diagnose and stage cancers have facilitated the development of sophisticated plans of treatment. This technique has produced improved patient survival rates, as well as cures for many pediatric malignancies.

The selection of antineoplastic agents used in treating a child with cancer is made primarily on the basis of the histology of the tumor and the extent of the disease. The dose and schedule of the drug administered are critical in achieving maximum benefit (Bertolone, 1997).

WEB SITES:

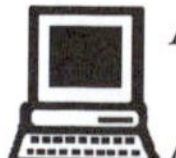

American Society of Pediatric Hematology/Oncology: *www.aspho.org*
Association of Pediatric Oncology Nurses: *www.apon.org*
Others: ______________________________

NURSING PLAN OF CARE

ANTINEOPLASTIC THERAPY

Focus Assessment

Subjective

- Interview the patient regarding his or her previous experience with chemotherapy.
- Determine the patient's level of knowledge regarding chemotherapy and cancer.

Objective

- Assess the patient for nausea and vomiting.
- Inspect the patient's oral cavity daily.
- Assess the patient's breath sounds.
- Monitor the patient's vital signs.
- Note the patient's type of cancer, length of illness, prognosis, and previous chemotherapy.
- Assess the patient's nutritional status.
- Review the patient's laboratory data.
- Assess the patient's urinary output and hydration level.

Patient Outcome Criteria

The patient will:

- Demonstrate stable weight or progressive weight gain toward a goal and be free of signs of malnutrition.
- Demonstrate normalization of laboratory values.
- Demonstrate that antinausea medications are effective.
- Comply with dietary restrictions.
- Display adequate fluid balance.
- Display moist mucous membranes.
- Demonstrate techniques to maintain and restore integrity of oral mucosa.
- Identify interventions for specific condition; prevent complications and promote healing as appropriate.
- Demonstrate adequate oxygenation of tissues by arterial blood gas values within patient's normal range.
- Be free of respiratory distress.
- Display appropriate range of feelings.
- Verbalize accurate information about diagnosis and treatment regimen.
- Initiate necessary lifestyle changes and participate in treatment regimen.

Nursing Diagnoses

- Altered nutrition less than body requirements, related to consequences of treatment

(continued)

(continued)

- Risk for noncompliance with dietary restrictions of chemotherapy related to no alcohol while taking methotrexate; no foods high in tyramines while taking procarbazine
- Risk for fluid volume deficit, related to excessive losses through vomiting, diarrhea, wounds, or impaired oral intake
- Oral mucous membrane altered, related to side effects of chemotherapeutic agents (antimetabolites)
- Risk for skin and tissue integrity impaired, related to effects of chemotherapy, immunologic deficit, altered nutritional state or anemia, presence of lesions, or drug extravasation
- Risk for gas exchange, impaired, related to alveolar membrane thickening (pulmonary fibrosis), altered blood flow, or decreased circulation or altered oxygen carrying capacity
- Fear and anxiety related to situational crisis, threat to or change in health and socioeconomic status, role functioning, interaction patterns, threat of death, separation from family
- Knowledge deficit related to lack of exposure or recall, information misinterpretation, myths, unfamiliarity with resources

Nursing Management

1. Monitor for side effects and toxic effects of chemotherapeutic agent.
2. Institute neutropenic and bleeding precautions when necessary.
3. Offer bland, easily digested diet.
4. Administer antiemetic medication.
5. Administer chemotherapeutic drugs in the late evening so the patient may sleep at the time emetic effects are greatest.
6. Monitor for adequate fluid intake, dehydration, and electrolyte imbalance.
7. Monitor for effectiveness of measures to control nausea and vomiting; assist patient in obtaining a wig or other head covering device as appropriate.
8. Offer six small feedings daily.
9. Ascertain that the I.V. is infusing well; dilute antineoplastic agents.
10. Administer appropriate antidotes per protocol and physician's orders if extravasation occurs.
11. Avoid using commercial mouthwash products that contain alcohol or phenol and may increase mucous membrane discomfort; use mouthwash made from warm saline and dilute solution of hydrogen peroxide or baking soda and water.
12. Administer analgesics and topical xylocaine jelly, antimicrobial mouthwash, or both (e.g., nystatin) as needed for stomatitis.
13. Monitor nutritional status and weight.
14. Minimize stimuli from noises, light, and odors, especially food.
15. Follow recommended guidelines for safe handling of parenteral antineoplastic drugs during drug preparation.

PATIENT EDUCATION

- Inform the patient and his or her family about how antineoplastic agents work on cancer cells.
- Instruct the patient and his or her family about the effects of chemotherapy on bone marrow functioning.
- Instruct patient and his or her family on ways to prevent infection (e.g., avoiding crowds and using good hygiene and handwashing techniques).
- Instruct the patient on the pretreatment hydration instruction sheet when appropriate.
- Instruct the patient to promptly report fever, chills, nosebleed, excessive bruising, tarry stools, severe headaches, or prolonged vomiting.
- Inform the patient to avoid aspirin products.
- Instruct the patient and his or her family to monitor for signs and symptoms of stomatitis and to perform good oral hygiene.
- Inform the patient to avoid temperature extremes while receiving chemotherapy.
- Inform the patient that hair loss is expected as determined by the type of chemotherapeutic agent.
- Instruct the patient to avoid hot, spicy foods.
- Instruct the patient and his or her family to monitor for organ toxicity as determined by the type of chemotherapeutic agent used.
- Discuss with the patient the possibility of sterility and other reproductive system impairments.
- Inform long-term survivors and their families of the possibility of second malignancies and the importance of reporting increased susceptibility to infection, fatigue, or bleeding.
- Instruct the patient to avoid scratching his or her skin.

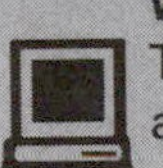

WEB SITES: Oncolink: *www.cancer.med.upenn.edu*
This site gives extensive information for patients, caregivers, and clinician. Cancer news, disease-oriented menu, causes and prevention, clinical trails, conferences, and psychosocial support form the University of Pennsylvania Cancer Center.

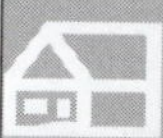

HOME CARE ISSUES

The most common antineoplastic agents given by the I.V. route for chemotherapy prescribed in the home are 5-FU and FUDR. Many other agents can be administered safely in the home care setting with the appropriate level of specialized clinical oncology support.

Common issues of concern in delivery of chemotherapy in the home are as follows:

PATIENT AND FAMILY EDUCATION

- Family members must understand the nature of the risk of handling cytotoxic drugs.
- It is the professional healthcare team's responsibility on behalf of the agency to provide education regarding safe practices in handling these drugs.
- Potential risks to persons who come in contact with chemotherapy drugs and associated safety measures should be discussed with patients and their families before the initial home chemotherapy treatment.
- The Joint Commission for the Accreditation of Healthcare Organizations (JCAHO) 1995 has guidelines for home care, which address the use of hazardous substances in the home setting.

ADMIXTURE

- Antineoplastic agents must be prepared in a biologic safety hood for protection during admixture; this task must be accomplished in a pharmacy.

TRANSPORT OF DRUG

- In the home care situation, the family or nurse often obtains antineoplastic agents. The drugs are labeled as cytotoxic, capped securely, and sealed and packaged in an impervious packing material for transport. The outside of the bags or bottles containing the prepared drug should be wiped with moist gauze. Entry ports should be wiped with moist alcohol pads and capped (OSHA, 1995).
- Transport should occur in sealed plastic bags and in containers designed to avoid breakage. The patient's family should be cautioned to protect the package from breakage and taught the necessary procedures if a spill occurs. Spill kits should be available in the home care setting.

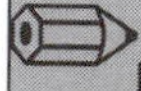

NOTE: Personnel involved in transporting hazardous drugs should be trained in spill procedures, including sealing off the contaminated area and calling for appropriate assistance (OSHA, 1995).

ADMINISTRATION

- The family member who will administer the drug must be taught safe handling of chemotherapeutic agents, use of latex gloves, and how to handle the tubing or infusion pump during delivery of drug.
- The area of the patient's home designated for preparation of drug should be apart from the family activity area and food preparation.
- Ceiling fans, if present, should be turned off.
- The work surface area should be one that can be cleaned, such as a card table.
- All family members should remain outside the rooms in which the drugs are prepared and administered, if possible. Children should be cared for outside the home on the day of chemotherapy.
- All supplies should be assembled on a disposable, absorbent, plastic-backed pad that is taped over the work surface area. Only syringes, needles, and I.V. sets with Luer lock fittings are used.
- Administering aerosolized hazardous drugs requires special engineering controls to prevent exposure to healthcare workers and others (OSHA, 1995).

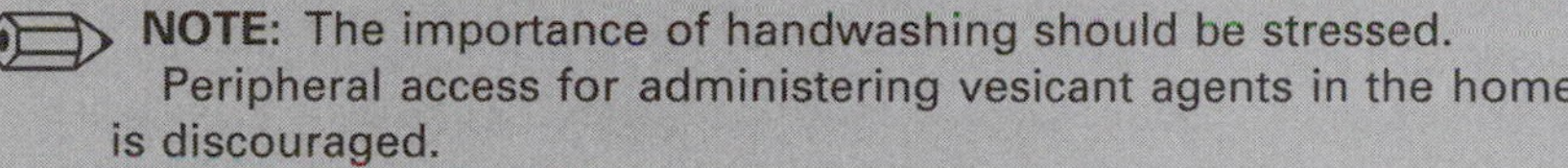

NOTE: The importance of handwashing should be stressed.
Peripheral access for administering vesicant agents in the home is discouraged.

DISPOSAL

- Needles, syringes, and breakable items not contaminated with blood or other infectious materials should be placed in a sharps container before being stored in the waste bag. Hazardous drug-related wastes should be handled separately from the trash and disposed of in accordance with the applicable Environmental Protection Agency (EPA) state and local regulations.

MONITORING

- Clinical monitoring of a patient receiving chemotherapy at home demands close attention. Clinical monitoring should include laboratory values, physical status, fluid status, and drug-related side effects and toxicities (Grace & Tomaselli, 1995).

DISPOSAL OF EXCRETA

- Cytotoxic activity of drugs and their metabolites can remain active in excreta for 48 hours or more. This special situation means that urine, feces, vomitus, and other excreta should be treated with caution, and the patient's family should wear gloves when handling excreta, linens, or tissues.
- It is suggested that the dilution in most sewer systems is adequate to decrease the risk to both the patient's family and the environment.
- Sheets and other laundry soiled with excreta should be washed twice and kept separate from other family laundry.

KEY POINTS

- The role of nurses in administering chemotherapy includes patient assessment and history, patient education, and knowledge of treatment objectives.
- The cell cycle includes the nonproliferative resting phase (G0), the presynthetic stage (G1), the interval after synthesis of DNA (G2), synthesis of DNA (S), and mitosis (M).
- Classifications of antineoplastic agents are either CCPS or CCPN.
- Key nursing interventions and assessments with alkylating drugs include monitoring the site for infiltration, CBC, platelets, and liver enzymes; administering antiemetics; assessing respiratory status and blood pressure; and prehydrating and assessing the oral cavity.
- Key nursing interventions and assessments with antimetabolite agents include assessing oral mucosa for stomatitis; and monitoring the CBC, platelets, liver enzymes, and renal function. The drug infusion should be stopped if the WBC count drops below 3000/µ/L.
- Key nursing interventions and assessments with anthracycline antibiotics include monitoring for possible hypersensitivity reactions; assessing the oral mucosa; assessing the infusion site frequently for infiltration (avoid extravasation); monitoring CBC count, platelets, cardiac enzymes, and ECGs; monitoring renal function; premedicating with dexamethasone, diphenhydramine, or cimetidine before the infusion of paclitaxel; and administering antiemetic agents.
- Key nursing interventions and assessments with hormones and hormone antagonist include assessing for mood swings and changes in psychological state; monitoring electrolytes when appropriate; monitoring blood pressure; assessing for signs of feminization with estrogens in males; assessing females for masculinizing effects with androgens; assessing for signs of phlebitis; encouraging low-salt diets; and monitoring weight.
- Key nursing interventions and assessments with biologic response modifiers include assessing emotional status; assessing for flulike symptoms; assessing CBC count, differential, platelets, electrolytes, and liver function before initiating therapy; assessing for presence of infection; and assessing cardiac and pulmonary function.
- Common side effects of chemotherapy include:
  1. Short-term complications such as venous fragility, alopecia, diarrhea, constipation, altered nutritional status, anorexia or taste alteration, and fatigue
  2. Acute side effects such as hypersensitivity or anaphylaxis, extravasation, stomatitis and mucositis, nausea and vomiting, and myelosuppression
  3. Toxic side effects involving the cardiac, neurologic, renal, and pulmonary systems
- Neutropenia predisposes patients to infection, and AGC of 1500 to 2000/µL puts patients at moderate risk for infection. An AGC lower than 500/µL places patients at severe risk for infection.
- With a platelet count below 50,000 /µL, there is a potential for bleeding. Thrombocytopenia places patients at risk for CNS and GI bleeding.
- Use meticulous sterile technique in accessing vascular devices.
- Assess vein patency with 10 to 20 mL of sodium chloride before infusing cytotoxic agents.

CHAPTER ACTIVITIES

COMPETENCY CRITERIA: Administration of Antineoplastic Therapy
COMPETENCY STATEMENT: Competent I.V. nurses will be able to administer I.V. chemotherapy and follow guidelines for dealing with cytotoxic drug.
Note: The cognitive (knowledge) information that is embedded within this performance-based competency includes cellular physiology and kinetics; classifications of antineoplastic agents, side effects and administration guidelines; and knowledge of routes of administration.

The competency *links* to the competency of infection control and central venous access management.

Performance	Skilled	Needs Education
Critical Action Statements		
1. Performs preinfusion assessment A. Assesses previous response to drug therapy B. Reviews laboratory data (CBC count, AGC, platelet) C. Interviews for patient history D. Performs physical assessment E. Calculates body surface area or dose based on height and weight		
2. Performs patient education before infusion		
3. Identifies correct dose, administration route, and rationale for administration A. Verifies I.V. access patency B. Checks medication dose with another nurse		
4. Verifies physician order		
5. Administers antineoplastic therapy following set protocol A. Gathers supplies need for drug administration B. Washes hands, dons gown and gloves, and sets up work area C. Checks patency by instilling 10 to 20 mL of sodium chloride D. Administers drug at prescribe rate E. Uses Luer-Lok connectors		

(continued)

(continued)

Performance	Skilled	Needs Education
Critical Action Statements		
5. *(continued)* F. Flushes tubing on completion of one drug before administering another drug G. Identifies the frequency of I.V. patency checks		
6. Monitors infusion for complications A. Infiltration and extravasation B. Infusion rate		
7. Discontinues antineoplastic therapy following set protocol A. Explains procedure, washes hands, gathers equipment B. Removes I.V. administration set and access needle for access device following agency policy C. Disposes of equipment using biohazard containers		
8. Documents performance of procedure and patient response		

EVALUATION CRITERIA

1. Return demonstration of administration techniques.
2. Demonstration of management of extravasation protocols.
3. Clinical preceptorship with clinical skills demonstrated with supervision.

CRITICAL THINKING ACTIVITY

1. In your facility, locate the protocol for extravasation. Is there a specific extravasation kit available on your unit?

2. How does your facility deal with neutropenic patients?

3. What criteria are used at your facility for competency in delivery of antineoplastic therapy?

4. How is new information distributed in your facility on the latest cancer pharmacological interventions?

POST-TEST

1. The goal of cancer immunotherapy is to:
   a. Produce remission
   b. Promote tumor-nonspecific immunity
   c. Stimulate immunocompetence in cancer patients
   d. Decrease the side effects of traditional chemotherapy
2. A side effect of anthracyclines is:
   a. Photosensitivity
   b. Cardiotoxicity
   c. Psychosis
   d. Neurotoxicity
3. A patient who is considered neutropenic and at risk for infection has an absolute granulocyte count (ABC) below:
   a. 10,000/µL
   b. 4000/µL
   c. 2000/µL
   d. 1000/µL
4. Pulmonary toxicity is associated with which of the following antineoplastic therapies?
   a. Bleomycin
   b. Paclitaxel
   c. Cisplatin
   d. Carboplatin
5. IP antineoplastic therapy delivers the drug directly into a(n):
   a. Artery
   b. Cavity
   c. Vein
   d. Ventricle
6. In a patient receiving doxorubicin (Adriamycin) via peripheral I.V. infusion, the nurse should monitor:
   a. The ECG
   b. Uric acid levels
   c. Potassium levels
   d. Abdominal girth
7. When planning nursing care for a patient receiving vincristine intravenously, the following nursing intervention should be considered:
   a. Restrict fluids during treatment.
   b. Limit the dosage of acetaminophen.
   c. Observe the I.V. site for drug infiltration.
   d. Place the patient on neutropenic precautions.
8. Which of the following is a major side effect of the alkylating agent carmustine?
   a. Bone marrow depression
   b. Numbness and tingling of extremities

   c. Elevated BUN
   d. Pulmonary toxicity
9. Before administering antimetabolites, the nurse should check the following laboratory data:
   a. Sodium and potassium
   b. BUN and creatinine
   c. Liver enzymes and amylase
   d. WBC count and platelets
10. Cancer patients who experience anemia and thrombocytopenia have traditionally been treated with:
    a. Antibiotic therapy
    b. Blood component therapy
    c. Corticosteroid therapy
    d. I.V. hydration therapy
11. Adverse effects of alkylating agents primarily are related to the:
    a. GI system
    b. Neurologic system
    c. Kidney
    d. Liver

REFERENCES

Angel, F.S. (1995). Current controversies in chemotherapy administration. *Journal of Intravenous Nursing,* 18 (1), 16–23.

Bertolone, K. (1997). Pediatric oncology: Past, present, and new modalities of treatment. *Journal of Intravenous Nursing.* 20 (3), 136–140.

Coleman, C. (1998). Overview of biotherapy and nursing considerations. *Journal of Intravenous Nursing.* 21 (6), 367–373.

Doyle, M. (1995). Oncology therapy. In Terry, J., Baranowski, L., Lonsway, R., & Hedrick, C. (eds.). *Intravenous Therapy: Clinical Principles and Practice.* Intravenous Nurses Society. Philadelphia: W.B. Saunders.

Falkenstrom, M,K. (1998). Pain management of the patient with cancer in the homecare setting. *Journal of Intravenous Nursing,* 21 (6), 327–335.

Giger, J.N., & Davidhizar, R.E. (1999). *Transcultural Nursing: Assessment and Intervention* (3rd ed.). St. Louis: Mosby.

Grace, L.A., & Tomaselli B.J. (1995). Intravenous therapy in the home. In Terry, J., Baranowski, L., Lonsway, R., Hedrick, C. (eds.). *Intravenous Therapy: Clinical Principles and Practice.* Intravenous Nurses Society. Philadelphia: W.B. Saunders.

Groenwald, S.G., Grogge, M.H., Goodman, M.S., & Yarbro, C.H. (1997). *Cancer Nursing: Principles and Practice* (4th ed.). Boston: Jones & Bartlett.

Ingwersen, K.C. (1996). Cell cycle kinetics and antineoplastic agents. In Barton-Burke, M., Wilkes, G., Ingwersen, K.C. (eds.). *Cancer Chemotherapy: A Nursing Process Approach* (2nd ed.). Sudbury, MA: Jones and Bartlett Publishers; 21–42.

Intravenous Nurses Society (1996). Administration of antineoplastic agents: position paper. *Journal of Intravenous Therapy,* 19 (2), 72–73.

Intravenous Nurses Society (1998). Standards of practice. *Journal of Intravenous Nursing Supplement.* Philadelphia: J.B. Lippincott.

Joint Commission on Accreditation of Healthcare Organizations. (1995). Standards for the accreditation of home care. Chicago: JCAHO.

Jordan, E. (1993). Preparing for hair loss. *Coping, 2*, 44–46.

Kuhn, M.A. (1998). *Pharmacotherapeutics: A Nursing Process Approach* (4th ed.). Philadelphia: F.A. Davis.

LaBell, L., O'Neil, K., & Bing, C.M. (1990). An overview of home healthcare programs. *Journal of Pharmacy Practice*, 3 (1), 4–10.

Lundquist, D., & Holmes, W. (1993). Documentation of neurotoxicity resulting from high-dose cytosine arabinoside. *Oncology Nursing Forum*, 20, 1409–1418.

Lydon, J. (1986). Nephrotoxicity of cancer treatment. *Oncology Nursing Forum*, 13 (2), 68–77.

Moraca-Sawicki, A.M. (1998). Antineoplastic chemotherapy. In M. Kuhn (ed.). *Pharmacotherapeutics: A nursing Process Approach* (3rd ed.). Philadelphia: F.A. Davis; 800–829.

Moran, P. (2000). Cellular effects of cancer chemotherapy administration. *Journal of Intravenous Therapy*, 23 (1), 44–51.

Nursing 97 (1997). Update 97: The latest on treatment of cancer fatigue. *Nursing 97*, (10) 44–45.

Oncology Nursing Society. (1992). Cancer chemotherapy guidelines: Pittsburgh: OSHA. (1995). *Controlling Occupational Exposure to Hazardous Drugs*. Department of Labor Docket No. CPL 2–2.

Otto, S. (1995). Advanced concepts in chemotherapy drug delivery: Regional therapy. *Journal of Intravenous Nursing*, 18 (4), 170–176.

Parker, S.L., Tong, T., Boldne, S. (1996). Cancer statistics. *Cancer Journal Clinic*, 46, 5–27.

Pharmacia, Inc. (1995). Package insert Zinecard (dextrazoxane for injection). Ohio Pharmacia Adria, Inc.

Phillips, L.D., & Kuhn, M. (1999). *Manual of Intravenous Drugs* (2nd ed.). Philadelphia: J.B. Lippincott.

Skeel, R.T. (1999). Biologic and pharmacologic basis for cancer chemotherapy. In Skeel, R.T. (ed.). *Handbook of Cancer Chemotherapy*. Philadelphia: Lippincott Williams & Wilkins, 3–20.

Skeel, R.T., & Ganz, P.A. (1999). Systematic assessment of the patient with cancer and long-term medical complications of treatment. In Skeel, R.T. (ed). *Handbook of Cancer Chemotherapy*. Philadelphia: Lippincott Williams & Wilkins, 34–56.

Smith, M.R., & Khan, N. (1999). Disorders of hemostasis and transfusion therapy. In Skeel, R.T. (ed). *Handbook of Cancer Chemotherapy*. Philadelphia: Lippincott Williams & Wilkins.

Tipton, J.M., & Skeel, R.T. (1995). Management of acute side effects of cancer chemotherapy. In Skeel, R.T. (ed.). *Handbook of Cancer Chemotherapy* (4th ed.). Philadelphia: Lippincott Williams & Wilkins.

Topuz, E., Aydiner, A., Saip, P., et al. (1997). Local complications associated with intraperitoneal chemotherapy. Meeting abstract. University of Istanbul, Institute of Oncology, Internet. Available: www.slip.net/mcdavis/database.

Weinstein, S. (2000). *Plumer's Principles and Practices Of Intravenous Therapy* (7th ed.). Philadelphia: J.B. Lippincott, 445–507.

Woodard, W.L., & Hogan, D.K. (1996). Oncologic emergencies: Implications for nurses. *Journal of Intravenous Nursing*, 19 (5), 256–263.

ANSWERS TO CHAPTER 13

Pre-Test

1. a, **2.** b, **3.** c, **4.** b, **5.** a, **6.** b, **7.** b, **8.** d, **9.** d, **10.** d, **11.** b

Post-Test

1. c, **2.** b, **3.** d, **4.** a, **5.** b, **6.** a, **7.** c, **8.** a, **9.** d, **10.** b, **11.** a

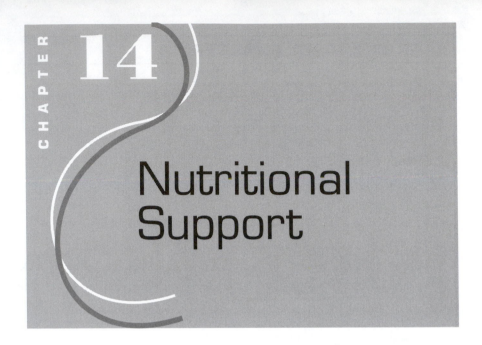

CHAPTER 14

Nutritional Support

Every careful observer of the sick will agree in this that thousands of patients are annually starved in the midst of plenty, from want of attention to the ways which alone make it possible for them to take food.

Florence Nightingale, 1859

CHAPTER CONTENTS

LEARNING OBJECTIVES

Upon completion of this chapter, the reader will be able to:

1. Define all terminology related to nutritional support.
2. Identify the goals of parenteral nutrition.
3. Identify the key elements of a nutritional assessment.
4. List the key points in administration of glucose, protein, and fat emulsions.
5. Describe the three major classifications of malnutrition.
6. Identify early candidates for nutritional support.
7. Identify the component used to treat essential fatty acid deficiency.
8. Describe the use of the additives heparin, insulin, and H_2 inhibitors to parenteral nutrition.
9. Describe three-in-one solutions.
10. List the key concepts of cyclic therapy.
11. Identify the TPN treatment plan for patients with renal or liver disease.
12. Identify key concepts of peripheral parenteral nutrition.
13. State nursing considerations related to the delivery of nutritional support.
14. Identify the complications related to nutritional support.
15. Use the nursing process in caring for a patient with nutritional support.

GLOSSARY

Amino acid Chief organic component of protein
Anergy Lack of immune response to an antigen
Anthropometry measurement Measurement of a part or whole of the body
Basal energy expenditure (BEE) The amount of energy produced per unit of time under "basal" conditions
BCAA Branched-chain amino acid
C-TPN Cyclic total parenteral nutrition
EFAD Essential fatty acid deficiency
Fat emulsion Natural product consisting of a mixture of neutral triglycerides of predominantly unsaturated fatty acids; permits inclusion of fat calories in the I.V. nutritional regimen
HPN Home parenteral therapy
Kwashiorkor Malnutrition characterized by an adequate calorie intake with inadequate amount of protein
Marasmus Malnutrition characterized by decreased intake of calories with adequate amounts of protein intake
Peripheral parenteral nutrition (PPN) Nutritional support via a peripheral vein; glucose limited to 10 percent
Refeeding syndrome Syndrome in which the body, during its bout with starvation, adapts to nutritional deprivation and compensates by decreasing basal energy requirements
Total parenteral nutrition (TPN) I.V. nutritional support delivered by central access; supplying glucose, protein, vitamins, electrolytes, trace elements, and sometimes fats to maintain the body's growth, development, and tissue repair
Total lymphocyte count (TLC) Integral component of the immune system
Total nutrient admixture (TNA) A three-in-one formula of amino acids, fats, and dextrose in one container

PRE-TEST

1. Parenteral proteins are supplied as:
   a. Synthetic crystalline amino acids
   b. Casein amino acids
   c. Immunoglobulins
2. To treat or prevent essential fatty acid deficiency, _____ is administered.
   a. Protein
   b. 10 percent dextrose
   c. Lipid emulsion
   d. Trace elements
3. During times of stress, ______ metabolism is radically altered.
   a. Protein
   b. Fat
   c. Carbohydrate
   d. Vitamin C
4. Which of the following may be added to total parenteral solutions?
   a. Regular insulin, heparin, and H_2 inhibitors
   b. Iron, vitamin K, and cimetidine
   c. Iron, heparin, and neutral protamine Hagedorn (NPH) insulin
   d. Regular insulin, vitamin K, and H_2 inhibitors
5. A solution of three-in-one admixture refers to the combination of _______, _______, and _______ in one solution container.
   a. Fat emulsion, dextrose, and amino acids
   b. Fat emulsion, vitamins, and electrolytes
   c. Fat emulsion, heparin, and insulin
   d. Dextrose, amino acids, and trace elements
6. Components of a nutritional assessment include:
   a. Dietary history
   b. Anthropometric measurements
   c. Diagnostic tests
   d. Physical examination
   e. All of the above
7. Total parenteral nutrition includes which of the following key elements?
   a. Carbohydrates
   b. Protein
   c. Fats
   d. Electrolytes and vitamins
   e. All of the above
8. The purpose of heparin added to the TPN solution is to:
   a. Enhance blood glucose levels
   b. Thin the TPN solution so it infuses easily
   c. Decrease incidence of subclavian vein thrombosis and fibrin sheath
   d. Prevent hyperglycemia
9. Criteria for PPN include:
   a. Good venous access

b. No fluid restrictions
c. Ability to tolerate fat emulsion therapy
d. Expectation that patient will resume oral feeding within 2 weeks
e. All of the above

10. Which of the following filters is used with total nutrition admixtures (three-in-one)?

a. 0.2 micron
b. 1.0 micron
c. 1.2 micron
d. 2.0 micron

● ● ●

NUTRITIONAL SUPPORT

Nutritional support nursing is the care of individuals with potential or known nutritional alterations. "Nurses who specialize in nutritional support use specific expertise to enhance the maintenance and/or restoration of an individual's nutritional health" (American Society for Parenteral and Enteral Nutrition [ASPEN], 1999). Nutrition support nursing encompasses all nursing activities that promote optimal nutritional health. Nursing interventions are based on scientific principles. The scope of practice includes, but is not limited to, direct patient care; consultation with nurses and other healthcare professionals in a variety of clinical settings; education of patients, students, colleagues, and the public; participation in research; and administrative functions (ASPEN, 1998).

It is important for nurses in all settings to respect the importance of adequate nutrition and the adverse effects of malnutrition. The goals of parenteral nutrition include:

1. To provide all essential nutrients in adequate amounts to sustain nutritional balance during periods when oral or enteral routes of feedings are not possible or are insufficient to meet the patient's caloric needs
2. To preserve or restore the body's protein metabolism and prevent the development of protein or caloric malnutrition
3. To diminish the rate of weight loss and to maintain or increase body weight
4. To promote wound healing
5. To replace nutritional deficits (Baranowski, 2000)

WEB SITES:
American Society for Parenteral and Enteral Nutrition:
www.clinnutri.org
Other:______________________________

CONCEPTS OF NUTRITION

Nutritional balance occurs when nutrients are provided in sufficient quantities for the maintenance of body function and renewal of these components. Nutritional balance is based on three factors: (1) intake of nutrients (quantity and quality), (2) relative need for nutrients, and (3) the ability of the body to use nutrients.

NUTRITIONAL DEFICIENCY

When nutritional deficiency exists, the body's components are used to provide energy for essential metabolic processes. For example, body stores of carbohydrates, fats, and protein are metabolized as energy sources in nutritional deficiency states. Carbohydrates are stored in the muscle and liver as glycogen. Adipose tissue is the body's long-term energy reserve of fat. Body protein is not stored in excess of the body's needs; therefore, use of body protein without replacement adversely affects total body function (Ford & Vizcarra, 1995).

MALNUTRITION

Malnutrition is a nutritional deficit associated with an increased risk of morbidity and mortality. Death from protein energy malnutrition and other nutritional deficiencies occurs within 60 to 70 days of total starvation in normal weight adults. Total starvation for less than 2 to 3 days in healthy adults is mainly glycogen and water losses (ASPEN, 1999). Starvation alters the distribution of carbohydrates, fats, and protein substrates. Brief starvation (24 to 72 hours) rapidly depletes glycogen stores and uses protein to produce glucose (gluconeogenesis) for glucose-dependent tissue. Prolonged starvation (longer than 72 hours) is associated with an increased mobilization of fat as the principal source of energy, reduction in the breakdown of protein, and increased use of ketones for central nervous tissue fuel. Stress in the form of pain, shock, injury, and sepsis intensifies the metabolic change seen in those with brief and prolonged starvation. Poor nutrition causes weight loss and generalized weakness, which affects the functional ability and quality of life (Wilson, 1996).

Three types of malnutrition have been defined and classified by an International Classification of Diseases (ICD) diagnostic code: marasmus, kwashiorkor, and mixed malnutrition. The outcome of nutritional assessment determines the category to which an undernourished person is assigned.

Marasmus

Marasmus is caused by a decrease in the intake of calories with adequate protein–calorie ratio. In this type of malnutrition, a gradual wasting of body fat and skeletal muscle takes place with preservation of visceral proteins. The individual looks emaciated and has decreased **anthropometric** measurements and **anergy** to common skin test antigens.

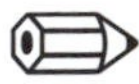 **NOTE:** Marasmus is associated with chronic illness and starvation.

Kwashiorkor

Kwashiorkor is characterized by an adequate intake of calories along with a poor protein intake. This condition causes visceral protein wasting with preservation of fat and somatic muscle. It is seen during a period of decreased protein intake as seen with liquid diets, fat diets, and long-term use of I.V. fluids containing dextrose. Loss of body protein is caused by depleted circulating proteins in the plasma. Individuals may appear obese and have adequate anthropometric measurements but decreased visceral proteins and depressed immune function.

Mixed Malnutrition

Mixed malnutrition is characterized by aspects of both marasmus and kwashiorkor. The person presents with skeletal muscle and visceral protein wasting, depleted fat stores, and immune incompetence. The affected person appears cachectic and usually is in acute catabolic stress. This mixed protein–calorie disorder has the highest risk of morbidity and mortality.

Effects of Malnutrition

The hazards of malnutrition on bodily function are decreased protein stores, albumin depletion, and impaired immune status. Without protein stores in the body, a deficiency of total body protein results first in decreased strength and endurance (loss of muscle mass) and ultimately in decreased cardiac and respiratory muscle function. Skeletal muscle wasting occurs in a ratio of about 30 to 1 compared with visceral protein loss. The loss of gastrointestinal (GI) function follows skeletal muscle wasting and is associated with hypoalbuminemia. Protein–calorie malnutrition is one of the most common causes of impairment of immune function. Both B- and T-cell–mediated immune functions are impaired, causing enhanced susceptibility to infections.

NUTRITIONAL ASSESSMENT

A nutritional assessment of high-risk patients supplies the physician and nurse with invaluable information regarding a patient's nutritional status (Table 14–1).

The nutritional assessment encompasses routine history taking with emphasis on dietary history, anthropometric measurements, diagnostic testing, and a complete physical examination (Blackburn-Capel, 1998).

INS STANDARDS The nurse's responsibility before administration includes review of the patient's height, weight, nutritional status, and diagnosis and current laboratory values (INS, 2000, 14).

The Joint Commission on the Accreditation of Healthcare Organizations (JCAHO, 1998) standards for both hospital and home care mandate nutritional assessment as part of the specific nutrition care standards emphasizing an interdisciplinary approach.

HISTORY

The history is divided into four major components: medical, weight changes, social, and dietary. The medical history should include a specific history of weight; chronic diseases; surgical history; presence of increased

TABLE 14-1

COMPONENTS OF A NUTRITIONAL ASSESSMENT

History
- Medical
- Social
- Dietary

Anthropometric measurements
- Skinfolds
- Height and weight
- Midarm circumference
- Midarm muscle circumference

Biochemical assessment
- Serum albumin and transferrin levels
- Serum electrolytes
- Total lymphocyte count
- Urine assays (creatinine, height index)

Energy requirements

Physical examination

Other Indices
- Nitrogen balance
- Indirect calorimetry
- Prognostic Nutritional Index (PNI)

losses, such as from draining wounds and fistulas; and factors such as age and drug, alcohol, and tobacco use. The social history affecting nutrient intake includes income, education, ethnic background, and environment during mealtime, along with religious considerations (Blackburn-Capel, 1998). The dietary history often provides clues as to the cause and degree of malnutrition. The components of a dietary history include appetite, GI disturbances, mechanical problems such as ill-fitting dentures, food allergies, medications, and food likes and dislikes.

AGE-RELATED CONSIDERATIONS: ELDERLY ADULTS

It is estimated that one in four elderly people is malnourished. Elderly people who are malnourished tend to have a longer and more expensive hospital stay.

Inadequate dietary intake in elderly people is multifaceted and includes physiologic changes in the GI tract, social and economic factors, drug interactions, disease, and excessive alcohol abuse. Poor dental health and missing teeth contribute to the malnutrition problem (Smeltzer & Bare, 2000).

CULTURAL AND ETHNIC CONSIDERATIONS: NUTRITION

Culture can determine the foods a patient eats and how they are prepared and served. Culture and religion together often determine if certain foods are prohibited and if certain foods and spices are eaten. When taking a dietary history, the nurse must be sensitive to culture and religious beliefs related to foods (Smeltzer & Bare, 2000).

ANTHROPOMETRIC MEASUREMENTS

Anthropometry is the measurement of a part or whole of the body. It is a method of determining body composition. To estimate the size of the body fat mass, a skinfold test is done on the triceps of the nondominant arm using a caliper. Along with the skinfold measurement, a midarm circumference and midarm muscle circumference evaluation are performed. The height and weight are also part of this evaluation, with serial weights providing helpful information related to the protein–calorie status of the person. To calculate the current weight as a percentage of the usual weight, use the following calculation:

% Ideal body weight (IBW) = [Current weight ÷ IBW] × 100

Weight loss is important because it reflects inadequate calorie intake. Weight loss indicates an increased loss of protein from the body cell mass in individuals who are malnourished. Current weight does not provide information about recent changes in weight; therefore, patients are asked about their usual body weight (UBW; Smeltzer & Bare, 2000).

% of UBW = (Current body weight/UBW) × 100

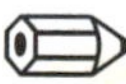 **NOTES:** A loss of 10% of the usual weight or a current weight less than 90% of IBW is considered to be a risk factor of nutrition-related complications (Ford & Vizcarra, 1995).

Mild malnutrition = 85 to 95 percent IBW
Moderate malnutrition = 75 to 84 percent IBW
Severe malnutrition = less than 75 percent IBW

In simple starvation, 20 percent loss of body weight is associated with marked decreases in muscle tissue and subcutaneous fat, giving the patient an emaciated appearance. Gross loss of body fat can be observed not only from appearance but also by palpating a number of skinfolds. When the dermis can be felt between the fingers on pinching the triceps and biceps skinfolds, considerable loss from body stores of fat has occurred. Protein stores can be assessed by inspection and palpation of a number of muscle groups, such as the triceps, biceps, and subscapular and infrascapular muscles. The long muscles in particular are profoundly protein depleted when the tendons are prominent to palpation.

BIOCHEMICAL ASSESSMENT

Several tests are available to assess patients' biochemical nutritional status. The anergy test is recommended for assessing immunologic response and involves the intradermal injection of antigens. Proper nutrition is a key to an intact immune system, and a lack of response to antigens is considered anergic and possibly indicates malnourishment.

Biochemical assessment reflects both the tissue level of a given nutrient and any abnormality of metabolism. Studies of serum protein, albumin, globulin, transferrin, retinol-binding protein, hemoglobin, serum vitamin A, carotene, and vitamin C can reflect the utilization of nutrients. Total lymphocyte count is also measured for the body's response immunologically.

Serum Albumin and Transferrin Levels

Albumin is a major protein synthesized by the liver. Approximately 40 percent of protein mass is in the circulation. The serum albumin concentration is normally between 3.5 and 5.0 g/dL. An albumin level of 2.8 to 3.2 g/dL represents mild protein depletion, 2.1 to 2.7 g/dL reflects moderate depletion, and less than 2.1 g/dL indicates severe depletion.

Serum transferrin is a beta globulin that transports iron in the plasma and is synthesized in the liver. Transferrin is present in the serum in concentrations of 250 to 300 mg/dL. The serum levels are affected by nutritional factors and iron metabolism. Levels lower than 100 mg/dL indicate severe depletion (Smelzter & Bare, 2000).

Prealbumin and Retinol-Binding Protein

Prealbumin functions in thyroxine transport and as a carrier for retinol-binding protein. Normal serum concentrations range from 15.7 to 29.6 mg/dL. Levels of 10 to 15 mg/dL reflect mild depletion, 5 to 9.9 mg/dL reflect moderate depletion, and a level lower than 5 mg/dL indicates severe depletion.

Total Lymphocyte Count

Immunologic testing is designed to assess nutritional deficiencies. The most commonly used test for the assessment of immunocompetence is the **total lymphocyte count (TLC).** The TLC is derived from the routine complete blood count (CBC) with differential. The TLC is calculated by means of the following formula.

$$\text{TLC} = \frac{\%\ \text{Lymph} \times \text{WBC}}{100}$$

A TLC between 1200 and 2000/μL indicates mild lymphocyte depletion; a TLC between 800 and 1199/μL indicates moderate lymphocyte depletion; and a TLC lower than 800/μL indicates severe lymphocyte depletion.

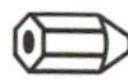 **NOTE:** TLC must be interpreted with caution because many other non-nutritional factors may contribute to decreased lymphocyte counts.

Serum Electrolytes

Serum electrolyte levels provide information about fluid and electrolyte balance and kidney function. The creatinine/height index calculated over a 24-hour period assesses the metabolically active tissue and indicates the degree of protein depletion, comparing expected body mass for height and actual body cell mass (Smeltzer & Bare, 2000).

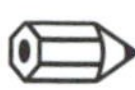 **NOTE:** Many nutrition teams have incorporated a Subjective Global Assessment into their practice. A disadvantage to the Subjective Global Assessment is that it is a subjective data collection and depends on the experience of the clinician collecting and interpreting the data (Wilson, 1996).

ENERGY REQUIREMENTS

Energy requirements are dependent on a number of factors, which include the body surface area (derived from height and weight), age, and gender. Total daily energy expenditure has three components: (1) **basal energy expenditure (BEE** or BMR); (2) energy expenditure related to an activity; and (3) specific dynamic action of food. Determination of energy needs can be determined from the BEE or resting metabolic expenditure. The BEE accounts for 65 to 75 percent of energy expenditure and may be measured or estimated (Kinney, 1990). The traditional method used to estimate BEE is the Harris-Benedict equation, which takes into consideration influence of patient's weight in kilograms, height in centimeters, age, and gender (Baranowski, 2000).

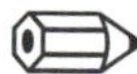 **NOTE:** A simpler, widely accepted method used to estimate daily adult caloric requirements is to use 30 to 35 cal/kg.

PHYSICAL EXAMINATION

The final phase of the nutritional assessment is a complete physical examination. Findings from a physical examination can reflect protein–calorie malnutrition along with vitamin and mineral deficiencies. The physical examination should include evaluation of the patient's hair, nails, skin, eyes, oral cavity, glands, heart, muscles, and abdomen, along with a neurologic evaluation and evaluation of delayed healing and tissue repair (Table 14–2). The physical examination should also include objective measurements of wound healing, grip strength, skeletal muscle function, and respiratory muscle function.

TABLE 14–2

PHYSICAL FINDINGS ASSOCIATED WITH DEFICIENCY STATES

Area Assessed	Physical Findings	Associated Deficiencies
Hair	Flag sign (transverse depigmentation of hair)	Protein, copper
	Hair easily pluckable	Protein
	Hair thin, sparse	Protein, biotin, zinc
Nails	Nails spoon shaped	Iron
	Nails lackluster, transverse riding	Protein–calorie
Skin	Dry, scaling	Vitamin A, zinc, essential fatty acids
	Flaky paint dermatosis	Protein
	Follicular hyperkeratosis	Vitamins A, C; essential fatty acids
	Nasolabial seborrhea	Niacin, pyridoxine, riboflavin
	Petechiae, purpura	Ascorbic acid, vitamin K
	Pigmentation, desquamation (sun-exposed area)	Niacin (pellagra)
	Subcutaneous fat loss	Calorie
Eyes	Angular blepharitis	Riboflavin
	Corneal vascularization	
	Dull, dry conjunctiva	Vitamin A
	Fundal capillary microaneurysms	Ascorbic acid
	Scleral icterus, mild	Pyridoxine
Perioral	Angular stomatitis	Riboflavin
	Cheilosis	
Oral cavity	Atrophic lingual papillae	Niacin, iron, riboflavin, folate, vitamin B_{12}
	Glossitis (scarlet, raw)	Niacin, pyridoxine, riboflavin, vitamin B_{12}, folate
	Hypogeusesthesia (also hyposomia)	Zinc, vitamin A
	Magenta tongue	Riboflavin
	Swollen, bleeding gums (if teeth present)	Ascorbic acid
	Tongue fissuring, edema	Niacin

(Continued)

TABLE 14-2

PHYSICAL FINDINGS ASSOCIATED WITH DEFICIENCY STATES *(Continued)*

Area Assessed	Physical Findings	Associated Deficiencies
Glands	Parotid enlargement	Protein
	Sicca syndrome	Ascorbic acid
	Thyroid enlargement	Iodine
Heart	Enlargement, tachycardia, high output failure	Thiamine ("wet" beriberi)
	Small heart, decreased output	Calorie
	Sudden heart failure, death	Ascorbic acid
Abdomen	Hepatomegaly	Protein
Muscles, extremities	Calf tenderness	Thiamine, ascorbic acid (hemorrhage into muscle)
	Edema	Protein, thiamine
	Muscle wastage (especially temporal area, dorsum of hand, spine)	Calorie
Bones, joints	Bone tenderness (adult)	Vitamin D, calcium, phosphorus (osteomalacia)
Neurologic	Confabulation, disorientation (Korsakoff's psychosis)	Thiamine
	Decreased position and vibratory senses, ataxia	Vitamin B_{12}, thiamine
	Decreased tendon reflexes, slowed relaxation phase	Thiamine
	Ophthalmoplegia	Thiamine, phosphorus
	Weakness, paresthesias, decreased fine tactile sensation	Vitamin B_{12}, pyridoxine, thiamine
Other	Delayed healing and tissue repair (e.g., wound, infarct, abscess)	Ascorbic acid, zinc, protein

OTHER INDICES

Nitrogen Balance

A sensitive indicator of the body's gain or loss of protein is its nitrogen balance. An adult is said to be in nitrogen equilibrium when the nitrogen intake from food equals the nitrogen output in urine, feces, and perspiration. The nitrogen balance is a measure of daily intake of nitrogen minus the excretion. It is used to assess protein turnover. A positive nitrogen balance indicates an anabolic state with an overall gain in body protein for the day. A negative nitrogen balance indicates a catabolic state with a net low of protein.

Negative nitrogen balance indicates that tissue is breaking down faster than it is being replaced. In absence of protein, the body converts protein to glucose for energy. This occurs with fever, starvation, surgery, burns, and debilitating diseases.

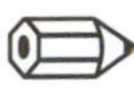

NOTE: Each gram of nitrogen loss in excess of intake represents the depletion of 6.25 g of protein or 25 g of muscle tissue (Smeltzer & Bare, 2000).

Indirect Calorimetry

The indirect calorimetry is a technique used in measuring the resting energy expenditure based on oxygen consumption and carbon dioxide production.

Prognostic Nutritional Index

The prognostic nutritional index (PNI) is an assessment technique that is based on four measures selected by analysis and computer-based stepwise regression that are then incorporated into a linear predictive model. The clinically important factors as determined by this analysis include the serum albumin concentration, serum transferrin, triceps skinfold thickness, and delayed hypersensitivity. This predictive model relates the risk of morbidity to nutritional status.

NUTRITIONAL REQUIREMENTS

Nutritional requirements are based on a basic formula that must contain all essential macro- and micronutrients for adequate energy production, support of synthesis, replacement, and repair of structural or visceral proteins; cell structure; production of hormones and enzymes; and maintenance of immune function. The basic design contains carbohydrates, protein, fat, electrolytes, vitamins, trace elements, and water.

CARBOHYDRATES

The I.V. source of carbohydrates is predominately dextrose. Glycerol, sorbitol, or fructose can provide other sources of carbohydrate calories. These are considered nondextrose carbohydrates and do not require insulin for metabolism. The nondextrose carbohydrates may require more energy in the metabolism process. Invert sugar and xylitol provide other sources of carbohydrate calories.

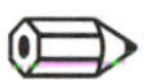 **NOTE:** 1 g carbohydrate = 4 kcal

Glucose

The major purpose of carbohydrates is to provide energy. Glucose provides calories in parenteral solutions. Carbohydrates also spare body protein. When glucose is supplied as a nutrient, it is stored temporarily in the liver and muscle as glycogen. When glycogen storage capacity is reached, the carbohydrate is stored as fat. When glucose is provided parenterally, it is completely bioavailable to the body without any effects of malabsorption.

When dextrose is administered rapidly, the solution acts as an osmotic diuretic and pulls interstitial fluid into the plasma for subsequent renal excretion. The nurse must be aware that when infusing 20 to 70 percent dextrose solutions, the rate must be kept within 10 percent of the prescribed order. (Table 14–3 provides a list of dextrose solutions, osmolarity, and kcal/L.) The pancreas secretes extra insulin to metabolize infused glucose. If 20 to 70 percent dextrose is discontinued suddenly, a temporary excess of insulin in the body may cause symptoms of hypoglycemia (Metheny, 1996).

Dextrose is usually administered concurrently with lipids for two reasons: (1) to prevent hyperglycemia and avert the need for extra insulin and (2) to reduce respiratory demands.

The number of dextrose calories in parenteral preparation may vary considerably, depending on the needs of the patient. The range may be from 400 to 5000 cal/d and depends on the age, weight, and clinical status of the patient along with laboratory determinations (Josephson, 1999).

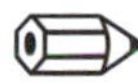 **NOTE:** Dextrose increases the metabolic rate, which in turn raises ventilatory requirements.

For peripheral infusions, a 10 percent or less dextrose concentration must be maintained at an isotonic or mildly hypertonic osmolarity to prevent vein irritation, damage to the vein, and thrombosis. Hypertonic concentrations of 20 percent and above

TABLE 14–3

DEXTROSE SOLUTIONS FOR TOTAL PARENTERAL NUTRITION

Solution (%)	g/L	kcal/L	mOsm/L
5	50	170	252
10	100	340	505
20	200	680	1010
30	300	1020	1515
40	400	1360	2020
50	500	1700	2525
60	600	2040	3030
70	700	2380	3535

must be administered through a central venous catheter (CVC) placed in the superior vena cava.

Dextrose Substitutes

When a patient has allergies to corn derivatives, invert sugar, alcohol sugars (sorbitol and xylitol), or fructose may be used in place of dextrose. Fructose and alcohol do not require insulin for peripheral utilization, but they have potentially dangerous side effects that are not associated with dextrose use. Severe toxic effects can occur with alcohol sugars, including lactic acidosis, hepatic failure, hyperuricemia, and depletion of liver adenosine triphosphate and inorganic phosphate.

FATS

Fat is a primary source of heat and energy. Fat provides twice as many energy calories per gram as either protein or carbohydrate. Fat is essential for the structural integrity of all cell membranes. Linoleic acid and linolenic acid are the only fatty acids essential to humans. These two acids prevent essential fatty acid deficiency (**EFAD**). Linoleic acid is necessary as a precursor of prostaglandins. It regulates cholesterol metabolism and maintains the integrity of cell walls. Signs and symptoms of EFAD include desquamating dermatitis, alopecia, brittle nails, delayed wound healing, thrombocytopenia, decreased immunity, and increased capillary fragility.

Lipid Administration

When fat is used as a calorie source in parenteral nutrition, there are less problems with glucose homeostasis, carbon dioxide (CO_2) production is lower, and hepatic tolerance to I.V. feedings may improve. Primarily, I.V. fats are supplied by safflower or soybean oil, with egg yolk phospholipids and glycerol to provide tonicity. Fat emulsions provide 1.1 kcal/mL (10% solution) or 2.0 kcal/mL (20% solution) (Metheny, 1996).

The initial rate of **fat emulsions** should be 1 mL/min for the first 15 to 30 minutes of the infusion. The rate may be increased to 2 mL/min subsequently.

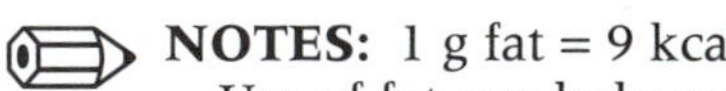
NOTES: 1 g fat = 9 kcal
Use of fat can help control hyperglycemia in stress states.

Complications associated with EFAD include impaired wound healing, platelet dysfunction, increased susceptibility to infection, and development of fatty liver. In patients with respiratory failure, the administration of fat can help decrease carbon dioxide excretion The primary purpose of fat emulsions in patients with TPN is to prevent or treat EFAD with infusion of two or three 500-mL bottles of 10 or 20 percent fat emulsions per week (Table 14–4 provides a listing of lipid emulsions for TPN.)

TABLE 14–4

LIPID EMULSIONS FOR TOTAL PARENTERAL NUTRITION

Manufacturer	Emulsion/ Percentage	Available	Osmolarity (mOsm/L)
Abbott	Liposyn II 10%	50/50 safflower oil, soybean oil	10% (1.1 kcal/mL) 276
	Liposyn II 20%	50/50 safflower oil, soybean oil	20% (2.0 kcal/mL) 258
	Liposyn III 10%	Soybean oil	10% (1.1 kcal/mL) 284
	Liposyn III 20%	Soybean oil	20% (2.0 kcal/mL) 292
	Liposyn III 30%	Soybean oil	30% (3.0 kcal/mL) 305
Clintec	Intralipid 10%	Soybean oil	10% (1.1 kcal/mL) 280
	Intralipid 20%	Soybean oil	20% (2.2 kcal/mL) 330
	Intralipid 30%	Soybean oil	30% (3.0 kcal/mL)
B. Braun	NutriLipid 10%	Soybean oil	10% (1.0 kcal/mL) 280
	NutriLipid 20%	Soybean oil	20% (2.0 kcal/mL) 330

Source: Gahart B.L., & Nazareno, A.R. (1999). *Intravenous Medications.* St. Louis: Mosby.

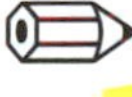 **NOTE:** Twenty percent fat emulsions are better utilized by the body.

To prevent EFAD, 2 to 4 percent of the total calorie requirement should come from linoleic acid (25 to 100 mg/kg/d). Ten percent of calories from soy or safflower oil emulsions should provide adequate linoleic acid to prevent EFAD.

A 1.2-micron filter must be used when infusing total nutrient admixtures (TNA). This filter was found to remove *Candida albicans* and to prevent passage of particulate and precipitates.

Administration sets that contain DEHP (Di(2-ethylhexyl) phthalate) plasticizers extract lipids from the set. It is recommended to use a separate administration sets, glass infusate containers, or special non-PVC (polyvinyl chloride) bags.

It is very important to carefully inspect fat emulsions for "breaking-out" (or "oiling out"), which is the separation of an emulsion visually. Do not use if there is an identifiable yellowish streaking or the accumulation of yellow droplets in the admixed emulsion.

PROTEIN

Protein is a body-building nutrient that functions to promote tissue growth and repair and replacement of body cells. Protein is also a component in antibodies, scar tissue, and clots. **Amino acids** are the basic units of protein. There are eight essential amino acids needed by adults that must be supplied by the diet: isoleucine, leucine, lysine, methionine, phenylalanine, threonine, tryptophan, and valine.

> **AGE-RELATED CONSIDERATIONS: NEWBORN INFANTS**
> Newborn infants require another amino acid, histidine. Premature infants also require cystine and tyrosine.

Parenteral proteins are elemental, providing a synthetic crystalline amino acid that does not cause an antigenic reaction. These proteins are available in concentrations of 3 to 15 percent and come with and without electrolytes. (Some amino acid solutions are presented in Table 14–5.) An increased need for protein by the body is usually reflected by an increase in excretion of urinary nitrogen, as evidenced by laboratory values.

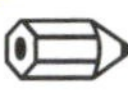

NOTE: Protein requirements for healthy adults are 0.8 percent g/kg/d; in critical illness states, the requirements are 1.2 to 2.5 g/kg/d. Protein sparing can be accomplished by administration of 100 to 150 g of carbohydrate daily.

ELECTROLYTES

Electrolytes are infused either as a component already contained in the amino acid solution or as a separate additive. Electrolytes are available in several salt forms and are added based on the patient's metabolic status.

The electrolytes necessary for long-term TPN include potassium, magnesium, calcium, sodium, chloride, and phosphorus. Potassium is needed for the transport of glucose and amino acids across cell membranes. Approximately 30 to 40 mEq of potassium is necessary for each 1000 calories provided by the parenteral route. Potassium may be given as potassium chloride, potassium phosphate, or potassium acetate salt. Serum potassium levels must be closely monitored during TPN administration.

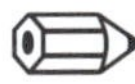

NOTE: Patients with impaired renal function may need decreased amount of potassium.

Other electrolytes included in nutritional support include:

- Magnesium sulfate at 10 to 20 mEq every 24 hours
- Calcium gluceptate, gluconate, or chloride at 10 to 15 mEq in 24 hours
- Sodium chloride, acetate, lactate, or phosphate at 60 to 100 mEq in 24 hours

TABLE 14–5

AMINO ACID SOLUTIONS FOR TOTAL PARENTERAL NUTRITION

Solution	Protein	Concen-tration (%)	Nitrogen (%)	Osmolarity mOsm/L (g/100 mL)
Abbott	Aminosyn	3.5	0.55	357
	Aminosyn II	3.5	0.55	308
	Aminosyn II	4.25	0.65	894
	Aminosyn	5	0.786	500
	Aminosyn II	5	0.786	438
	Aminosyn	7	1.10	700
	Aminosyn II	7	1.10	800
	Aminosyn	8.5	1.33	850
	Aminosyn II	8.5	1.3	742
	Aminosyn	10	1.57	875
	Aminosyn II	10	1.57	1000
	Aminosyn III	15	2.3	1300
	Stress formulation: Aminosyn-HBC	7	1.12	665
Clintec Nutrition	Travasol	3.5	0.591	450
	Travasol with electrolytes	3.5	0.591	450
	Travasol	5.5	0.924	575
	Travasol	8.5	1.42	890
	Travasol	10	1.68	970
	Travasol with electrolytes	8.5	0.924	575
	Novamine	15	2.37	1388
	Stress formulation: BranchAmin	4	0.443	316
B. Braun	FreAmine III	3	0.46	300
	FreAmine III	8.5	1.42	810
	FreAmine III	10	1.57	950
	FreAmine III with electrolytes	3	0.46	405
	TrophAmine	6	0.93	525
	TrophAmine	10	1.55	875
	ProcalAmine	3	0.46	735
	Stress formulation: FreAmine HBC	6.9	0.97	620
	Hepatic formulation: HepatAmine	8	1.2	785

- Phosphorus sodium or potassium at 20 to 45 mEq in 24 hours
- Chloride is provided based on acid–base status

Electrolytes must be individually compounded and can be highly variable in the patient receiving TPN. Choice of each of the above salts depends on renal and cardiac functioning, disease-specific needs, acid–base balance, and any abnormal losses during the course of illness.

VITAMINS

Vitamins are necessary for growth and maintenance, along with multiple metabolic processes. The fat- and water-soluble vitamins are needed for patients requiring TPN. Recommendations for the daily administration of I.V. multivitamins are provided in Table 14–6.

Controversy exists over the exact parenteral vitamin requirements for patients receiving TPN. Certain disease states can alter vitamin requirements, and the sequelae of vitamin deficiency can be catastrophic to very ill patients. Vitamin K is not a component of any of the vitamin mixtures formulated for adults. Maintenance requirements can be satisfied by administering vitamin K, 5 mg per week, intramuscularly.

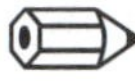 **NOTE:** Sufficient vitamin K is found in lipids; if a patient receives daily lipid supplementation, vitamin K injections are not needed.

TRACE ELEMENTS

Trace elements (also called microelements) are found in the body in minute amounts. Basic requirements are very small, measured in milligrams. Each trace element is a single chemical and has an associated deficiency state. The many functions of trace elements are often synergistic (Metheny, 1996).

Zinc contributes to wound healing by increasing the tensile strength of collagen; copper assists in iron's incorporation of hemoglobin. The other trace elements (i.e., selenium, iodine, fluorine, cobalt, nickel, and iron) all

TABLE 14–6

DAILY VITAMIN RECOMMENDATIONS FROM THE AMA

Vitamin	Amount
A	3300 IU
D	200 IU
E	10 IU
Ascorbic acid (C)	100 mg
Folic acid	400 μg
Niacin (B_3)	40 mg
Riboflavin (B_2)	3.6 mg
Thiamine (B_1)	3.0 mg
Pyridoxine (B_6)	4.0 mg
Cyanocobalamin (B_{12})	5.0 μg
Pantothenic acid (B_5)	15 mg
Biotin (B_7)	60 μg

have been identified as beneficial. Table 14–7 provides recommendations for the daily trace elements.

PARENTERAL NUTRITION MEDICATION ADDITIVES

In addition to combining amino acids, dextrose, fats, electrolytes, vitamins, and trace elements, medications such as insulin, heparin, and histamine 2 (H_2) inhibitors are commonly added to TPN solutions. A variety of other medications are compatible with TPN solutions, including some anti-infective agents. Adding medications with TPN solutions depends on various factors, including the physical compatibility of the admixed components, the chemical stability of the drug, the retention of drug concentration over time, and the bioactivity of the components after admixture.

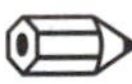 **NOTE:** Always check current information about drug compatibility with TPN solutions.

Compatibility is always an issue whenever two agents are combined. Parenteral solutions should be used immediately after mixing or else refrigerated. Stability of the admixed component dictates the appropriate length of time that the solution may be refrigerated. The parenteral solutions must be infused within 24 hours or discarded (INS, 1998, 42).

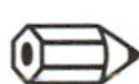 **NOTE:** Piggybacking medications directly into TPN solutions is generally not recommended because of the guidelines that a designated port be used only for nutritional support.

Insulin

Hyperglycemia is the most common complication of TPN therapy. Hyperglycemia is caused by the high concentration of glucose in the TPN solutions. Insulin is considered to be chemically stable in parenteral nutrition. By adding regular insulin to the parenteral admixture, some patients benefit from the enhanced blood glucose levels. Insulin is responsible for adequate metabolism of carbohydrates. Insulin also has a lipolytic effect and an increased muscle uptake of amino acids

NOTE: Only regular insulin is appropriate for I.V. administration.

TABLE 14–7

DAILY TRACE ELEMENTS RECOMMENDATIONS FROM THE AMA

Trace Element	Amount
Zinc	2.5 to 40 mg
Copper	0.5 to 1.5 mg
Chromium	10 to 15 μg
Manganese	0.15 to 0.8 mg

Heparin

Heparin in doses of 1000 to 3000 U/L is sometimes added to parenteral nutrition solutions to decrease potential formation of a fibrin sleeve, which may lead to venous thrombosis. Concerns related to the possibility of heparin-induced thrombocytopenia have decreased this practice (Baranowski, 2000).

Histamine 2 (H_2) Inhibitors

Cimetidine, Pepsid, Reglan, or Zantac can be added to the TPN solution as a prophylactic measure against development of stress ulcers.

ADMIXTURE COMPLICATIONS

Admixture complications involve the formation of precipitates in the formula. The Food and Drug Administration (FDA) has issued a safety alert regarding the hazards of precipitation associated with parenteral nutrition (1994). Two deaths and at least two cases of respiratory distress have been reported as being related to infusion of three-in-one TPN admixtures containing precipitate of calcium phosphate. Because of the potentially life-threatening events, caution should be taken to ensure that precipitates have not formed in any parenteral nutritional admixtures.

The FDA suggests the following steps to decrease the risk of additional injuries:

1. The amounts of phosphorus and calcium added to the admixture are critical. The solubility of the added calcium should be calculated from the volume at the time the calcium is added and should not be based on the final volume.
2. Some amino acid injections for TPN admixtures contain phosphate ions. These phosphate ions and the volume at the time the phosphate is added should be considered.
3. The line should be flushed between the addition of any incompatible components.
4. A lipid emulsion in a TNA admixture obscures the presence of a precipitate. Add calcium before the lipid solution.
5. A filter should be used when infusing either central or peripheral parenteral nutrition (PPN). Standards of practice vary, but the following is suggested: 1.2-micron air-eliminating filter for lipid-containing admixtures or a 0.22-micron air-eliminating filter for nonlipid-containing admixtures.
6. Parenteral nutrition admixture should be administered within the following time frames:
   - If stored at room temperature, start within 24 hours after mixing.
   - If stored at refrigerated temperatures, start within 24 hours of rewarming.
7. If symptoms of acute respiratory distress, pulmonary embolus, or interstitial pneumonitis develop, stop the infusion immediately and thoroughly check solution for precipitates.

MODALITIES FOR DELIVERY OF NUTRITIONAL SUPPORT

Modalities for nutritional support include enteral nutrition, PPN, TPN, TNA, and cyclic therapy. There are also specialized parenteral formulas that can be used for patients in renal or liver failure or in stress formulas. Figure 14–1 provides an algorithm for determining the choice of nutritional support.

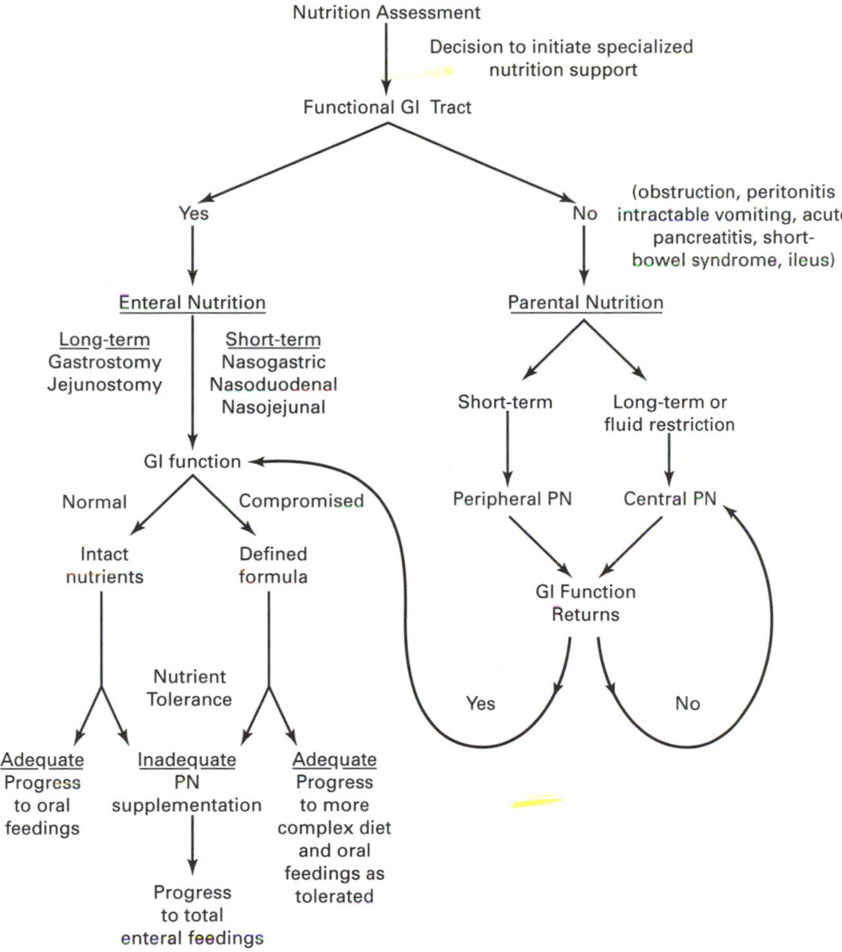

FIG. 14–1. Routes to deliver nutritional support to adults: Clinical decision algorithm. This clinical decision algorithm outlines the selection process for choosing the route of nutritional support in adult patients. Major considerations for selecting the feeding route and nutritional support formula include gastrointestinal function, expected duration of nutrition therapy, aspiration risk, and the potential for or the actual development of organ dysfunction.

NUTRITIONAL SUPPORT

Patients who are good candidates for nutritional support are those who suffer from a multiplicity of problems. Their clinical course can be complicated by malnutrition and depletion of body protein (Fig. 14–2).

The indications for TPN in adults include a 10 percent deficit in preillness body weight; an inability to take oral food or fluids within 7 days after surgery; and hypercatabolic situations, such as major infections with fever and burns. Other conditions that have shown an efficacy for nutritional support include short gut syndrome, enterocutaneous fistulas, renal failure, and hepatic failure (Table 14-8).

Candidates for TPN within the home care environment include patients (1) whose intake is insufficient to maintain an anabolic state; (2) whose ability to ingest food orally or by tube is impaired; (3) who are uninterested in ingesting or unwilling to ingest adequate nutrients; (4) who have underlying medical conditions that preclude their being fed orally or by tube; and (5) whose preoperative and postoperative nutritional needs are prolonged (Smeltzer & Bare, 2000).

> **AGE-RELATED CONSIDERATIONS: PEDIATRICS**
>
> The leading use of nutritional support in the pediatric population is for the support of infants with inadequate absorptive surface owing to congenital defect or loss from necrotizing enterocolitis.

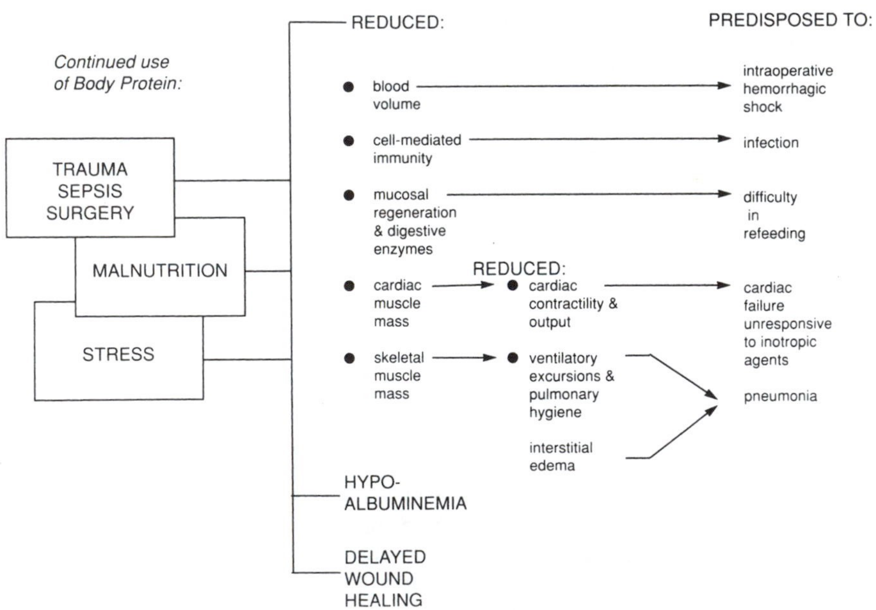

FIG. 14–2. Body protein depletion.

TABLE 14-8

CANDIDATES FOR TOTAL PARENTERAL NUTRITION

Chronic weight loss
- Malnutrition
- Anorexia nervosa
- Anorexia of cancer
- Cancer malabsorption syndrome
- Chronic vomiting and diarrhea
- 10% of preillness weight loss

Serum albumin below 3.5 g/dL
- Bowel surgery
- Short-bowel syndrome
- Massive bowel resection

Conditions requiring bowel rest
- Acute pancreatitis
- Bowel fistulas
- Inflammatory bowel disease
- Obstruction
- Paralytic ileus
- Peritonitis

Malabsorption of enteral therapy

Excessive nitrogen loss
- Abscesses
- Fistulas
- Infections
- Wounds

Hypermetabolic states
- Burns
- Critical illness

Multiple trauma

Hepatic or renal failure

Coma

ENTERAL NUTRITION

Enteral nutrition includes the ingestion of food orally and the nonvolitional delivery of nutrients by tube into the GI tract. Patients who are good candidates for enteral tube feeding are those who will not, should not, or cannot eat but who have a functional GI tract.

Advantages of enteral tube feeding include the following:

1. Maintenance of GI structure and functional integrity
2. Enhanced utilization of nutrients
3. Ease and safety of administration
4. Lower cost

Disadvantages include:

1. Contraindicated for patients with diffuse peritonitis, intestinal

obstruction, intractable vomiting, paralytic ileus, or severe diarrhea that makes metabolic management difficult.
2. Not recommended during the early stages of short bowel syndrome or presence of severe malabsorption (ASPEN,1999).

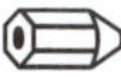

NOTE: Enteral tube feeding is considered safer than parenteral nourishment because mechanical, infectious, and metabolic complications are usually less severe than those encountered with parenteral nutrition.

Use the parenteral route only when a patient is at risk of malnutrition from not eating, a trial of enteral nutrition has failed, or when a patient has severely diminished intestinal function because of underlying diseases or treatment is anticipated.

Key Points in Delivery of Enteral Nutritional Support

1. The GI tract must be functioning.
2. The nutrition program should be tailored to meet lifestyle needs.
3. Potential candidates for enteral tube feeding should be evaluated by a multidisciplinary team of healthcare professionals.
4. The patient must be monitored for:
   - Formula intolerance (gastric residuals every 4 to 8 hours)
   - Stools (frequency and consistency)
   - Tube tolerance (placement and maintenance checks)
   - Effectiveness (weight gain, nutrient intake)
   - Laboratory tests

Complications Associated with Enteral Nutrition

1. Incorrect tube placement
2. Occlusion of feeding tube
3. Pulmonary aspiration of feeding
4. Tracheoesophageal fistula
5. Acute sinusitis
6. Otitis media
7. Diarrhea
8. Metabolic imbalances: hypoglycemia, hyperglycemia, hyperosmolar nonketotic dehydration, EFAD

PERIPHERAL PARENTERAL NUTRITION

Parenteral nutrition support is used to nourish patients who either are already malnourished or have the potential for developing malnutrition and who are not candidates for enteral nutrition (ASPEN, 1999). PPN was first proposed in the early 1970s as a "nitrogen-sparing" therapy.

The ASPEN (1998) practice guidelines may be used to provide partial or total nutritional support for up to 2 weeks in selected patients who cannot ingest or absorb oral or enteral tube-delivered nutrients or in those for whom central vein parenteral nutrition is not feasible.

Generally, PPN provides dextrose in percentages below 20 percent with 500 mL of amino acids and fat emulsions via a peripheral line. This therapy maintains the nutritional state in patients who can tolerate relatively high fluid volume, those who usually resume bowel function and oral feeding within a few days, and those who are susceptible to catheter-related infection of central venous TPN. PPN can be delivered by an over-the-needle catheter or by a peripherally inserted central line. Osmolarity factors of the solution must be considered when delivering PPN (INS, 1998, 30).

INS STANDARDS When parenteral nutrition is administered in final concentrations of 10 percent or lower or 5 percent protein or lower, the solution should not be administered peripherally for longer than 7 to 10 days unless supplementation with oral or enteral feeding is provided to ensure adequate nutrition (INS, 2000, 74).

The delivery of PPN involves both advantages and disadvantages. Advantages of PPN include:

1. Avoids insertion and maintenance of a central catheter
2. Delivers less hypertonic solutions than central venous TPN
3. Reduces the chance of metabolic complications from that of central venous TPN
4. Increases calorie source, along with fat emulsion

Disadvantages of PPN include:

1. Cannot be used in nutritionally depleted patients
2. Cannot be used in volume-restricted patients because higher volumes of solution are needed to provide adequate calories
3. Does not usually increase a patient's weight
4. May cause phlebitis owing to the osmolarity of the solution

A standardized ordering sheet is used to specify the protein, calories, and electrolyte content of each solution tailored to the client. Standard PPN includes the following basic formula:

> 100 to 150 g of dextrose with 1.0 to 1.5 g amino acids/kg (final concentrations of 1.75 to 3.5% amino acids and 5 to 10 percent dextrose), along with 500 mL of 10 or 20 percent lipids and electrolytes, trace elements, and vitamins.

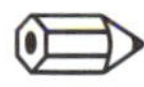

NOTE: Prolonged infusions should be limited to solutions that are lower than 900 mOsm/L. Reports have shown that with the use of three-in-one solutions, a higher osmolality may be tolerated. No greater than 10 percent final concentration of dextrose should be infused peripherally (ASPEN, 1999).

TOTAL PARENTERAL NUTRITION

Parenteral nutrition via central vein is used to provide nutrients at greater concentrations and smaller fluid volumes than is possible with PPN. Central venous access can be maintained for prolonged periods (weeks to years) with a variety of catheters that must be surgically placed and maintained. Central I.V. nutrition support is referred to as TPN. It reverses starvation and adequately achieves tissue synthesis, repair, and growth.

TPN solutions infused through a central vein are highly concentrated and range from 1800 to 2000 mOsm/kg with final additives compared with 300 mOsm/kg in plasma. TPN is usually administered at rates of no more than 200 mL/h (Baranowski, 2000).

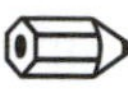

NOTE: Central I.V. nutrition has been administered in the home setting successfully for periods as long as 19 years (ASPEN, 1999).

INS STANDARDS Parenteral nutrition requires final filtration and an electronic infusion device for administration (INS, 2000, 74).

The delivery of TPN involves both advantages and disadvantages. Advantages include:

1. Dextrose solution of 20 to 70 percent administered as a calorie source
2. Useful for long-term use (usually longer than 3 weeks)
3. Useful for patients with large caloric and nutrient needs
4. Provides calories; restores nitrogen balance; and replaces essential vitamins, electrolytes, and minerals
5. Promotes tissue synthesis, wound healing, and normal metabolic function
6. Allows bowel rest and healing
7. Improves tolerance to surgery
8. Is nutritionally complete

Disadvantages include:

1. May require a minor surgical procedure for insertion of a tunneled catheter or implanted port
2. May cause metabolic complications, including glucose intolerance, electrolyte imbalances, and EFAD
3. Fat emulsions may not be used effectively in some severely stressed patients (especially burn patients)
4. Risk of pneumothorax or hemothorax with central line insertion procedure

INS STANDARDS After parenteral nutrition solutions are prepared, they should be used immediately or refrigerated.

The length of time that the solution may be refrigerated is based on stability of the admixed components (INS, 1998, 30).

After they are hung, parenteral nutrition solutions must be infused or discarded within 24 hours (INS, 2000, 74).

All parenteral nutrition solutions should be filtered during administration with a 0.2-micron filter. When lipid emulsion is added to these solutions, a 1.2-micron filter should be used (INS, 1998, 30).

Parenteral nutrient lines, whether central or peripheral, should be dedicated to these solutions. With the exception of lipid emulsions, it is preferred that no I.V. push or piggyback medication be added to these lines (INS, 1998, 30).

TOTAL NUTRIENT ADMIXTURES

Total nutrient admixtures (TNAs) are systems that are combinations of dextrose, amino acids, and fat emulsions in one container. Referred to as total nutritional admixture, all-in-one solutions, or three-in-one solutions, this product combines fat, amino acids, and dextrose in one container. The formula is provided in a 3-L container that infuses over 24 hours. Lipids are mixed with dextrose and amino acid solution in the pharmacy. This solution is white and has a nonreflective surface, making precipitation difficult to observe. These admixtures have been shown to be stable and well tolerated by patients via central line administration. Compounding of lipids, amino acids, and dextrose solutions raises the pH of the formula.

Total nutrient admixtures must be administered through a 1.2-micron filter because of the mean particle size of fat droplets (Fig.14–3). There is a potential that cholestasis may develop and that long-chain triglycerides may depress the immune system. Catheter occlusion resulting from fat deposits has been reported with long-term use of this therapy. Limited data exist on the compatibility and stability of TNA with various products and concentration.

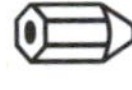

NOTE: The most common organism in TNA is *Candida albicans*. Bacterial or fungal growth may be enhanced by admixture of fat

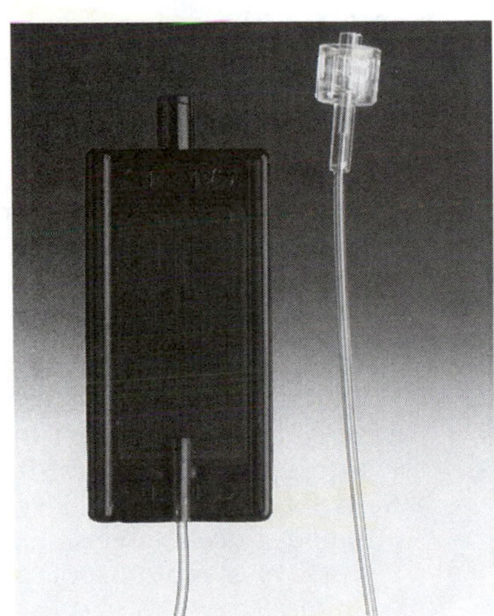

FIG. 14–3. Lipipor TNA filter set for total nutrient admixture administration with 1.2-μm air-eliminating filter. (Courtesy of Pall Corporation, Port Washington, New York.)

emulsions with dextrose and amino acid solutions. The solutions should be observed for pink discoloration and for separation of oils in the three-in-one admixture.

CYCLIC THERAPY

For patients requiring long-term parenteral nutritional support, **cyclic TPN (C-TPN)** is widely used. This therapy delivers concurrent dextrose, amino acids, and fat over a regimen of reduced time frame, usually 12 to 18 hours, versus a 24-hour continuous infusion.

Dehydration can occur when fluid requirements are not met. Monitoring should include pulse, orthostatic blood pressures, examination of mucous membranes, skin turgor, and laboratory tests such as blood urea nitrogen (BUN), creatinine, hematocrit, and albumin.

Symptoms of excess fluid administration should be monitored, such as weight gain resulting in edema or infusion-related shortness of breath. If too much fluid is administered during the cyclic period, the time frame should be extended. Using the C-TPN regimen requires twice the manipulations as continuous TPN; therefore, the risk of sepsis associated with central line manipulation must be considered.

Key Points in the Delivery of C-TPN

1. This therapy is indicated for patients stabilized on continuous TPN.
2. This therapy is indicated for long-term parenteral nutrition.
3. The patient's cardiovascular status must be able to accommodate large fluid volume during the cyclic phase.
4. For patients without complications such as glucose intolerance or a precarious fluid balance, a 12-hour cycling regimen can be used.

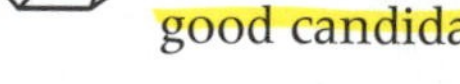

NOTE: The patient who is septic or metabolically stressed is not a good candidate for C-TPN.

Advantages include:

1. Prevents or treats hepatotoxicity induced by continuous TPN
2. Prevents or treats EFAD in patients on fat-free TPN 3
3. Improves quality of life by encouraging normal daytime activities and enhances psychological well-being

Disadvantages include:

1. Patients must be observed for symptoms of hypoglycemia, hyperglycemia, dehydration, excessive fluid administration, and sepsis associated with central-line manipulation.
2. Hyperglycemia can develop during the peak C-TPN flow rate. Blood glucose levels should be checked whenever the patient displays symptoms of nausea, tremors, sweating, anxiety, or lethargy.

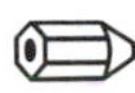

NOTE: Blood glucose should be checked 1 hour after tapering off C-TPN initially until stable.

SPECIALIZED PARENTERAL FORMULAS

Some parenteral formulas are designed to meet the needs of patients with specific disease states such as renal and liver failure and general stress conditions such as trauma, burns, and sepsis.

Renal Formulas

Patients in renal failure who are in need of parenteral nutrition minimal quantities of essential amino acids enhance urea utilization and improve nephron repair. The amino acid L-histidine enhances amino acid utilization in those with uremia. Formulas used for patients in renal failure should not contain nonessential amino acids. Standard crystalline amino acid solutions contain both essential and nonessential amino acids.

Renal preparations decrease the rate of blood urea nitrogen formation and minimize deterioration of serum potassium, magnesium, and phosphorus (Josephson, 1999).

Common preparations include Aminess 5.2 percent, Aminosyn-RF 5.2 or 5.4 percent, and NephrAmine. These formulas are contraindicated in the presence of severe, acid–base and electrolyte imbalances or hyperammonemia.

Hepatic Formulas

Solutions high in branched-chain amino acids (BCAA) are designed for liver disease. Patients with chronic liver disease have elevated levels of aromatic amino acids and depressed levels of **BCAA.** Most commonly these formulas are limited to patients with encephalopathy. The administration formulas high in BCAA would seem to be beneficial; however, as with formulas for renal failure, controversy exists.

Common preparations include BranchAmin, HepatAmine, and Novamine 15 percent. These formulas are contraindicated in patients who are anuric.

Stress Formulas

Patients with infection; sepsis; and the trauma of burns, surgery, shock, and blunt or penetrating injuries often become hypercatabolic. In this situation, an increase nitrogen excretion caused by altered protein metabolism occurs. Severely stressed patients need more protein to meet increased nutritional needs, so high metabolic stress formulas, which are similar to hepatic formulas, are available for this patient population. This group of patients has a predilection to break down BCAA in the muscles. Formulas with high BCAA replenish those depleted in the stressed patient (Josephson, 1999). Examples of stress formulas include Aminosyn-HBC, BranchAmin, FreAmine HBC, and Novamine 15 percent.

PARENTERAL NUTRITION IN THE PEDIATRIC PATIENT

Pediatric patients receiving PPN or TPN usually fall into two major categories:

- Those with congenital or acquired anomalies of the GI tract
- Those with intractable diarrhea (Weinstein, 1997)

Total parenteral nutrition must be monitored in the pediatric patient to meet the demands of growth and development. Children have a high basal metabolic rate per unit of body weight, an increased evaporative fluid loss, and immature kidneys. Infants and young children need additional amino acids, which are nonessential in adults. The amino acids required for infants and children include histidine, tyrosine, cystine, and taurine. Special amino acid formulas are available to meet these needs (Ford & Vizcarra, 1995).

Assessment

Nutritional assessment of pediatric patients uses standard growth curves. Calculation of the ratio of weight to height indicates wasting, and calculation of the ratio of height to age indicates stunting of growth. Anthropometric measurements are used as gauges of somatic protein and fat stores. Visceral protein stores are evaluated by determining serum albumin, serum transferrin, prealbumin, and retinol-binding protein levels.

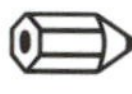

NOTE: Pediatric requirements for I.V. nutrition follow general guidelines and are based on protein, calorie, and fluid needs per kilogram of body weight.

The nurse must monitor the child's physical status, including reporting abnormal findings of temperature spikes, inappropriate glucose spills, chills, rashes, irritability, and decreased level of consciousness. Serum level of various chemistry and hematology tests are assessed daily for the first week and then decreased to a weekly schedule for the stable hospitalized or home TPN patients.

Another area of assessment includes psychological support. Most TPN patients are infants who are acutely ill and deprived of maternal warmth and comfort. Cuddling and holding the child should be encouraged, along with allowing the parents to participate in their child's care (Weinstein, 1997).

Monitoring

Many children require long-term support at home. Monitoring includes many of the same parameters as for adults. The monitoring during initiation of parenteral nutrition includes daily weight, strict intake and output, daily electrolytes until stable, serum glucose measurements every 8 to 12 hours, serum triglycerides and free fatty acid levels weekly, and liver function test biweekly.

In addition, children require evaluation of growth determinations including weight, height, head circumference, and anthropometric measurements for the duration of the therapy.

NOTE: The predominant complication associated with parenteral nutrition in infants is cholestasis.

When a child if first started on TPN, the percentage of dextrose infused is gradually increased from 5 percent to a maximum of 20 to 25 percent via a central line, according to caloric needs and tolerance of the child. Depending on caloric expenditure based on stress levels, lipids may be provided biweekly or daily.

NOTE: Because of the high-risk behaviors of children, catheter sepsis rate in children may rise as high as 10 percent because of increased risks (e.g., teething children have been known to bite the TPN catheter).

COMPLICATIONS OF PARENTERAL NUTRITION

Complications associated with parenteral nutrition are divided into four groups: (1) mechanical or technical (involving catheters, pumps, and other apparatus for administration), (2) infections, (3) metabolic, and (4) nutritional (Table 14–9). Complications may be minimized by appropriate monitoring and nursing interventions.

Mechanical or Technical (Catheter-Related)

Pneumothorax

Pneumothorax results when injury occurs during catheter placement. Blood, air, or infusion of fluid collects in the pleural cavity. Care must be taken to assess catheter placement before infusion of TPN. Assess for sharp chest pain, decreased breath sounds, changes in vital signs, and respiratory status. If pneumothorax has occurred, it is evident on a chest radiogram.

Air Embolism

Passage of air into the heart can occur during insertion of the central line or during catheter maintenance. All connections should be taped and procedures strictly followed for tubing changes along with dressing management techniques. Change tubing during patient's expiratory respiratory phase. Apply an occlusive dressing over the site after the catheter has been removed.

Vein Thrombosis

Long-term central catheterization can cause vein thrombosis in the superior vena cava or its tributaries. Use of a silicone catheter decreases the risk of thrombogenic factors. Pulmonary emboli can be a secondary

TABLE 14–9

COMPLICATIONS ASSOCIATED WITH NUTRITIONAL SUPPORT

Mechanical/ Technical Complications Complication/Etiology	**Symptoms**	**Treatment**	**Prevention**
Air Embolism Cause: When line is interrupted and air is inspired while the line is open	Cyanosis, tachypnea, hypotension churning heart murmur (classic sign)	Immediately place patient on left side and lower the head of the bed; this may keep the air within the apex of the right ventricle until it is reabsorbed; administer oxygen	Line placement by appropriately trained personnel; use care in injection cap changes; do not use scissors near catheter
Vein Thrombosis Causes: Mechanical trauma to vein, TPN osmolarity, hypercoagulopathy	Swelling or pain in one or both arms, shoulders, or neck; increased anterior chest venous pattern, external jugular distension; or fluid leaking from arm May be asymptomatic	Diagnosis may be made by arm venography, contrast studies, MRI, and radionucleotide study Treatment is controversial and depends on extent of thrombus Conservative treatment without removal consists of anticoagulants Discontinuation of catheter	Tip placement in SVC not upper arm or subclavian Early recognition of symptoms
Catheter Malposition Cause: Catheter inadvertently advanced into an incorrect vein during placement Can occur spontaneously after insertion caused by coughing or vomiting	Swelling of arm or neck, pain, difficulty flushing catheter, difficulty infusing TPN Ear gurgling sound	Reposition with guidewire under fluoroscopy or remove Reposition the patient before flushing line	Not always possible to prevent Follow techniques to prevent malposition Always use radiography to confirm tip placement

Metabolic Complications			
Altered Glucose Metabolism Hypoglycemia: Rebound Cause: Abrupt cessation of TPN	Diaphoresis, irritability, nervousness, shakiness	Administer dextrose or decrease insulin Maintain I.V. at constant rate	Maintain steady rate of infusion; wean gradually
Hyperglycemia Cause: Carbohydrate intolerance, insulin resistance, rapid TPN delivery, diabetes, sepsis, traumatic stress	Increased serum glucose, acetone breath, anxiety, confusion, dehydration, polydipsia, polyuria, malaise	Decrease dextrose TPN concentration or decrease rate administer insulin per sliding scale	Accurate glucose monitoring, gradual TPN rate, increase stable TPN infusion rate
Hyperammonemia Cause: Liver disease where ammonia is shunted past the liver and accumulates in blood	Asterixis (flapping tremor), lethargy, neurologic changes, altered ECG, vomiting, coma	Limit protein intake, enemas and antibiotics to revert growth of ammonia-producing bacteria in intestines	Accurate monitoring of serum ammonia level, monitoring of protein intake for patients with liver disease
Hypernatremia Cause: Water deprivation or loss, excessive TPN administration, profuse diaphoresis, diabetes insipidus, vomiting, diarrhea	Serum Na elevated to 145 mEq/L; urine specific gravity elevated to 1.015; thirst; elevated temperature; dry, swollen tongue; sticky mucous membrane; lethargy	Gradually decrease serum sodium levels to prevent cerebral edema Administration of water	Monitor serum electrolytes I and O, assess for insensible losses

(Continued)

TABLE 14–9

COMPLICATIONS ASSOCIATED WITH NUTRITIONAL SUPPORT *(Continued)*

Mechanical/ Technical Complications Complication/Etiology	Symptoms	Treatment	Prevention
Metabolic Complications			
Hypokalemia Cause: Alkalosis caused by shift of K into cells, GI losses, diuretic therapy, TPN, steroid administration, osmotic diuresis, anorexia	Serum K below 3.5 mEq/L, anorexia, fatigue, muscle weakness, decreased gastric motility, postural hypotension, ECG changes	TPN supplementation; replace GI losses	Monitor serum potassium, strict I and O, assess for digitalis toxicity
Hyperkalemia Cause: Renal impairment, iatrogenic-induced, TPN, metabolic and respiratory acidosis, tissue damage	Serum K elevated above 5.5 mEq/L ECG changes, cardiac arrest, muscular weakness, flaccid muscles, intestinal colic, diarrhea	Reduce TPN volume of K, cation exchange resins, dialysis	Accurate monitoring of K accurate I and O
Hypomagnesemia Cause: GI losses, refeeding after starvation, renal disease, TPN administration	Apprehension, depression, apathy, neuromuscular hyperexcitability, tremors, PVCs, tachycardia, ventricular fibrillation	Parenteral supplementation	Monitor serum Mg, assess for neuromuscular changes
Hypophosphatemia Cause: TPN supplementation without adequate phosphorus replacement, burns, malabsorptive states, and starvation	Apprehension, irritability, seizures, decreased RBCs, muscle weakness, insulin resistance	I.V. supplementation in the TPN	Monitor serum Mg levels

Hypocalcemia Cause: Vitamin D deficiency, insufficient calcium or magnesium intake, malabsorption, pancreatitis	CNS irritability, confusion, muscle cramps in extremities, muscle spasms, laryngeal spasms, seizures, tetany	Supplement TPN with calcium or I.V. calcium, correct magnesium or phosphate deficiencies	Accurate serum chemistry levels, avoid calcium-depleting medications, maintain adequate calcium intake
Infections			
Sepsis Cause: Skin contamination at insertion site, hub, and tubing junction from hands of healthcare professionals; homogenous seeding from other sources	Chills, fever, malaise, elevated WBC count, diarrhea, tachycardia, tachypnea, flushing hypotension	Remove catheter or replace catheter over guidewire Antibiotics Administer oxygen Prepare to treat for septic shock	Maintain aseptic technique Aseptic dressing changes Use 0.22-micron filter
Nutritional Alterations			
Refeeding Syndrome Cause: Occurs during initial phase of TPN Body during its bout of starvation has adapted somewhat to nutritional deprivation: decreased basal energy requirements Causes electrolyte shift	Cardiorespiratory complications edema, hypernatremia, hypokalemia, hypomagnesemia, hypophosphatemia	Can be averted by starting TPN gradually and gradually increasing rate	Monitor patient response to TPN

(Continued)

TABLE 14–9

COMPLICATIONS ASSOCIATED WITH NUTRITIONAL SUPPORT ***(Continued)***

Mechanical/ Technical Complications Complication/Etiology	Symptoms	Treatment	Prevention
Nutritional Alterations			
Essential Fatty Acid Deficiency Cause: Deficient intake	Minimal symptomatology until long term, soft tissue calcification, hypocalcemia, and tetany Numbness and tingling of the mouth and fingers	Fat emulsion supplementation in TPN or with intermittent infusions	Accurate calculation of protein and fat and CHO ratios to maintain a positive nitrogen balance
Altered Mineral Balance Cause: Result of deficiencies caused by malnourishment or starvation	Chromium: elevated serum lipid levels, insulin resistance, glucose tolerance Copper: hypochromic microcytic anemia, neutropenia Iron: fatigue, glossitis, hypochromic microcytic anemia Manganese: CNS changes Selenium: Cardiomyopathies Zinc: Alopecia, apathy, confusion, poor wound healing	Supply adequate supplementation in TPN	Monitor for abnormal laboratory values

Altered Vitamin Balance Cause: Disease processes can alter vitamin requirements TPN must supply the needed fat- and water-soluble vitamin supplements	Vitamin A: Dry, scaly, rough, cracked skin; decreased saliva; impaired digestion; diarrhea Vitamin D: Decreased serum calcium or phosphorus levels Vitamin E: RBC hemolysis Vitamin K: Delayed clotting Vitamin B_1: Increased serum and urine lactate or pyruvate levels, anorexia, confusion, fatigue, painful calf muscle Vitamin B_2: Glossitis, stomatitis, dermatitis, photophobia Vitamin B_3 (Niacin): Dermatitis, glossitis, diarrhea, dementia Vitamin B_{12}: Anorexia, depression dyspnea, memory lapses, delirium, hallucinations Folic acid: Macrocytic anemia, diarrhea, glossitis Vitamin C: bleeding gums, petechiae, depression	Provide vitamin supplements in TPN	Monitor for symptoms and assess for deficits

complication of vein thrombosis. Thrombolytic therapy is of benefit when flow rates are affected owing to thrombus formation, as is the use of heparin added to the infusate to prevent thrombosis. The physician should be notified if thrombosis is suspected.

Catheter Malposition

This complication can occur during introduction of the catheter. If there is difficulty in passage of the catheter, cardiac arrhythmias during insertion along with irregularities of flow of infusate could indicate malposition of the catheter. Check dressing at least every 4 hours for signs of inadvertent displacement. Report suspected catheter malposition to the physician promptly.

Metabolic

Complications associated with metabolic imbalances when administering TPN are either avoidable or controllable.

Altered Glucose Metabolism: Rebound Hypoglycemia

Rebound hypoglycemia condition is caused by abrupt cessation of TPN. Maintain a steady rate of infusion, and wean gradually when discontinuing usually prevents with condition. The patient exhibits diaphoresis, irritability, nervousness, and shaking. The infusion can be decreased by one half the rate for 1 to 2 hours if needed. This usually is not necessary if the patient is eating.

Altered Glucose Metabolism: Hyperglycemia

Hyperglycemia is a common metabolic occurrence with TPN because of the high dextrose concentrations included in the admixture. Other factors that put the patient at risk for hyperglycemia are the presence of overt or latent diabetes mellitus, older age, sepsis, hypokalemia, and hypophosphatemia.

Conditions of stress result in decreased glucose tolerance and hyperglycemia in up to 25 percent of patients on TPN. Infusion of large amounts of glucose can also unmask latent diabetes, making hyperglycemia one of the most common complications encountered with parenteral nutrition. Other considerations when infusing formulas containing high concentrations of glucose is the potential effect of carbohydrate metabolism on respiration. Metabolism of carbohydrates results in increased production of carbon dioxide that must be compensated for by increased minute ventilation. This could precipitate respiratory failure in patients with preexisting respiratory disease or interfere with weaning from mechanical ventilation.

Factors that predispose a patient to glucose intolerance include:

- Presence of overt or latent diabetes mellitus
- Older age

- Pancreatitis
- Hypokalemia
- Hypophosphatemia
- Thiamine or B_6 deficiency
- Some antibiotics
- Steroids
- Conditions of stress, such as sepsis or surgery, result in decreased glucose tolerance and hyperglycemia in as many as 25 percent of TPN patients

Nursing considerations include:

1. Begin TPN infusion at a slow rate (40 to 60 mL/h).
2. Gradually increase the rate 25 mL/h until the maximal infusion rate is achieved.
3. Maintain a steady state of infusion (TPN must stay within 10 percent of prescribed rate).
4. Use a rate control device to monitor the infusion.
5. Monitor serum blood sugar every 6 hours, particularly during the first week of infusion.
6. Record fluid intake and output accurately every 8 hours.
7. Measure hourly urine output if urinary losses are above 250 mL/h.
8. Check body weight daily using the same scale. The ideal weight gain for patients receiving TPN is approximately 2 lb per week.
9. Monitor vital signs at regular intervals. Look for signs of hypovolemia.

Essential Fatty Acid Deficiency

Lipid administration is important for delivery of essential fatty acids. If the regimen for nutritional support does not include a calorie source from fats, the patient is at risk for EFAD. Fats may be administered in amounts that supply 30 to 50 percent of the calories. By adding fats to the nutritional support, CO_2 production can be decreased and other metabolic complications may be avoided.

Hyperammonemia

Ammonia accumulates in the blood in those with liver disease. An elevated blood ammonia level is a common finding in infants and children receiving TPN. High protein intake may lead to elevated ammonia levels. Arginine is important in the urea cycle, and a deficiency of this amino acid may contribute to the development of hyperammonemia.

Limiting protein intake, enemas, and antibiotics to prevent growth of ammonia-producing bacteria in the intestines may help. Monitor the serum ammonia levels and limit the essential protein in the TPN solution (Josephson, 1999).

NOTE: In adults, the most common laboratory finding is that of elevated transaminase levels; the most common abnormality is liver steatosis. Cholestasis and gallbladder disease are potential complications of long-term TPN.

Electrolyte Imbalances

Major electrolyte imbalances associated with TPN can occur if excessive or deficient amounts of electrolytes are supplied in the daily fluid allowance. These include imbalances of sodium, potassium, magnesium, phosphate, or calcium.

- Sodium: Hypernatremia: To maintain homeostasis, the sodium ion is driven from the intracellular space into the extracellular space. This compensatory mechanism tries to combat the extracellular anion loss (Metheny, 1996). This shift can cause hypernatremia.
- Potassium: Hypokalemia: Potassium is also driven into the intracellular space during TPN. Serum potassium can become depleted with an inadequate supply of this electrolyte along with the use of insulin in the TPN solution. Insulin administration further intensifies intracellular potassium.
- Potassium: Hyperkalemia: A high potassium blood level can occur with renal impairment, iatrogenic-induced, or with metabolic and respiratory acidosis when potassium shifts out of the cells. Interventions include reducing the amount of potassium ion in the TPN solution.
- Magnesium: Hypomagnesemia: The magnesium electrolyte also is driven into the intracellular space during TPN administration. This condition is less common than hypophosphatemia or hypokalemia in patients receiving TPN (Metheny, 1996). This electrolyte should be included in TPN solution compounding. Hypomagnesemia is a common imbalance in critically ill and less acutely ill patients. This condition is often overlooked.
- Phosphate: Hypophosphatemia: Adenosine triphosphate (ATP) is required for all cell energy production. Protein synthesis begins when TPN is administered and phosphate is driven into the intracellular space as a component of ATP. Therefore, a deficiency of phosphate can occur. Include phosphate in TPN supplementation.
- Calcium: Hypocalcemia: Because of the fact that most patients receiving parenteral nutrition are malnourished and have low serum albumin levels, their total serum calcium levels are usually also below normal. The hypocalcemia is not physiologically significant and does not usually result in paresthesias or other signs of tetany. The usual TPN solution contains 5 to 10 mEq/L of calcium.

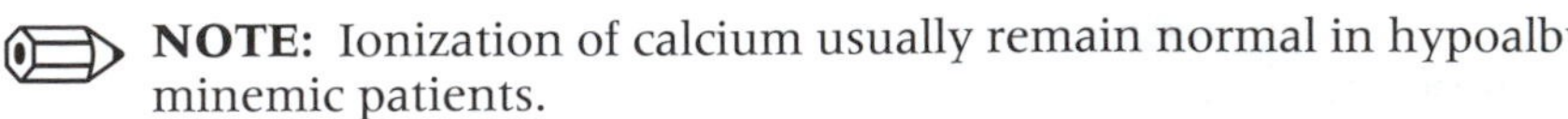

NOTE: Ionization of calcium usually remain normal in hypoalbuminemic patients.

Nursing considerations include:

1. Observe for signs and symptoms of hypophosphatemia, hypokalemia, hypomagnesemia, and hypernatremia. (See Chapter 4 for a review of signs and symptoms.)
2. Chemistry panel should be drawn every 3 days to check electrolyte levels.

Infectious and Septic Complications

When TPN is provided by a central line, there are concerns related to the contamination of the CVC, as discussed in Chapter 12. Catheter-related sepsis is a serious complication of central TPN therapy. This complication is preventable with strict aseptic techniques.

Patients undergoing TPN are often immune compromised as a result of malnutrition; these patients are highly susceptible to infection. The origin of TPN catheter-related sepsis is most often the site itself; infection related to contaminated infusates is rare because of meticulous admixing protocols.

Catheter-Related Sepsis

Catheter-related infections or sepsis may result from skin contaminants at the insertion site, hub and tubing/device junction contamination, from the hands of health care professionals, and homogenous seeding from other sources (e.g., lungs, urine, abdomen, wounds).

Options for management of catheter-related sepsis include exchange of the catheter over the guidewire and removal of the catheter. The decision is determined by the patient's clinical status, culture results, and the nature of the offending organism (Weinstein, 1997).

Nursing considerations include:

1. Maintain aseptic technique in catheter maintenance and administration of TPN.
2. Aseptic dressing changes should be done every 48 to 72 hours if nontransparent occlusive dressing is used; every 4 to 7 days, depending on institutional policy, if transparent dressing is used. (See Chapter 12 for dressing management.)
3. Use of a 0.22-micron inline antimicrobial filter is recommended for TPN lines, except when lipid emulsion is added to these solutions, at which time a 1.2-micron filter should be used (INS, 1998, 30).

Nutrition Alterations

Refeeding Syndrome

Refeeding syndrome is a complication that can occur during the initial phases of TPN. This occurs when the body, during its bout with starvation, adapts to nutritional deprivation and compensates by decreasing basal energy requirements. This initiation of nutritional support, especially if it is undertaken too aggressively, can result in an electrolyte shift from the plasma to the intracellular fluid. Cardiorespiratory complications can occur. The result of refeeding syndrome is manifested by edema, hypernatremia, hypokalemia, hypomagnesemia, and hypophosphatemia.

After the body has reestablished normal albumin and electrolyte balances, the refeeding processes are reversed. Refeeding syndrome can be avoided by initiating TPN slowly, then gradually increasing the rate while carefully monitoring the patient's response and serum electrolyte levels (Josephson, 1999).

Altered Mineral Balance

Mineral imbalances are usually the result of deficiencies, the cause being malnourishment or starvation and insufficient supplementation in the parenteral nutrition source. The most common deficiencies include chromium, copper, iron, manganese, selenium, and zinc (Josephson, 1999).

Altered Vitamin Balance

Vitamin requirements can be altered by disease processes. The parenteral nutrition must supply the needed fat-soluble and water-soluble vitamin supplements. During illness, vitamin deficiencies can produce serious consequences for which the nurse must assess. (Josephson, 1999).

DISCONTINUATION OF NUTRITIONAL SUPPORT

Before discontinuation of parenteral or enteral nutritional support, one of the following criteria shall be applicable:

- Parenteral nutrition should not be discontinued until nutrient requirements can be met by enteral or oral nutrients.
- Enteral nutrition should not be discontinued until nutrient requirements can be met by oral nutrients.
- Parenteral or enteral nutrition support should be discontinued whenever the patient's medical condition, especially complications, indicates.
- Parenteral or central nutrition support should be terminated when the physician judges that the patient no longer benefits from the therapy. The decision to discontinue support must be made according to accepted community standards of medical care and in compliance with applicable law (ASPEN, 1998).

ETHICAL CONSIDERATIONS

Today, nutrition plays a fundamental role in religious, cultural, and ethnic traditions and has evolved in most societies as a symbol of caring and comfort relationships. The decision to commence, withhold, or withdraw nutritional support is often a controversial issue (Breier, 2000).

Areas in which ethical decisions occur in nutritional support include unconscious patients, patients receiving critical care, home care patients, and patients with cancer. I.V. nurses have an important professional responsibility to uphold ethical principles in the planning and delivery of parenteral nutritional care. Implications for practice include, but are not limited to:

1. Being familiar with the basic legal and ethical principles
2. Clarifying personal values related to euthanasia, use of life-sustaining treatments, pain, advance directives, terminal disease, and the prolongation of life
3. Recognizing the basis for conflicting legal judgments in cases associated with removal of nutritional support
4. Participating in the formalizing of standards of care and establishing departmental polices and procedures to guide decision-making for parenteral support of malnourished, terminally ill or incompetent patients
5. Deliberating a course of action for individual cases that places the ultimate interests of the patient above all other considerations
6. When appropriate, providing information to physicians and surgeons, caregivers, and patients to assist them in making informed decisions regarding the use of various feeding modalities
7. Participating in the deliberations of hospital ethics committees
8. Using published guidelines as a basis for ethical decision making (Breier, 2000)

Nurses should make decisions and perform actions on behalf of patients receiving nutrition support in an ethical manner. Nurses should be guided by individual state practice laws and the ANA standards of Clinical Nursing Practice (ASPEN, 1999). This includes maintaining patient confidentiality; acting as a patient advocate; administering care in a nonjudgmental, nondiscriminatory, and culturally sensitive manner; and delivering care that preserves and protects patient autonomy, dignity, and rights (JCAHO, 1999).

Nurses should work with an interdisciplinary healthcare team to resolve moral, ethical, and legal dilemmas while developing appropriate resolutions (JCAHO, 1998).

STANDARDS OF PRACTICE FOR NUTRITIONAL SUPPORT

Standards of practice related to nutritional support have been addressed by ASPEN (1998) and the INS (2000). Presented here are the accepted Standards of Practice related to nutritional support. Parenteral nutrition volume is based on patient tolerance.

Implementation Standards

Parenteral formulations shall be prepared according to established guidelines for safe and effective nutritional therapy (Fig. 14–4).

1. Parenteral formulations shall be sterile.
2. Parenteral formulations should be stored at 4°C.
3. Policies should be established limiting additions to the parenteral feeding formulations after they are infusing.
4. Patients or responsible persons shall receive education and demonstrate competence in access route care in home care situations.

Monitoring Standards

Patients should be monitored for therapeutic efficacy, adverse effects, and clinical changes that might influence specialized nutritional support. The potential for serous complications with TPN is unacceptably high unless careful monitoring is conducted by experienced clinicians. Protocol for monitoring TPN is included in Table 14–10 (ASPEN, 1998).

1. Protocols shall be developed for periodic review of the patient's clinical and biochemical status.
2. Routine monitoring should include nutrient intake; review of current medications; signs of intolerance to therapy; weight changes; biochemical, hematologic, and other pertinent data, including clinical signs of nutrient deficiencies and excesses; adjustment of therapy; changes in lifestyle; psychosocial problems; and changes in home environment.
3. Assessment of patient's major organ functions should be made periodically (ASPEN, 1998).

Nutritional Standards

1. Weigh the patient daily (may be decreased to two to three times per week in stable patients).
2. Evaluate nitrogen balance weekly (or as needed to determine adequacy of protein intake).
3. Albumin, transferrin, transthyretin (prealbumin), or retinol-binding protein may be measured as needed to assess visceral protein status.
4. Total lymphocyte count and anergy panels may be used to monitor changes in immune function.
5. Creatinine height index may be used to monitor somatic protein status.

ADULT TAILORED TPN SOLUTION ORDERS

TAILORED SOLUTION
- 1000 ml -

A 24 hour supply of TPN solution compounded by pharmacy will reflect changes with the next bottle made unless otherwise noted.

Amino Acids
_____% ❑ Aminosyn _______% Final concentration
❑ Aminosyn RF_____ml
❑ Heptamine _____ml

Dextrose _______ % Final concentration
_______ cc

	Additions	PHARMACY USE
Na Chloride	mEq	
Na Acetate	mEq	
Na Phosphate°	mM*	
K Chloride	mEq	
K Acetate	mEq	
Mg Sulfate	mEq	
Ca Gluconate	mEq	
Insulin, regular	Units	
Adult Tace-Element Solution° Multivitamin Infusion° Famotidine	_____ _____ _____	To be added per 24 hours

TAILORED SOLUTION: FLOW RATE _____________ ml/hr.

FAT EMULSION _____% Volume_____ ml Frequency_____ Flow Rate_____ ml/hr.

* Monitoring Note
Na Phosphate contains (per ml):
Na+ 4.4 mEq, and P 3 mM
K Phosphate contains (per ml):
K+ 4.4 mEq, and P 3 mM

° Recommended Dosage:
MVI-12 . . . . .1 unit/day
Adult Trace Element Solution. . . . . . .5 ml/day

Physician Signature ______________________________ M.D. Date __________

FIG. 14–4. Adult-tailored TPN solution orders. (Courtesy of Enloe Medical Center.)

TABLE 14–10

SUMMARY OF MONITORING PARENTERAL NUTRITION THERAPY

Before initiation of therapy by central line:
- Check placement of catheter tip by radiography

After initiation of TPN:
- Start TPN infusion slowly
- Check temperature and vital signs every 6 hours
- Monitor blood sugar every 6 hours initially, then once a day
- Maintain strict intake and output
- Check weight daily
- Decrease TPN solutions gradually
- Change TPN and lipid administration sets every 24 hours

Metabolic monitoring
- Liver function: Periodically monitor liver enzyme, bilirubin, triglyceride, and cholesterol level
- Electrolyte profile daily, then twice a week
- Serum profiles weekly at first calcium, AST, ALT, alkaline phosphatase, BUN and creatinine, PT, PTT; and then monthly
- Trace elements initially, then every 3 months with long-term TPN

Nutritional monitoring
- Serial weight daily until stable
- Serum albumin twice a week
- Assess nitrogen balance with a 24-hour urine collection
- Check albumin, transferrin, prealbumin, or retinol-binding protein
- Check total lymphocyte count and anergy panels
- Check creatinine height index to monitor protein

NURSING PLAN OF CARE

ADMINISTRATION OF TPN

Focus Assessment

Subjective
- History of weight loss
- History of disease and malnourished state
- Biographic data
- Past health history
- Allergies and medications

Objective
- Vital signs, especially temperature
- Level of consciousness
- Skin turgor
- Weight gains or losses
- Tissue edema

(continued)

(continued)

- Ratios of urinary output to intake
- Oral mucous membranes
- Serum blood glucose levels

Patient Outcome Criteria

The patient will:

1. Stabilize weight and gradually increase to within 10 percent of ideal weight
2. Be free of infection; afebrile.
3. Gain weight at a rate of 1 lb every 3 weeks, increasing to 1 lb every 2 weeks.
4. Display moist skin and mucous membranes, stable vital signs, individually adequate urinary output, and no edema.
5. Verbalize understanding of condition or disease process and individual nutritional needs.
6. Correctly perform necessary procedures and explain reasons for the actions.
7. Demonstrates skill in managing the TPN regimen.

Nursing Diagnoses

- Altered nutrition less than body requirements related to chewing or swallowing difficulties; anorexia; nausea; vomiting; difficulty or inability to procure foods
- Altered health maintenance related to poor dietary habits, with perceptual or cognitive impairment
- Altered nutrition (greater than body requirement) related to imbalance of intake versus activity expenditure
- Altered tissue perfusion (peripheral) related to infusion of irritating solution

Nursing Management

1. Assist with insertion of central line.
2. Insert peripheral I.V. central catheter per agency protocol.
3. Ascertain correct placement of I.V. central catheter by radiography before beginning TPN.
4. Maintain central line patency and dressing per agency protocol.
5. Monitor for infiltration and infection.
6. Check the PPN or TPN solution to ensure correct nutrients are included as ordered.
7. Maintain sterile technique when preparing and hanging TPN solution.
8. Keep infusion within 10 percent of prescribed rate.
9. Use an infusion pump for delivery of TPN solutions.
10. Avoid rapidly replacing lagging TPN solutions.
11. Monitor daily weight.
12. Monitor intake and output.
13. Monitor serum albumin, total protein, electrolyte, glucose and chemistry profile.

(continued)

(continued)

14. Monitor vital signs.
15. Monitor blood sugar every 6 hours.
16. Administer insulin as ordered, to maintain serum glucose in the designated range as appropriate.
17. Report abnormal signs and symptoms associated with TPN to the physician and modify care accordingly.
18. Maintain standard precautions.

PATIENT EDUCATION

The patient receiving enteral nutrition, PN, or TPN will need education, periodic assessment, and retraining as needed.

- Inform the patient about the purpose and duration of the projected nutritional support.
- Instruct the patient on the product hang time.
- Educate the patient and caregiver about management of the access device.
- Instruct the patient receiving enteral feedings about clean techniques for handling the tube, maintaining the access site, and flushing the tube to maintain patency.
- Inform the patient about complications associated with TPN administration, including:
  - Metabolic complications such as hypoglycemia and electrolyte imbalances (recognize and respond to these complications)
  - Mechanical or procedural problems (catheter or tube occlusion, leakage, breakage, or dislodgement)
  - Equipment malfunction or breakage
  - Infusion contamination precipitate or in homogeneity (recognize and report signs and symptoms of localized or systemic infectious process)
- Provide 24-hour phone numbers for home care agency or physician so that patient or caregiver can access professional help.

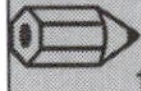

NOTE: Refer to Home Care Issues for further educational information for the home care patient.

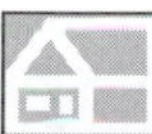

HOME CARE ISSUES

Home parenteral nutrition (HPN) has been well established over the past 10 years and should be instituted and supervised by a multidisciplinary team with knowledge and expertise (ASPEN, 1998). Patients and their families can be taught to safely administer I.V. admixtures, and they can be monitored in a home setting. Hospital-to-home transition can be a difficult task. Keep in mind that the day of discharge is usually physically and emotionally stressful; the home care nurse should be in attendance for starting the TPN infusion at home.

Before home therapy for nutritional support is initiated, a baseline electrolyte chemistry panel, magnesium and phosphorus levels, and a CBC should be obtained within 7 days of discharge. Home safety must be determined before discharge from the hospital. Successful home therapy depends on several factors:

1. Medical stability
2. Emotional stability
3. Patient's lifestyle
4. Intellectual ability (client or primary caregiver)
5. Visual acuity
6. Manual dexterity
7. Home environment:
   - Dry storage space for supplies
   - Refrigerator large enough to store admixtures
   - Clean low-traffic area for procedure preparation
   - Electronic outlets for any electronic equipment

The patient or caregiver and home environment should be suitable for safe delivery and monitoring of HPN (ASPEN, 1998).

Advantages of home treatment for nutritional support are that it involves lesser expense than treatment in the hospital; it allows the patient to remain in a familiar, comfortable surrounding, thereby decreasing the confusion associated with age-related environment changes; in many cases, it allows the patient to return to normal activities; and it is associated with a lower risk of acquiring a nosocomial infection. HPN is usually cycled or given over a 12- to 16-hour period, and most of the administration occurs during the sleeping hours (Grace & Tomeselli, 1995). In addition, a person's control over his or her body and the self-care responsibility increase self-esteem (Weinstein, 1997).

The home education process should include but not be limited to:

1. Verbal and written instructions of appropriate procedures
2. Demonstration and return demonstration of procedures by primary caregiver

(continued)

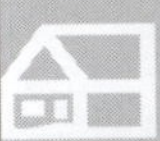

HOME CARE ISSUES *(continued)*

3. Evaluation and documentation of competency
4. Self-monitoring instruction
5. Limitations of physical activity
6. Emergency intervention and problem-solving techniques
7. Care of infusion equipment, solutions, and supplies
8. Disposal of supplies
9. Expectations of home care and medical and nursing follow-up

Home care training must be individually designed according to the individual's capabilities. Assessment of the patient's physical and emotional status before each teaching session aids in determining goals for that session. A minimum number of people should be involved with each teaching session to limit distractions and anxiety.

Because complex treatments such as ventilators, I.V. infusions and chemotherapy are being administered in home and outpatient settings, nutritional assessment of the patient in these settings is important (Smeltzer & Bare, 2000).

The patient or caregiver shall receive education and demonstrate competence in the preparation and administration of home parenteral nutrition support.

1. Instruction should be given on:
   - Proper storage of formulated and admixed parenteral feeding formulations
   - Inspection of home parenteral nutrition containers and contents
   - Aseptic technique required for the admixture procedure and administration via access device
   - Use of parenteral infusion equipment
   - Proper disposal of used containers, tubing, and needles
   - Drug–nutrient and nutrient–nutrient interactions
   - Medication information and administration
2. Educational material tailored to the patient and the therapy is provided to the patient/caregiver for use at home.
3. Patient or caregiver education should include periodic reassessment and retraining as needed.
4. Patient or caregiver should receive education and demonstrate competence in recognition and riptide response to complications.
   - Able to recognize and respond to indications of potential metabolic complications
   - Should be able to recognize mechanical and procedural problems that include, but are not limited to, catheter or tube occlusion, leakage, breakage or dislodgement; equipment malfunction or breakage; infusate or precipitate contamination or inhomogenicity
   - Able to recognize and report signs and symptoms of a localized or systemic infectious process
   - State when and whom to contact when complications occur

KEY POINTS

- Candidates for nutritional support include those with:
  - Altered catabolic states
  - Chronic weight loss
  - Conditions requiring bowel rest
  - Excessive nitrogen loss
  - Hepatic or renal failure
  - Hypermetabolic states
  - Malabsorption states
  - Malnutrition
  - Multiple trauma
  - Serum albumin levels below 3.5 g/dL
- Nutritional deficiencies fall into three categories: marasmus, kwashiorkor, and mixed malnutrition
- Effects of malnutrition include a decrease in protein stores, albumin depletion, and impaired immune status.
- Nutritional assessment includes:
  - History (medical, social, and dietary)
  - Anthropometric measurements (weight, skinfold tests, midarm circumference)
  - Biochemical assessments (serum albumin serum transferrin, prealbumin and retinol-binding protein, total lymphocyte counts, serum electrolytes)
  - Energy requirements
  - Physical examination
  - Other Indices (nitrogen balance, indirect calorimetry, prognostic nutritional index)
- Parenteral nutrition is an admixture of water, carbohydrates, amino acids, lipids, electrolytes, multivitamins, and minerals formulated to meet an individual patient's needs
- Modalities for delivery of nutritional support include:
  - Enteral nutrition
  - Peripheral nutrition
  - Parenteral nutrition
  - TPN
  - TNA
  - Cyclic therapy
- Peripheral parenteral nutrition, delivered into a peripheral vein, is indicated for patients who need a complete nutrient source but are not depleted, consist of a 2 to 5 percent amino acid solutions in combination with 5 to 10 percent dextrose. Fat emulsions of 10 to 20 percent may be combined or administered separately. This therapy is delivered for a limited time, usually 2 weeks.
- Total parenteral nutrition, delivered by central line, is the I.V. administration of hypertonic glucose (20 to 70%) and amino acids (3.5 to 15%), along with all additional components required for complete support.
- Nutritional support must be filtered with a 0.22-micron filter, except for when lipids are added to TNAs, which must have a 1.2-micron filter.
- Complications of parenteral nutrition include:
  - Mechanical or technical complications
  - Metabolic complications
  - Complications associated with infections
  - Nutritional complications

CHAPTER ACTIVITIES

COMPETENCY CRITERIA: Nutritional Support
COMPETENCY STATEMENT: Competent I.V. nurses will be able to demonstrate competency in administration of nutritional support.
Note: The cognitive (knowledge) information that is embedded within this performance-based competency includes aseptic technique, knowledge of CVC design and catheter tip location, AND recognition of signs and symptoms of complications of nutritional support.

This competency *links* to the competency of infection control, initiation of peripheral and central lines, AND management of I.V. therapy equipment.

Performance	Skilled	Needs Education
Critical Action Statements		
1. Initiates PPN A. Verifies correct PPN solution B. Identifies patency of peripheral line C. Prepares appropriate equipment, including filters D. Administers 10% dextrose or less AND 5% protein solutions in peripheral site		
2. Initiates TPN A. Verifies correct TPN solution B. Prepares correct equipment, including filter, using sterile technique C. Uses aseptic technique for accessing central line D. Verifies placement and irrigates with sodium chloride E. Attaches I.V. tubing and begins infusion at prescribed rate		
3. Documentation and patient education A. Documents procedure B. Educates patient or significant others about PPN or TPN		

(continued)

(continued)

Performance	Skilled	Needs Education
Critical Action Statements		
4. Maintains TPN infusion A. Washes hands and follows standard precautions B. Ensures that the correct solution is infusing at the prescribed rate C. Identifies the dressing change interval for VAD D. Ensures that daily weight and strict I and O are obtained and documented E. Identifies specific temperature requiring physician notification F. Performs blood sugar monitoring every 6 hours G. Reviews laboratory data to identify abnormalities		

EVALUATION CRITERIA

1. Observation of management of nutritional support by preceptor.
2. Review of documentation.

CRITICAL THINKING ACTIVITY

1. Check your agency policy and procedure manual for guidelines for monitoring the patient on TPN. Is there a set policy, and how are these procedures documented?

2. You check your patient on TPN at the beginning of the shift and find that the fat emulsion has a 0.22-micron filter attached in the line in which it is infusing. What do you do?

3. A patient has had a blood glucose level of 100 mg/dL during the course of the first 48 hours of TPN. The next time you check the blood sugar, it is 240 mg/dL. What could be the reason for this sudden increase in blood sugar? How would you begin to check for the problem?

4. The physician has ordered cyclic TPN for 12 hours for your patient who has been stabilized on nutritional support for 2 weeks. How would you explain this therapy to the patient? Upon discharge, what kind of guidelines would you provide?

POST-TEST

1. H_2 Inhibitors are added to parenteral nutrition to:
   a. Decrease incidence of vein thrombosis
   b. Act as a prophylactic measure against development of stress ulcers
   c. Increase muscle uptake of amino acids
   d. Increase the tensile strength of the collagen
2. Insulin is added to parenteral nutrition for:
   a. Enhancing blood glucose levels
   b. Metabolism of carbohydrates
   c. Lipolytic effect
   d. All of the above
3. Which of the following key concepts is true of TNAs?
   a. Solution must be changed every 8 hours.
   b. Precipitation may be difficult to observe.
   c. Solution must be administered through a 0.22-micron filter.
   d. Risk of contamination increases because of twice the manipulations of the system.
4. The key point(s) in delivery of PPN would be that the:
   a. Patient will resume oral intake within 2 weeks.
   b. PPN maintains patient nutritional state only.
   c. Osmolarity of the solution is a major consideration.
   d. All of the above
5. The advantage(s) of home care nutritional support include:
   a. Increased control of one's body
   b. Decreased risk of acquiring a nosocomial infection
   c. Continuation of normal routine
   d. All of the above
6. The type of malnutrition that most commonly occurs in the acutely ill hospitalized patient is:
   a. Kwashiorkor
   b. Marasmus
   c. Mixed malnutrition
   d. Anorexia nervosa
7. How many kilocalories does a 20 percent lipid emulsion provide?
   a. 1.0
   b. 1.1
   c. 2.0
   d. 2.2
8. All of the following are metabolic complications associated with TPN administration **EXCEPT:**
   a. Hypoglycemia
   b. Hypocalcemia
   c. Hyperkalemia
   d. Refeeding syndrome

9. Which of the following are the three essential nutrients included in parenteral nutrition required for anabolism and tissue synthesis?
   a. Trace elements, protein, and fats
   b. Protein, carbohydrates, and fats
   c. Fats, electrolytes, and carbohydrates
   d. Vitamins, electrolytes, and protein
10. All of the following are considered anthropometric measurements **EXCEPT:**
   a. Midarm muscle circumference
   b. Weight
   c. Skinfold thickness
   d. Serum transferrin

REFERENCES

American Society for Parenteral and Enteral Nutrition (1999). Guidelines for the use of parenteral and enteral nutrition in adult and pediatric patients. Internet. Available: 1999/2000.

American Society for Parenteral and Enteral Nutrition (1998). *The A.S.P.E.N. Nutrition Support Practice Manual.* American Society for Parenteral and Enteral Nutrition.

A.S.P.E.N. Board of Directors (1995). Standards of Practice: Standards for nutrition support: Hospitalized patients. *Nutrition in Clinical Practice,* 10 (12), 208–219.

A.S.P.E.N. Board of Directors (1999) Standards for home nutrition support. *Nutrition in Clinical Practice,* 14 (96), 151–161.

Baranowski, L. (2000). Parenteral nutrition. In Corrigan, A.M., Pelletier. G., & Alexander, M. (eds.). *Intravenous Nurses Society: Core Curriculum for Intravenous Nursing.* Philadelphia: Lippincott. 331–394.

Blackburn-Capel, J. (1998). Nutritional assessment: Determining metabolic needs of the TPN patient. Intravenous Nurses Society Annual Conference. Houston, Texas.

Breier, S.J. (2000). Ethics and total parenteral nutrition: *Issues for Intravenous Nurse Professionals.* 23 (1), 52–57.

Ford, C.D. & Vizcarra, C. (1995). Parenteral nutrition. In Terry, J., Baranowski, L., Lonsway, R., & Hedrick, C. (eds.). *Intravenous Therapy: Clinical Principles And Practices.* Philadelphia: W.B. Saunders, pp. 219–245.

Grace, A., & Tomaselli, B. (1995). Intravenous therapy in the home. In Terry, J., Baranowski, L., Lonsway, R., & Hedrick, C. (eds.). *Intravenous Therapy: Clinical Principles and Practices.* Philadelphia: W.B. Saunders, pp. 505–534.

Intravenous Nursing Society (2000). Revised standards of practice. Philadelphia: Lippincott Williams & Wilkins.

Josephson, D.L. (1999). *Intravenous Infusion Therapy for Nurses: Principles and Practice.* Albany: Delmar Publishers.

Joint Commission on Accreditation of Healthcare Organizations (JCAHO)(1998). *Comprehensive Accreditation Manual for Hospital and Home Care. Improving Organization Performance.* Oakbrook Terrace, IL: 267–294.

Kinney, J.M. (1990). Clinical biochemistry: Implications for nutritional support. *Journal of Parenteral and Enteral Nutrition,* 14 (5S), 148–156.

Kuhn, M. (1998). *Pharmacotherapeutics: A Nursing Process Approach* (4th ed.). Philadelphia: F.A. Davis.

Metheny, N.M. (1996). *Fluid and Electrolyte Balance: Nursing Considerations* (3rd ed.). Philadelphia: J.B. Lippincott.

Smeltzer, S.C., & Bare, B.G. (2000). Health assessment. *Brunner & Suddarths's Textbook of Medical-Surgical Nursing.* Philadelphia: Lippincott, pp. 60–67.

Weinstein, S.M. (2000). *Plumer's Principles & Practice of Intravenous Therapy* (7th ed.). Philadelphia: Lippincott Williams & Wilkins.
Wilson, J.M. (1996). Nutritional assessment and its application. *Journal of Intravenous Nursing,* 19(6), 307–314.

ANSWERS TO CHAPTER 14

Pre-Test

1. a, **2.** c, **3.** c, **4.** a, **5.** a, **6.** e, **7.** e, **8.** c, **9.** e, **10.** c

Post-Test

1. b, **2.** b, **3.** b, **4.** d, **5.** d, **6.** a, **7.** c, **8.** d, **9.** b, **10.** d

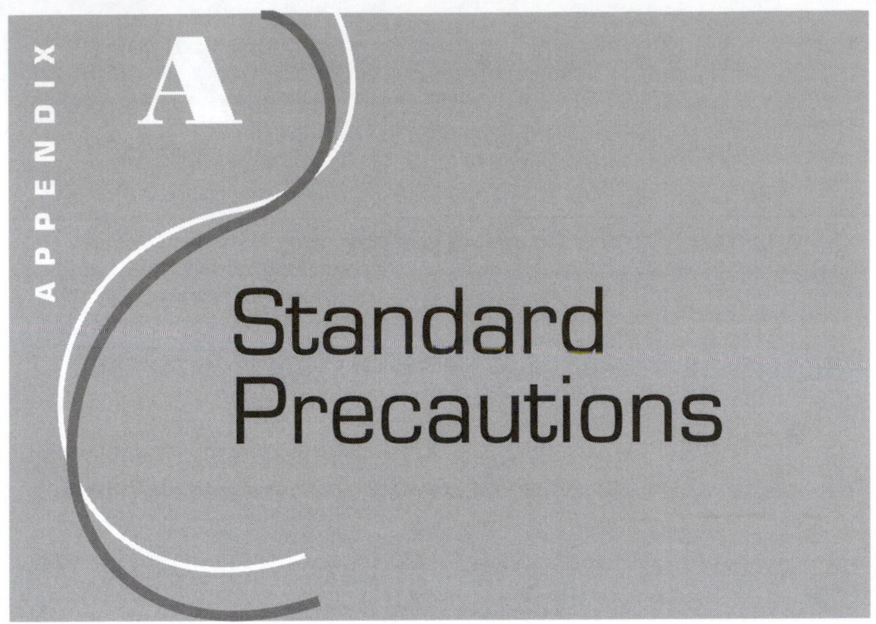

Standard precautions are a combination of Universal Precautions and body substance isolation practices. This approach to infection control is a two-tiered system. In the first tier, the same practices are used on all hospital patients regardless of their specific diagnosis or presumed infection status.

Standard precautions apply to: (1) blood; (2) all body fluids; (3) excretions and secretions (sweat is exempted from this listing); (4) nonintact skin; and (5) mucous membranes.

In the second tier, the precautions are designed for specific patients who are known or suspected to be infected with organisms that are highly transmissible.

Category IB 9: Strongly recommended for all hospitals and reviewed as effective by experts in the field and a consensus of HICPAC based on strong rationale and suggestive evidence, even though definitive scientific studies have not been done.

TIER ONE

I. STANDARD PRECAUTIONS

A. HAND WASHING

1. Wash hands after touching blood, body fluids, secretions, excretions, and contaminate items, whether or not gloves are worn.
2. Wash hands immediately after gloves are removed, between

patient contacts, and when otherwise indicated to avoid transfer of microorganisms to other patients or environments.
3. Use plain soap for routine handwashing (non-antimicrobial).
4. Use an antimicrobial agent or waterless antiseptic agent for specific circumstances as defined by infection control.

B. GLOVES

1. Wear gloves (clean, non-sterile gloves are adequate) when touching blood, body fluids, secretions, excretions and contaminated items.
2. Put on clean gloves just before touching mucous membranes and non-intact skin.
3. Change gloves between tasks and procedures on the same patient after contact with material that may contain a high concentration of microorganisms.
4. Remove gloves promptly after use, before touching non-contaminated items, and environmental surfaces, and before going to another patient, and wash hands immediately to avoid transfer of microorganisms to another patient or environments.

C. MASK, EYE PROTECTION, FACE SHIELD

1. Wear a mask and eye protection or a face shield to protect mucous membranes of the eyes, nose, and mouth during procedures and patient-care activities that are likely to generate splashes or sprays of blood, body fluid, secretions, and excretions.

D. GOWN

1. Wear a gown (a clean, non-sterile gown is adequate) to protect the skin and to prevent soiling of clothing during procedures and patient-care activities that are likely to generate splashes or sprays of blood, body fluids, secretions or excretions.
2. Remove soiled gown promptly, as soon as possible and wash hands to avoid transfer of microorganisms to other patients or environments.

E. PATIENT-CARE EQUIPMENT

1. Handle used patient-care equipment soiled with blood, body fluids, secretions, and excretions in a manner that prevents skin and mucous membrane exposures, contamination of clothing and transfer of microorganisms to other patients and environments.

2. Ensure that reusable equipment is not used for the care of another patient until it has been cleaned and reprocessed appropriately.
3. Ensure single use items are discarded properly.

F. ENVIRONMENTAL CONTROL

1. Ensure that the hospital has adequate procedures for the routine care, cleaning and disinfection of environmental surfaces, beds, bed-rails, bedside equipment, and other frequently touched surfaces.

G. LINEN

1. Handle, transport, and process used linen soiled with blood, body fluids, secretions and excretions in manner that prevents skin and mucous membrane exposures and contamination of clothing, and that avoids transfer of microorganism to other patients and environments.

H. OCCUPATIONAL HEALTH AND BLOODBORNE PATHOGENS

1. Take care to prevent injuries when using needles, scalpels, and other sharp instruments or devices; when handling sharp instruments after procedures; when cleaning used instruments; and when disposing of used needles.
2. Never recap used needles, or otherwise manipulate them using both hands, or use any other technique that involves directing the point of a needle toward any part of the body; rather use either a one-handed "scoop" technique or a mechanical device designed for holding the needle sheath.
3. Do not remove used needles from disposable syringes by hand, and do not bend, break, or otherwise manipulate used needles by hand.
4. Place used disposable syringes and needles, scalpel blades and other sharp items in appropriate puncture-resistant containers, which are located as close as practical to the area in which the items were used, and place reusable syringes and needles in a puncture-resistant container for transport to the reprocessing area.
5. Use mouthpieces, resuscitation bags, or other ventilation devices as an alternative to mouth-to-mouth resuscitation methods in areas where the need for resuscitation is predictable.

I. PATIENT PLACEMENT

1. Place a patient who contaminates the environment or who does not (or cannot be expected to) assist in maintaining appropriate hygiene or environmental control in a private room.
2. If a private room is not available, consult with infection control professionals regarding patient placement or other alternatives.

TIER TWO

II. AIRBORNE PRECAUTIONS

In addition to Standard Precautions, use Airborne Precautions, or the equivalent, for patients known or suspected to be infected with microorganisms transmitted by airborne droplet nuclei. Category IB

A. PATIENT PLACEMENT

1. Place the patient in a private room.
2. Monitor negative air pressure in relation to the surrounding areas.
3. Six to twelve air changes per hour.
4. Appropriate discharge of air outdoors or monitored high-efficiency filtration of room air before the air is circulated to other areas in the hospital.
5. Keep the room door closed and the patient in the room.
6. When a private room is not available, place the patient in a room with a patient who has active infection with the same microorganism, unless otherwise recommended.

B. RESPIRATORY PROTECTION

1. Wear respiratory protection (N95 respirator) when entering the room of a patient with known or suspected infectious pulmonary tuberculosis.
2. Susceptible persons should not enter the room of patients known or suspected to have measles (rubeola) or varicella (chicken pox) if other immune caregivers are available.
3. If susceptible persons must enter the room of a patient known or suspected to have measles or varicella, they should wear respiratory protection (N95 respirator). Persons immune to measles or varicella need not wear respiratory protection.

C. PATIENT TRANSPORT

1. Limit the movement and transport of the patient from the room to essential purposes only.
2. If transport or movement is necessary, minimize patient dispersal of droplet nuclei by placing a surgical mask on the patient.

III. DROPLET PRECAUTIONS

A. PATIENT PLACEMENT

1. Place in private room.
2. If a private room is not available, place the patient in a room with a patient who has active infection with the same microorganism but with no other infection.
3. When a private room is not available and placement with another patient is not achievable, maintain spatial separation of at least 3 feet between the infected patient and other patients and visitors.
4. The door may remain open.

B. MASK

1. In addition to wearing mask as outlined under Standard Precautions, wear a mask when working within 3 feet of the patient.

C. PATIENT TRANSPORT

1. Limit the movement and transport of the patient from the room to essential purposes only. Mask the patient if possible.

IV. CONTACT PRECAUTIONS

A. PATIENT PLACEMENT

1. Place the patient in private room.
2. If a private room is not available, place the patient in a room with a patient who has active infection with the same microorganism but with no other infection.
3. When a private room is not available and placement with another patient is not achievable, consider the epidemiology of the microorganism and the patient population.

B. GLOVES AND HAND WASHING

1. In addition to wearing gloves as outlined in Standard Precautions, wear gloves when entering the room.
2. Change gloves after having contact with infective material that may contain high concentrations of micro-organisms (fecal material and wound drainage).
3. Remove gloves before leaving the patient's room and wash hands immediately with an anti-microbial agent or waterless antiseptic agent.

C. GOWN

1. In addition to wearing a gown as outlined in Standard Precautions, wear a gown when entering the room if you anticipate that your clothing will have substantial contact with the patient, environmental surface, or items in the patient's room, or if the patient is incontinent or has diarrhea, an ileostomy, a colostomy, or wound drainage not contained by a dressing.
2. Remove the gown before leaving the patient's environment.

D. PATIENT TRANSPORT

1. Limit the movement and transport of the patient from the room to essential purposes only.
2. If the patient is transported out of the room, ensure that precautions are maintained.

E. PATIENT-CARE EQUIPMENT

1. When possible, dedicate the use of non-critical patient-care equipment to a single patient to avoid sharing between patients.

Source: Garner, J.S. (1996). Hospital Infection Control Practices Advisory Committee. Guideline for Isolation Precautions In Hospitals. Public Health Service, US Department of Heath and Human Services, Centers for Disease Control and Prevention, Atlanta, GA.

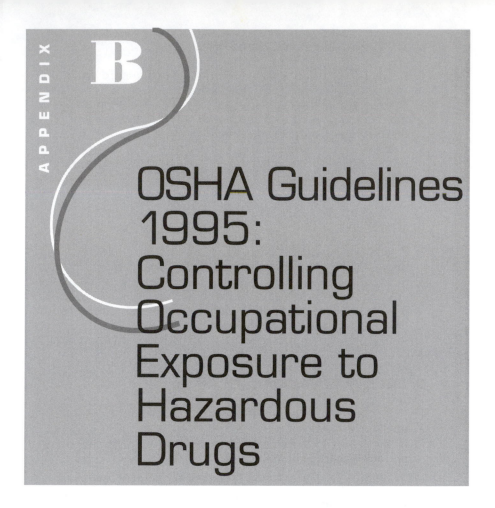

Appendix B: OSHA Guidelines 1995: Controlling Occupational Exposure to Hazardous Drugs

The Occupational Safety and Health Administration (OSHA) established guidelines for the management of cytotoxic (antineoplastic) drugs in the workplace in 1986. At that time engineering controls and personal protective equipment (PPE) were not standardized. Practices have improved, but the problems associated with administration of chemicals still exist.

In 1995, OSHA revised its work practice guidelines to incorporate hazardous drugs (HDs) in addition to the cytotoxic drugs covered in the 1986 guidelines. The recommendations apply to all practice settings in which employees are occupationally exposed to HDs. Anesthetic agents are not included in the review. There are four drug characteristics that are considered hazardous:

1. Genotoxicity
2. Carcinogenicity
3. Teratogenicity or fertility impairment
4. Serious organ other toxic manifestations at low doses

TABLE 1

DRUGS CONSIDERED AS HAZARDOUS

Altretamine	Cyclosporine	Ifosamide	Mitoxantrone
Aminoglutethi-mide	Cytarabine	Interferon-A	Nafarelin
L-Asparaginase	Dacarbazine	Isotretinoin	Pipobroman
Azathioprine	Daunorubicin	Leuprolide	Plicamycin
Bleomycin	Diethylstilbestrol	Levamisole	Procarbazine
Busulfan	Doxorubicin	Lomustine	Ribavirin
Carboplatin	Estradiol	Mechlore-thamine	Streptozocin
Carmustinel	Estramustine	Medroxyproges-terone	Tamoxifen
Catinomyin	Ethnyl estradiol	Mestrol	Testolactone
Chlorambucil	Etoposide	Melphalan	Thioguanine
Chloramphenicol	Floxuridine	Mercaptopurine	Thiotepa
Chlorotrianisene	Fluorouracil	Methotrexate	Uracil mustard
Chlorozotocin	Flutamide	Mitomycin	Vidarabine
Cisplatin	Ganciclovir	Mitotane	Vinblastine
Cyclophosphamide	Hydroxyurea		Vincristine
	Idarubicin		Zidovudine

I. ENVIRONMENTAL PROTECTION

A. Risks to personnel working with HDs are by three main routes: aerosols, dermal absorption, and ingestion.
B. Manipulations that can cause splattering, spraying, and aerosolization include withdrawal of needles from drug vials, drug transfer via syringes and needles or filter straws, breaking open ampules, and expulsion of air from a drug-filled syringe.
C. HD preparation should be performed in a restricted, preferably centralized area.
D. Signs restricting the access of unauthorized personnel are to be prominently displayed.
E. Smoking, drinking, applying cosmetics, chewing gum, and eating where these drugs are prepared, stored, or used also increases the chance of exposure.
F. The use of Class II or III Biologic Safety Cabinets (BSC) that meet the current National Sanitation Foundation Standard should minimize exposure to HDs during preparation. If a BSC is unavailable (such as in private practice office), the sharing of a cabinet or sending the patient to a center where HDs can be prepared in a BSC is an alternative solution. Alternatively, preparation can be performed in a facility with a BSC and the drugs transported to the area of administration.

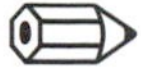

NOTE: Use of a dedicated BSC where only HDs are prepared is prudent medical practice. Use of a horizontal BSC is contraindicated in the preparation of HDs.

G. The cabinet should be cleaned according to the manufacturer's recommendations. Decontamination most frequently is done weekly, as well as whenever spills occur or when cabinet requires moving.
H. Decontamination should consist of surface cleaning with water and detergent followed by thorough rinsing. The use of detergent is recommended because there is no single accepted method of chemical deactivation for all agents.

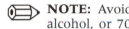

NOTE: Avoid use of quaternary ammonium cleaners, ethyl alcohol, or 70% isopropyl alcohol. Spray cleaners should also be avoided because of the risk of spraying the HEPA filter.

I. Cleaning should proceed from the least to the most contaminated areas. All materials from the decontamination process should be handled as HDs and disposed of in accordance with federal, state, and local laws.
J. Procedures for spills and emergencies, such as skin or eye contact, should be available to workers.

II. PERSONAL PROTECTIVE EQUIPMENT

A. BASIC PRECAUTIONS

1. All PPE must be donned before work is started in the BSC.
2. All items necessary for drug preparation should be placed within the BSC before work is started.
3. Extraneous items should be kept out of the work area.

B. GLOVES

1. The thickness of gloves used in handling HDs is more important than the type of material. Latex gloves are best and should be used for preparation of HDs unless the drug product manufacturer specifically stipulates that some other glove provides better protection. Thicker, longer latex gloves that cover the gown cuff are recommended for use with HDs.
2. Gloves with minimal or no powder are preferred, since the powder may absorb contamination.
3. Individuals with latex allergy should consider the use of vinyl or nitrile gloves or glove liners.
4. Double-gloving is recommended if it does not interfere with an individual's technique.
5. All gloves are permeable to some extent. They should be changed regularly (hourly) or immediately if they are torn.

C. GOWNS

1. A protective disposable gown made of lint-free, low-permeability fabric with a closed front, long sleeves, and elastic or knit cuffs should be worn.
2. The cuffs should be tucked under the gloves.

D. RESPIRATORY PROTECTION

1. A NIOSH approved respirator should be worn when a BSC is not currently available.
2. The use of respirators must comply with OSHA's Respiratory Protection Standard, including selection, fit testing, and worker training.

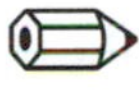

NOTE: Surgical masks are not appropriate, since they do not prevent aerosol inhalation.

E. EYE AND FACE PROTECTION

1. Eyeglasses with temporary side shields are inadequate protection.
   a. Use a respirator with a full face piece.
   b. Use a plastic face shield or splash goggles complying with American National Standards Institute regulations.
   c. Eyewash facilities should be made available.

F. DISPOSAL OF PPE

1. All gowns, gloves, and disposable materials used in preparation should be disposed of according to the hospital's hazardous drug waste procedures.
2. Goggles, face shields, and respiratory equipment may be cleaned with mild detergent and water for reuse.

G. WORK EQUIPMENT

1. Syringes and I.V. sets with Luer-lock fittings should be used for HDs.
2. Syringe size should be large enough so as not to be full when the entire drug dose is present.
3. All syringes and I.V. bags containing HDs should be labeled with a distinctive warning label.

NOTE: The following are special handling/disposal precautions

4. A covered disposable container should be used to contain excess solution. A covered sharps container should be in the BSC.
5. HD-labeled plastic bags must be available for all contaminated materials (including gloves, gowns, and paper liners).
6. Preparation of HDs must be carried out in a BSC on a disposable plastic-backed paper liner.
7. All needles used in the course of preparation must be placed in sharps containers for disposal without being crushed, clipped or capped.
8. Drug administration sets should be primed within the BSC.
9. Vials
   a. The use of large-bore needles (No. 18 or 20) avoids high-pressure injections through syringes of solution in vials; however many large-bore needles are more likely to drip. Multiuse dispensing pins are recommended to avoid these problems.
   b. Venting devices such as filter needles or dispensing pins permit outside air to replace the withdrawn liquid.
   c. Another technique is to add diluent slowly to the vial by alternatively injecting small amounts and allowing displaced air to escape into the syringe. This air should not be expelled into room air because it may contain drug residue. It should either be injected into a vacuum vial or left in the syringe to be discarded.
   d. The drug should be cleared from the needle and hub of the syringe before separating to reduce spraying or separation.
10. Ampules
    a. Ampules with dry material should be gently tapped down before opening to move any material in the top of the ampule to the bottom quantity.
    b. A sterile gauze pad should be wrapped around the ampule neck before breaking the top.
    c. If adding a diluent, inject slowly down the inside wall of the ampule. Tilt the ampule to ensure that all the powder is wet before agitating.
    d. After the solution is withdrawn from the ampule with a syringe, the needle should be cleared of solution by holding it vertically with the point upward; the syringe should be tapped to remove air bubbles.
11. Transport of HDs
    a. The outside of bags or bottles containing the prepared drug should be wiped with moist gauze.
    b. Entry ports should be wiped with moist alcohol pads and capped.
    c. Transport should occur in sealed plastic bags and transported in containers designed to avoid breakage.

d. Any HDs that are shipped are subject to EPA regulation as hazardous waste.

III. DRUG ADMINISTRATION

A. PERSONAL PROTECTIVE EQUIPMENT

1. The National Study Commission on Cytotoxic Exposure has recommended that personnel administering HDs wear gowns, latex gloves, and chemical splash goggles or equivalent safety glasses.
2. NIOSH-approved respirators should be worn when administering aerosolized drugs.

B. ADMINISTRATION KIT

1. Protective and administration equipment may be packaged together and labeled as a HD administration kit. The kit should include:
   a. Personal protective equipment
   b. Gauze (4 × 4) for cleanup
   c. Alcohol wipes
   d. Disposable plastic-backed absorbent liner
   e. Puncture-resistant container for needles and syringes
   f. Thick sealable plastic bag (with warning label)
   g. Accessory warning labels

C. WORK PRACTICES

1. Hands should be washed before donning and after removing gloves.
2. Gowns or gloves that become contaminated should be changed immediately.
3. Employees should be trained in proper methods to remove contaminated gloves and gowns.
4. Infusion sets and pumps that should have Luer-lock fittings should be observed for leakage during use.
5. A plastic-backed absorbent pad should be placed under the tubing during administration to catch any leakage.
6. Sterile gauze should be placed around any push sites.
7. Priming I.V. sets or expelling air from syringes should be carried out in a BSC.
8. Syringes, I.V. bottles, and bags and pumps should be wiped clean of any drug contamination with sterile gauze.
9. Dispose of administration sets intact.

10. Waste bag should follow HD disposal requirements.
11. Protective goggles should be cleaned with detergent and properly rinsed.
12. Nursing stations where cytotoxic drugs will be administered should have spill and emergency skin and eye decontamination kits available.

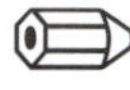

NOTE: The increased use of HDs in the home environment necessitates special precautions. Employees involved in home care delivery should follow the above work practices and employers should make administration and spill kits available.

D. AEROSOLIZED DRUGS

1. In the case of pentamidine, engineering controls include treatment booths with local exhaust ventilation designed specifically for its administration.
2. Ribavirin can be administered in isolation rooms with separate HEPA-filtered ventilation systems via endotracheal tube.
3. Both isolation and ventilation are used for volatile HDs.

E. CARING FOR PATIENTS RECEIVING HDS

1. The Bloodborne Pathogens Standard provides guidelines for universal precautions, which must be observed to prevent contact with blood or other potentially infectious materials.
2. Personnel dealing with excreta, primarily urine, from patient who have received HDs in the last 48 hours should be provided with and wear latex or other appropriate gloves and disposable gowns, to be discarded after each use whenever contaminated.
3. Eye protection should be worn if splashing is possible.
4. Linen soiled with blood or other potentially infectious materials as well as contaminated with excreta must be managed according to the Bloodborne Pathogens Standard. Linen should be placed in specially marked laundry bags and placed in a labeled impervious bag.
5. Any reusable item should be washed twice with detergent by personnel wearing double latex gloves and a gown.

IV. WASTE DISPOSAL

A. EQUIPMENT

1. Thick, leak-proof plastic bags, colored differently from other hospital trash bags, should be used for routine accumulation and collection of used containers, discarded gloves, gowns, and other disposable material.

2. Needles, syringes, and breakable items not contaminated with blood or other potentially infectious materials should be placed in a sharps container before being stored in the waste bag. Those contaminated with blood **must** be placed in a sharps container.
3. The waste bag should be kept inside a covered waste container clearly labeled **HD Waste Only.**

B. HANDLING

1. Personnel disposing of HD waste should wear gowns and protective gloves when handling waste containers.

C. DISPOSAL

1. Hazardous drug-related wastes should be handled separately from other hospital trash and disposed of in accordance with applicable EPA, state, and local regulations.
2. Disposal can occur at either an incinerator or a licensed sanitary landfill for toxic wastes.

D. SPILLS

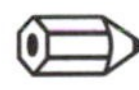

NOTE: Incidental spills and breakages should be cleaned up immediately by a properly protected person.

1. *Personnel contamination cleanup*
   a. Immediately remove the gloves or gown.
   b. Immediately cleanse the affected area with soap and water.
   c. Flood an affected eye at an eyewash station for 15 minutes.
   d. Obtain medical attention.
   e. Document the exposure in the employee's medical file.
2. *Cleanup of small spills (less than 5 mL)*
   a. Liquids should be wiped with absorbent gauze pads; solids with wet absorbent gauze.
   b. Spill areas should be cleaned three times using detergent solution followed by clean water.
   c. Any broken glass fragments should be picked up with a small scoop (never the hands) and placed in a sharps container.
   d. Contaminated reusable items, such as glassware and scoops, should be treated as previously outlined under reusable items.
3. *Cleanup of large spills*
   a. The area should be isolated.
   b. For spills larger than 5 mL liquid, spread is limited by gently covering with absorbent sheets or spill-control pads or pillows.
   c. If powder is involved, damp cloths or towels should be used.

   d. Protective apparel including respirators should be used as with small spills when there is any suspicion of airborne powder or that an aerosol has been or will be generated.
   e. All contaminated surfaces should be thoroughly cleaned three times with detergent and water.
4. *Spills in the BSC*
   a. Extensive spills within a BSC necessitate decontamination of all interior BSC surfaces after completion of the spill cleanup.
5. *Spill kits*
   a. Spill kits should be clearly labeled.
   b. The American Society of Hospital Pharmacists (ASHP) recommendations:
      (1) Chemical splash goggles
      (2) Two pairs of gloves
      (3) A low-permeability gown
      (4) Two sheets (12 × 12 inches)
      (5) 250-mL and 1-liter spill control pillows
      (6) Sharps container
      (7) Small scoop to collect glass fragments
      (8) Two large HD waste-disposal bags

V. STORAGE AND TRANSPORT

A. STORAGE AREAS

1. Limit authorized personnel to access to areas where HDs are stored.
2. Facilities used for storing HDs should not be used for other drugs.
3. Warning labels should be applied to all HD containers.

B. RECEIVING DAMAGED HD PACKAGES

1. Damaged shipping cartons should be opened in an isolated area or a BSC by a designed employee wearing double gloves, a gown, goggles, and appropriate respiratory protection.
2. Broken containers and contaminated packaging mats should be placed in a sharps container and then into HD disposal bags.

C. TRANSPORT

1. HDs should be securely capped or sealed and placed in sealed clear plastic bags.
2. Personnel involved in transporting HDs should be trained in spill procedures, including sealing off the contaminated area and calling for appropriate assistance.

VI. MEDICAL SURVEILLANCE

A. MEDICAL EXAMINATIONS

1. Employees who will be working with HDs in the workplace should have a pre-placement medical examination including an initial evaluation consisting of history, physical examination, and laboratory studies.
2. Examinations should be updated on a yearly basis or every 2 to 3 years.
3. Postexposure evaluation is tailored to the type of exposure.
   a. For cytotoxic drugs, the skin and mucous membranes
   b. For aerosolized HDs, the pulmonary system
4. Exit examinations and laboratory evaluation should be guided by the individual's history of exposures.
5. The examining physician should consider the reproductive status of employees and inform them regarding relevant reproductive issues.

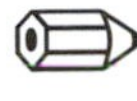

NOTE: Spontaneous abortion and congenital malformation excesses have been documented among workers handling some hazardous drugs without currently recommended engineering controls and precautions.

VIII. HAZARD COMMUNICATION

Employers shall develop, implement, and maintain at the workplace a written hazard communication program for employees handling or otherwise exposed to chemicals, including drugs that represent a health hazard to employees.

VII. TRAINING AND INFORMATION DISSEMINATION

A. EMPLOYEES MUST BE INFORMED OF THE REQUIREMENTS OF THE HAZARD COMMUNICATION STANDARD, INCLUDING:

1. Any operation or procedure in their work area where drugs that present a hazard are present
2. Location and availability of the written hazard communication

B. EMPLOYEE TRAINING

1. Methods and observations that may be used to detect the presence or release of HDs
2. Physical and health hazards of the covered HDs in the work area

3. The measures employees can take to protect themselves from hazards
4. The details of the hazards communication program developed by the employer, including an explanation of the labeling systems.

Source: US Department of Labor (1995). Controlling occupational exposure to hazardous drugs. Occupational Safety and Health Administration, Instruction CPL 2-2, 21-1 to 21-31.

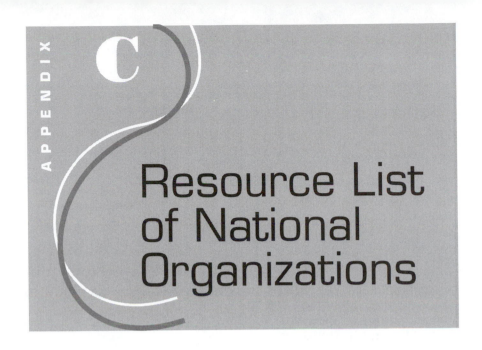

APPENDIX C
Resource List of National Organizations

AMERICAN ASSOCIATION OF CRITICAL CARE NURSES (AACN)
101 Columbia Avenue
Aliso Viejo, CA 92656-1491
1-800-899-2226
http://www.aacn.org

AMERICAN SOCIETY OF PAIN MANAGEMENT NURSES
11512 Allecingie Parkway
Richmond, VA 23235

AMERICAN SOCIETY FOR PARENTERAL AND ENTERAL NUTRITION—NURSE'S COMMITTEE
8630 Fenton Street, Suite 412
Silver Springs, MD 20910-3803

ASSOCIATION OF NURSES IN AIDS CARE
704 Stoney Hill Road, Suite 106
Yardley, PA 19067
(215) 321-2371

ASSOCIATION FOR PROFESSIONALS IN INFECTION CONTROL AND EPIDEMIOLOGY
1061 16th Street NW
Washington, DC 20016

ASSOCIATION OF PEDIATRIC ONCOLOGY NURSES
Suite 3A
11512 Allecingie Parkway
Richmond, VA 23235

CENTERS FOR DISEASE CONTROL AND PREVENTION
1600 Clifton Road
Atlanta, GA 30333
http://www.cdc.gov

INTRAVENOUS NURSES SOCIETY
Fresh Pond Square
10 Fawcett Street
Cambridge, MA 01238
(617) 489-5202
http://www.ins1.org

NATIONAL ASSOCIATION FOR PRACTICAL NURSE EDUCATION AND SERVICE, INC. (NAPNES)
1400 Spring Street, Suite 310
Silver Springs, MD 20910

ONCOLOGY NURSING SOCIETY
501 Holiday Drive
Pittsburgh, PA 15220
(412) 921-7373
http://www.ons.org

SOCIETY FOR VASCULAR NURSING (SVN)
309 Winter Street
Norwood, MA 02062

TRANSCULTURAL NURSING SOCIETY
http://www.tcns.org

APPENDIX

D

Summary of Recommended Procedures for Maintenance of Intravascular Catheters, Administration Sets, and Parenteral Fluids

SUMMARY OF RECOMMENDED PROCEDURES FOR MAINTENANCE OF INTRAVASCULAR CATHETERS, ADMINISTRATION SETS, AND PARENTERAL FLUIDS

Frequency of Catheter/ Device Change	Frequency of Dressing Change	Frequency of Administration Set Change	"Hang Time" for Parenteral Fluids	Use of Antimicrobial Ointments
		Peripheral Venous Catheters		
In adults, change catheter and rotate site every 48-72 hours. Replace catheters inserted under emergency conditions within 24 hours.	Leave dressings in place until the catheter is removed or changed, or the dressing becomes damp, loosened, or soiled.	Change intravenous tubing, including "piggyback" tubing, no more frequently than at 72-hour intervals.	Do not leave parenteral nutrition fluids hanging >24 hours.	*No recommendation* for the routine application of antimicrobial ointments to catheter site.
In pediatric patients, *no recommendation* for the frequency of catheter change or for the removal of catheters inserted under emergency conditions.		*No recommendation for* intravenous tubing changes beyond 72-hour intervals. Change tubing used to administer blood, blood products, or lipid emulsions within 24 hours of completing the infusion.	*No recommendation* for the "hang time"" of intravenous fluids other than parenteral nutrition fluids.	

Peripheral Arterial Catheters and Pressure-Monitoring Devices				
In adults, change catheter and rotate insertion sites every 4 days. In pediatric patients, *no recommendation* for the frequency of catheter change.	Leave dressing in place until the catheter is removed or changed, or the dressing becomes damp, loosened, or soiled.	Change intravenous tubing, including "piggyback" tubing, no more frequently than at 72-hour intervals.	Do not administer dextrose-containing solutions or parenteral nutrition fluids through the pressure monitoring circuit. Use only heparinized normal saline.	*No recommendation* for the routine application of antimicrobial ointments to catheter site.
Replace disposable or reusable transducers at 96-hour intervals. Replace other components of the system, including the tubing, continuous-flush device, and flush solution at the time the transducer is changed.		*No recommendation* for intravenous tubing changes beyond 72-hour intervals.	*No recommendation* for the "hang time" of heparinized normal saline.	

(Continued)

SUMMARY OF RECOMMENDED PROCEDURES FOR MAINTENANCE OF INTRAVASCULAR CATHETERS, ADMINISTRATION SETS, AND PARENTERAL FLUIDS *(Continued)*

Frequency of Catheter/ Device Change	Frequency of Dressing Change	Frequency of Administration Set Change	"Hang Time" for Parenteral Fluids	Use of Antimicrobial Ointments
Midline Catheters				
No recommendation for the frequency of catheter change.	Leave dressing in place until the catheter is removed or changed, or the dressing becomes damp, loosened, or soiled.	Change intravenous tubing, including "piggyback" tubing, no more frequently than at 72-hour intervals. *No recommendation* for intravenous tubing changes beyond 72-hour intervals. Change tubing used to administer blood, blood products, or lipid emulsions within 24 hours of completing the infusion.	Do not leave parenteral nutrition fluids hanging >24 hours. *No recommendation* for the "hang time" of intravenous fluids other than parenteral nutrition fluids.	*No recommendation* for the routine application of antimicrobial ointments to catheter site.
Central Venous Catheters (Nontunneled Catheters and Tunneled Catheters [Hickmans, Groshongs, Ports])				
Do not routinely change percutaneously inserted (nontunneled) central venous catheters either by rotating insertion sites or by guidewire-assisted catheter exchange.	Leave dressing in place until the catheter is removed or changed, or the dressing becomes damp, loosened, or soiled.	Change intravenous tubing, including "piggyback" tubing, no more frequently than at 72-hour intervals.	Do not leave parenteral nutrition fluids hanging >24 hours.	Do not routinely apply antimicrobial ointments at catheter insertion.

No recommendation for frequency of change of tunneled catheters, totally implantable devices (i.e., ports), or the needles used to access them.	*No recommendation* for the frequency of routine changes of dressing used on catheter site.	*No recommendation* for intravenous tubing changes beyond 72-hour intervals. Change tubing used to administer blood, blood products, or lipid emulsions within 24 hours of completing the infusion.	*No recommendation* for the "hang time" of intravenous fluids other than parenteral nutrition fluids.	
Peripherally Inserted Central Venous Catheters				
Change at least every 6 weeks. *No recommendation* for frequency of change when the duration of therapy is expected to exceed 6 weeks.	Leave dressing in place until the catheter is removed or changed, or the dressing becomes damp, loosened, or soiled. *No recommendation* for the frequency of routine changes of dressing used on catheter site.	Change intravenous tubing, including "piggyback" tubing, no more frequently than at 72-hour intervals. *No recommendation* for intravenous tubing changes beyond 72-hour intervals. Change tubing used to administer blood, blood products, or lipid emulsions within 24 hours of completing the infusion.	Do not leave parenteral nutrition fluids hanging >24 hours. *No recommendation* for the "hang time" of intravenous fluids other than parenteral nutrition fluids.	Do not routinely apply antimicrobial ointments at catheter insertion.

(Continued)

SUMMARY OF RECOMMENDED PROCEDURES FOR MAINTENANCE OF INTRAVASCULAR CATHETERS, ADMINISTRATION SETS, AND PARENTERAL FLUIDS *(Continued)*

Frequency of Catheter/ Device Change	Frequency of Dressing Change	Frequency of Administration Set Change	"Hang Time" for Parenteral Fluids	Use of Antimicrobial Ointments
Central Arterial Catheters (Pulmonary Artery Catheters)				
Change catheter at least every 5 days.	Leave dressing in place until the catheter is removed or changed, or the dressing becomes damp, loosened, or soiled. *No recommendation* for the frequency of routine changes of dressing used on catheter site.	Change intravenous tubing, including "piggyback" tubing, no more frequently than at 72-hour intervals. *No recommendation* for intravenous tubing changes beyond 72-hour intervals.	*No recommendation* for the "hang time" of intravenous fluids other than parenteral nutrition fluids.	Do not routinely apply antimicrobial ointments at catheter insertion.
Central Hemodialysis Catheters				
No recommendation for the frequency of catheter change.	Leave dressing in place until the catheter is removed or changed, or the dressing becomes damp, loosened, or soiled. *No recommendation* for the frequency of dressing change.	*Not applicable.* (Do not use hemodialysis catheters for purposes other than hemodialysis [e.g., administration of fluids, blood/ blood products, or parenteral nutrition].)	*Not applicable.* (Do not use hemodialysis catheters for purposes other than hemodialysis [e.g., administration of fluids, blood/blood products, or parenteral nutrition].)	Apply povidone-iodine ointment to the insertion site before and after hemodialysis.

Umbilical Catheters				
No recommendation for frequency of catheter change.	*Not applicable*	Change intravenous tubing, including "piggyback" tubing, no more frequently than at 72-hour intervals. *No recommendation* for intravenous tubing changes beyond 72-hour intervals. Change tubing used to administer blood, blood products, or lipid emulsions within 24 hours of completing the infusion.	Do not leave parenteral nutrition fluids hanging >24 hours. *No recommendation* for the "hang time"of intravenous fluids other than parenteral nutrition fluids.	*No recommendation* for the routine application of antimicrobial ointnents to the catheter site.

***Source:** From Department of Health and Human Services. *Intravascular Device-Related Infections Prevention: Guideline Availability.* Bethesda, MD: Centers for Disease Control and Prevention, 1995, with permission.

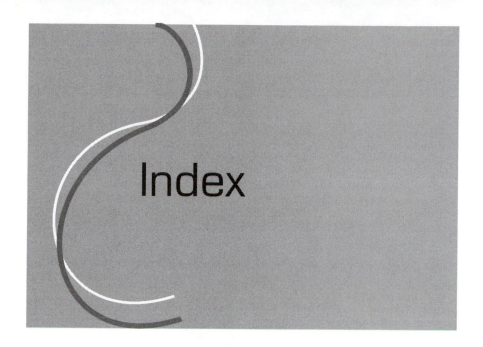

Index

An "f" following a page number indicates a figure; a "t" following a page number indicates a table.